INTERNATIONAL DICTI[ONARY] OF PSYCHOTHERA[PY]

The *International Dictionary of Psychotherapy* is a systematized compendium of the numerous psychotherapies that have evolved over the past 30 years. With contributions from over 350 experts in the field, it highlights the diverse schools of psychotherapy, tracing their histories and traditions, while underlining their specific strengths in dealing with human behaviours, feelings and perceptions in the contemporary world.

The book traces eight principal paradigms: psychodynamic, behavioural, existential-humanistic, body-expression, systemic-relational, cognitive, interactional-strategic and eclectic. It presents to the expert and non-expert reader an array of models that grew from a specific paradigm, sharing the same fundamental epistemology and therapeutic strategies. This is accomplished through a reader-friendly approach that presents clear definitions of the key constructs of each paradigm, and transversal concepts that are common to the diverse practices of psychotherapy.

The *International Dictionary of Psychotherapy* provides a clear picture of the numerous types of psychotherapeutic treatments and their applications, while offering a close examination of the efficacy and evaluative methods developed as a result of numerous debates and research carried out within the psychotherapeutic community.

It represents an essential resource for psychotherapeutic and psychoanalytic practitioners and students, regardless of background or creed.

Giorgio Nardone is Director of the Post Graduate School of Brief Strategic Psychotherapy, located in Arezzo, Italy, and of the School of Managerial Training in Communication and Strategic Problem Solving, located in Arezzo and Florence, Italy. He is co-founder, along with Paul Watzlawick, of the Centro di Terapia Strategica where he conducts work as a psychotherapist, professor and researcher. He has authored and co-authored nearly 30 publications, many of which have been translated from Italian into English, Spanish, French, Russian and Japanese.

Alessandro Salvini is Scientific Director of the Psychology and Psychotherapy Institute "Psicopraxis" of Padua and School of Specialization in Psychotherapy-Interactive. He was formerly Professor of Clinical Psychology at the University of Padua and President of the College of Professors of Clinical Psychology of Italian Universities. He is the author of numerous scientific publications, including eight books.

INTERNATIONAL DICTIONARY OF PSYCHOTHERAPY

Edited by Giorgio Nardone and Alessandro Salvini

Routledge
Taylor & Francis Group
LONDON AND NEW YORK

First published 2019
by Routledge
2 Park Square, Milton Park, Abingdon, Oxon OX14 4RN

and by Routledge
52 Vanderbilt Avenue, New York, NY 10017

Routledge is an imprint of the Taylor & Francis Group, an informa business

British Library Cataloguing-in-Publication Data
A catalogue record for this book is available from the British Library

Library of Congress Cataloging-in-Publication Data
Names: Nardone, Giorgio, 1958- author. | Salvini, Alessandro, author.
Title: International dictionary of psychotherapy / Giorgio Nardone and Alessandro Salvini. Other titles: Dizionario internazionale di psicoterapia. English
Description: Milton Park, Abingdon, Oxon ; New York, NY : Routledge, 2019. |
Identifiers: LCCN 2018047521 (print) | LCCN 2018047958 (ebook) | ISBN 9780429024788 (Master eBook) |ISBN 9780367110949 (hardback) | ISBN 9780367110932 (pbk.) | ISBN 9780429024788 (ebk)
Subjects: LCSH: Psychotherapy—Dictionaries.
Classification: LCC RC475.7 (ebook) | LCC RC475.7 .N3713 2019 (print) | DDC 616.89/1403—dc23
LC record available at https://lccn.loc.gov/2018047521

ISBN: 978-0-367-11094-9 (hbk)
ISBN: 978-0-367-11093-2 (pbk)
ISBN: 978-0-429-02478-8 (ebk)

Typeset in Bembo
by Swales & Willis Ltd, Exeter, Devon, UK

CONTENTS

CONTRIBUTORS

Editors: Giorgio Nardone, Alessandro Salvini
International Advisors: Mony Elkaïm, Camillo Loriedo, Pio E. Ricci Bitti, John Sommers-Flanagan, Jeffrey H. Zeig

CONTRIBUTORS

Paradigms

Marianna Mazza, Piero Petrini, Michel Botbol, Luigi Janiri (*psychodynamic paradigm*)

Paolo Meazzini (*behavioural paradigm*)

Irivin D. Yalom (*existential-humanistic paradigm*)

Luciano Rispoli (*expressive-corporeal paradigm*)

Jean-Jacques Wittezaele (*interactional-strategic paradigm*)

Padraic Gibson (*relational-systemic paradigm*)

Mario Antonio Reda, Maria Francesca Pilleri (*cognitive paradigm*)

John Sommers-Flanagan, Rita Sommers-Flanagan, Veronica I. Johnson (*eclectic paradigm*)

Appendix «Empirical research in psychotherapy»

Gianluca Castelnuovo, Enrico Molinari, Giorgio Nardone, Alessandro Salvini

Models

Alexander James F., Anchisi Roberto, Anderson Harlene, Andolfi Maurizio, Andreas Steve, Anger Katharina, Anger-Diaz Barbara, Arciero Giampiero, Battaglini Irene, Beck Judith S., Benelli Ezio, Boccalon Roberto, Brizzi Saro, Caruso Sergio, Chiari Gabriele, Corti Luca, Cresti Alida, Cruciani Paolo, Dattilio Frank M., De Coro Alessandra, De Monte Ettore, Delicato Ninfa, Dèttore Davide, Di Ciaccia Antonio, Di Pietro Mario, Durando Stefania, Fizzotti Eugenio, Formica Ivan, Ganda Gianluca, Giangrasso Barbara, Gilligan Stephen G., Giuliani Massimo, Giusti Edoardo, Guadagno Marie E., Hoffmann-Bisinger Ilka R., Jedlowski Milena, Keeney Bradford, Kessler Susanne, Liccione Davide,

Longhin Luigi, Loriedo Camillo, Lo Savio Giovanni, Lo Verso Girolamo, Madanes Cloe, Mazzoli Giansecondo, Miselli Giovanni, Moderato Paolo, Moselli Patrizia, Nardi Bernardo, Nardone Giorgio, Novellino Michele, Pagliaro Gioacchino, Patrizi Patrizia, Petruccelli Filippo, Portelli Claudette, Quattrini Giovanni Paolo, Rawson Penny, Ray Wendel A., Rispoli Luciano, Robbins Michael S., Rolla Enrico, Romagnoli Domenico, Rosati Ottavio, Rosselli Massimo, Rossi Nicolino, Schmidt Gunther, Selekman Matthew D., Shapiro Francine, Sirigatti Saulo, Solomon Roger M., Spagnuolo Lobb Margherita, Stein Murray, Tamburello Antonino, Voltolin Adriano, Wubbolding Robert E., Zeig Jeffrey K., Zito Salvatore, Zucconi Alberto.

Entries

Adenzato Mauro, Anchisi Roberto, Anger Katharina, Anger-Diaz Barbara, Antonelli Giorgio, Antonetti Silvana, Ardito Rita B., Aschieri Filippo, Attianese Antonio, Aversa Luigi, Balbo Marina, Ballardini Maria, Balsamo Maurizio, Bani Marco, Barabuffi Alessio, Barbuto Florinda, Barsotti Alessandra, Bartoletti Alessandro, Battaglini Irene, Beck Judith S., Bella Andrèe, Bellantoni Domenico, Bellotti Franco, Benelli Chiara, Benelli Ezio, Benvenuti Anna, Bergomi Sara, Bianchi Laura, Bianconi Alessandra, Birkas-Kovats Dezsoe, Blasi Stefano, Bonzanini Ruggero Ioris, Bordin Elena, Borgo Stefania, Borgogno Franco, Boria Giovanni, Boschi Stefano, Bottone Mario, Bracciodieta Lorenzo, Brizzi Saro, Bruni Francesco, Bruzzone Daniele, Cagnoni Federica, Cairo Elisabetta, Cambrini Loredana, Cannavina Anna, Caponeri Massimo Adolfo, Caramalli Claudia, Carrera Giuseppina, Carta Stefano, Caruso Amedeo, Casonato Marco, Cassullo Gabriele, Castelnuovo Gianluca, Casula Consuelo, Cavaleri Pietro Andrea, Cavallari Giorgio, Celi Fabio, Cerioli Luciano, Cervari Paolo, Chiodi Lata M., Chiodini Moira, Cigoli Vittorio, Cirillo Stefano, Cirlà Mario, Cocchi Angelo, Conrotto Francesco, Copelli Cristina, Coradeschi Davide, Corti Ilaria, Corti Luca, Couyoumdjian Alessandro, Cresti Alida, Cruciani Paolo, D'Ambrosio Mario, Dazzi Nino, De Antoniis Simona, De Bei Francesco, De Coro Alessandra, De Marinis Donatella, De Monte Ettore, De Paolis Daniele, De Renzis Giovanni, Defilippi Pier Giuseppe, Desideri Giada, Dèttore Davide, Di Ciaccia Antonio, Di Nucci Franco, Di Pietro Mario, Dodet Maurizio, Dorella Antonio, Drazien Muriel, Durando Stefania, Erba Germana, Fanelli Cristiana, Fassina Simona, Federici Susanna, Fellin Lisa Chiara, Ferrara Antonio, Ferrucci Piero, Filoni Rosaria, Fina Nadia, Fiumanò Marisa, Fois Fabio, Formica Ivan, Fossi Giordano, Fossi Stefania, Francesetti Gianni, Frank Eric C., Furman Ben, Gaffuri Maria, Ganda Gianluca, Garcia-Rivera Teresa, Garzonio Marco, Gasparini Carla, Gay Marco, Gazzillo Francesco, Genchi Manuela, Geyerhofer Stefan, Giachi Elena, Giangrasso Barbara, Giuliani Massimo, Guglielmotti Federica, Guido Stefania, Harwood Mark T., Hybarger Chad, Iapoce Angiola, Iberni Elisabetta, Ioppolo Fabrizio, Isardi Lina, Jedlowski Milena, Kakaraki Dimitra, Kaufman Gianni, Keeney Bradford, La Scala Marco, Lai Giampaolo, Lenzi Silvio, Leone Guglielmotti Raffaella, Liccione Davide, Lingiardi Vittorio, Liverano Antonella, Lo Savio Giovanni, Lo Verso Girolamo, Longhin Luigi, Loriedo Camillo, Luci Monica, Luisetti Elena, Luzi Valerio, Manca Maria Luisa, Manfrida Gianmarco, Mangini Enrico, Marks Isaac, Mazzeschi Susanna, Melli Gabriele, Meluzzi Alessandro, Menafro Mariarosaria, Meneghelli Anna, Meringolo Patrizia, Meroni Bruno, Milanese Roberta, Miselli Giovanni, Moderato Paolo, Molgora Sara, Molinari Enrico, Montanari Claudia, Montano Antonella, Mordazzi Paolo, Moselli Patrizia, Mosticoni Roberto, Munari Franca, Nanetti Franco, Nardi Bernardo, Nardone Giorgio, Nebbiosi Gianni, Neri Claudio, Nicasi Stefania, Novellino Michele, Orifiammi Paola, Ortu Francesca, Pagliaro Gioacchino, Pagnini Francesco, Palmieri Gaspare, Panizza Sandro, Parmeggiani Luisa, Parmeggiani

Michela, Pecorara Rossana Silvia, Pedon Arrigo, Perfetto Giuseppe, Pergolizzi Francesca, Persico Anna Silvia, Petracca Cristina, Petruccelli Filippo, Pietrabissa Giada, Pilleri Maria Francesca, Pilò Francesca, Poerio Vincenzo, Poggiolini Daniela, Poletto Anna Elisabetta, Portelli Claudette, Presti Giovambattista, Procacci Michele, Putti Simonetta, Quattrini Giovanni Paolo, Quesito Franco, Rainieri Barbara, Rampin Matteo, Ratti Giuliana, Reda Mario Antonio, Rezzonico Giorgio, Ricci Marina Luisa, Rinaldi Benedetta, Roberti Alessio, Rolla Enrico, Romagnoli Domenico, Rombolà Corsini Giuseppe, Rosati Ottavio, Rosselli Massimo, Rossi Pier Luigi, Sacco Giuseppe, Sagliaschi Samanta, Salles Virginia, Salvini Alessandro, Santabbondio Daniela, Santori Enrico D., Sarno Lucio, Sassaroli Sandra, Scabini Eugenia, Sciaky Riccardo, Selvaggi Laura, Selvini Matteo, Sibilia Lucio, Simonelli Barbara, Sirigatti Saulo, Sluzki Carlos E., Smiraglia Stanislao, Soriani Bellavista Massimo, Sorrentino Anna Maria, Spagnuolo Lobb Margherita, Speranza Anna Maria, Symington Joan, Szasz Thomas, Tallerini Antonio Giovanni, Tamburello Antonino, Thanopulos Sarantis, Tibaldi Marta, Tomm Karl, Trapanese Enzo Vittorio, Vadalà Giuseppe M., Valerio Paolo, Veronesi Ilaria, Versaci Rosa, Vigneri Matilde, Vincelli Francesco, Vitelli Roberto, Vitolo Antonio, Voltolin Adriano, Wittezaele Jean-Jacques, Yalom Irvin, Yapko Michael D., Zeig Jeffrey K., Zerbetto Riccardo, Zetti Marta, Zucconi Alberto.

EDITORIAL BOARD

Text editing and supervision: Giorgio Nardone, Alessandro Salvini, Roberta Milanese.

Scientific advisors: Patrizia Meringolo, Enrico Molinari, Stanislao Smiraglia.

Managing board

Roberta Milanese (*board coordinator and manager; interactional-strategic paradigm*), Alessandro Bartoletti (*eclectic and expressive-corporeal paradigm*), Federica Cagnoni (*cognitive-behavioural paradigm*), Gianluca Castelnuovo (*systemic-relational*), Valerio Luzi (*psychodynamic paradigm*), Claudette Portelli (*humanistic-existential paradigm*), Elisa Valteroni (*REFERENCES*).

Editorial staff

Debora Crippa, Giulio De Santis, Bernardo Paoli

Editor entry contributors

Aceti Serena, Aloe Gaetano, Balbi Elisa, Balzani Tiziana, Bannella Federica, Barsotti Alessandra, Bartoletti Alessandro, Belluomini Alessandra, Benedusi Manuel, Bertoncelli Sara, Bolmida Mauro, Bonsangue Monica, Bonzanini Ruggiero Ioris, Bottini Roberto, Cagnoni Federica, Cantafio Lucia Rosa, Castelnuovo Gianluca, Cecchetti Sara, Chiodini Moira, Da Ros Tania, D'Ascanio Nicola, De Antoniis Simona, De Santis Giulio, Desideri Giada, Di Carlo Flavia, Di Virgilio Barbara, Faccio Elena, Fantappiè Cecilia, Farinella Lara, Filella Nicoletta, Gerboni Emilio, Giannotti Samantha, Igochina Olga, Iudici A., Lacagnina Alida, Licari Giuseppe, Liguoro Dalila, Luzi Valerio, Malagola M. Piera, Maniotti Luisa, Mariotti Roberta, Martino Elisa, Mascolo Giammario, Masera Andrea, Massironi Carlo,

Mazzeschi Susanna, Mazzucchelli Emma, Meneghin Patrizia, Milanese Roberta, Mordazzi Paolo, Muriana Emanuela, Nardone Giorgio, Olocco Mara, Pagliai Marco, Pagliaro Gioacchino, Panturco Matteo, Paoli Bernardo, Perissutti Roberto, Pettenò Laura, Portelli Claudette, Quarato Maria, Rampin Matteo, Ratto Chiara, Ravasio Antonio, Romaioli Diego, Rosciglione Giovanna, Salvini Alessandro, Smiraglia Stanislao, Soriani Bellavista Massimo, Vallarino Andrea, Verbitz Tiziana, Verdesca Maria Teresa, Vulcano Giulietta.

ENGLISH EDITION

Translation contributors: Michele Salvagno, Sharon Vella Camilleri, Claudette Portelli.

Editing contributors: Roberta Milanese, Giovanni Albertini, Michela Olivieri, Michele Salvagno.

INTRODUCTION

Giorgio Nardone and Alessandro Salvini

The term psychotherapy appeared in writing for the first time in 1892, coined by Bernheim, (even though it had been used by Felkin two years earlier) who wrote a book entitled *Psychotherapeutic Hypnotism*, referring to a healing process that took place not on the patient's sick body but on his "psyche". However, 2,300 years prior to this, a famous sophist, Antiphon, had already edited the first manual of psychotherapy, titled *The Art of Consolation*.

As he had affirmed in one of his works, "nothing exists that cannot be cured by words". As reported by Plutarch and Xenophon, he had taken up, in his city of Corinth, a true and proper profession as a psychotherapist, curing the ill through the use of his rhetoric. Even Hippocrates, the first doctor, besides the use of remedies, used words and gestures as therapeutic antidotes. After all, Hippocrates was the nephew of Gorgias, the most celebrated of the sophists, who, by chance, had defined therapy as the combination of "touch, remedy and words".

Hence one can say that the history of psychotherapy as a healing discipline began here, curing people through different practices without the use of drugs or surgical intervention, but by working on the relationship, through the use of dialogue and therapeutic action.

Psychotherapy can neither be subsumed into medicine, even though it cures physical pain such as somatisations, nor by shamanism, even though there are often therapeutic changes that might seem magical. This healing process distinguishes itself as unique, since it is neither related to biology and medicine, nor to beliefs and magic. As Antiphon and Hippocrates first suggested, the therapeutic power of words and actions elicit a process of change in the perceptions, which in turn change emotions, reactions and the meaning of events and the experiences of sufferings endured. Even though it shares theories, instruments and applications with psychology and psychiatry, psychotherapy distinguishes itself from them. As we know well, psychology deals with the study of human beings and their healthy or unhealthy, normal or abnormal, individual or social, mental or behavioural manifestations, while psychiatry, being a branch of traditional medicine, deals with medical treatments to mental disorders, such as the use of drugs, surgical interventions and other physical means. Psychotherapy, even though it deals practically with the same pathologies as psychiatry, focuses on methods that are purely psychological, such as the use of dialogue, behavioural and mental prescriptions, communication and interpersonal relationships, introspection and training, which define it in its own unique way.

Doubtless, great merit goes to Freud and psychoanalysis for the widespread interest in psychotherapy in our modern world, offering an alternative to medical and psychiatric interventions. However, today, we have numerous different types of psychotherapies, which have brought this discipline a long way in its evolution, producing many different therapies, and can often seem highly divergent. However, even though there are many different psychotherapeutic approaches, as Jeffrey K. Zeig (Zeig and Munion, 1990) underlines, there is a fundamental agreement on the definition of the concept that marks the characteristics and the applications of psychotherapy as a proper autonomous discipline; that even though it evolved from psychology and medicine it became an "emergent quality" that defined itself from both sciences. Just like water, which is the synthesis of hydrogen and oxygen, psychotherapy took another form and property, becoming totally different from its original components. Psychotherapy today represents theoretical practices that define it as a unique and independent profession.

With over a century of intellectual effort from extraordinary masters in the field (who were often attacked by numerous other disciplines, such as traditional psychiatry), the psychotherapy community has progressively assembled a wealth of wisdom, practices and multi-disciplinary projects, which has made psychotherapy flourish and become one of the most significant cultural enterprises of modern times. The psychotherapy community has managed to free individuals from ideological, ethnocentric and normative dogmas, and transformed clients' relationships with themselves, others and their world.

Driven by the competing aspects of its various approaches, psychotherapy has become a cultural and social movement, which has gained growing acceptance as a result of its practical effects. Distinguishing itself from psychiatry and psychology, psychotherapy, with its various models, theories and practices, has also, in many countries, undergone a process of regulation to become a legalized profession. Legal recognition has rendered psychotherapy a scientific practice and allowed it to become a warranted profession, within a plurality of recognised models and paradigms.

For example, legal registration in Italy, which has legitimized the existence of various specific and diverse competencies of psychotherapists, has managed to avoid: (a) the intrusion of practices that do not "own scientific knowledge"; and (b) the subordination and confusion between the profession of psychotherapist and that of other professional figures, who employ a mindset and practices that are incompatible with psychotherapy at an epistemological level.

Today, various schools of specialization in psychotherapy exist in Italy, which are officially recognized as training institutes, reserved for medical and psychology graduates, which adhere to specific therapeutic approaches. This has created a sort of map of the different psychotherapeutic approaches, which has made our efforts in compiling this dictionary easier. Unlike in other Western countries, the Italian context does not confer a superordinate status upon any one model of therapy, as one might encounter in France or Belgium. Neither does the Italian context follow the reductionist process of "manualization", which is fundamental to the psychotherapeutic milieu in the United States. In certain cases, the supporters of such positions, who for years have obstructed psychotherapy, today claim to regulate and control it by assimilating it into a mere therapeutic procedure.

Misconceptions can also be dictated by lack of knowledge regarding the real scientific foundations of psychotherapy and/or the conviction that human actions, with their diversities and problems, can be totally reduced to the competence of a single profession, which often ends up being overvalued. While various research has demonstrated that psychotherapy was created to fill these lacunae, the conviction that psychotherapy can be assimilated or subordinated to another discipline or professional practice can lead to this error, since it shares a similar language to that used by other sciences.

Psychotherapy is a clinical practice informed by the use of communication that is not mere transfer of information, but is a use of language and action that brings about change. Thus it maintains an epistemology and mentality that is different from other disciplines. It is not reductionist and positivist, but follows a hermeneutic and pragmatic tradition.

The intent of this dictionary is to highlight the autonomy of psychotherapy as a science and a profession that differs from academic and experimental psychology which are oriented towards the inquiry and knowledge of mental processes in experimental contexts. Psychotherapy is oriented towards the modification of a person's behaviours, feelings and perceptions in a specific temporal context.

The primary aim of this text is to bring to light how the international psychotherapy community has evolved in the past 30 years and to place in the foreground the acquired knowledge of this profession, which often goes beyond its own clinical field.

As this dictionary manages to convey, psychotherapy is often asked to face a multiplicity of situations and thus requires the use of a whole array of information: from implicit knowledge, such as common sense, explicit knowledge derived from social anthropology, neurobiological disciplines and more. Other forms of psychotherapy require knowledge of logic, linguistics, philosophy, science and critical literature.

The psychotherapy movement and community have generated knowledge directed towards the *know-how* of things, such as the use of narratives, performative language and other communication skills that are capable of significantly influencing the way a person feels, perceives, remembers and acts. These are competencies and skills that psychotherapy has, today, even rendered accessible to other professions. Over the years, psychotherapists have provided many useful forms of training and teaching to doctors and other practitioners who need to help patients to change their diets and their lifestyles, and, of course, to gain their compliance with treatment. Psychotherapists have assisted psychologists, sociologists and other experts in communication to acquire informative and persuasive methods to use in their work when they need to practice intrapersonal and cultural influence.

Throughout this dictionary, through the work of its various contributors, it is clear that even though each type of psychotherapy places a different emphasis on how to resolve a client's or patient's problem, change cannot be achieved without the use of the clients own language, the utilisation of their unique social and existential system of reference and their active participation. Through the superb collaboration of the most qualified representatives of the entire international psychotherapy community, it has been possible to put together the principal paradigms that constitute the growing diversity and richness of the numerous models of psychotherapy.

The style for this dictionary was selected to convey to the reader a collection of models, which, even though they have different expressions, all grew from a specific paradigm, sharing the same fundamental epistemology and therapeutic strategies.

The reader, who may not be well acquainted with the international position of psychotherapy and of its schools and traditions, might be surprised to learn that the same tree might produce fruit that is similar yet so different one from the other.

It is appropriate to remind the reader that this differentiation is provided by the particular form of knowledge and practice reflected by the various strategic solutions put into play by each specific model, such as mental states, psychological processes, autobiographical reconstructions, free association, cognitive schemas, attempted solutions and others, in the treatment of the different types of human suffering.

From our point of view, even though certain models are similar, they are not identical and thus cannot be integrated into a singular theoretical definition. If we assume, metaphorically, that every territory requires a different map and that some maps are more suitable than others, it would be erroneous to want to fuse the different models together in a sort of unitary theory of treatment for psychological disorders.

As Sommers-Flanagan and Sommers-Flanagan (2004) demonstrate, these diverse models of psychotherapy have their own reasons for existing, and it is their own unique and respective paradigmatic, theoretical and practical criteria (objectives and methods, etc.) that give them legitimacy. Just like the elements in a toolbox, which are meant to be used to resolve different problems, the same applies to the various psychotherapies that have evolved.

This dictionary is essentially a photograph of the geography of psychotherapeutic practices, strategies, skills and procedures. This is not a mere review of the different perspectives, but rather an exposition of the fundamental paradigms lying within the diverse psychotherapeutic models and their original technical and practical characteristics.

While this dictionary provides an overview of different forms of psychotherapy, it also exposes a kind of golden thread that connects and unites (even though it does not unify) the various models. Thus, what might seem heterogeneous and scarily incomprehensible to the naked eye, actually reveals a number of commonalities in psychotherapy. It is possible to assume a position, which the philosophers of science call "plurality", according to which, a certain event can be shaped through different cognitive and practical processes, where the legitimacy of a particular practice is awarded by the nature of the event and the objectives that are supposed to be reached.

Now that we have specified this premise, we can give a unitary and prototype definition of psychotherapy.

> With the term psychotherapy, we mean a coherent and specific system of psychological practices, which are guided by specific theories of the mind and of human behaviour, which are meant to resolve a certain class of emotional, cognitive and relational problem/s, being symptomatic or not.

We recognize psychotherapists to be those qualified professionals who hold a dual role as clinicians and researchers, following a theory of the mind and certain related protocols for treatment. In other words, we define a psychotherapist as a professional who assumes all of the theoretical and practical commitments specific to his/her model of reference, which is characterized by a dialogical practice, through which it is possible to resolve problematic, disturbing relationships one might hold with oneself, others or the world. From a social and clinical point of view, such relationships are dysfunctional and symptomatic, while, from a subjective point of view, they produce suffering and discomfort in one's life. A common claim shared by all psychotherapeutic models is the importance of theoretical and technical training that qualifies a psychotherapist.

We hope that by now it has became clear to the reader that the purpose of this project, originating from the idea of offering a well-defined mapping of the specific properties of psychotherapy, is to highlight the professional individuality of each model, by setting forth the different theoretical constructions and practices that coexist within them.

With this aim in mind we decided to avoid giving authors/contributors any rigid editorial criteria to follow, knowing that the different paradigms hold their own different languages. In this way we were able to offer to the reader, not only the possibility of discriminating between the numerous psychotherapeutic models but also of recognizing their specific characteristics and use of language. In fact, we believe that it would have been reductive to require, for example, the behaviourist model and the psychodynamic model to use a common language, because the former uses a language that is based on objectivity, while the latter uses a language that is based on symbolism.

We believe that the dictionary not only respects the different theoretical and practical prerogatives of each model but it also remains loyal to the respective and distinctive lexical and communicational commitments of each of the different models.

This dictionary distinguishes itself from other editorial attempts to give an exposition of psychotherapies (Zeig and Munion, 1990; Ford and Urban, 1998; Sommers-Flanagan and Sommers-Flanagan, 2004), both for:

a) The structure of the dictionary, which is meant to provide a rapid reader-friendly consultation and;
b) The specific format, which divides the psychotherapies into epistemological paradigms written and amended by internationally renowned experts in each specific approach. It then goes deeper, to present the different theoretical-practical models with their specific constructs and techniques. Moreover, the editorial board thought it appropriate to introduce key words, which are common transverse concepts shared by the different approaches.

Finally, we felt the need to end this dictionary with an evaluation of the relative literature related to the efficacy of psychotherapy. In fact, this pluralistic work could not be complete if a single methodology were used to present the different forms of psychological treatment. We wanted to take some distance from the arrogant position that has been adopted in recent decades by various authors, who, in line with what is considered "the evidence-based" movement, have inflicted, from medical psychiatry onto psychotherapy, a decisively reductionist manualised nosography. Our intention has been to provide to the reader with a clear picture of the numerous types of psychotherapeutic treatment and their application, while offering a close examination of the efficacy and evaluative methods developed as a result of numerous debates carried out within the psychotherapeutic sphere.

We have tried throughout to avoid limiting our presentation to mere statistical measurement and evaluation procedures that are contaminated by rigid methodological criteria, which fail to take into account the real potential of operative knowledge. Our intention is to underline how this can provide vitality and constant evolution to psychotherapy, as well as practical validity, self-correction and ongoing improvement. From our point of view, this is an imperative prerogative for the construction of scientific knowledge that is free from traditional dogmas and from in vogue ideologies.

REFERENCES. Ford D.H., Urban H.B., *Contemporary models of psychotherapy*, 1998; Hersen M., Sledge W., *Encyclopedia of psychotherapy*, 2002; Sommers-Flanagan J., Sommers-Flanagan R., *Counseling and psychotherapy theories in context and practice: skills, strategies and techniques*, 2004; Unterstein M., (ed.), *Sofisti: testimonianze e frammenti*, 1949; Zeig J.K., Munion W.M., (eds.), *What is psychotherapy?: Contemporary perspectives*, 1990.

THE EIGHT PARADIGMS

And their respective theoretical-applicative models

PSYCHODYNAMIC PARADIGM

M. Mazza, P. Petrini, M. Botbol, and L. Janiri

THE UNCONSCIOUS. From the topographic point of view, Freud introduced the division of three systems, namely the Unconscious, Preconscious and Conscious. The concept of the unconscious in Freud has a descriptive sense, referring to all that is not in the sphere of consciousness and that includes the preconscious and, in a dynamic sense, referring to those ideas that possess a dynamic character and that remain excluded from consciousness through their intensity and activity. The dynamic unconscious is related to an intrapsychic conflict between different antagonistic forces that prevents it from its access to consciousness (Freud, 1914). In his work entitled "The unconscious" (1915) Freud offers the theory of an unconscious constituted by drive representations and thing presentations: Freud hypothesizes that these more primitive drive- and thing- representations become linked eventually to word presentations in the preconscious and the conscious. In the beginning there is a mixture of drive representations, memory traces and thing representations, and then the linking with word presentations in the preconscious and conscious mind occurs.

The notion of unconsciousness in its simple descriptive sense is disputed. We are able to know and recall things that are not at the moment conscious to us, in the sense of their not being in our immediate awareness. Because a conception present to consciousness can become absent, and after an interval present once again without its return being a result of perception, we tend, as Freud has explained, to speak of such conception as unconsciously present in our mind (Blass, 2014). Freud's notion of the unconscious goes far beyond this descriptive sense of the term and refers to something much more substantive and specific. It includes certain kinds of motivational forces, which for dynamic reasons are barred from consciousness, and ideas that are inherently latent from earliest times, but which shape our experience and the way we perceive the world. The unconscious is regarded as the ground of psychic reality, the location of psychopathology and the object of analytic action (Blass, 2014).

Freud claimed that only some part of the unconscious can be known by the symbolic traces it leaves on our conscious, waking life. Freud (1915) delineated this portion when he noted that some unconscious instinctual impulses are "highly organized, free from self-contradiction", relatively indistinguishable in structure from those that are conscious or preconscious, and yet "they are unconscious and incapable of becoming conscious".

The psychoanalytic setting and method provide a unique arena in which the duality of mental life can emerge and be recognized. Archaeological analysis is based on the patient's associations guided by his resistances to his unconscious wishes. By virtue of his free-floating attention, the analyst can gain access to this repressed material. The structure and multiple meanings of the unconscious aspect of experience can be traced. We perceive the present through the lens of unconscious, psychic reality (LaFarge, 2014). The analytic relationship exists in a dual aspect, as both a conscious contemporary experience with an object in the external reality and an unconscious relationship, existing in phantasy and memory, evoked by this external reality. Memories are always at least in part memories of phantasies (Freud, 1899). In the analytic situation, transference and countertransference represent an interplay of the contemporary relationship between analyst and patient and the reverberating system of unconscious phantasy and phantasy-shaped memory. The analyst's own unconscious makes an important contribution to conscious experience with the patient, and the recognition that the analyst's experience is also stimulated by unconscious aspects of the patient's experience leads to the understanding that the analyst's countertransference is an important source of information about the patient. Unconscious elements arising from both the analyst and the patient enter the analysis through the medium of the analyst's associations and reverie (Racker, 1957). The analytic setting provides a space where shifting dramas, shaped by a reverberating system of contemporary interactions between analyst, patient and unconscious experiences can become alive in words and action. At the same time the setting is invested with unconscious phantasies (LaFarge, 2014).

In his *New Introductory Lectures to Psycho-Analysis* (1933) Freud uses for analytic treatment the metaphor of "chemical precipitations", to explain the possibility for the mind of triggering processes in which various elements are transformed, thereby creating a new product.

In Freud's clinical treatment of hysteria, the supremacy of psychic reality over external reality directed his focus of interest to understanding repressed phantasies that manifest themselves in somatic phenomena (Garcia de Barros, 2012). Phantasies are understood in Freud's work to be the product of ego's fantasizing function: their form is imposed by the organization of the ego and its defensive requirements. Once the phantasy content has been repressed, it becomes a content of potential desire and is added to the repressed material and subjected to the primary process (Laplanche and Pontalis, 1968). In her paper "The nature and function of phantasy" Susan Isaacs (1948) provided a theoretical systematization of the concept of unconscious phantasy. She specifically refers to the more primitive strata of psychic life, constituted of phantasies that are correlated with bodily experiences. These phantasies represent life and death drives aimed at the maternal object, fulfil the imaginary satisfaction of desires and take the place of defence mechanisms. With relational experience and maturity these phantasies are gradually organized into specialized functions that form the basis for all the symbolic activities of mental processing (Garcia de Barros, 2012). Segal (1994) distinguishes between more primitive phantasies, which are characteristic of the paranoid-schizoid position and appear in more primitive symbolic forms, and phantasies that appear as proper symbol formations, and are characteristic of the depressive position. She suggests that thought derives from the act of fantasizing: at the onset of mental activity, unconscious phantasy performs the functions that are subsequently replaced by thought. The concept of unconscious phantasy, central to psychoanalytic theory, has undoubtedly been particularly important in Melanie Klein's work. According to Isaacs's postulation regarding oral, anal and genital primary phantasies that are expressed through sensations, feelings and images, Klein (1957) called "memories in feelings" the emotional experiences of the first few months of life that long precede language acquisition and emerge in the transference. Matte-Blanco (1988), by discussing the microscopy of the deepest unconscious layers, indirectly provides an explanation of the implicit concepts of Klein's work. He suggests that two irreconcilable logics are determinant, to varying degrees, for the psychic process: one is asymmetrical and characteristic of the conscious system, based on the principle of non-contradiction, while the other is the symmetrical logic of the unconscious. The properties of the unconscious system according to Freud are: timelessness, displacement, substitution of external reality by psychic reality, lack of contradiction between two opposite drives and condensation, all of them stemming from two principles governing the logic of unconscious: generalization and symmetry. Matte-Blanco classifies the bi-logical structures constituting the entire psychic life into strata that are differentiated by the greater or lesser amount of thought processes accordant with one or the other of the logics present in that stratum. The first layer, virtually conscious and governed by the asymmetrical logic, is followed by two further layers with increasing degrees of symmetry until the fourth and final layer, which is virtually unconscious. According to Matte-Blanco, Kleinian investigation is particularly directed at the third and fourth layers of this continuum (Garcia de Barros, 2012). For LaFarge (2014), unconscious phantasy is the term that best captures the specific and substantive sense of the unconscious: it is an organization of unconscious wishes, fears and beliefs relating to the self, objects and part-objects that shape our inner reality and determine our experience, behaviour and the dramas we find ourselves repeating throughout our lives. Being fundamentally unconscious, it is only through the lived repetition of the unconscious phantasies that they can be known. In analysis the lived repetition is the transference process and hence transference is an essential feature of the analytic practice.

DRIVE (INSTINCT). Sigmund Freud's theory of drives (called "instincts" in the Standard Edition) evolved throughout his life and work. In *Three Essays on the Theory of Sexuality* (1905d) Freud wrote: "The concept of instinct is one of those lying on the frontier between the mental and the physical". Freud also indicates that the first experiences of pleasure are derived from bodily needs necessary to the conservation of life, such as the oral activities of babies that are linked to feeding. It is only at a second stage that the sexual functions find relative autonomy in relation to the self-preservative instincts. The drive is characterized by its source, its pressure, its aim and its object. Freud initially described a class of drives known as the life instincts and believed that these drives were responsible for much of behaviour. Eventually, he came to believe that these life instincts alone could not explain all human behaviour. Freud determined that all instincts fall into one of two major classes: the life instincts (Eros) or the death instincts (Thanatos). The life instincts, often called sexual instincts, are those dealing with basic survival, pleasure, reproduction and, more generally, any type of bond between or among objects. These instincts are essential for sustaining the life of the individual as well as the continuation of the species. The energy created by the life instincts is known as libido.

In his "The theory of the instincts" in *An Outline of Psycho-Analysis* (1938) Freud discussed the fact that instincts can change and alter their goals (by displacement) and can also substitute for one another by passing the energy of one instinct onto another. The libido has the characteristic of being mobile, and Freud accepts that it has undeniable somatic sources, but it flows into the ego from various bodily organs. The diversity of the instincts, their alterations and manifestations unlinked to any single bodily zone show that Freud understands instincts and complex instincts as not being reducible to a causal determinism (Moya and Larrain, 2016).

The concept of the death instincts was initially described in Freud's book *Beyond the Pleasure Principle*, in which he proposed that "the goal of all life is death" (1920). He noted that after people experience a traumatic event, such as war, they often reenact the experience. He concluded that people hold an unconscious desire to die, but that the life instincts largely temper this wish. In Freud's view, self-destructive behaviour is an expression of the energy created by the death instincts. When this energy is directed outward onto others, it is expressed as aggression and violence. The notions of binding and unbinding are crucial. Affect and representation become bound to each other as one goes from the Unconscious system to the Preconscious-Conscious. In the Unconscious, energy is unbounded and mobile, and the rules of the primary process such as displacement and condensation dominate. The pleasure principle reigns, there is an absence of thinking and a predominance of visual and sense impressions. Words are used as objects and there is no sense of time. In the Preconscious-Conscious system energy becomes bounded, leading to the creation of a temporal sequence and a delay of motor discharge through secondary process thinking. In *Beyond the Pleasure Principle* the binding of affects and representations becomes a characteristic of the life drives themselves, in contrast to the death drives.

The death instinct cannot fully express itself because it is mingled and fused with the libidinal drive. Only when a defusion occurs does it manifest itself through unambiguous psychopathological states. Under normal circumstances, the death drive is subsumed by the aim of bringing the living organism back to a quiet state. In fact it works silently outside consciousness and beyond every possibility of being represented in the unconscious. The compulsion to repeat, the nature of primary masochism, the resistance to treatment and the merciless aspect of Superego would all be expressions of the death instinct (De Masi, 2015).

The disjunction between drives and representations follow different vicissitudes in Freud's meta-psychological papers. This disjunction enables Freud to provide a model for understanding different psychopathologies. In hysteria the affect is discharged whilst the ideational content is repressed. In obsessional neurosis the ideational content is rejected and transformed, and the affect disappears via the mechanisms of isolation and reaction formation. In phobias the ideational content is displaced and the quantitative element is transformed into anxiety. Later Freud described a drive that does not correspond to any representation but expresses itself in the repetition compulsion. This is at the basis of Green's (1999) formulations on the negative, the dimension of blank spaces without representations, and that of mental structures where representations have disappeared. So the role of the analyst is not that of interpreting what is already in the mind of the patient, but rather that of inaugurating the symbolic domain and the world of representations.

Freud understands the death instinct in two apparently incompatible ways: on the one hand, as a catastrophic occurrence, destructive and self-destructive for the ego; on the other one, as a quiet return to the state of nirvana. Green (2001) develops Freud's idea regarding the desire for life versus the desire for death and nirvana. Green believes that the desire for an object is central to the human psyche. But when this desire fails, a possible solution is a primary identification, the "narcissistic identification", in which the ego fuses with the object. In this process the ego begins to develop a sense of self-sufficiency and in this state remains isolated. Green calls this state "death narcissism": the living desire is coming under the influence of the desire for death, which seeks withdrawal to an inert and insignificant nirvana.

Green does not accept the idea that the death drive is a tendency towards completely reducing tension so as to attain the inorganic state. However, he uses Freud's central idea that the death drive is an attempt to return to a previous state and this drive is conservative or regressive. Roussillon asserts that the return to the previous state is a defence against a passively experienced return. This can happen when a child's insufficient adaptation to the first environment and to the mother's care causes the baby to experience states of psychic death. The memory traces from this primitive agony are subjected to a repetition compulsion that functions in such a way that the agony cannot be integrated and symbolized. Roussillon (2013) recently described traumatic situations in which certain particular features of the responses and reactions of the environment to the individual's drive impulses have impeded the integration and processing of them. As a consequence, destructiveness is manifested to an even greater degree. In these clinical situations binding of the drives is very difficult to set up and ambivalence, rather than being expressed as a conflict, tends to generate paradoxical patterns that imprison the individual in various kinds of existential deadlock. De Masi (2015) affirms that pleasure does not depend only on the defence of the self against the demands of external reality, or on drive discharge. In its production, the destructive mechanisms, directed against the subject's own self or others, seem as efficacious as those involved in the survival of the individual through self-affirmation and satisfaction of the drives.

DREAMS. In 1900 Sigmund Freud published his grandiose work *The Interpretation of Dreams*. In Freud's theory, dreams represent "the royal road to a knowledge of the unconscious". Dreams are disguised fulfillments of repressed wishes, a representation of unconscious desires, thoughts and motivations. Freud also described two different components of dreams: manifest content and latent content. Manifest content is the actual images, thoughts and content contained within the dream, while the latent content is the hidden psychological meaning of the dream. During dream analysis, the person in therapy shares the manifest content of the dream with the therapist. After specific symbols are pulled from the manifest content, the therapist utilizes free associations to facilitate the exploration of repressed material. The analysis of dreams must come to grips with what Freud calls "the dream-work". Analysis is thus concerned with process, rather than content, as it is the process that reveals the workings of the unconscious. Freud locates four main aspects to the dream-work, the means by which the hidden wish becomes expressed. These four aspects account for how wishes and desires become structured and organized unconsciously: condensation (condenses many different ideas into one element); displacement (replaces a latent element by a well-concealed allusion to it, so the psychical emphasis is shifted from an important element to a relatively trivial one); considerations of representability or figurability (transform thoughts into visual elements); secondary revision (makes something whole and more or less coherent out of the distorted product of the dream-work).

In subsequent works Freud would modify his initial assertion regarding dreams as mental activity assigned the function of guarding sleep, thus intervening in the allucinatory fulfillment of repressed unconscious desires (Vincour Fischbein and Miramon, 2015). In "Lecture XVII: The sense of symptoms" in *Introductory Lectures on Psycho-Analysis* (1915–1916) Freud proposes that symptoms, dreams and faulty operations reveal a meaning that is linked with the lived experience of the subject.

In *Beyond the Pleasure Principle* (1920) Freud postulates that the exceptions to dreams as wish-fulfillments may not be exceptions to the rule, but may be dreams whose traumatic genesis is more marked than in others. Years later (1938) he specified that, in the case of the traumatic neuroses, the dream is an attempt to get rid of a disturbance of sleep by means of a wish-fulfillment. Here emerges a new Freudian conception of the dream-work as serving an anti-trauma function with the aim of maintaining psychic integrity (Vincour Fischbein and Miramon, 2015).

Bion (1992) affirmed that the function of dreaming can be understood as a mental construct to be digested by the metabolic function of emotional experience. In such perspective dreams acquire the status of "α-thoughts": they are the raw material in the function of learning from emotional experience. According to Bion, dreams may manifest as "dream-transformations" in the patient, in the analyst and in the treatment, and dreaming gives a sense of the process. The dream-work is an attempt to achieve common sense as a part of the synthesizing function of the dream (Vincour Fischbein and Miramon, 2015).

Botella (2014) focuses on the theory that not only do dreams contain an unrepresented memory, but also the dream-work can be a model for constructing memories. A "regredience" of thought processes allows access to be gained to early psychic zones beyond represented memories. In such a perspective, archaeological psychoanalysis can be complemented by transformational analysis.

THE OEDIPUS COMPLEX. In Freud's theory the access to genitality and to the choice of a sexual object in adult life depends fundamentally on one's adequately overcoming the Oedipus complex. Although Freud had previously alluded to the oedipal situation, in a letter to Ferenczi dated

28 June 1908 the oedipal theme is first addressed under the heading "Oedipus complex". Freud underlines the oedipal conflict as the "nuclear complex of every neurosis" (1909) and in *Totem and Taboo* (1912–1913) he localizes this complex in the inheritance of mankind. Freud suggests the existence of a primal horde whose primal father had monopolized the women of the horde, forced his sons into sexual abstinence and expelled them. The frustrated sons got together and killed the primal father but they felt guilty about the murder and did not realize their former incestuous wishes. This event would have been imprinted on the phylogenic heritage of mankind, and, because Freud considered ontogenesis as a recapitulation of phylogenesis, the oedipal situation of an individual would repeat these dynamics (Zepf *et al.*, 2016). Subjects' identities and psychopathologies, as well as their intersubjective and social relations, are structured at their foundation around this complex.

Childhood genital organization is linked both to the apex of the Oedipus complex and its dissolution. Before this phase boys display an affectionate identification with their fathers and are not rivalrous with them regarding their mothers. Wishes and phantasies characteristic of the Oedipus complex emerge during the phallic phase and betray a double orientation derived from our innate bisexuality: the boy child wants to take the father's place as the mother's love object (positive or active Oedipus complex), or he wants to stand in for the mother as the object of the father's desires (negative or passive Oedipus complex) (Hartke, 2016). Concerning girls, Freud sees their pre-oedipal links with their mothers as more important and protracted than those of boys. Instead of a castration complex they develop castration denial and penis envy. The most important consequence for girls' later development is to abandon their mother as love object and replace her with their father. This finally introduces them to the Oedipus complex while, in the boy, the fear of castration destroys the Oedipus complex (Freud, 1925).

Melanie Klein (1945) places the complex's origin in the second year of life. The early manifestations of the Oedipus complex begin with the infant's relationship with the breast and are present during the first year of life. For Freud libidinal wishes, phallic phase and castration anxiety are the foundation of oedipal issues. For Klein, the bedrock is believed to be destructive fantasies, the primary relationship with the mother's breast and other anxieties more primitive than castration anxiety (Hartke, 2016). The oscillation between two primary objects, father's penis and mother's breast, both in boys and girls, is responsible for an intimate interaction between the positive and negative Oedipus complex. For Klein the development of the Superego and the Oedipus complex are intertwined, and this point of view no longer sees the Superego as heir to the Oedipus complex, as Freud would have it. The combined parent figure, characteristic of paranoid-schizoid position, is the fantasy that one's parents, or their sexual organs, are united and give the parents mutual and permanent oral, anal and genital gratification. Klein emphasizes the importance of undoing the combined parent figure to achieve an adequate evolution of the complex: being able to distinguish the two parents allows children to understand their parent's relationship and is the precondition to unite them in a loving fashion (Hartke, 2016). Winnicott (1969) firmly agreed with the Freudian theory that the Oedipus complex belonged developmentally to the phase after infancy. Thus, despite his agreement with Klein's views about female sexuality, he distances himself from her radical rewriting of the Freudian theory. He outlined that the father has a structuring role on the mind of the baby, and that this is also connected to the place of the father in the mother's mind: that is, not only the baby's father but also his mother is important for his mental development. Winnicott believed that the Oedipus complex is not only a story about the child's desires but inevitably includes the sense of the relationship between parents, that is, the primal scene also includes the child's reality perception of the link between his parents. The complex is elaborated with his conscious and unconscious phantasies about that relationship and his part in it (Joyce, 2016).

TRANSFERENCE AND COUNTERTRANSFERENCE. In the last chapter of *Studies on Hysteria* (Breuer and Freud, 1895) transference gets its first mention. At this point Freud considered transference to be a mere impediment to treatment. In 1905 he postulated that the analysis of transference is the principal factor involved in the therapeutic action of psychoanalysis: "Transference, which seems ordained to be the greatest obstacle to psycho-analysis, becomes its most powerful ally" (1905e). Freud saw transference as being aspects of the patient's early history being repeated, transferred in his relationship with the analyst. Through the phenomenon of transference, the past repeats itself in the present and in a psychoanalysis it becomes "a piece of real life". Freud also outlined that "we must treat the patient's illness not as an event of the past, but as a present-day force". The shifting of analytic focus from external reality to psychic reality was later deepened and extended by Klein's discovery of a whole inner realm of objects, an unconscious world within that is in interplay with external reality. Melanie Klein took this further, showing how aspects of the very early relationship of the child with his parents were internalized and built up his inner world of objects, and that aspects of these inner objects were projected into the relationship with the analyst forming the transference.

Christopher Bollas (1987), in an early contribution, described the creation of an internal space within the analyst for the reception of the patient's unconscious transference material. Recently Ogden (2014), taking up Winnicott's masterful analysis of "Fear of breakdown" (1971), considers the transference as a form of fantasy activity that is a means of thinking for the first time, in relation with the analyst, about emotional events of the past that were too disturbing to be experienced at the time when they occurred.

Psychoanalysis differs from other treatments in that it utilizes the therapist's subjectivity: the analyst observes inwards to register his or her emotional reactions with the patient. These reactions are summarized as countertransference (Salomonsson, 2012). Winnicott (1949) remarks that the analyst may reach and manage his love and hate in reaction to the actual personality and behaviour of the patient. Freud (1912) suggested that the analyst should turn his unconscious like a receptive organ towards the transmitting unconscious of the patient. The many controversies surrounding the definition, significance and technical use of countertransference begin with the word itself, invented by Freud. Countertransference is both a hindrance and a tool for understanding the patient. It must be seen as ubiquitous, and it must be seen as non-pathological (Greenberg, 2012). The analyst is not only required to diagnose and to make interventions; he has to observe himself as part of what occurs in the interaction between transference and countertransference. And the analyst does not only react but is also influenced by many factors: his fundamental attitude, his individual life and learning history, situation-specific feelings (Wegner, 2014). Heimann (1950) and Rosenfeld (1987) accorded an important status to the countertransference analysis as a diagnostic tool.

Sandler (1976) includes in the concept of transference not only the illusory perception of the other, but also the unconscious attempts to manipulate the other to act out predetermined roles in order to enact a repetition of preceding experiences or relationships, so it is inevitable that the analyst will also enter into the part assigned to him by the patient. The analyst will identify unconsciously with the internal object with whom the patient is trying to repeat, in the transference, a significant situation from the past. The analysis of the countertransferential reactions and, in particular, those intense, chaotic and disturbing emotions, from which the analyst can only disentangle himself in the après-coup through a careful and patient work on the countertransference, allows him to distinguish between what belongs to the patient and what belongs to him (Rosenfeld, 1987).

The intensity of certain countertransferential feelings can be traced back to pathological defences, to unresolved conflicts and to the analyst's "blind spots" (Freud, 1912). The process of working through such feelings must therefore take place in the double direction of self-analysis, which allows him to find, inside himself, the parts of himself that remain unanalyzed (Russo, 1998).

Ogden (1995) very clearly describes the relationship between the subjectivity of the analyst and that of the patient and emphasizes the role of the analyst's reverie during the session. Ogden relies on Bion's concept of reverie, that is, everything that goes on in the mind of the analyst during the session. He includes all kinds of daydreams and fantasies, not just those that seem to be related to the patient's material.

There is in psychoanalysis an ongoing theoretical articulation of the relationship between the intrapsychic and the interpsychic. The concepts of countertransference and projective identification include identifying what is going on in the analyst's mind in order to formulate an understanding of the patient's internal world. Winnicott has emphasized the role of the environment in the constitution of the psyche itself. The notion of transitionality is at the junction between inside and outside. Bion has conceptualized the transformational role of the environment. He has indicated the way in which the maternal function of containing thoughts and feelings is internalized and enables the creation of mental space and the development of thought. Green (1999) suggests the concept of framing structure as being at the origins of representation. When holding her infant, the mother leaves the impression of her arms on the child, which constitutes the framing structure that, in her absence, contains the loss of the perception of the maternal object. The negative hallucination of the mother and of the mother's body is, therefore, a precondition for thought and capacity to symbolize. Laplanche (1989) has suggested that infantile sexuality develops under the influence of the parental and primarily maternal "enigmatic signifiers" imprinting the mother's unconscious on the child's erogenous zones, along with the erotic link she has with the father and with the father's own unconscious.

Transference today is understood to be transference based on the past, coming from the present, here and now, transference that transports (Green, 2011). Green describes transference as a double act: it addresses the word and it addresses the object: through the act of verbalization all psychic movements get translated. Observing the transference-countertransference relationship in her clinical work, Alvarez de Toledo (1996) noticed that the act of speaking, in addition to the common function of communicating thoughts, both in its associative and interpretative aspects, serves as a vehicle for actualizing primary unconscious phantasies. Through projective identification, these phantasies reach the psychoanalyst's mind in the form of feelings, emotions and images, often separated from the content of the patient's verbal communication. The author suggests that the psychoanalyst's countertransference reaction is due to the primary origin of these phantasies, revealed through the nonverbal aspects of speech in the relationship with the psychoanalyst.

VERTICAL AND HORIZONTAL PARADIGMS. The vertical and horizontal paradigms cross the experience of the analytic relationship in a complex way, as in a Cartesian graph, and both contribute not only to understanding, but also to accomplishing the therapeutic process.

The vertical paradigm is the traditional paradigm, characterized by an asymmetric analytic relationship shifted on the patient's side, with particular focus on instincts, transference, internal objects. The analyst as a person is the object of the patient's transference, the analyst-mirror, or the "subject supposed to know" described by Lacan (1964): he is in the analytic situation to observe, infer, participate only in order to understand and treat. Analytic work develops through the historical-temporal dimension of "there and then", from the patient's childhood, by probing the past for searching traumas, significant events, damaged relations, oedipal patterns, primal scenes, early relational modes. The theory is to give sense to data gathered by the analyst and thus it must be a strong theory (instincts, sex, dreams) that is an integral part of the setting, among the analyst's tools.

The analyst is swinging between helping a "natural" recomposition of the analyzed elements and reconstructing missing pieces, between the tasks of the chemist and those of the archaeologist, through the transference's analysis and the analysis of the resistances and the interpretation.

In the horizontal paradigm the patient's past is re-experienced and corrected, not only through what Greenberg (1981) calls "participation with" by the therapist, namely empathic participation, but also and especially through "participation in", namely the therapist's temporary identification with figures of the patient's past, due to the therapist's predisposition based on past experiences (so called "enactment"). In any case, the starting point of the therapist's interventions should always be what the therapist feels (Bacciagaluppi, 2012), and there are more symmetric positions of analyst and patient. The analyst's contributions to the relationship become central, from countertransference to therapist's transference, from projective identification to projective counteridentification, from countertransference's acting to enactment. The analytic scene takes place in the "here and now" of the couple's living situation, in a confrontation between two unconscious attitudes. The "here" refers primarily to what is going on between the two participants in the room, but in addition it conveys the immediate, often concrete, reality of the individual's experience, which may, for example, be focused on his body, or the analyst's room-body. The "now" implies a sense of time, not just past and future, but an awareness of the patient's situation at the moment, one that is dynamic, never static, and that changes from moment to moment. This kind of work of course not only involves an awareness about what is going on immediately in the patient but is necessarily dependent on the analyst's sensitivity, so far as is possible, to what is being evoked in himself (Joseph, 2013).

The analytic process is based upon a work of construction: "analyst and patient build up together one of the possible histories, based on phenomena that take place in their relationship" (Riolo, 1999). Construction is *ex novo* and is a shared construction of stories, narratives, representations or mental contents and mainly psychic structures; what is particularly important in the analysis of severe patients (borderline and psychotic), in order to change the subject's mental functioning. The process is no longer a path, even of the transference neurosis, but becomes a sort of metabolism.

INTERSUBJECTIVITY AND FIELD. The concepts of intersubjectivity and otherness are relevant to psychoanalysis in terms of both the construction of subjectivity and the form the analytic relationship is deemed to assume. Notions such as the analyst as a mirror, analytic neutrality, the rule of abstinence, and the transference and countertransference are some of the issues discussed in the context of the pluralism of psychoanalysis today (Glocer Fiorini, 2016). In Freud's works the role of the mother as the first other encountered in the initial situation of helplessness constitutes the root of the construction of subjectivity. The Oedipus myth describes the shaping and structuring of subjectivity, showing how wishes and rivalries concerning the parents ultimately lead to various kinds of identifications and object choices. The formation of the Superego as an expression of the voices of parents, educators and culture draws attention to certain theoretical aspects that inevitably include other persons (Glocer Fiorini, 2016).

The patterns of experience that organize the psyche of the analyst and the patient determine the confrontation of their subjectivities in the analytic situation. Their interaction gives rise to the intersubjective matrix, that will be at the origin of changes in the patient's psyche. Although the intersubjective phenomena was approached and formulated in different ways in South America and in European countries, a truly intersubjective turn has affected the psychoanalytic world in the last 60 years (Bohleber, 2010). Developmental research has shown how the childlike self emerges from reciprocal regulation and recognition processes in the primary relationships. Modern research into early mentalization processes postulates a self that can only materialize by being mirrored by the psyche of the primary object. William and Madeleine Baranger (1961) have been developing the field theory of the analytical situation: dynamics and power of the "analytical field" are determined by an underlying unconscious fantasy. Field is a place in which the circularity of the interaction therapist–patient is fully expressed, and is the origin of everything relational. The idea of a field is primarily that of an affective, social or cultural environment able to nourish and sustain, or in any way influence, also negatively, individuals and relations in its context and dependent on it. The field in such a theoretical frame denotes the situation of two persons who are inextricably linked and complementary during this situation, and involved in the same dynamic process; the individuals, engaged and immersed in the field they produce by interacting, are to be distinguished from it, which qualifies as a third element with independent dynamics. The unconscious phantasies of the analytic pair confer a specific meaning on the bi-personal field that indicates the degree of urgency imposed on the moment-to-moment interpretation. Bezoari and Ferro (1992) associate the concept of the bi-personal field with Bion's (1962) theory of the container–contained relationship, the constitution of the apparatus for thinking and the importance of psychoanalyst's mind in obtaining maximum productivity in each session. The sum of the observational standpoints of psychoanalyst and patient in relation to the field constitutes what is known as an affective "olograph" because of the similarity in the depth perception that results from the association between two images of the same object viewed from different angles.

Harry Stack Sullivan (1953) developed his theory of interpersonal psychiatry, a relationship in which each member is involved as a part of an interpersonal field and not as a separate entity, in processes influenced by the field and, in turn, influencing it. Ferro (1999) has theorized his own concept of "bi-personal field", in which the participants converge to give rise to a new entity, which is more than the sum of the two individual fields. Psychoanalysis is going towards a relational perspective that, considered as a whole, shows some common ground based upon: theory of intersubjectivity, enactment, "corrective emotional experiences", role responsiveness, hermeneutic-constructivist model, two-person psychology, contemporary psychoanalysis.

Ogden (1994) terms the product of the unconscious interplay the "analytic third", a third subjectivity, generated by the analyst and analysand. According to Ogden, both individual subjectivities (patient/analyst) will be encompassed by a third unconscious subject of the analysis, created conjointly in a very specific form of projective identification, with constantly shifting contents. It constitutes an intersubjective analytic third that the author calls "subjugating third", having the characteristic of encompassing the individual subjectivities of the participants (Ithier, 2016). In de M'Uzan's (2013) work intersubjectivity implies the depersonalization of the analyst: the analyst should be prepared to experience a certain vacillation of his/her identity and allows the analysand to invade his/her psychic space, triggering what he calls "paradoxical thoughts". These are thoughts existing in a potential state of the analysand, who will be led to elaborate them with the analyst's help. A sort of new organism may emerge, a "psychological chimera", which has its own models of function (Ithier, 2016). Ithier (2016) designs this chimera as a "mental squiggle", referring to the famous "squiggle" game described by Winnicott (1971): the drawing made by the analyst and the child, then by the child and the analyst, produces the concrete representation of a new character born from the unforeseen encounter of their unconscious processes. Here, once again, the intersubjective interaction between the two members of the pair appears, as well as an openness to the unconscious.

According to L. Russo (2000) two levels of affectivity coexist in the analytic relation: the one pertains to the origins, the fusional link to the mother, before any representation and individual issue. It is mimetic, archaic, contagious, may be lived in the present, and coincides with the idea of a structural unconscious and primitive states of mind (the Bion's protomental); the other, expressing itself in the separate dimension of the differentiated subject–object relationship, open to representations and words, diachronic, liable to be remembered and told, coincides with the idea of the repressed unconscious, in the oedipal area. At this latter level, transference as a re-edition takes place, whereas at the former level, analyst and patient build up a story by itself, independent of their respective stories.

REFERENCES. Alvarez de Toledo LG., *The analysis of "associating", "interpreting", and "words"*, in «The International Journal of Psychoanalysis», 1996, 77; Bacciagaluppi M., *Paradigms in psychoanalysis: An integration*, 2012; Baranger M., Baranger W., *The analytic situation as a dynamic field*, in «The International Journal of Psychoanalysis», 1961, 89; Bezoari M., Ferro A., *Elements of a model of the analytic field*, in «Rev Psychoanal», 1992, 47; Bion W.R., *Cogitations*, 1992; Bion W.R., *The psychoanalytic study of thinking: II A theory of thinking*, in «The International Journal of Psychoanalysis», 1962, 43; Blass R.B., *Introduction to "How and why unconscious phantasy and transference are the defining features of psychoanalytic practice"*, in «The International Journal of Psychoanalysis», 2014, 95; Bohleber W., *Destructiveness, intersubjectivity and trauma: The identity crisis of modern psychoanalysis*, 2010; Bollas C., *Expressive uses of the countertransference. Notes to the patient from oneself*, in «Contemporary Psychoanalysis», 19, 1, 1987; Botella C., *On remembering: The notion of memory without recollection*, in «The International Journal of Psychoanalysis», 2014, 95; Breuer J., Freud S., *Studies on hysteria*, in *The Standard Edition*, 1895, II; De Masi F., *Is the concept of the death drive still useful in the clinical field?* in «The International Journal of Psychoanalysis», 2015, 96; Ferro A., *The bi-personal field: Experiences in child analysis*, 1999; Freud S., (1920), *Beyond the pleasure principle*, in *The Standard Edition*, 18; Freud S. (1909), *Five lectures on psycho-analysis*, in *The Standard Edition*, XI, 1953–1974; Freud S. (1905e), *Fragment of an analysis of a case of hysteria*, in *The Standard Edition*, VII, 1953–1974; Freud S. (1915–1916), *Introductory lectures on psycho-analysis (part III)* in *The Standard Edition*, XVI, 1953–1974; Freud S. (1933), *New introductory lectures on psycho-analysis*, in *The Standard Edition*, XII, 1953–1974; Freud S. (1914), *On the history of the psychoanalytic movement. Papers on metapsychology and other works: The unconscious*, in *The Standard Edition*, XIV, 1953–1974; Freud S. (1912), *Recommendations to physicians practicing psycho-analysis*, in *The Standard Edition*, XII, 1953–1974; Freud S. (1899), *Screen memories*, in *The Standard Edition*, III, 1953–1974; Freud S. (1925), *Some psychological consequences of the anatomical distinction between the sexes*, in *The Standard Edition*, XIX, 1953–1974; Freud S. (1938), *The theory of the instincts*, in *An outline of psychoanalysis*, in *The Standard Edition*, XXIII, 1953–1974; Freud S. (1915), *The unconscious*, in *The Standard Edition*, XIV, 1953–1974; Freud S. (1905d), *Three essays on the theory of sexuality*, in *The Standard Edition*, VII, 1953–1974; Freud S. (1912–1913), *Totem and taboo*, in *The Standard Edition*, XIII, 1953–1974; Garcia de Barros I., *The Latin American contribution to the psychoanalytic concept of phantasy*, in «The International Journal of Psychoanalysis», 2012, 93; Glocer Fiorini L., *Intersubjectivity, otherness, and thirdness: A necessary relationship*, in «The International Journal of Psychoanalysis», 2016, 97; Green A., *Borderline cases: From private madness to death and destruction drives*, in «French Rev Psychoanal», 2011, 75, 2; Green A., *Life narcissism, death narcissism*, 2001; Green A., *The work of the negative*, 1999; Greenberg J., *Commentary on José Bleger's theory and practice in psychoanalysis: Psychoanalytic praxis*, in «The International Journal of Psychoanalysis», 2012, 93; Greenberg J., *Prescription or description: Therapeutic action of psychoanalysis*, in «Contemporary Psychoanalysis», 1981, 17; Hartke R., *The Oedipus complex: A confrontation at the central cross-roads of psychoanalysis*, in «The International Journal of Psychoanalysis», 2016, 97; Heimann P., *On countertransference*, in «The International Journal of Psychoanalysis», 1950, 31; Isaacs S., *The nature and function of phantasy*, in «The International Journal of Psychoanalysis», 1948, 29; Ithier B., *The arms of the chimeras*, in «The International Journal of Psychoanalysis», 2016, 97; Joseph B., *Here and now: My perspective*, in «The International Journal of Psychoanalysis», 2013, 94; Joyce A., *Infantile sexuality: Its place in the conceptual developments of Anna Freud and Donald W. Winnicott*, in «The International Journal of Psychoanalysis», 2016, 97; Klein M. (1957), *Envy and gratitude and other works 1946–1963*, 1975; Klein M., *The Oedipus complex in the light of early anxiety*, in *The writings of Melanie Klein*, 1945; Lacan J. (1964), *The four fundamental concepts of psychoanalysis*, in *The seminars of Jacques Lacan*, XI, 1977; LaFarge L., *How and why unconscious phantasy and transference are the defining features of psychoanalytic practice*, in «The International Journal of Psychoanalysis», 2014, 95; Laplanche J., Pontalis J.-B., *Fantasy and the origins of sexuality*, in «The International Journal of Psychoanalysis», 1968, 49; Laplanche J., *Towards a general theory of seduction*, in *New foundations for psychoanalysis*, 1989; M'Uzan de M., *During the session. Considerations on the analyst's mental functioning*, in *Death and identity*, 2013; Matte-Blanco I., *Thinking, feeling and being: Clinical reflections on the fundamental antinomy of human beings and world*, 1988; Moya P., Larrain M., *Sexuality and meaning in Freud and Merleau-Ponty*, in «The International Journal of Psychoanalysis», 2016, 97; Ogden T., *Analyzing forms of aliveness and deadness of the ransference-countertransference*, in «The International Journal of Psychoanalysis», 1995, 76; Ogden T., *Fear of breakdown and the unlived life*, in «The International Journal of Psychoanalysis», 2014, 95, 2; Ogden T., *The analytic third: Working with intersubjective clinical facts*, in «The International Journal of Psychoanalysis», 1994, 75; Racker H., *The meanings and uses of countertransference*, in «The Psychoanalytic Quarterly», 1957, 26; Riolo F., *Il paradigma della "cura"*, in «Rivista di Psicoanalisi», XLV, 1999, 1; Rosenfeld H., *Impasse and interpretation: Therapeutic and anti-therapeutic factors in the psychoanalytic treatment of psychotic, borderline, and neurotic patients*, 1987; Roussillon R., *The function of the object in the binding and unbinding of the drives*, in «The International Journal of Psychoanalysis», 2013, 94; Russo L., *L' indifferenza dell'anima*, 2000; Russo L.,

Sul contro-transfert, in « Rivista di Psicoanalisi», 1998, 44; Salomonsson B., *Psychoanalytic case presentations in a weaving thoughts group: On countertransference and group dynamics*, in «The International Journal of Psychoanalysis», 2012, 93; Sandler J., *Countertransference and role-responsiveness*, in «International Review of Psychoanalysis», 1976, 3; Segal H., *Phantasy and reality*, in «The International Journal of Psychoanalysis», 1994, 75; Sullivan H., *The interpersonal theory of psychiatry*, 1953; Vincour Fischbein S., Miramon B., *Theoretical trajectories: Dreams and dreaming from Freud to Bion*, in «The International Journal of Psychoanalysis», 2015, 96; Wegner P., *Process-oriented psychoanalytic work in initial interviews and the importance of the opening scene*, in «The International Journal of Psychoanalysis», 2014, 95; Winnicott D.W. (1969), *The use of an object in the context of Moses and Monotheism*, in Winnicott C., Shepherd R., Davis M. (eds.), *Psychoanalytic explorations*, 1989; Winnicott D.W., *Fear of breakdown*, in «Int Rev Psychoanal», 1971, 1; Winnicott D.W., *Hate in the countertransference*, in «The International Journal of Psychoanalysis», 1949, 30; Winnicott D.W., *Therapeutic consultations in child psychiatry*, 1971; Zepf S., Ullrich B., Seel D., *Oedipus and the Oedipus complex: A revision*, in «The International Journal of Psychoanalysis», 2016, 97.

BEHAVIOURAL PARADIGM

P. Meazzini

THE FIRST GENERATION. During the 1950s, psychoanalysis, in all its ramifications, was the elective psychotherapy. There were no opposing views: just some lunatic, as English people say, tried to confute some psychoanalytic hypothesis, but with little success. However, that decade revealed the shallowness in which "the joyous psychoanalytic war machine" (as it was called by A. Salter (1952)) could wreck. On the one hand, "client-centered therapy" started to take shape. This approach was also among the first to conduct empirical research in clinical psychology. On the other hand, "behavioural therapy" developed in those years. These were two very different points of view but both were potential subverters of the stagnant psychoanalytic vision. In all truth, the emergence of behavioural therapy is not only linked to the crypticism and to the alleged ineffectiveness of psychoanalysis (not yet proven at that time); above all, it depended on a way of coping with psychopathological problems by adopting a view that was, at that time, in some ways opposite in respect to the established tradition (Meazzini, 1980, 1955).

The main names, which formed the first generation of behavioural therapists, are basically three. In 1952, Hans Eysenck (not to be confused with Michael Eysenck, a brilliant cognitive psychologist), affected the psychological culture of that period by taking the risk of publishing an article (1952) in which he stated that psychodynamic therapies were producing inadequate results, below those obtained by control groups without treatment. The effect of this article was disruptive: the uproar was so deafening that Eysenck risked losing his job at the Maudsley Institute of Psychiatry (personal communication). It should be noted that Eysenck's article was not free of methodological flaws, but its publication had two main consequences. On the one hand, it showed that "the emperor has no clothes", that is, it was stated that psychodynamics, in all its forms, does not work. On the other hand, it opened a line of research aiming at measuring the impact of different psychotherapies in respect of the disorders experienced by subjects (this was called *outcomes and process research* and it led to meta-analytic research). Eysenck's "allergy" to psychoanalysis was always present in his work as a researcher and essayist. This culminated in *Decline and Fall of the Freudian Empire* (1985), which was an ironically corrosive libel. Precisely for this reason, it was never translated into Italian, given the complacent attitude of Italian publishers and press towards smoky but fascinating theories. However, Eysenck was not the only

"Pasdaran" of the era. To his credit, two vital contributions for the future development of behavioural therapy need also to be mentioned: one is the writing of the first manifesto of this therapy, which was written together with S. Rachman (Eysenck and Rachman, 1965). In this text, psychodynamics was compared to a point of view that was, in some ways, diametrically opposite. In fact, much of the literature about the unconscious, preconscious, etc., was considered as fiction; the importance of a subject's past was denied; these concepts were replaced by the courageous focus on the here-and-now and on the need to formulate assumptions, theories and therapeutic strategies that could undergo scientific scrutiny. The second contribution is the development of a very articulate theory of personality. This theory started from sources that were historically distant in time and arrived to explain two fundamental personality attitude pairs: extraversion–introversion and neuroticism–stability, to which Eysenck added psychoticism. However, despite his efforts, his personality theory did not have a significant influence on behavioural therapy.

The second main author of the first generation of behavioural therapists is J.Wolpe, which was the only real therapist in the behavioural triad of the 1950s. His support of Eysenck's manifesto was not dictated by theoretical dissatisfactions, but by therapeutic failures. Wolpe, South African by birth, received a mandate by his government to intervene on World War II veterans to help them to overcome their painful psychological disorders and to integrate them back into society (Wolpe, 1958; Wolpe and Lazarus, 1966). Wolpe tried to achieve these results using the only existing therapy at the time, namely, psychodynamic psychotherapy: his failure was very frustrating. For this reason, he searched for other ways and he discovered, with some surprise, the existence of more promising possibilities. The approaches that persuaded him the most were the theory of C. Hull, which was dominant in the psychology of that time, and the line of research initiated by J. Masserman, who was interested in studying the evolution of neuroses (as they were called at that time) of dogs. Wolpe was prompted by the interesting data arising from this line of research; first, he worked on states of anxiety and phobia in animals (cats) and then he applied the most beneficial strategies to man. The theoretical basis of his work, derived from C. Sherrington, was later disproved by neurophysiological research. However, from a practical viewpoint, Wolpe elaborated one of the most used and effective strategies in behavioural therapy: "systematic desensitization", which is applicable to all the disorders that today are known as generalized anxiety disorders. Equally important was his commitment to developing another intervention strategy: assertive training, for which he owes a debt to Salter. Assertive training was created to help people with social phobia to overcome relational discomfort, but this method has found numerous applications in other clinical areas and in non-therapeutic fields. In particular, it was adopted in schools, where it became a stimulus to producing curricula designed to teach students social skills and pro-sociality, and in organizations, where it became a must in management training.

The third and perhaps brightest member of the first generation of behaviourists is B.F. Skinner (Skinner, 1938, 1953, 1973). He was not as brilliant a theorist as Eysenck nor therapist as Wolpe: he was a rigorous scientist and an intriguing author. His *Walden Two* cannot be forgotten. In this utopian novel, he outlined a future society organized under the laws of learning discovered and experimented by Skinner himself. Beyond his literary "digressions", Skinner's contributions to behavioural therapy were numerous. He solved a long-standing problem in the methodology of clinical and applied psychology by responding positively to this question: "Is it possible to produce scientifically reliable results by working on a single subject rather than on groups?". The answer to this question was a research methodology and a therapeutic intervention called, today, "single-subject experimental design". This very important methodology solved a question concerning the outcome of therapeutic interventions, which can be summarized in this way: Are the results truly the product of a therapeutic intervention, or only one of the many non-specific factors involved during that time period? This methodology could finally make a clean sweep of the attempts made by world famous psychologists (Piaget above all) to create a solid experimental basis to their theoretical building, which was often obtained by observing a single subject. It is worth mentioning a strong methodological statement made by Skinner: it is more favourable to dedicate 100 hours to studying a single subject rather than an hour to 100 subjects. The advent of the "single-subject" methodology has had significant implications both for the world of research and psychotherapy: it was highlighted that in both these areas it is possible to test theories and hypotheses by using the tools developed by experimental science. One of the most promising achievements of the manifesto of Boulder, a town in Colorado where the most important deans of faculty of psychology gathered in the 1950s, was to define the mission of clinical psychologists and psychotherapists. In short, this category of clinicians should have included in their competence the typical rigour of scientific researchers on the one hand, and the ability to understand others, a fundamental prerequisite in every psychotherapy approach, on the other. However, Skinner is not only known for this important methodological innovation; he is unanimously considered the leading theoretician of learning. Thanks to his research, several laws that govern behaviour were discovered; terms as reinforcement, reinforcement programmes, learning without errors, etc., are now part of so-called general psychology. Equally remarkable were the deductions made by Skinner and his students, which were then tested on an applicative level, starting from his research and discoveries made in laboratory: this is what is known as Applied Behaviour Analysis (ABA). This is a series of strategies aiming at identifying and, where necessary, modifying the existing relationships between a behaviour and the situations that precede and follow its appearance. These strategies subvert the view according to which behaviours would be the result of internal cognitive mechanisms and unconscious processes; they show how it is the environment that needs to be changed in order for its modification to cause a change in behaviour. This shocking reversal of perspective was accepted due to three observations; first observation: working on a behavioural level means obtaining more explicit and verifiable data than those referring to a cognitive universe and even more than those referring to the unconscious, whose exploration is anchored to a game of metaphors and inferences; second observation: behaviour does not consist only of visible actions – including language – but also of covert responses, which are accessible to the person who experiences them. These responses are based on the laws that govern people's public behaviour. In this case, the expression used is *covert conditioning* (Cautela, 1986); third observation: similar considerations can be applied to the concept of environment, which does not only refer to external stimuli, but also to stimuli internal to the person, such as thoughts, emotions, etc. (Galeazzi and Meazzini, 2003). For example, a thought can be stimulated by an emotional event or by a previous thought and it can be, in turn, reinforced by another emotional event or by another thought. ABA has been and continues to be applied to the understanding and treatment of many disorders concerning adults and developmental age subjects. This approach has found its maximum effectiveness in the rehabilitation field. A reassuring aspect of ABA, and of interventions that were inspired by it, is the constant focus on verifying the impact of the adopted strategies. This is another difference in respect to the traditional clinical case report, where it is difficult, if not impossible, to exclude the possibility that clients' changes are the direct consequence of the strategy adopted. Finally, a considerable merit of the first generation of behavioural therapists is the creation of an environment that enabled a wide and rapid dissemination of this therapy. First, it spread in the Anglo-Saxon culture and then throughout the world; in many countries (Northern Europe) it has reached a prominent position within the diversified universe of psychotherapy. Of course, there were exceptions – France and Italy in particular, where psychoanalytic thought and Marxist ideology were strong. Moreover, the latter was a resolute opponent of any cultural input coming from the USA.

THE MIDDLE GENERATION. The following generation brought really unorthodox and interesting changes. The greatest impact was determined by the cognitive revolution that spread both in experimental and clinical psychology, although the two approaches were and still are very different.

A. Bandura was the most important author among those who accepted the behaviourist manifesto, although he expanded the boundaries of behavioural therapy. In chronological order, the first of his merits (Bandura, 1969) was the analytical and thorough presentation, Teutonic in breadth and depth, of *behaviour modification* (an American expression indicating behavioural therapy). The most interesting element for the behavioural therapists in that period was the clarity used to express his belief that the therapies based on in-vivo exposure and performance have a greater effectiveness and efficiency than the therapies based on verbal communication. All the strategies based on these elements, such as exposure, desensitization etc., particularly useful in the treatment of social phobia and agoraphobia, benefited from this validation. Another contribution was the introduction of a theoretical and practical approach, which he called "social learning theory". His theoretical effort was based on the attempt to identify a free zone between psychodynamic theories and strictly behaviourist theories derived from Skinner. In an important article (Bandura, 1977), he expressed his disappointment towards psychodynamic theories, as they were obsessively focused on considering internal processes the ultimate causes of human behaviour. According to him, these could be identified only through a dubious and confused inferential method: "the attribution of behaviour to inner forces can perhaps be likened to early explanatory schemes in other branches of science". The disappointment expressed in respect of the behavioural perspective represented by Skinner was more mitigated. This was criticised "for providing an incomplete rather than an inaccurate account of human behaviour". Starting from these criticisms aimed at two opposing interpretations of human behaviour, Bandura developed his theory along three directions. The first one is epistemological and it is called circular determinism: a now widely shared belief according to which "psychological functioning is best be understood in terms of a continuous reciprocal interaction between behaviour and its controlling conditions". Among the factors that make this interaction possible, there are intra-individual processes and cognitive processes in particular. He analysed them – this is the second direction – in the light of the HIP (human information processing) model. Finally, the concept of self-efficacy is of central importance and it represents the pivotal point of the latest research conducted by Bandura and his group. Self-efficacy is based on the concept of expectancy, that is, a set of expectations that people develop towards different segments that compose their psychological and, more broadly, existential reality. Two classes of expectancies are particularly interesting: the first one refers to efficacy expectations in their strict sense; namely, it concerns the probability of generating a particular behaviour or performance that people assign to themselves. Surely these probabilities depend on the proportion of successes and failures experienced by people during their ontogenetic development and how they were interpreted and evaluated. The second class concerns results and not behaviour, that is, it contains expectancies closely linked to the probability that people assign to themselves of obtaining rewarding results through the production of behaviours. Finally, it is important to remember the hundreds of studies of other authors who have scrutinized in detail the phenomenon of modelling (learning by imitation), a process by which a person learns or unlearns new behavioural patterns by observing another person who takes on the role of the model. These strategies are particularly effective in solving problems arising during the developmental age. Therefore, they have become a fundamental element of many psychotherapies directed to this group of clients. In this second generation, Bandura excels on a theoretical and experimental level. However, the research conducted by M. Seligman on depression appear more interesting on a therapeutic level. These studies (1972) gave life to the concept of helplessness and gave rise to some very effective behavioural treatments, especially when combined with cognitive therapy (Beck's approach in particular). Moreover, Seligman should also be remembered for another aspect that could lead to the emergence of a new paradigm in the already crowded universe of psychology: positive psychology. Among other things, this approach is changing the way of looking at people and of intervening on them by focusing not only on healing but also on a significant improvement in people's quality of life.

Another author, with a more circumscribed importance than Seligman, is D. Meichenbaum. Initially, he was interested in the application of Skinnerian techniques on clients in developmental age. Later, he developed a new technique, called "self-instructional training" (Meichenbaum and Goodman, 1971). Thanks to this method, hyperactive children could control their behaviour by giving proper instructions to themselves. However, his most important contribution (Meichenbaum, 1985) was a new strategy aiming at controlling stress, known as *stress inoculation training*. Different behavioural techniques can be found in it, such as Jacobson's relaxation, systematic desensitization, etc. The original aspect of this strategy – derived from the theory of L. Lurja and his belief that language can also be used to guide and control human behaviour – is the identification of internal dialogue. This is represented by the words that people direct to themselves: depending on its characteristics, internal dialogue can make a difficult situation of the subject heavier or can lighten it; the task of the therapist is to change it and to make it useful for overcoming stress. Finally, there is one more strategy: *problem solving therapy*, based on an obvious observation: many psychological problems are the result of people's inability to make the best use of their intellectual resources to solve them. G. Spivack's group (Spivack and Shure, 1974; Spivack *et al.*, 1976) was among the first to develop and implement problem solving strategies. They applied them to subjects of developmental age with social adjustment problems. D. Mahoney (1977) and T. D'Zurilla (1986) extended their application to psychological disorders such as stress, relationship problems, agoraphobia, depression, etc. An Italian version of problem solving therapy was proposed by Meazzini (2009a, 2009b), who perfected the algorithm on which this strategy is based. The main steps are the perception of the problem, its acceptance and description, the generation of alternatives, the identification of the consequences, the assessment of the consequences, the taking of decisions and their implementation.

CONCLUSION. In its original form, behavioural therapy no longer exists. The Skinnerian version survives only or mainly in the United States, due to a group of "guardians" who want to maintain the sacred fire of their master. What an unhappy fate for a scientist to be transformed into a guru! In the rest of the world, it has become an integral part of cognitive-behavioural therapy, to which it contributed with a good number of intervention strategies and a rigorous scientific approach. This new model is constantly under a process of refinement and change: there are always interesting innovations subjected to scientific scrutiny. In recent years, there has been an unpredictable alliance with Buddhist thought, which has given rise to significant innovations, like mindfulness training models, action commitment therapy and compassion therapy. The world of science is a graveyard full of crosses, that is, theories that after an initial wave of interest showed so many gaps that they were abandoned; it is too early to say what the fate of these theories will be.

REFERENCES. Bandura A., *Principles of behaviour modification*, 1969; Id., *Self efficacy: Toward a unifying theory of behavioural change*, in «Psychological Review», 1977, 84; Cautela J., *The covert conditioning handbook*, 1986; D'Zurilla T.J., *Problem solving therapy*, 1986; Eysenck H.J., *The effects of psychotherapy: An evaluation*, in «Journal of Consulting Psychology», 1952, 16; Id., *Decline and fall of the Freudian empire*, 1985; Eysenck H.J., Rachman S., *The causes and cures of neurosis*, 1965; Galeazzi A., Meazzini P., *Mente e comportamento*, 2003; Mahoney M.J., *Personal science: A cognitive-learning therapy*, in A. Ellis, R. Grieger (eds.), *Handbook of rational therapy*, 1977; Meazzini P., *Il comportamentismo: una storia culturale*, 1980; Id., *La terapia del comportamento: una storia*, 1995; Id., *Mi stresso, quindi sono*, 2009a; Id., *Problemi quotidiani*, 2009b; Meichenbaum D., *Stress inoculation training*, 1985; Meichenbaum D., Goodman J., *Training impulsive children to talk to themselves: A means of developing self control*, in «Journal of Abnormal Psychology», 1971, 77; Salter A., *Conditioned reflex therapy*, 1949; Id., *The case against psychoanalysis*, 1952; Seligman M.E.P., *Learned helplessness*, 1972; Skinner B.F., *The behaviour of organism*, 1938; Id., *Science and human bevavior*, 1953; Id., *Studi e ricerche*, 1959; Id., *About behaviourism*, 1973; Spivack G., Shure M.-B., *Social adjustment of young children: A cognitive approach to solving real life problems*, 1974; Spivack G., Platt J.J., Shure M.-B., *The problem solving approach to adjustment*, 1976; Wolpe J.J., *Psychotherapy by reciprocal inhibition*, 1958; Wolpe J.J, Lazarus A., *Behaviour therapy techniques*, 1966.

EXISTENTIAL-HUMANISTIC PARADIGM

I. Yalom

BASIC ASSUMPTIONS. This rather modern paradigm resides on an ancient idea that considers each human being has a unique set of potentials that yearn to be realized. Aristotle's "entelechy" referred to the full realization of potentiality. The fourth cardinal sin, sloth or accidie, has been interpreted by many thinkers as "the sin of failing to do with one's life all that one knows one can do". This is a key concept in the writings of almost every modern humanistic or existential theorist or therapist. Although it has been given many names, such as self-actualization, self-development, development of potential, growth, autonomy and so on, the underlying concept is simple: each human being has an innate set of capacities and potentials and, furthermore, has a primordial knowledge of these potentials. One who fails to live as fully as he or she can, experiences a deep, powerful feeling which I refer to as "existential guilt".

Karen Horney's mature work is based solidly on the concept that, under favourable conditions, the human being will naturally develop his or her intrinsic potential just as an acorn will develop into an oak tree. Horney's major work, *Neurosis and Human Growth*, is subtitled *The Struggle Towards Self-Realization.* Psychopathology, in her view, occurs when adverse circumstances inhibit a child from growing towards the realization of his or her own possibilities. The child then loses sight of its potential self and develops another self-image: "an idealized self" towards which it directs its life energies. She speaks of the sense of alienation, of being split from what one really is, which results in one's overriding one's genuine feelings, wishes and thoughts.

Thus, existential-humanistic therapies view the patient in human rather than behavioural or mechanistic terms. Humanistic and existential approaches share a belief that people have the capacity for self-awareness and choice, and therapy can help this process (Rogers, 1961).

It is my belief that the vast majority of experienced therapists, regardless of adherence to some particular ideological school, employ these existential-humanistic insights and approaches. All competent therapists realize, for example, that an apprehension of one's finiteness can often catalyse a major inner shift of perspective, that it is the relationship that heals, that patients are tormented by choice, that a therapist must catalyse a patient's "will" to act, and that the majority of patients are bedevilled by a lack of meaning in their lives.

Existential-humanistic therapists may employ any of a large variety of techniques used in other approaches in so far as they are consistent with basic existential presuppositions and a human, authentic therapist–patient encounter.

HISTORICAL EVOLUTION. This paradigm is considered to be the "third force" in therapy, as an alternative to the Freudian psychoanalytical and behavioural approaches. This movement began to rumble in the late 1950s, it surfaced and coalesced in the 1960s and it rode madly off in all directions at once in the 1970s. Academic psychology had by the 1950s been long dominated by two major ideological schools. The first, and by far the longest dominant, was a scientific positivistic behaviourism. The second was Freudian psychoanalysis. A minor voice first heard in the late 1930s and 1940s belonged to abnormal and social psychologists who coexisted uncomfortably in the experimental psychology bastions. Gradually those personality theorists (for example, Gordon Allport, Henry Murray and Gardner Murphy and later George Kelly, Abraham Maslow, Carl Rogers and Rollo May) grew uncomfortable with the limitations of both the behaviouristic and the analytic schools. They felt that both of these ideological approaches to the person excluded some of the most important qualities that make the human being human – for example, choice, values, love, creativity, self-awareness, human potential.

In 1950 they formally established a new ideological school which they labelled "humanistic psychology". Humanistic psychology, referred to as the rise of the "third force" in psychology, became a robust organization with growing membership rolls and an annual convention attended by thousands of mental health professionals. In 1961 the American Association of Humanistic Psychology founded the *Journal of Humanistic Psychology*, which has included on its editorial board such well-known figures as Carl Rogers, Rollo May, Lewis Mumford, Kurt Goldstein, Charlotte Buhler, Abraham Maslow, Aldous Huxley, and James Bugental.

The fledgling organization made some early attempts to define itself. In 1962 it formally stated:

> Humanistic Psychology is primarily concerned with those human capacities and potentialities that have little or no systematic place, either in positivist or behaviourist theory or in classical psychoanalytic theory: e.g., love, creativity, self, growth, organism, basic need-gratification, self-actualization, higher values, being, becoming, spontaneity, play, humor, affection, naturalness, warmth, ego-transcendence, objectivity, autonomy, responsibility, meaning, fairplay, transcendental experience, psychological health and related concepts.

In 1963 the association's president, James Bugental, suggested five basic postulates:

- Man, as man, supersedes the sum of his parts (that is, a man cannot be understood from a scientific study of part-functions);
- Man has his being in a human context (that is, man cannot be understood by part-functions which ignore interpersonal experience);
- Man is aware (and cannot be understood by a psychology which fails to recognize man's continuous, many-layered self-awareness);
- Man has choice (man is not a bystander to his existence; he creates his own experience;
- Man is intentional (man points to the future; he has purpose, values and meaning.

Much in these early manifestos – anti-determinism, the emphasis on freedom, choice, purpose, values, responsibility, the dedication to appreciating the unique experiential world of each individual – is of great importance in the existential frame of reference. But by no means is the American field of humanistic psychology synonymous with the Continental existential tradition; there is a fundamental difference in accent. The existential tradition in Europe has always emphasized human limitations and the tragic dimensions of existence. Perhaps it has done so because Europeans have had a greater familiarity with geographic and ethnic confinement, with war, death and uncertain existence. The United States (and the humanistic psychology it spawned) bathed in a Zeitgeist of expansiveness, optimism, limitless horizons and pragmatism. Accordingly, the imported form of existential thought has been systematically altered. Each of the basic tenets has a distinct New World accent. The European focus is on limits, on facing and taking into oneself the anxiety of uncertainty and non-being. The humanistic psychologists, on the other hand, speak less of limits and contingency than of development of potential, less of acceptance than of awareness, less of anxiety than of peak experiences and oceanic oneness, less of life meaning than of self-realization, less of apartness and basic isolation than of I–Thou and encounter.

In the 1960s the counterculture with its attendent social phenomena – such as the free speech movement, the flower children, the drug culture, the human-potentialists, the sexual revolution – engulfed the humanistic psychological movement. Soon the association conventions developed aspects of a carnival. The big tent of human psychology was, if nothing else, generous and soon included a bewildering number of schools barely able to converse with one another even in an existential Esperanto. Gestalt therapy, transpersonal therapy, encounter groups, holistic medicine, psychosynthesis, Sufi, and many, many others pranced into the arena. The new trends have value orientations that bear significant implications for psychotherapy. There is an emphasis on hedonism ("if it feels good, do it"), on anti-intellectualism (which considers any cognitive approach as "mind fucking"), on individual fulfilment ("doing your own thing", "peak experiences"), and on self-actualisation (a belief in human perfectibility is common to most humanistic psychologists, with the major exception of Rollo May, who is more deeply grounded in the existential philosophical tradition).

These proliferating trends, especially the anti-intellectual ones, soon effected a divorce between humanistic psychology and the academic community. Humanistic psychologists in established academic positions felt uneasy about the company they were keeping and gradually disaffiliated themselves. Fritz Perls, himself far from an advocate of discipline, expressed great concern about the "turner-ons", the "anything goes", the "instant sensory awareness" approach, and eventually the three figures who supplied humanistic psychology with its initial intellectual leadership – May, Rogers and Maslow – grew deeply ambivalent about the irrational trends and gradually decreased their active sponsorship.

Existential psychotherapy thus has a hazy relationship with humanistic psychology. They share many basic tenets, however, and many humanistic psychologists have an existential orientation; among them Maslow, Perls, Bugental, Buhler and, especially, Rollo May, while there remains a group of relatives whom I shall refer to as "humanistic psychoanalysts" and who split off early from the genealogical branches. The major voices in this group – Otto Rank, Karen Horney, Erich Fomm and Helmuth Kaiser – were all trained in the European Freudian psychoanalytic tradition but emigrated to American: and all, with the exception of Rank, made their major contributions while immersed in the American intellectual community. Each objected to Freud's instinct-powered model of human behaviour and each suggested important correctives. Though the work of each was far-ranging, each, for a period of time, turned his or her attention to some aspect of existential therapy. Rank, whose contributions have been brilliantly augmented by latter-day interpreter Ernest Becker, emphasized the importance of the will and of death anxiety; Horney, the crucial role of the future as an influencer of behaviour (the individual is motivated by purpose, ideals and goals rather than shaped and determined by past events); Fromm has masterfully illuminated the role and fear of freedom in behaviour; while Kaiser has dealt with responsibility and isolation.

In addition to these major branches of philosophers, humanistic psychologists and humanistically oriented psychoanalysts, the genealogical tree of existential therapy contains an important segment constituted by the great writers who, no less fully than their professional brethren, explored and explicated existential issues. Thus, the voices of Dostoevsky, Tolstoy, Kafka, Sarte, Camus and many other distinguished teachers were of great influence. Great literature survives, as Freud pointed out in his discussion of Oedipus Rex, because something in the reader leaps out to embrace its truth. The truth of fictional characters moves us because it is our own truth. The truth of fictional characters is ultimately highly self-revelatory. Thornton Wilder once wrote: "If Queen Elizabeth or Frederick the Great or Ernest Hemingway were to read their biographies, they would exclaim, 'Ah – my secret is still safe!' But if Natasha Rostov were to read *War and Peace* she would cry out, as she covered her face with her hands: "How did he know? How did he know?"

LIMITATIONS OF EMPIRICAL PSYCHOTHERAPY RESEARCH. Existential-humanistic originating therapies are like a homeless waif who was not permitted into the better academic neighborhoods. The lack of academic support from academic psychiatric and psychology has significant implications for the field of existential therapy, since academically dominated institutions control all the vital supply routes that influence the development of the clinical disciplines: the training of clinicians and academicians , research funding, licensure, and journal publication.

It is worth taking a moment to consider why the existential approach is so quarantined by the academic establishment. The answer centres primarily on the issue of the basis of knowledge – that is, how do we know what we know? Academic psychiatry and psychology, grounded in a positivist tradition, value empirical research as the method of validating knowledge.

The basic tenets of existential therapy are such that empirical research methods are often inapplicable or inappropriate. For example, the empirical research method requires that the investigator study a complex organism by breaking it down into its component parts, each simple enough to permit empirical investigation. Yet this fundamental principle negates a basic existential principle. A story told by Viktor Frankl is illustrative:

Two neighbours were involved in a bitter dispute. One claimed that the other's cat had eaten his butter and, accordingly, demanded compensation. Unable to resolve the problem, the two, carrying the accused cat, sought out the village wise man for judgement. The wise man asked the accuser, "How much butter did the cat eat". "Ten pounds," was the response. The wise man placed the cat on the scale. Lo and behold! It weighed exactly ten pounds. "Mirabile dictu!" he proclaimed. "Here we have the butter. But where is the cat?"

Where is the cat? All the parts taken together do not reconstruct the creature. A fundamental humanistic credo is that "man is greater than the sum of his parts". No matter how carefully one understands the composite parts of the mind – for example, the conscious and the unconscious, the superego, the ego and the id – one still does not grasp the central vital agency, the person whose unconscious (or superego or id, or ego) it is. Furthermore, the empirical approach never helps one to learn the meaning of this psychic structure to the person who possess it. Meaning can never be obtained from a study of component parts, because meaning is never caused, it is created by a person who is superordinate to all his parts.

But there is in the existential approach a problem for empirical research even more fundamental than the one of "Where is the cat?" Rollo May alluded to it when he defined existentialism as "the endeavor to understand man by cutting below the cleavage between subject and object which has bedeviled Western thought and science since shortly after the Renaissance" (May, 1984).

The existential position challenges the traditional Cartesian view of the world full of objects and subjects who perceive the objects. Obviously, this is the basic premise of the scientific method: there are objects with a finite set of properties that can be understood through objective investigation. The existential position cuts below this subjective–objective cleavage and regards the person not as a subject who can, under the proper circumstances, perceive external reality but as a consciousness who participates in the construction of reality. To emphasize this point, Heidegger always spoke of human being as dasein. Da (there) refers to the fact that the person is there, is a constituted object (an "empirical ego"), but at the same time constitutes the world (that is, is a "transcendental ego"). Dasein is at once the meaning giver and the known. Each dasein therefore constitutes its own world; to study all beings with some standard instrument as though they inhabited the same objective world is to introduce monumental error into one's observations.

It is important to keep in mind, however that the limitations of empirical psychotherapy research are not confined to an existential-humanistic orientation in therapy; it is only that they are more explicit in the existential-humanistic approach. In so far as therapy is a deeply personal, human experience, the empirical study of psychotherapy of any ideological school will contain errors and be of limited value.

In my opinion the proper method of understanding the inner world of another individual is the "phenomenological" one; to go directly to the phenomena themselves, to encounter the other without "standardized" instruments and presuppositions. So far as possible one must "bracket" one's own world perspective and enter the experiential world of the other. Such an approach to knowing another person is eminently feasible in psychotherapy: every good therapist tries to relate to the patient in his manner. That is what is meant by empathy, presence, genuine listening, non-judgemental acceptance, or an attitude of "disciplined naivety" to use May's felicitous phrase. Existential therapists have always urged that the therapist attempt to understand the private world of the patient rather than to focus on the way the patient has deviated from the "norms". But this phenomenological approach, which by definition is non-empirical, raises staggering and yet unsolved problems for the researcher who struggles to achieve high scientific standards in his or her work.

In spite of these reservations, my professional training has compelled me to consider the extant research for each of the four basic existential concerns – death, freedom, isolation and meaninglessness. And, of course, careful research can shed light on several important areas of inquiry.

Yet there are still other domains where knowledge must remain intuitive. Certain truths of existence are so clear that logical argument or empirical research corroboration seems highly gratuitous. Karl Lashley, the neuro-psychologist, is said to have once commented: "If you teach an airedale to play the violin, you don't need a string quartet to prove it".

In my work, I have tried to present a paradigm, a psychological construct, that offers the clinician a system of explanations – a system that permits him or her to make sense out of a large array of clinical data and to formulate a systematic strategy of psychotherapy (Yalom, 1980, 2008, 2003; Yalom and Leszez, 2005). It is a paradigm that has considerable explanatory power; it is parsimonious (that is, the assumptions rest on experience that may be intuitively perceived by every introspective individual). Furthermore, it is a humanistically based paradigm, consonant with the deeply human nature of the therapeutic enterprise. But it is *a* paradigm, not *the* paradigm – useful for some patients, not for all patients: employable by some therapists, not by all therapists. The existential-humanistic orientation is one clinical approach among other approaches. It re-patterns clinical data but, like other paradigms, has no exclusive hegemony and is not capable of explaining all behaviour. The human being has too much complexity and possibility to permit that it do so.

Existence is inexorably free and thus, uncertain. Cultural institutions and psychological constructs often obscure this state of affairs, but confrontation with one's existential situation reminds one that paradigms are self-created, wafer-thin barriers against the pain of uncertainty. The mature therapist must, in the existential-humanistic theoretical approaches, as in any other, be able to tolerate the fundamental uncertainty.

REFERENCES. Horney K., *Neurosis and human growth*, 1950; May R., *The discovery of being: Writings in existential psychology*, 1984; Rogers C., *On becoming a person: A therapist view of psychotherapy*, 1961; Yalom I.D., *Existential Psychotherapy*, 1980; Id., *Staring at the sun: Overcoming the Terror of death*, 2008; Id., *The gift of therapy: An open letter to a new generation of therapists and their patients*, 2003; Yalom I.D., Leszcz M., *The theory and practice of group psychotherapy*, 2005.

BODY-EXPRESSION PARADIGM

L. Rispoli

HISTORY. It was in the 1920s that Wilhelm Reich first elaborated his hypothesis on the existence of connections between the psyche and the soma that were extremely deep and complex, so much so that it became indispensable for psychotherapy to also work on the body.

Actually, Freud's formulations had already underlined that it was necessary to take into account the processes of the body when studying the functional processes of the psyche. In accordance with the scientific model of the time, this aspect was presented in Freud's theory of the drives as "Biologism". Also, after Freud, much attention was dedicated to the body sphere in relation to the healthy development of the child.

However, it was no longer possible to keep on considering the body as important only in relation to the initial stages of the history of a person. The body is there during the therapeutic relationship itself, in the processes of interaction and communication; even if the therapeutic model only provides for concentrating on the verbal, symbolic or fantasmatic aspects. The body is present in the silences, in the tone of the voice, in the movements, in the positions of the therapist and of the patient in the setting. One talks and acts with one's body, even if in an implicit or unconscious manner. Further, during the therapy, the bodies of both patient and therapist are totally present. That is why, throughout its history, clinical psychology has acknowledged the importance of the body, even if only indirectly and implicitly. Interest in the body has induced many researchers to look into this vast and fascinating sphere, though few have actually accessed it: on the contrary, it is the body that finds its way into a technique, sometimes in some theoretical considerations, or in the notes of certain authors.

One needs only think of the active technique of S. Ferenczi (1920, 1926, 1930), the corrective emotional experience of F. Alexander (1956), of the *holding* and *psyche-soma* of D.W. Winnicot (1965, 1958), the concept of primary love of M. Balint (Balint, 1952; Balint and Balint, 1968), and, to continue, of the formulation of the Self by H. Kohut (1971, 1977, 1978) and D.N. Stern (1985) and the theories on *haptonomie* by B. This and F. Veldman (1985). Other examples come from behaviourism (with its concepts, such as *modelling* and *flooding*), from the Gestalt (with its interest in the way the body represents itself, and how it represents itself to the others), from the studies by J.H. Schultz (Schultz and Luthe, 1959) on somatic autogenous training, from cognitivism (with the concepts of *feedback* on a psycho-physiological level), from systemic therapy (with its techniques of "family sculpting").

THE CURRENTS IN BODY PSYCHOTHERAPY. Reich theorized the direct approach to the body in therapy (although working methods at the time were very limited), supporting the necessity of interventions aimed at modifying the muscle and the neurovegetative conditions that otherwise continued to act on the patient, bringing him back to his state of illness. His concept of *functional identity* between psyche and *soma* led to further research and formulations.

A whole lot of experimentation originated from there: a movement that led the way towards new techniques and interesting discoveries known as body-psychotherapy. It is important to outline, however, that the privileged dimensions in this area were experimentation, laboratory work and the approach to innovation. This often resulted in a lack of development of the theoretical field and the chaotic presence of contrasting models, usually isolated and centred on themselves. With all that, the field contributed many interesting points, which now are part of the development and the history of psychotherapy, but which would have needed a profound theoretical reorganization. This unfortunately never took place due to the reticence to compare notes and meet other authors, other schools and especially scientific researchers: as a result there are many different isolated models, some of which even have contrasting theoretical bases, while most are self-referential.

Within these models many different lines of thought stand out. Among the best known followers of Reich, A. Lowen (1958, 1967, 1972) defined the relationship between emotions and parts of the body, observing in this a number of mechanisms parallel to the psychic ones; Lowen developed the "typologies" of character outlined by Reich, aiming his therapy at reaching a "loosening" through intense positions and movements. Many are the contributions of other authors, though they may not be as well known. In the American group: E. Reich (1977) with his work on newly born babies; J. Pierrakos (1974) with his energy centre; the *orgonomy* of E.F. Baker (1969); the *radix* of C.R. Kelley (1978); the theory of movement of N. Bull; the primal therapy of D. Casriel (1976) and A. Janov (1970); the postural integration of I. Rolf (1977); the psycho-motor theory of A. Pesso (1969); the body of R. Kurtz and H. Prestera (1976) and Kurtz (1990); M. Sharaf on vegetotherapy (1983); rebirthing by L. Orr and J. Leonard (Leonard and Laut, 1983); movement by M. Feldenkrais (1991); postural integration by J. Painter (1986); the researches on body and spirituality by D. Johnson (1977, 1994); the relationship between body and word by G. Downing (1996); the theories on the development of human beings by S. Keleman (1975, 1987); the trauma theory of P. Levine (1992). From Central and South America we shall remember also: J. Ajuriaguerra (1962) on relaxation and body tone; R. Estrada Villa for his detailed studies on Reichian therapy. Body psychotherapy evolved in a number of branches: the eutonia of G. Alexander (1985), psycho-peristalsis by G. Boyesen (1985); the movements of M. Alexander (1969); the Norwegian school of vegetotherapy of O. Raknes (1970), N. Waal (1955), A. Bulow-Hansen (see Bunkan 1982), H. Thornquist and B.H. Bunkan (1982) and B. Blumenthal; the works of D. Boadella (1986, 1987), with the concepts of embryonic layers (*ectoderm,* mesoderm and endoderm); the theoretical contributions of H.G. Petzold (1977) on integrative therapy; T. Bertherat's antigymnastique (Bertherat and Bernstein, 1977); J. Stathman's (1989) unitive psychology; J. Donnars's trance (1985); B. Dolto's psychodynamic of the skin (1976); F. Lewin (Lewin, 1998) and C. Lewin-Gros's Biodynamics; the Psychoorganic analysis of P. Boyesen and A. Fraisse (1994); body-centred psychotherapy by Y. Maurer (1987); somatoanalysis by R. Meyer (1991); J. Liss's biosystemics (Liss and Stupiggia, 1994); W. Davis's energy charge (1997); L. Marcher's psycho-corporeal dynamics (1989); M. Meignant's amourology (1992); C. Lubrano's vegetotherapy and the social area (1994). For a theoretical and critical point of view read L. Rispoli's contributions, which lead to the development of an entirely new area, that of "Functional" psychology, modern Functionalism, in its many complex aspects: the theory of child development, the theory of the person, the etiopathogenetic theory, the theory of treatment, the study of the therapeutic process, and finally the theory of the technique (Rispoli, 1993, 2003, 2004).

Nowadays we can talk of an area of Functionalism that stems not only from the various researches conducted on the body–mind relations, but also from the studies of early functionalism (the School of Chicago), from the recent discoveries on the prenatal and neonatal life, in the studies on neuroscience and psychophysiology, from the theories of the Self.

PSYCHOSOMATIC AND SOMATOPSYCHIC. What really happens in psychotherapy when one focuses on the body and works on it (touching it, moving it, changing its postures and the way it moves, massaging it in certain ways)?

It is not just that new techniques are added to other psychotherapeutic models, but the existing models are radically transformed. When psychotherapy began working on and with the body, 70 years ago, a number of occurrences, reactions, processes were evidenced, which, at the time, had not yet been examined. The effects of the psychotherapeutic work on the body are intense and visible: they are emotional but also psychophysiological. To explain these phenomena it became necessary to formulate a new theory of the person's functioning, different from the existing ones. The main point is the realization that when physical contact is used with the patient the theoretical framework of reference needs to be changed considerably.

In order to explain how the work at body level directly makes old experiences surface, one should start by thinking that in all probability it is not true that the processes we call "mental" (symbolic, elaborative) control all our "life processes". On the other hand, one must also admit that body processes influence thought, mental patterns and representations, and that it is possible that the body processes are autonomous when they become disconnected from the state of original integration. Sometimes it is the body that makes it possible to retrieve the processes of symbolization that otherwise would not surface. We must think in terms of a sort of "body memory", a peripheral memory consisting of the permanent traces of past experiences: repeated and habitual postures, permanent alterations of perception thresholds, chronic modifications of basic muscle tone, movements that become sculpted in time. We must also consider that emotions somehow "stratify" in various areas of the body when the child experiences his earliest relations with his surroundings (with positive or negative results).

The child feels and expresses his emotions with his whole body, living an experience in full, already in the early stages of his life. Therefore he will feel, for example, tenderness with the touch of the hands and the stroke of a cheek; but also with his back when he is picked up and held in someone's arms, in his legs when he relaxes, against a soft tummy and when he makes eye contact with someone. It is therefore difficult to hold on to the idea of a stage when the mouth is the centre of attention and pleasure, of another stage when everything moves to a different part of the body, and so on. On the contrary, in every part of the body one can identify the "layers" of several emotional feelings. Some are the emotions that were openly expressed in childhood, but, in some cases the child might also block or hold back those he has not lived serenely and are not accepted by the adults (doing so with his body: by clenching his fists, stiffening his legs, holding his breath and blocking his neck) or he may be induced by his adults to exaggerate others (by intensifying the posture of the shoulders or of the bust in the expression of strength, fright or weakness); in these parts of the body one will then find, in a pre-eminent and "external" manner, those painful experiences. When those parts of the body are touched and moved, the "superficial layer" of the old negative and painful experience will surface, the one that covers the deeper layer of positive feelings (connected with the pleasant movements that involved that part of the body).

THE PROBLEM OF EXPRESSING, NOT JUST OF ANALYZING. The crucial theoretical point is still whether to analyze (elaborate) or express. For a long time the belief was that to make the body act in psychotherapy could produce a short-circuit of experiences, emotions, elaborations; that in this way one operated outside the boundaries of analysis and elaboration (*acting out*). This was because the theoretical knowledge at the time had not yet discovered that the body is capable of producing intense and visible effects over the mind. Once this knowledge had been acquired, researchers started to realize that the body is not a reflex of the mind, that it is not only important as a symbolic representation, and consequently that working with the body in psychotherapy is not an escape from the elaboration but it is part of the elaboration itself, as a whole. Having reached this first important theoretical stage, another essential point still remained to be cleared. Some researchers, anchored to other clinical models, suggested that the experiences of the body involvement should be analyzed according to the same theories used to analyze dreams or any other experience in psychodynamic psychotherapy. However, in this way, any work conducted with the body would still remain an everyday experience of life: I do something (play a sport, have sexual intercourse, go for a walk, have a massage, etc.) and afterwards my sensations, my experiences, are analyzed. There would be no point to reason about the body in psychotherapy in such a case. For the use of the body to have a sense in psychotherapy, one has to be convinced that a direct intervention on the body produces real change, not only sensations and experiences to be analyzed; in other words, it is to be assumed that one of the factors of change consists in expressing oneself. It is not a question of relieving emotions, nor of finding a creative expression, but of expressing with one's whole self (and therefore also with one's body) emotional states and modalities of relation that are essential in our lives.

CHANGE. How does change take place? This is one of the most delicate points that need to be clarified: the theories on body therapies and expressive therapies are almost never really clear on this point. Actually, it seems sufficient to "express", to "move the body" because the body is the "truth", to regain "spontaneity" of movements and body expression. In fact expressive therapies often make use of expressive-creative techniques such as painting, dancing, writing. However, if the body is allowed to move and the person is to express himself freely (the way he is used to), what nearly always happens is that the same altered life processes are repeated, the ones that the person lives in his everyday life. If anger surfaces when he moves with strength it is because, in the reaction expressed, a parasitic anger insinuated itself into that person, an anger that does not allow him to live the expression of strength in full. When he moves, this person will just retrace and repeat this alteration (when he does not enhance it).

The Functional thought (Functional psychotherapy) has fully clarified this point with the theorization of a new factor of change consisting in the "reconstruction of the old Basic Experiences of the Self". Therefore the point is not that one should move or express – because in most cases this means falling back onto the old "tracks" – the altered and stereotyped life processes that have become repetitive and disconnected from the surrounding reality. The real aim is to work towards real changes, breaking old patterns and changing the way the body moves, the way experiences and emotions are expressed: even if one chooses to express oneself through modalities known as creative (dancing, authentic movement, painting, sculpture, music), the aim – since also in this case the existing dysfunctions will surface – is still to achieve a real change, induced and focused (in order to be considered "therapeutic"). The ultimate issue is to reconstruct the old experiences suppressed by the alteration, to retrace them, but at the same time to open them towards a sound and unaltered mode.

WORK ON THE BODY. The examples that follow serve to further clarify the concept of a therapy that also acts on the body of the patient and with changes not represented by the classical factors of change (the symbolic elaboration or turning what was not conscious into conscious), but by new factors of change. It is, however, important to point out that to make them comprehensible in their scientific and theoretical basis, these examples have been developed from the point of view of the "Functional thought", in other words the theory that has opened the way to the new area of modern Functionalism, which can certainly not be defined as the area of body psychotherapy.

a) *Altered movements.* Movements (the "Function of movement" to be more precise) can become chronically accelerated and fast, without pause and jerky, when the child is not helped to keep his calm, his capacity to stop, to feel what he is living, to savour it in full. Many children nowadays suffer from hyperactivity disorder (as school teachers are well aware) because they are exposed to an excessive number of stimuli in every field: toys that are increasingly noisy, bright and moving, videogames requiring speed and continuous small movements, frantic and explosive movies, an excess of extra school activities, of visual and sound stimuli and, last but not least important, they are always in a hurry. The movements of the child, therefore, tend to become frantic and ceaseless, also when not necessary: at school, for example, restless children get up and move all the time, they cannot remain seated even for five minutes. This alteration of movement has very serious consequences on the life of the child and on the other "Functions of the self": on his cognitive and imaginative abilities, which become increasingly inadequate, on his emotions which tend to become confused, with greater difficulties as regards his self-esteem and with a general state of anxiety and restlessness. When one Function is altered and stereotyped, it winds round itself in a short circuit, it becomes "disconnected" from the other Functions. Therefore, if no action is taken directly, it remains altered. It is no use telling a hyperkinetic child to stop, to slow down: his will, if applied on its own, can no longer control his movements, nor can imagination alone, nor being aware of the alteration, or the surfacing of memories of old situations that brought on the alteration. It is essential to act directly on the "movement" Function. Therefore, only a therapy whose method is to act also on the body can cure (step by step) the alteration of the movements, re-establishing the quiet and the calmness that has been lost, while a purely verbal therapy can recover all this with difficulty. It is of course important to act on all the other Functions, because the problem is caused not only by the movements: it is the whole Self that has been altered and therefore the action must involve the whole Self, so that all the Functions cooperate in re-establishing a very important Basic Experience in life: that of "just being". But the key work is clearly on the movement, with specific techniques of deep massage aimed at the direct modification of the lay-out of the muscle and its basic tension, with specific exercises, which the patient is required to repeat many times as "homework", with research and recovery, also with memories and guided imagery, of smooth movements and calm.

b) *Anxiety and the neurovegetative system.* If a person is continuously anxious, as a further example, he will surely tend towards chronic sympathetictonia. This means that the autonomic nervous (neurovegetative) system remains stuck mainly at alarm level and that all the internal organs innervated by this system behave as they would in a situation of danger, even if there is no danger. The blood pressure rises, the blood vessels contract, letting the blood flow to the brain and the muscles, the heart rate increases, digestion and bowel movement stop to allow the person to take quick action in danger, and so on. It is no use telling the person to calm down because the sympathetictonia turns into a mechanism that can no longer be controlled by the will, it cannot be changed, even by induced positive emotions or by opening memories and elaborating the experience of fear. The only possibility is to act directly on the neurovegetative system, on some of the "body" Functions (though no Function is purely a body Function), such as breathing (the most important regulator of the autonomic systems in our body), the deep muscle tone, postures. By restoring deep and spontaneous diaphragmatic breathing it is possible to combat chronic anxiety very well. But also "opening" postures that are closed and shrunken, or loosening chronically contracted muscles is a great help in restoring calm and serenity.

c) *Pain perception thresholds.* Some people feel pain at the slightest touch. One is not born with such low perceptive thresholds, it is not a natural characteristic: what happened then in the course of their lives? Probably because they felt they were continuously under threat during their childhood, the physiological Function "perceptive threshold" altered progressively and the tendency to feel a strong pain remained trapped inside them. Those who suffer from this Functional alteration feel that they are always in danger of being "attacked", they feel exposed to a threatening world, where the slightest thing can bring pain. Only by employing specific techniques of physical contact (integrated by a deep intervention on the emotions of tranquillity and on the feeling of protection) can these perceptive alterations be untangled and normal feelings restored.

CONCLUSION. All this helps us to realize that working with the body in psychotherapy is an important and precious resource that cannot be rejected. But in order to use the new potentiality, obtaining genuine results without damaging the patient, a new basic theory was needed, a theory that can explain what happens in psychotherapy within the body and with the body, what alterations are present and how to overcome them; a theory that takes into account the most recent scientific developments, that considers the person as a whole being, psyche and body as a whole, with all his cognitive, emotional, symbolic planes; but also motor and posture; as well as physiological, sensorial, perceptive planes, including the breathing systems, the neurovegetative system and the neuroendocrine one. This theory has to take into account the clinical practice developed over the years, in order not to repeat what has already been done. The theory that accomplished this is the Functional theory, which leads to modern Functionalism. Nowadays, thanks to the Functional thought, we know precisely what happens when a person moves in a certain way, or breathes in a certain way, or has certain postures, or feels some specific sensations in his body, or has a certain perception about his surroundings. It is possible to analyze whether these Functions are still mobile and integrated or whether they are already altered and in what way. As a consequence it is also possible to know what happens when action is taken on these altered Functions: touching, moving or making the body move, encouraging a certain way of breathing, making the person assume certain postures; therefore it is possible to guide the therapeutic intervention through a determined and precise project, which only a complex and advanced theory of the mind–body processes could support. This deep knowledge of the mind–body mechanism is the new frontier of very important battles for the health of human beings.

REFERENCES. Ajuriaguerra J., *Le corps comme relation*, «Revue Suisse de psychologie», 1962, ii, 2; Alexander F., *Psychoanalysis and psychotherapy*, 1956; Alexander G., *Eutony: The holistic discovery of total person*, 1985; Alexander M., *The resurrection of the body*, 1969; Baker E.F., *Man in the trap*, 1969; Balint M., *Primary love and psycho-analytic technique*, 1952; Balint M., Balint E., *Thrills and regression*, 1968; Bertherat T., Bernstein C., *The body has its reasons*, 1977; Boadella D., Liss J., *La psicoterapia del corpo*, 1986; Boadella D. *Biosintesi*, 1987; Boyesen G., *Entre psyché et soma, introduction à la psychologie biodynamique*, 1985; Bunkan B.H., Thornquist E. (1982), *Psychomotor therapy: An approach to the evaluation and treatment of psychosomatic disorders*, in Bunkan B.H., Thornquist E., Radøy L., *Psykomotorist behandling. Festskrift til Aadel Bülow-Hansen*, 1982; Casriel D., *A scream away from- happiness*, 1976; Davis W., *Biological foundation of the schizoid process*, in «Energy and Character», 1997, 28, 1; Dolto B., *Le corps entre les mains*, 1976; Donnars J., *La transe, technique d'épanouissement personnel*, 1985; Downing G., *The body and the word in psychotherapy*, 1996; Feldenkrais M., *Awareness through movement: Easy-to-do health exercises to improve your posture, vision, imagination and personal awareness*, 1991; Ferenczi S. (1920), *The further development of an active theory in psychoanalysis*, in J. Suttie *Final contributions to the theory and techniques of psychoanalysis*, 1930; Id. (1926), *Contra-indications to the "active" psycho-analytical technique*, in J. Suttie *Further contributions to the theory and technique of psycho-analysis*, 1980; Id. (1929), *The principle of relaxation and neocatharsis*, in E. Mosbacher *Final contributions to the problems and methods of psychoanalysis*, 1980; Fraisse A., *La fontaine de feu*, 1994; Janov A., *The primal scream. Primal therapy: The cure for neurosis*, 1970; Johnson D., *The Protean body: A rolfer's view of human flexibilty*, 1977; Johnson D., *Body, spirit and democracy*, 1994; Keleman S., *Your body speaks its mind*, 1975; Keleman S., *Embodyng experience*, 1987; Kelley C.R., *Orgonomy, bioenergetics and radix: The Reichian movement today*, 1978; Kohut H., *The analysis of the self*, 1971; Kohut H., *The restoration of the self*, 1977; Kohut H., *The search for the self, Volume I* (1950–1978), 1978; Kurtz R., Prestera H., *The body reveals*, 1976; Kurtz R., *Body-centred psychotherapy*, 1990; Leonard J., Laut P., *Rebirthing: The science of enjoying all your life*, 1983; Lewin F., *La psychologie biodynamique ou la joie retrouvée*, in «Solstice» 1998, 8; Levine P., *Transforming trauma: The body as healer*, in Sheets-Johnstone M. (ed.), *Giving the body its due*, 1992; Liss J., Stupiggia M., *La terapia biosistemica*, 1994; Lowen A., *The language of the body*, 1958; Lowen A., *The betrayal of the body*, 1967; Lowen A., *Depression and the body*, 1972; Lubrano C., *Gli adolescenti e la psicoterapia corporea*, in «Quaderni di Psicoterapia Corporea», 1994; Marcher L., *The bodynamic character structure model*, in «Energy and Character», 1989, 20, 1; Maurer Y., *Körperzentrierte Psychotherapie*, 1987; Meignant M., *Amourologue*, 1992; Meyer R., *Le corps aussi, de la psychanalyse à la somatanalyse*, 1991; Painter J. W., *Deep bodywork and personal development*, 1986; Pesso A., *Movement in psychotherapy*, 1969; Petzold H. G., *Psychotherapie und Körperdynamik*, 1977; Pierrakos J., *The core of Man*, 1974; Raknes O., *Wilhelm Reich and orgonomy*, 1970; Reich E., *Emotional first aid*, in «Energy and Character», 1977, 8, 3; Rispoli L., *Psicologia Funzionale del Sé*, 1993; Rispoli L., *Il sorriso del corpo e I segreti dell'anima*, 2003; Rispoli L., *Esperienze di Base e sviluppo del Sé*, 2004; Rolf I., *Rolfing: The Integration of human structures*, 1977; Sharaf, M.. *Fury on Earth: A biography of Wilhelm Reich*, 1983; Schultz J.H., Luthe W., *Autogenic training: A psychophysiologic approach to psychotherapy*, 1959; Stattman J., *The creative trance*, 1989; Stern D.N., *The interpersonal world of the child*, 1985; This B., Veldman F., *L'haptonomie*, Document de travail, 1985; Thornquist E., Bunkan B.H., *Hva er psykomotorist behandling*, 1982; Waal N., *A special technique of psychotherapy with on autistic child*, in Caplan G. (ed.) *Emotional problems of early childhood*, 1955; Winnicott D.W., *Through paediatrics to psychoanalysis*, 1958; Winnicott D.W., *The maturational process and the facilitating environment*, 1965.

INTERACTIONAL-STRATEGIC PARADIGM

J.J. Wittezaele

As Einstein pointed out, there is no "neutral" observation; any observation is driven and supported by specific theoretical premisses that orient the look of the observer. *Paradigms* are theoretical premises or models of reference that allow scientists to "map" the phenomena they are studying and to problematize them. In the interactional and strategic approach, the theoretical models of reference are drawn from cybernetics and the general theory of systems. Beyond this systemic view of human beings – shared with other models based on the same epistemological foundations –, the interactional and strategic approach relies on an original explanatory model of the creation of psychological problems within human interactions, as well as on a theory of the therapeutic communication that enables us to solve them.

THE BIRTH OF THE INTERACTIONAL PARADIGM. The paradigm that guided the scientific development up to the end of the 19th century was particularly formalized by Descartes in his famous 1637 work, *The Discourse on Method.* Descartes postulated that a neutral observer can view the surrounding world with an impartial eye and that it is possible to investigate the functioning of a complex phenomenon by isolating each of its variables and by altering them one by one while keeping the others stable, in order to determine the specific role of each of them within the overall phenomenon. The Cartesian approach thus suggested the possibility of knowing the intrinsic "nature" of each element. Thanks to these methodological principles, the so-called hard sciences underwent an extraordinary development and their technological progress has been unequalled. The social sciences did not remain immune to this new cultural model: they studied human behaviour, as if man could be isolated from his environment and even from parts of his own body (the liver, skin, blood, etc.). It is from this very perspective that the nature of the human being and the inner determinants of his behaviour were studied.

Thomas Kuhn (1962) has shown that scientific progress goes through "critical phases" during which the traditional paradigms are questioned because they do not allow an understanding of certain facts or for certain problems that researchers are facing to be resolved. This destiny has been shared by the Cartesian paradigm as well. Since the beginning of the twentieth century, some scientists have shown that the Cartesian paradigm ignores a whole series of essential characteristics of life, properties generated by the links between different entities or between the components of those entities. Around the 1940s, researchers in various fields started to examine these problems and conceived methodological tools in order to approach these phenomena from a comprehensive perspective. It became possible to analyze and understand the functioning of organized and "self-regulated" phenomena, that is, phenomena able to sustain a functioning equilibrium by correcting by themselves the modifications generated by inner or outer changes, having thus some autonomy from their environment. The insistence of the Cartesian approach on the *nature* of the elements of a whole could give an account of the phenomena having a *linear causality*, but left aside the relations between these very elements; it could not be applied to self-regulated phenomena in which the effect provoked by one element will correct the cause, in function of the goal to be reached or the purpose of the phenomenon itself (phenomena having a *circular causality*: the effect, in turn, modifies the cause) (Wiener, 1948). Cybernetics and the general theory of systems elaborated new methodological tools, making possible the study of certain characteristics of phenomena that had gone unnoticed up to that point; in particular their organization, structural dynamics and the regulation between those organized wholes and the environment in which they live (Ashby, 1956; Von Bertalanffy, 1968; Von Foerster, 1974, 1990). This stimulated interest in biologists, who study living organisms, but also in sociologists and anthropologists, who found in these two theoretical models a more adequate method to give an account of the social regulations between and within different communities. This new point of observation changed the way of considering human behaviour: the unity of analysis shifted from an isolated human being to the dynamics of the interactions between man and his environment. This *process* became the object of study.

THE STUDY OF COMMUNICATION AND CONTROL. The focus was now on what happens between individuals, that is, on the information that is exchanged, how this information is coded and decoded and on how it controls the behaviour of individuals. Cybernetics was a new discipline: the science of communication and control. From the 1950s onwards, a group of researchers (G. Bateson, E. Goffman, R. Birdswhistel, E.T. Hall and others), relying on concepts drawn from cybernetics and the general theory of systems, proposed and developed a view of communication phenomena that broke with the traditional "telegraphic" model: a transmitter sends a message to a receiver who decodes it (Heims, 1991). Following Norbert Wiener, the father of cybernetics, who viewed the universe as "a myriad of messages to whom it may concern" (1948), these researchers made communication the very matrix of behaviour: we are immersed in a flow of information that models us, that create a dynamic and evolutive network that very often determines us without us knowing it. Our "personal score" (to use the "orchestral" metaphor of communication) is largely determined by that of our partner, family, culture, and the verbal aspects of communication are largely conditioned by the non-verbal information we continuously receive from our environment. The British anthropologist Gregory Bateson (1904–1980) took part in the development of cybernetics. He got interested in these questions during field work in New Guinea, where he noticed that individual and historical approaches to human behaviour left a whole series of such behaviour unexplained, and that, taking into account the interactions between tribes or between members of a tribe, generated very different explanatory hypotheses (Bateson, 1936). He emphasized that the exchanges of information (the interactions) are structured and that they participate in defining "relationship rules" between partners, which will then limit, "frame", their subsequent exchanges and generate individual behaviours that are incomprehensible outside of this very frame. For example, let's take the custom of *Potlatch* (a ceremonial and cultural ritual based on giving, in North American Natives but also in various ethnic groups of the Pacific Ocean), which governs the relationships between certain tribes. This relational rule implies that when the tribe A pays a visit to a neighbouring tribe B, the tribe A must offer a gift. When the second tribe in turn visit the first one, they will have to bring another gift that is "at least as important" as the gift they received. Bateson noticed that this rule could lead to an outbid or an escalation, to the point that certain tribes may have to offer goods in a way that challenged their own survival. Bateson elaborated the following reasoning: if, in his way of approaching phenomenon, the researcher takes only into account the behaviours within one of the two tribes, he may be led to consider a partial hypothesis (such as: this tribe has suicidal tendencies!), whereas if the observation encompasses both tribes and their relationship, the explanation takes up a totally different dimension. If the information exchanged between the elements of a complex system allows for their stability, one can say that the behaviour of these individual elements is "controlled" by the whole. The explanation of the behaviour of an element must therefore take into account these overall influences. If, when studying the phenomenon of tides, one limits one's observation to the sea water, one will be led to conceive explanatory hypotheses postulating the existence of an "inner force" able to periodically attract and repell the mass of water. But if one looks at the Earth, the sea water, the moon and their interactions simultaneously, the explanation will clearly be different.

THE STUDY OF COMMUNICATION PARADOXES: THE "BATESON PROJECT". Imbued with the concepts of cybernetics, Bateson tried to build up a new science of man, integrating the interactional view (Bateson, 1972, 1979). He obtained a research budget for a study on the "effects of paradoxes on behaviour". This research was based on the discovery that various logical levels exist in human communication, as is the case in a chess game where the level of the exchange of moves between two players can be distinguished from the level of the rules of the game, which is a more abstract, more general level that offers a "frame" for the different moves. Similarly, the exchange of direct messages in human communication takes place within a context that defines the relational rules between the communicating partners. The question motivating Bateson's research can be summarized as follows: what happens if the rules of the game, apparently logical and sensible at a general level, prevent, in fact, every concrete initiative of the players in an implicit way? In order to carry out his research, Bateson recruited several colleagues: the psychiatrists Don D. Jackson, John Weakland, William Fry and Jay Haley. In order to check their effects, they researched all the situations presenting different levels of communication – the so-called *paradoxes*, as defined by B. Russel and A. Whitehead in their *Theory of Logical Types*. Bateson was particularly skilled in surrounding himself with brilliant people and chose the psychiatrist Don D. Jackson, an expert in pathological familiar homeostasis, as a member of his group. Thanks to his vital contribution, the first studies on paradoxical communication in psychotic patients' families were therefore conducted in the nearby Mello Park Hospital. Why did those patients have frequent crises after their parents visits? How is communication structured within these families? The studies, which aimed to answer those questions, gave birth to the *double bind theory*, which describes a communication system that forces the individual who is subject to that system to behave in an "abnormal" way (Sluzki and Ransom, 1976). Let us imagine a relationship between a mother and her child. Every time the child takes an initiative, her mother punishes him; so, the child "learns" to avoid the punishment (this is the implicit "rule of the game" between his mother and himself at the relational level). This rule being established, the mother will then force the child to act spontaneously: "Hey, when will you stop clinging to me all the time, do something!" The child "knows" that if he takes an initiative he will be punished, but he must obey his mother's direct command, otherwise he will be punished. Since this context is blocking any "normal" way out (if he obeys the relational message, he disobeys the direct command, and vice versa), the child must then resort to "abnormal" conduct in order to find some ways out (ignore all messages, receive all messages at the same level, invent an imaginary world in which ways out can arise . . .); in short, the symptoms that are usually described as an expression of a disturbed mind become desperate attempts to find solutions to an environment that does not allow it. This double bind theory marked a decisive turning point in the approach to mental illness. One would not try anymore to treat a sick psyche, but to modify the structure of communication within a "pathological" family system: it is no longer the individual that has to be treated – it is the relation!

This theory, published in 1956, was the materialization of the systemic paradigm in the world of psychotherapy, and it marked the beginning of systemic family therapies. The interactional approach claims that individuals develop through communication. A good management of communicational phenomena between the individual and his environment allows the person to feel well. On the other hand, a bad relationship with the environment can make life difficult, disturb the mind, modifiy the way we perceive our environment, alter our image of the world and our self-image, and even make us doubt deeply on our identity; in brief, *communication is the matrix of mental health.*

"CONSTRUCTING A REALITY". In the midst of all this, how does an individual succeed in constructing an identity for himself, in giving a meaning to his relation with the world? While showing the essential importance of communication, cybernetics could not ignore the relation that connects the researcher to his object of study. To say it with Heins von Foerster: "in order to write a theory of the brain, you need a brain". So, we have come full circle: one cannot isolate the researcher from his objects of study; one has to take this relativism into account in order to approach the study of the "Pattern that Connects": this led the study of human behaviour to adopt a *constructivist* point of view of reality.

The individual is part of numerous systems that control his behaviour, that shape him in some ways (we are transformed by our family relationships and by our culture), but he is also linked to his environment by a reflexive consciousness structured around language (where words *stand for* things). In addition to the adaptative learnings that occur while man interacts with his environment, "man knows that he knows", as Bateson used to say. To put it simply, let's say that if man lives his life, he also thinks it. But this thinking system is biased because, as the eye cannot see itself, it is difficult for the individual to see his active participation in the interactional process and so he tends to perceive his own behaviour as a reaction to the behaviour of others. In a way, he *punctuates* his interactions from his own point of view. The reality he reflexively knows is thus nothing other than a personal construction and represents an absolute reality only for himself. The lessons each person draws from her own history, her experiences – widely influenced by culture and the various social pressures – reflect these different biases but constitute at the same time the conscious reference points she uses to "think" her life.

Despite the influences of the systems he belongs to, man has nevertheless a relative autonomy that makes him a builder of meaning, a builder of reality. These two inseparable aspects of the human being – *systemic and constructivist* – simultaneously allow the provision of a full account of the complexity of man and of the many "psychological" difficulties he may encounter. The union of both systems can indeed give rise to more or less important discrepancies: for example, one can think that it is necessary to control the behaviour of a rebellious teenager – because all of our previous decoding and the social pressures lead us to that conclusion – and act in that direction even if this control results in an ever stronger rebellion; or one can struggle with depression and exhort oneself to be active (because we believe that "only willpower will get us out of it!") even if these efforts lead us to even more failures and to a worsening of our condition. So, when we try to relieve a person's psychological suffering, we need to perceive both the interactional process between the individual and his environment (what he does concretely, how he reacts to the signals of the environment) and the reflexive decoding he makes out of them, the "construction of the world" that goes with it. Like any language, this construction of the world has a structure of its own: the *meaning* ascribed to the element of knowledge (and which depends on the context), the *generalizations* and abstractions drawn from the previous experiences, their "logical" organization – in particular the *causal* links a person can establish between the various parts of her experience ("if I do A, I could get B"), as well as the related emotions that allow the individuals to head towards what is favourable to themselves and to avoid what could harm them, to look for pleasant situations and to protect themselves against dangers. This aspect of communication is widely used by psychotherapists in their work: "reframing", rephrasing, metaphors, aphorisms, are some of the many means available to help patients construct "more functional realities".

PRAGMATICS OF COMMUNICATION AND PSYCHOTHERAPY. A particular aspect of communication has been a decisive factor in the practical applications of cybernetics and of the theory of systems, especially in therapy. In addition to its "informative" aspect (the relation to a former event, which refers to the question of "meaning", that is, to *semantics*), every message is at the same time an order, a command, an incentive to react. Each and every received message implies a reply; one can attempt to mask it, one can try to hide the effect of the message, but receiving a message inexorably generates a reaction. As Paul Watzlawick summarized it: "one cannot not communicate". This "injunctive" aspect of communication stimulated research in the field of "pragmatics of communication", that is, the study of the effects of communication on behaviour. The main question is not "What is the meaning of this message?" in absolute terms, but "What is the effect of this message on the person one is communicating with?" (Watzlawick *et al.*, 1967)

A number of teams were set up throughout the world to work out therapeutic intervention techniques to modify the relationships within families where one or several members presented pathological symptoms. It was with this aim that Don D. Jackson created the Mental Research Institute (MRI) in Palo Alto in 1959. Virginia Satir, Paul Watzlawick, Richard Fish joined him, as well as John Weakland and Jay Haley, at the end of the "Bateson project" (Watzlawick and Weakland, 1977; Wittezaele and Garcia, 1992). Within the framework of their research on paradoxes, the latter two were in contact with Milton H. Erickson, a hypnotherapist with original and iconoclastic therapeutic methods.

When starting to treat patients and their families, they drew their inspiration from Erickson's methods (that were efficient but not very formalized), who was obtaining amazingly quick therapeutic results thanks to his strategic use of language. The efficacy of therapeutic communication became crucial: how to construct therapeutical interventions so that they have the desired impact on the patient and his family (Watzlawick, 1976, 1981, 1990)?

The crossbreeding of Erickson's unrestrained clinical creativity and Bateson's rigorous theoretical approach generated an original model of intervention, whose cornerstone – the concept of *attempted solution* – reflected its cybernetical epistemological premisses and laid the foundations of a real *theory of change*.

THE "ATTEMPTED SOLUTIONS": THE TARGETS OF THERAPEUTIC INTERVENTIONS. By applying the discoveries of cybernetics, the strategic psychotherapists do not focus their work on searching in the past for the "causes" of problems. The reason for this choice is the systemic principle of *equifinality* that shows that every behaviour is overdetermined and that the same cause does not necessarily generate the same effects (a good example is the phenomenon of resilience). It is the way of dealing with the difficulty that is inadequate, in other terms, the vicious circle of regulation between the individual and the problematic situation: regardless of its origin, a problem can persist only if the efforts to solve it have been and are ineffective (Watzlawick *et al.*, 1974).

We know that certain events in the past can leave an individual with deep wounds. A person can experience dramatic situations but one can never know if these events will cause this person to live the rest of her life in a black hole or if, alternatively, they will lead her to develop extraordinary capacities: the reactions of family members, their comments, their responses, can completely modifiy the impact of painful experiences in children. The same is true for adults. We sometimes hear people saying things like: "You can never recover from being raped, from a divorce, from being abandoned, from incest, lack of a father, loss of a child . . ." We notice today that these final comments, expressed as an absolute truth, can cement the ineluctability of the prediction. Overcoming these terrible experiences is possible; one has the right to want to enjoy one's life without these experiences preventing us from doing so: the keys to the solution of the problem created in the past are not buried in the past. Rather, they are in the present, in the way we deal with the memory of the past, in the way we react today. In short, we can say that the past remains present if the present reinforces the past. It is by curing the present that we allow patients to heal from their past. This is done, not by having patients becoming aware of the impact of their past experience, but by helping them to find solutions to the difficulties generated from the past in their present life. Moreover, it is not because the problem originated in a distant past that the solution will take time: old problems can be solved in a few sessions. This is the daily experience of psychotherapists who work with strategic approaches.

The aim of the treatment is therefore to stop the ineffective attempted solutions that, instead of solving the problem, worsen the situation due to a process of *escalation*. Giorgio Nardone has suceeded in systematizing certain large classes of "attempted solutions". For instance, on the basis of his therapeutical results, he proved that a systematic avoidance of a frightening situation can lead to a phobic problem; that a repeated effort to fall asleep leads to insomnia; that repeatedly exerting one's willpower to get rid of symptomatic behaviour can create a compulsion; that an excessive effort to fight against the craving for food can lead to bulimia; that the will to control an undesired behaviour can cause its exacerbation; etc. Any difficulty, be it personal, relational, familial, can be analyzed in this way. It is by studying the solutions to the problems that we can learn how the problems function (Nardone, 1996). Thanks to this methodological evolution, psychotherapy becomes a technological process where the solution matches the problem. The so-called psychopathologies become dysfunctional models of perceiving the reality that have to be replaced by functional ones. It is therefore no longer necessary to use a normative view of psychological difficulties; we only have to follow the patient in his desire to evolve. Moreover – and this is without doubt the most revolutionary aspect of this approach –, the therapist doesn't have to know what is good or not for his patient in the absolute: the very inefficient efforts of the patient are what indicates the way to the solution, which is a U-turn, a 180-degree reverse move compared to the direction of the attempted solutions. The therapist is no longer the gardian of moral order or of normality; he becomes an agent of change at his patient's service (Cagnoni and Milanese, 2009; Nardone, 2003; Nardone and Portelli, 2005; Nardone and Watzlawick, 1993, 2005: Nardone *et al.*, 2005; Nardone and Salvini, 2007; Nardone and Balbi, 2015).

THE IMPORTANCE OF COMMUNICATION IN THERAPEUTIC PROCESSES. The psychotherapist's aim is thus clear: to use all the resources of communication to ensure that his patient gives up his attempted solutions, so that the system can find a creative way to regulate itself.

If, on the one hand, the Palo Alto model is of great simplicity, close to a working drawing, and is therefore a fantastic *complexity reducer* to approach, and work with, ,human problems, on the other hand the implementation of the therapeutic interventions demands a complex expertise. In effect, the therapist must apply the most efficient techniques and the most refined communication strategies to make the patient give up his usual attempted solutions, towards which he is most of the time inexorably pulled by all his former learnings and construction of the world. The more rigid the patient's vision of the world, the more necessary for the therapist to be persuasive. The communication mode plays an essential role in implementing an intervention for change, and the resources of language become crucial.

In this way, the therapist has to be skilled in creating a secure relational context, in handling the techniques of change (in particular the counter-paradox, as in the *prescription of symptom* technique), in being ingenious enough to imagine prescriptions, the "tasks" or concrete experiences that, when implemented by the patient, will inevitably lead him to renounce his habitual attempted solutions. These concrete experiences, prescribed by the therapist, will allow the patient to reframe his perception of the problem, his own cognitive interpretation of the problematic situation. They are therefore constructed with great care, in order to serve as a "corrective emotional experience" (Alexander and French, 1946), allowing the patient to live and feel his own problematic situation in a way he never did before (Nardone and Milanese, 2018). From a theoretical perspective, the primary aim of each of these strategies is to stop the attempted solutions that maintain the problem. Contrary to widespread views in the field of psychotherapy, change precedes awareness: "if you want to see, you must learn to act", said the cybernetician Heinz von Foerster (1991). The interactional and strategic approach thus offers an eminently pragmatic method, where change doesn't involve the awareness of the "causes" of the problem but rather the concrete implementation of a new strategy to handle the difficulties. When change becomes effective and persistent, it produces at the same time a more functional reorganization at the cognitive, emotional, behavioural and relational levels, providing the individual with a greater adaptative flexibility to face a constantly changing environment (Wittezaele, 2003, 2008).

REFERENCES. Alexander F., French T.M., *Psychoanalytic therapy*, 1946; Ashby W.R., *An introduction to cybernetics*, 1956; Bateson G., *A survey of the problems suggested by a composite picture of the culture of a New Guinea tribe drawn from three points of view*, 1936; Id., *Steps to an ecology of mind: Collected essays in anthropology, psychiatry, evolution, and epistemology*, 1972; Id., *Mind and nature: A necessary unity*, 1979; Von Bertalanffy L., *General System Theory*, 1968; Cagnoni F., Milanese R., *Cambiare il passato*, 2009; Von Foerster H. (ed.), *Cybernetics of cybernetics*, 1974; Id., *Ethique et cybernétique de second ordre*, a lecture at the international Congress «Systèmes et thérapie familiale», 1990; Heims S.J., *The cybernetics group*, 1991; Kuhn Th.S., *The structure of scientific revolutions*, 1962; Nardone G., *Brief Strategic Solution-oriented therapy of phobic and obsessive disorders*, 1996; Id., *Cavalcare la propria tigre*, 2003;

Nardone G., Balbi E., *The logic of therapeutic change*, 2015; Nardone G., Milanese, R., *Il cambiamento strategico*, 2018; Nardone G., Portelli C., *Knowing through changing*, 2005; Nardone G., Verbitz T., Milanese R., *Prison of food*, 2005; Nardone G., Watzlawick P., *The art of change*, 1993; Nardone G., Watzlawick P., *Brief Strategic Therapy*, 2005; Nardone G., Salvini A., *The strategic dialogue*, 2007; Sluzki C.E., Ransom D.C., *Double bind: The foundation of the communicational approach to the family*, 1976; Watzlawick P., *How real is real? Communication, disinformation, confusion*, 1976; Id., *The invented reality*, 1981; Id., *Munchausen's pigtail: Or psychotherapy and reality*, 1990; Watzlawick P., Beavin J.H., Jackson D. D., *Pragmatics of human communication*, 1967; Watzlawick P., Weakland J.H., Fisch R., *Change: Principles of problem formation and problem resolution*, 1974; Watzlawick P., Weakland J.H., (eds.), *The interactional view: Studies at the mental research institute*, 1977; Wiener N., *Cybernetics*, 1948; Wittezaele J.J., *L'homme relationnel*, 2003; Id. (ed.), *La double contrainte*, 2008; Wittezaele J.J., Garcia T., *À la recherche de l'école de Palo Alto*, 1992.

SYSTEMIC-RELATIONAL PARADIGM

Padrail Gibson

Systemic family therapy emerged in the mid to late 1950s, although its roots can be traced back to the late nineteenth century and early twentieth century with the development of social work, group theory and later with the work of the child guidance movement (Boscolo *et al.*, 1987; Hoffman, 1981). There are multiple and complex historical contributions to the development of the model, many emanating from research on schizophrenia, communication and systems theory, (Watzlawick *et al.*, 1967; Ackerman, 1958) and numerous other socio-cultural sources (Jones, 1993).

Over time systemic family psychotherapy has gone through a number of different evolutions and borrowed from theories such as general systems theory (Wiener, 1948) and, later, cybernetics, particularly in the 1980s (although this influence has been significantly diluted through the introduction of social constructionism in more recent times) (Gergen, 1999; Boscolo and Bertrando, 1996).

The most significant contribution the family therapy movement has made to psychotherapy theory and practice was the paradigmatic shift in the understanding of of human distress. While there are many and varied models under the umbrella of "contemporary family therapy", lying at the heart of them all is the shift from the individual as the focus of treatment to the focus on the "person in relationship" as the treatment system (Boscolo and Bertrando, 1996; Gergen, 1999).

This shift in how the self of the patient and his/her distress is conceptualized has moved from the individual as the container of pathology, to the family or systems surrounding the individual. More recently (Boscolo and Bertrando, 1996; Jones, 1993; Madanes, 1984; White, 1990) there has been a return towards the individual and the notion of the "narrative self" (Freeman and Combs, 1996) and "dialogical self" (Boscolo and Bertrando, 1996; Gergen, 1999; White, 1990) or more specifically, a focus on how people are guided by the narrative they and others hold about them and their problem.

CHILD GUIDANCE MOVEMENT. The child guidance movement set out to challenge the conception that those with mental illness were suffering with a problem that was chronic and long-term. Because children and community-based treatment was the focus of the work it was inevitable that parents would be centre stage to the process of short-term psychiatric involvement. This new focus on the parent–child interaction had a distinct influence on family research and practice at that time, and pushed further the concept that psychopathology was not essentially an individualist "fact" and, as a result, the treatment of mental health problems was pushed into the environment of the child and their relationship with their parents (Ackerman, 1966; Freeman and Combs, 1996).

COMMUNICATION, SYSTEMS THEORY, CYBERNETIC INFLUENCE AND THE MENTAL RESEARCH INSTITUTE. While the child guidance and the family therapy movements were growing they began to challenge the prevailing theories of traditional psychotherapy; this was greatly aided by the introduction of cybernetics, systems and communication theory as a way of conceptualizing relationship problems.

Systems, cybernetics and communication theory shifted the focus of treatment from the individual to the mutually influential and circular nature of human relationships, paying close attention to feedback and self-organizing aspects of human interaction (Nardone and Ray, 2009).

Human behavior motivations and actions, according to these new theories, were not an outcome of a mysterious, internal, intra-psychic world, but were an outcome of their interaction with the world around them, their relationships and their communication with their significant social system (Anderson and Goolishan, 1992).

The establishment of the Bateson group in the USA and their study of human communication beginning around 1957 (a precursor to the work that would later evolve at the Mental Research Institute, in Palo Alto, CA) (Nardone and Ray, 2009) can be seen as being responsible for the introduction of principles from anthropology into psychiatry. Anthropological observations where the rules are few and simple (Watzlawick *et al.*, 1967) called upon the clinician to observe, in as objective a way as possible, the empirical effects of human interactions.

Using cybernetics and systems theory as a guiding context for their work, the group at the MRI, including influences from Gregory Bateson, Don Jackson, Paul Watzlawick, Jay Haley and John Weakland among others, led to the creation of a strategic model of therapy (Nardone and Ray, 2009). Originally working on pathological communication patterns in schizophrenic transaction, those connected to the Bateson Group, the MRI and later the Brief Therapy Center, published seminal papers in the field of human communication and brief therapy (Watzlawick *et al.*, 1967), inspiring many clinicians and models throughout the world, including the Solution Focused therapy model (De Shazer, 1985) and Nardone's Advanced Brief Strategic Therapy (Nardone and Portelli, 2007).

THE MILAN GROUP. Beginning in Italy in the 1970s, a group, informed by Gregory Bateson's work and initially directly supervised by Paul Watzlawick, which included Giuliana Prata, Mara Selvini Palazzoli, Luigi Boscolo and Gianfranco Cecchin, began their work with families. Each member of the group had formerly worked as a psychiatrists or psychoanalyst and the group went on to develop a model of therapy that would eventually become known as Milan Family Therapy. The Milan group and its mode of treatment had a significant effect in the family therapy field (Boscolo *et al.*, 1987; Hoffman, 1981).

The goal of Milan therapy was to seek to address those recurrent and complex behaviours and family interactions (or what they called games) with the use of strategic interventions (Boscolo and Bertrando, 1996). Their focus, in their latter phase, became less on directive and paradoxical interventions and they began to place emphasis on the types of questions and hypotheses being used by the therapist.

They also developed the use of circular questions, or questions that connected meaning and behaviour, connected patterns across time, questioned, directly and indirectly, relationships, intentions and patterns, among other things. This meant a fundamental shift in therapy from a hermeneutic or interpretative approach common in psychoanalysis, to a more rhetorical process (Boscolo and Bertrando, 1996).

The positive connotation of problematic behaviours and how these behaviours may (or may not) be useful for the individual and others in the family was also a central aspect of their work. The Milan team began to use more indirect means and, as mentioned below, their approach became more collaborative and focused more on what came to be known as a second-order approach to doing therapy (Madanes, 1984).

CULTURE AND GENDER. With the development of the feminist critique of many aspects of social agencies and other theories, family therapy itself came under the "microscope", with many therapists and academics in the field exploring the effects of power, gender, class, ethnicity and sociocultural background, on therapy and the therapeutic relationship (Burck and Daniel, 1999).

Family therapy began to evolve its approach to include many aspects of these critiques, incorporating them in to analyses of cases and into practice (Hoffman, 1988).

Along with the concern about gender biases, there was a greater recognition within the discipline of family therapy of the disparity in the social status of ethnic minorities and the effect these aspect of a person's position in society had on behaviour and meaning (Ho *et al.*, 2004; Hare-Mustin, 1978). Postmodernist thinking also had an impact here, challenging the status quo and what was dubbed as taken for granted knowledge (Burr, 1999), and foregrounding the influence of the therapist on the family and that of gender, power, history and the social context in which the family was embedded. This movement has had a significant impact on how contemporary family therapy is understood (Boscolo and Bertrando, 1998).

POSTMODERNISM. With the growing recognition of postmodern thinking entering the social sciences, family therapists began to question the expert position of therapist; their privileged position was also called into question, as was the validity of any theory used in therapy. Introducing the idea of "not knowing" were Andersen and Goolishan (1998). Not knowing had the effect of placing the client as expert in the therapy system; and the therapist was relegated to the person who asks searching or reflexive questions of the client, but they were to avoid offering directives or making specific interventions. The sceptical and non-interventionist approach had a significant effect on the field and how therapy was conducted.

The growing movement in the social sciences known loosely as postmodernism, or the general critique of anything seen as modernist or expert, or knowing, has provided a backdrop for current training and writing in the field of family therapy and has informed much of the narrative therapy field that has developed in recent times (Freeman and Combs, 1998) – a movement that places the primary emphasis of treatment on the stories people tell themselves and other about themselves and their problems. In this form of therapy emphasis is on replacing the narrative of the problem-saturated discourse that people live by with a more liberating and less problem-saturated conversation (White and Epston, 1990).

Historical overview of systemic family therapy and its most significant figures

1950s

In the 1950s Norbert Wiener coined the term "cybernetics"; his interest was primarily in feedback, information processing and the way these f+unction to regulate simple and more complex systems, essentially guided by the maxim that cybernetics was the science of control and communication in man and machines. A giant in the field, and without whom the field may have stagnated, was the English anthropologist Gregory Bateson, (whose father William Bateson coined the term genetics). Bateson, through his relationship with Don Jackson can be seen as the person who introduced anthropological principles into psychiatry. Using anthropology as a backdrop Bateson and Jackson decided that rules should be few and simple – those of basic, empirical observation in the here and now. This shift, along with work on communication, moved the focus of attention in the field onto observable, here-and-now data-gathering, thus eschewing the psychoanalytic principles of retrospective psychotherapy.

Ludwig von Bertalanffy (1969) held the belief, like Kurt Lewin, "that in any system the whole is greater than the sum of its parts" and that studying the relationship between the constituent parts of a system was a better way of understanding how the system functioned and how we could help it function better. Don Jackson had worked with John Weakland and Jay Haley who, having joined forces with Gregory Bateson, were studying communication patterns, and, in 1956, he published the seminal paper "Towards a theory of schizophrenia". It was Jackson who also introduced Cannon's biological notion of homeostasis into family therapy through the publication of his paper, "The question of family homeostasis".

At this stage in the history of family therapy, Ivan Boszomenyi-Nagy was also studying schizophrenic transaction in numerous clinical sites in the USA. Alongside these developments in the study of schizophrenia, Murray Bowen in the USA was proposing the ideas of individuation in families and the notion that problems arise in people's lives due to their inability to individuate effectively from their family of origin. Working in Baltimore on schizophrenia, and the effect marital relations may have on it, was Theodore Lidz, a significant and often absent figure in the literature on the field. Later in the decade, developing Lidz' work on schizophrenia, Carl Whittaker and colleagues developed a treatment for chronic and resistant schizophrenia.

1957 saw the foundation of the Mental Research Institute, in Palo Alto California, and as mentioned earlier, this institute (MRI), became a conduit for so many seminal ideas and thinkers of that time, including the later development of the Brief Therapy project, which saw the introduction to the field of Paul Watzalwick and William Fry. (Heinz Von Foerster, the cybernetician most associated with the field of family therapy would, in admiration of Paul, say that he was "an invention of Paul Watzlawick", such was his influence in introducing cybernetics to the field).

1960s

By the 1960s the book, *Families of the Slums* had been published by Salvador Minuchin and he had taken on the Child Guidance Clinic in Philadelphia. Virginia Satir was working at the MRI, leading the charge that we all had the capacity to grow and change; also Nathan Ackerman had developed his own clinic in New York at this point.

1970–1980s

From the 1970s onwards, family therapy began to flourish in Europe and the USA and discreet and differing schools of therapy emerged. Among these were the strategic model introduced by Haley and Madanes; the existentialist model developed by Carl Whitaker in Philadelphia; the structural approach pioneered by Salvador Minuchin; and Bowen's family of origin therapy. At this time, also, we see the development of what would later became known as the Milan Team, closely developed by Mara Selvini Palazzoli, Gianfranco Checcin, Guilana Prata and Luigi Boscolo. Trained in psychoanalysis, they had become dissatisfied with the psychoanalytic approach and initially began adopting the work of Paul Watzlawick from the Brief Therapy Group and the work of the MRI, but later, through the publication of Gregory Bateson's *Mind and Nature* in 1973, would use a more aesthetic approach to working with families as the context for treatment.

REFERENCES. Ackerman, N.W., *The psychodynamics of family life,* 1958; Id., *Treating the troubled family,* 1966; Anderson, H., Goolishian, H. (1992). *The client is the expert: A not-knowing approach to therapy,* in S. McNamee, K.J. Gergen (Eds.), *Inquiries in social construction: Therapy as social construction* (pp. 25–39); Boscolo, L., Cecchin, G., Hoffman, L., Penn, P., *Milan systemic family therapy: Conversations in theory and practice,* 1987; Boscolo, L., Bertrando, P., *Systemic therapy with individuals,* 1996; Burck, C., Daniel G. (2009),

Mirrors and reflections: Processes of systemic supervision; Burr, V. (1995), *An introduction to social constructionism*; de Shazer, S., *Keys to solution in brief therapy*, 1985; Freedman, J., Coombs, G. (1998), *Narrative therapy: The social construction of preferred realities*; Freeman J., Combs, G., *Narrative therapy*, 1996; Gergen, K. J., *An invitation to social construction*, 1999; Hare-Mustin, R.T. (1978), *A feminist approach to family therapy*, in «Family Process», 17, 181–194; Ho, M.K., Rasheed, J.M., Rasheed, M.N., *Family therapy with ethnic minorities* (2nd ed.), 2004; Hoffman, L., *Foundations of family therapy*, 1981; Hoffman, L. (1988), *A constructivist position for family therapy*, in «Irish Journal of Psychology», 1, 1; Jones, E., *Family systems therapy: developments in the Milan systemic therapies*, 1993; Madanes, C., *Behind the one-way mirror: Advances in the practice of strategic therapy*, 1984; Nardone, G., Portelli, C., *Knowing through changing*, 2007; Ray, W.A., Nardone. G. (2009), *Paul Watzlawick: Insight may cause blindness and other* essays; Von Bertalanffy, L., *General systems theory*, 1969; Watzlawick, P., Beavin, J., Jackson, D., *Pragmatics of human communication: A study of interactional patterns pathologies and paradoxes*, 1967; White, M., Epston, D. *Narrative means to therapeutic ends*, 1990; Wiener, N. (1948), *Cybernetics*, in «Scientific American», 179, 14–18.

COGNITIVE PARADIGM

M.A. Reda and M.F. Pilleri

The cognitive paradigm started to take shape in the 1960s in opposition to behaviourism (Watson, 1913) and thanks to the evolution of other sciences, especially physics (cybernetics and system theory) and ethology. The systematization and dissemination of the concepts proposed by cognitivism is usually dated back to 1967, when U. Neisser published his famous text entitled *Cognitive Psychology*. However, in the previous years, other works adopting a cognitive approach had already been published (Piaget, 1937, 1949; Ellis, 1958; Miller *et al.*,1960).

According to cognitivists, individuals organize their beliefs from birth through their interaction with the environment; these beliefs become progressively susceptible to modification through new experiences (piagetian mechanisms of assimilation and accommodation). Thus, man is seen as an "active explorer" of his environment, a problem-solver that elaborates his theories, and no longer as a passive individual in front of reality. In fact, man is considered as an "information processor", as a computer that stores and processes the data he receives. According to Neisser (1967), the work of psychologists in understanding cognitive processes is similar to the work of a technician who tries to find out how a computer has been programmed.

The cognitive paradigm was also applied to the field of psychotherapy. Cognitive psychotherapy developed in the 1970s (classical empiricist cognitivism) as cognitive behavioural therapy and evolved over the years in various theoretical paradigms, which shared the comparison with developments and theories of other disciplines. In Italy, the schools of cognitive psychotherapy are represented today by cognitive-constructivist therapies and by those developed from post-rationalist cognitivism. This was initially introduced by V. Guidano by giving particular prominence to emotional narratives, in their dynamic processes related to the problems connected to personal identity. The theoretical framework of the first-generation cognitive therapy, formalized thanks to the systematisations of A.T. Beck (1967, 1970), was based on the postulate that cognitions determine behaviour. This assumption was already expressed in the writings of Epicurus, the Stoics, and especially Epictetus, according to which men are not distressed by situations but by their views on them. "Neuroses" were therefore considered the result of thoughts and ideas (more or less realistic) derived from erroneous learnings determining perceptual alterations, evaluative exaggerations, fallacious deductions, dogmatic concepts. For example, the essential concepts for the pathogenesis of depression include evaluative exaggerations and negative ideas concerning themselves, the world and the future (Beck, 1967). Patients are not aware of their "automatic" thoughts, of their internal dialogue, and the therapist's task is to support them in their path to awareness. Different procedures were used for this purpose (behavioural techniques, derived from classical and operant conditioning, are still used as a therapeutic aid), but all of them were aimed at rectifying cognitive distortions and at replacing them with more realistic and adaptive thoughts (for example, explaining to patients that their despair was not determined by an unsolvable situation, but by their interpretations, by their tendency to give particular value only to some specific events). During the therapy, cognitive distortions were brought to light in order to replace them with more realistic and useful interpretations. Under the guidance of the therapist, patients could analyze the links between their interpretations and their underlying emotional states, to examine whether their conclusions were truly realistic. During this research, developmental antecedents have become important (and they are still considered essential), as they allow therapists to shed light on patients' current cognitions and cognitive schemas. In summary, the strategies of the first cognitive psychotherapists took shape through the following stages: helping the patient to become aware of their thoughts; transmitting the epistemological principles of cognitive therapy (for example, that the perception of reality is not the same for all individuals and that psychological processes can alter perception and understanding of reality); assessing the reasonableness of cognitions to determine which of them need to be changed; verifying the degree of adaptability to the changes.

In the 1980s, thanks to M.J. Mahoney (1974) and, in Italy, to V. Guidano and G. Liotti (1979) and M.A. Reda (1986), cognitive-constructivist therapies began to spread; these are rooted in G.A. Kelly's psychology of personal constructs (1955). Cognitive-constructivist authors do not reject many of the assumptions outlined in early cognitive theories and they continue to give particular emphasis to developmental antecedents and to the problems connected to attachment. However, these authors no longer evaluate knowledge in objective terms, but rather through personal processes of representation (each mind constructs its own representation of reality). With the transition from classical cognitivism to constructivist cognitivism, emotions perceived in a negative way become a cornerstone to understand cognitive processes: moreover, the participatory style of the therapist becomes crucial. In classical cognitivism, the attitude of the therapist is detached; whereas in constructivist cognitivism, it is empathetic and aware of facing a multiform processual reality. This reality evolves constantly in building personal meanings and it has necessarily a *raison d'être*, that is, its own functionality. In this sense, a person "in compensation" is someone who adjusts and who is flexible to different situations, who generates explanations that allow them to integrate disruptive events into their emotional narrative (Piaget's mobile balance, characterizing adaptive mechanisms).

The process of knowledge (as well as its construction and organization) begins at birth and continues throughout a person's development, allowing individuals to construct their own knowledge (both of themselves and the world). This system organizes itself in the course of its evolution and it undergoes continuous transformations to maintain balance. Therefore, it is not possible to speak of right or wrong cognitive modes, but rather of "organizations of personal meaning", which can have a more or less high degree of adaptability against external or internal perturbing situations. For some people, it will be easier to accept emotional fluctuations and to find a progressive balance thanks to the flexibility of their organizational structure (organizations with a high degree of adaptability). For other people, a restructuring is needed in special circumstances that cause intense emotional swings, to prevent a deep crisis in the development of knowledge. According to the constructivist perspective, people are never in a static situation of normality or pathology, but rather in a dynamic situation of balance–imbalance. Therapists need to understand this dynamic, during the therapeutic interaction, through a person's "emotional narrative". This can be more or less confused or rigid, but always indicative of a particular way of being (personal identity).

In some individuals, emotional distress cannot be integrated into their narrative, and for this reason it induces a situation of imbalance (Reda, 1986). Emotional distress is very often related to a person's need for personal change and renewed adaptation in front of affective, social, environmental interactions (attachments, separations, losses, etc.). Therefore, in a clinical setting, the conversation with the therapist is an important instrument, which is often used with maieutic method, to help the other person to "deliver the truth" (this dialogical mode can also be found in the first cognitivism). Through clinical conversations, the therapist can also capture "dysregulated" emotions and meanings. In fact, in addition to verbal communication, an analogic communication is used during the session (through gestures, facial expressions, posture, the rhythm of the voice) that expresses a person's deepest emotions. This double aspect of communication allows the therapist to examine the emotions and to know the patient's ability to rebalance their emotional and cognitive flow within their emotional narrative. Personal restructuring takes place through a therapeutic process that takes into account the developmental and attachment characteristics of subjects, and their way of experiencing emotions and constructing their own personal systems. During this process, patients are helped to identify their emotional activation states and to contextualize them with respect to their immediate experience, in order to construct alternative and more adaptive narratives. In fact, with the help of the therapist, patients reconstruct the operating patterns that gradually organized themselves (the way of thinking used by patients is taken into account, in addition to the emotional-sensory nucleus around which they have structured their sense of uniqueness and identity). Moreover, the history of a patient's development is analyzed to identify which reconstructions can be used to decode all the emotions, whether positive or negative. Thanks to the awareness of emotions, it is possible to produce internal changes which make individuals more "functional" against systemic perturbations (in the system of affections, work, etc.) that happen in the cycle of life. The therapeutic relationship is of great importance in this process of reconstruction as co-causal factor of change.

Understanding the organization of personal meaning of patients as well as their "dysregulated" emotions and cognitions, allows therapists to help them to make connections between their sensory and cognitive experiences and, in this way, to increase the level of flexibility and adaptability of their organization of personal meaning (patients are helped to construct a coherent and self-referred emotional narrative). This restructuring happens through a guiding mind of reference (the therapist) who, through the sharing of his/her situation, helps patients to feel understood. Feeling understood and being able to share one's own emotions and meanings is made possible by the relationship with the therapist, whose disclosure (information that therapists give about themselves) comes into contact with the patient through a relationship of reciprocity, which is primarily emotional. This relationship allows patients to recover a congruent emotional narrative (dysregulated emotions and meanings appear to re-regulate). The sharing of emotions and meanings of the patient is not achieved by exerting a pedagogical role or by assuming them to be inconsistent and irrational, but by accepting and sharing their personal characteristics and meanings. Within a cognitive-constructivist therapeutic relationship, the therapist's strategically oriented disruptive role is essential, in addition to the reciprocal relationship therapist–patient. This role facilitates the restructuring of the emotional narrative (therapists facilitate the reorganization that people make of their life story). The perturbing activity of the therapist consists in helping patients to understand why a too rigid narrative scheme caused, or is causing, that kind of imbalance, which takes the form of a symptom. A patient's self-awareness is the basis, or better, the stimulus that allows the comparison with different personal meanings or narratives. This facilitates the process of flexibilization that allows patients to exit from an excessive egocentricity.

REFERENCES. Beck A.T., *Depression: Clinical, experimental, and theoretical aspects*, 1967; Id., *Cognitive therapy: Nature and relation to behaviour therapy*, in «Behaviour Therapy», 1970, 1; Ellis A., *Rational psychotherapy*, in «Journal of General Psychology», 1958, 59; Guidano G., Liotti G., *Elementi di psicoterapia comportamentale*, 1979; Kelly G.A., *Personal construct psychology*, 1955; Mahoney M.J., *Cognition and behaviour modification*, 1974; Miller G., Galanter E., Pribram K., *Plans and the structure of behaviour*, 1960; Neisser U., *Cognitive psychology*, 1967; Piaget J., *The construction of reality in the child*, 1937; Id., *Traité de logique*, 1949; Reda M.A., *Sistemi cognitivi complessi e psicoterapia*, 1986; Watson J.B., *Psychology as the behaviourist views it*, in «Psychological Review», 1913, 20.

ECLECTIC PARADIGM

J. Sommers-Flanagan, R. Sommers-Flanagan and V.I. Johnson

The eclectic paradigm in psychotherapy is an historical and worldwide phenomenon and movement with many variations on a common theme. This chapter describes the eclectic paradigm as well as its rationale, history, current status and future directions.

THE ECLECTIC PARADIGM AS PHENOMENON AND MOVEMENT. The eclectic paradigm has a long and storied history in psychology and psychotherapy. Beginning in the 1930s, and perhaps before, strong debate emerged over whether psychology should adopt a pure theoretical system or a general eclectic paradigm. David Klein (1930), an early promoter of the eclectic model, stated:

> the system-builder tends to ignore facts at variance with his [her] favorite principle, or else in Procrustean fashion he [she] mangles them to fit the system. Might it not be preferable in the interests of psychological progress, if a choice has to be made, to mangle the system and preserve the integrity of the facts, or better yet, give up systems entirely, and have a single science of psychology?
> (p. 496)

In contrast, Richard Husband (1934) claimed that to be eclectic was to be logically unsound:

> It is the contention of this paper that such a procedure is logically unsound. Any psychological system, no matter what it is, is founded on certain fundamental premises. These premises must be compatible with each other, and all one's theories must follow them out consistently. Otherwise one is accepting a certain premise (monism for example) only in part and rejecting it elsewhere.
> (p. 380)

The basic argument – whether to retain theoretical purity or combine divergent ideas and techniques from various theories – has continued in many venues throughout the world for the past 80 years. Eclectically oriented theorists emphasize practical reality: therapeutic technique should be flexible because it needs to work for all clients who seek help, despite their many distinct multicultural, international and individual differences. Echoing Husband's (1934) position, theoretical purists counter that psychotherapeutic techniques should be logically sound and internally consistent with fundamental theoretical premises.

The eclectic paradigm is an evolving phenomenon and a strong contemporary movement within psychotherapy practice and research. From lowly beginnings, it has become a prominent perspective, particularly among American psychotherapists and theorists, and is a growing international force as well.

Historical and contemporary context

We begin our short review of the history and evolution of the eclectic paradigm with a few comments on theoretical purity.

Theoretical purity

Movements in psychotherapy are often stimulated and inspired by disagreement, conflict, and opposition (Sommers-Flanagan and Sommers-Flanagan, 2004). This was certainly true for the eclectic paradigm, as it emerged primarily in contrast and opposition to ideological purity. Even Freud, in reaction to his own narrow formulations of classical psychoanalysis, acknowledged the need for psychoanalytic psychotherapy as a necessary alternative to address individual patient differences.

In the first half of the twentieth century, proponents of three dominant theoretical paradigms – psychoanalysis, behaviourism and humanism/existentialism – were in great conflict with one another. Many theorists and practitioners parted ways to join one camp or another, while a few notable exceptions made efforts to combine or integrate various theoretical perspectives. An early example of theoretical integration was Dollard and Miller's (1950) efforts to integrate behaviourism and psychoanalysis.

Ideological purity, when taken to extremes, can turn into ideological dogmatism or theoretical fundamentalism. Within psychotherapy, nearly everyone knows at least a few theoretical fundamentalists who advocate their particular approach as constituting the truth, while considering all others as inefficient, destructive or heresy. Such rigidity has contributed to an eclectic response.

The eclectic response

Frederick Thorne is generally known as the grandfather of eclecticism. Writing in the 1950s and 1960s, he contended that psychotherapy was often guided by the psychotherapist's theoretical needs, rather than the client's therapeutic needs. He produced very interesting and relevant material on structuring the psychotherapy session and role induction (Thorne, 1959). Interestingly, also during the 1950s and 1960s, but on the other side of the Iron Curtain, Ferdinand Knobloch of Czechoslovakia, created an eclectic approach to psychotherapy (Knobloch and Knobloch, 1979).

Early status

Although eclecticism has been both lauded and criticized over the years, only recently have psychotherapy students and practitioners been able to openly embrace eclecticism without experiencing professional contempt or critique. This extremely negative view of eclecticism may have developed, in part, due to aggressive criticism of eclectic approaches in the professional literature. For example, Hans Esyenck famously referred to eclecticism as a "mish-mash of theories, a hugger-mugger of procedures, a gallimaufry of therapies" with no systematic rationale for treatment application (Eysenck, 1970, p. 145). Interestingly, despite Eysenck's disdain for eclectic approaches, his renowned review of psychotherapy efficacy (1952) identified 7,293 cases treated by eclectic means with a 64 per cent "cure" or recovery rate. He reported that eclectic approaches were more effective than psychoanalytic approaches and evaluated eclectic psychotherapy treatment nearly ten times as often as other approaches. Apparently, this "hugger-mugger of procedures" was remarkably common long before it was overtly fashionable.

Syncretism

Despite its negative early status, eclectic paradigmatic perspectives have become more popular among practicing psychotherapists. This may be due in part to certain distinctions made within the eclectic approach. In the early 1990s, Lazarus (1992) distinguished his particular approach (technical eclecticism) from whimsical, unreasoned, or even impulsive eclecticism by referring to the latter as *syncretism* (Lazarus, 1992, p. 12). Syncretism is now viewed as nearly universally unacceptable. In contrast, eclecticism is positively defined as a systematic procedure where psychotherapists choose their specific approaches based on "the client, setting, problem, and the nature of the counselor's skills" (Lazarus and Beutler, 1993, p. 384).

ECLECTIC PARADIGM MODELS. Within the eclectic paradigm, there are four predominate perspectives worldwide. These perspectives include (a) technical eclecticism, (b) theoretical integration, (c) common factors and (d) assimilative integration.

Technical eclecticism

Technical eclecticism, originally defined by Lazarus (1967), is a form of psychotherapy that combines two or more procedures or techniques with no regard for their varied theoretical roots. From Lazarus's perspective, technical eclecticism is an actuarial approach that focuses on predicting or discovering which specific techniques work best for which clients, problems and circumstances. Technical eclecticism is consistent with the contemporary evidence-based–practice movement.

Several specific approaches to technical eclecticism are currently practiced. A sampling includes: (a) Multimodal therapy (Lazarus, 1997); and (b) Systematic eclectic psychotherapy (Beutler, 1991).

Common factors

In the 1940s, writers and practitioners began identifying factors common to effective psychotherapy across various theoretical orientations. Alexander and French (1946) were among the first to boldly claim that a single therapeutic principle was common to all psychotherapies. They stated:

> In all forms of . . . psychotherapy, the basic therapeutic principle is the same: To re-expose the patient, under more favorable circumstances, to emotional situations which he [she] could not handle in the past. The patient, in order to be helped, must undergo a corrective emotional experience suitable to repair the traumatic influence of previous experiences.
>
> (Alexander, 1946, p. 66)

Jerome Frank was another early proponent of common factors in psychotherapy. Based on cross-cultural studies of healing processes, he proposed four common psychotherapy factors: a warm and empathic relationship between healer and sufferer, a special setting accompanied by positive expectations, a rationale for health and illness, and a culturally sanctioned treatment procedure (Frank, 1961).

Currently, many writers and researchers advocate a common factors model (Hubble *et al.*, 1999; Wampold, 2001). They often believe that practitioners should be trained to provide the "common core" of psychotherapy factors (similar to Frank's common factors) rather than in the application of theoretically driven techniques.

Psychotherapy integration

Psychotherapy integration involves integration of two or more theories at a conceptual level. Although originally defined as theoretical eclecticism (Lazarus, 1967), this approach is more commonly referred to as psychotherapy integration.

Psychotherapy integration is the most ambitious approach within the eclectic paradigm. For the integration to be complete, it must include "theoretical integration at all related levels, such as theories of personality and psychopathology, worldviews, and metatheoretical and epistemological assumptions" (Lampropoulos, 2001, p. 7). True theoretical integration is a most challenging enterprise.

Over the past two decades, many approaches to psychotherapy have claimed integrative status. A sampling of these include cyclical psychodynamics (Wachtel, 1997), dialectical behaviour therapy (DBT) (Linehan, 1993), eye-movement desensitization reprocessing (EMDR) (Shapiro, 2002), developmental counselling and therapy (DCT) (Ivey 1991), the transtheoretical model (Prochaska and DiClemente, 2005), the supraparadigmatic integrative model (Opoza, 1997), and multitheoretical psychotherapy (Brooks-Harris, 2008).

Assimilative integration

Stanley Messer (1992, 2008) introduced the concept of assimilative integration, an approach emphasizing that practitioners primarily adhere to a single theoretical orientation, but then, as needed, add techniques from other perspectives to supplement their work. For example, a behaviourally oriented therapist might decide, on occasion, to integrate a Gestalt two-chair technique into a therapeutic repertoire.

Assimilative integration is a less rigorous compromise to complete theoretical integration. Many approaches described as theoretical integrations may be more appropriately placed in the assimilative integration camp. For example, Marsha Linehan's DBT approach is primarily cognitive-behavioural, but can be viewed as having assimilated Hegelian and Buddhist philosophical principles.

Eclectic and integrative issues and conflicts

Not surprisingly, there are fractures and disagreement within the eclectic paradigm and psychotherapy integration movement. These disagreements range from simple classification challenges (e.g. Is the transtheoretical model most appropriately defined as an eclectic, integrational or second-order integration)? Other disagreements are more conceptual or philosophical. For example, Coscollà *et al.*, (2006) propose that theoretical integration represents a form of modernity, whereas technical eclecticism is postmodern in nature. They contend that, for many, the purpose of theoretical integration is to build an all-encompassing unified theory of everything.

Nichols (2001) views theoretical integration differently:

> An integrative therapist cannot tolerate simply being "a true believer" who sees no need to do any further searching in order to understand something. That is, an integrative therapist needs to embody an ability to tolerate ambiguity.
>
> (Nichols, 2001, p. 290)

Clearly, although tolerating ambiguity may be part and parcel of the eclectic paradigm, it is anathema to theoretical purists. To the extent that integrationists demand complete theoretical compatibility to exist under their theoretical umbrella, they do begin, as Coscolla *et al.* (2006) suggest, to occupy the same modernist space as the original theoretical purists.

THE ECLECTIC PARADIGM WORLDWIDE. Recent studies of psychotherapists in the United States show that, for every category of mental health practitioner, identification with an eclectic or integrative orientation is more common than any other single orientation (Norcross and Goldfried, 2005; Norcross and Prochaska, 1988). This finding is less typical in Europe where psychoanalytic approaches remain dominant in many countries. However, similarly to trends in the United States, much research conducted in 2008 indicates that eclectic and integrational approaches are gaining popularity.

Concerning Central Europe, Caspar (2008) reported:

> The most influential theories and orientations guiding psychotherapeutic work in Switzerland are psychodynamic, humanistic, cognitive-behavioural and systemic. In Germany, the dominant orientations are . . . psychoanalytic/psychodynamic and, increasingly, cognitive-behavioural.

Vasco (2008) reported on the current state of psychotherapy in Portugal. Like other countries, psychoanalysis and cognitive-behavioural techniques are most prominent and integrative techniques have gained popularity in recent years. Vasco's explanation for this shift towards more integrative techniques is simple: "a growing number of therapists are more interested in providing 'quality therapy' than in defending the 'faith' of a specific theoretical orientation" (2008, p. 72).

Two important studies investigated the situation outside Europe. In Argentina, Muller (2008) reported on psychotherapy practice trends over a five-year period. Traditionally a nation of psychoanalytically oriented psychotherapists, Muller reported 39.8 per cent of psychotherapists practicing within the eclectic paradigm. Based on the research questions and responses, it appeared that many surveyed psychotherapists operate from an assimilative integration perspective with psychoanalysis as the base theory from which they incorporate other techniques and models. Psychoanalytic, humanistic psychotherapies, and more recently cognitive-behavioural and family therapies are utilized in Japan (Iwakabe, 2008). However, psychotherapy is a relatively new endeavour in Japan, and traditional "talk therapy" techniques have been adapted to fit the culture. Iwakabe (2008) uses the term "cultural integration" to describe these adaptations, which take two forms: modifying techniques to be more culturally acceptable and sensitive, and developing theoretical concepts and techniques more congruent with Japanese worldview and practices.

In sum, the current literature on psychotherapy practice across the globe reflects a growing movement towards the eclectic paradigm. Definitions vary regarding what constitutes an integrative or eclectic practice, but the overall theme is one of combining complementary components of multiple theories in a thoughtful and purposeful way to best meet the needs of the clients served.

A sampling of organizations committed to educating and supporting psychotherapy integration and eclecticism include the Society for the Exploration of Psychotherapy Integration, the International Academy of Eclectic Psychotherapists, and the World Association of Eclectic Hypnotherapists. It is likely that organizations supporting the eclectic paradigm exist in most countries where psychotherapy services are prevalent. Publications focusing on the eclectic paradigm include (a) *International Journal of Eclectic Psychotherapy*, (b) *Journal of Psychotherapy Integration* and (c) *Integrative Psychological & Behavioural Science.*

FUTURE DIRECTIONS. The future of psychotherapy in general and the eclectic paradigm in particular is likely to be characterized by conflict, fragmentation and intermittent rapprochement. This is both frustrating and beneficial. As Mahoney (2008) has noted: "[There is a] need for a balanced appreciation of the 'essential tension' that must be reverently protected in the developmental dynamics of science. There is wisdom in tradition, just as there can be wisdom in innovation." We believe that tradition and innovation can coexist and that in its coexistence the eclectic paradigm will move forwards and serve the individual needs of all clients more effectively.

REFERENCES. Alexander F., French T.M., *Psychoanalytic therapy: Principles and application*, 1946; Beutler Larry E., *Selective treatment matching: Systematic eclectic psychotherapy*, in «Psychotherapy: Theory, Research, Practice, Training», 1991 28, 3; Brooks-Harris J., *Integrative multitheoretical psychotherapy*, 2008; Caspar F., *The current status of psychotherapy integration in Germany and Switzerland*, in «Journal of Psychotherapy Integration», 2008, 28, 1; Coscollà A., Caro I., Àvila A., Alonso M., Rodrìguez S., Orlinsky D., *Theoretical orientations of Spanish psychotherapists: Integration and eclecticism as modern and postmodern cultural trends*, in «Journal of Psychotherapy Integration», 2006, 16, 4; Dollard J., Miller N.E., *Personality and psychotherapy: An analysis in terms of learning, thinking, and culture*, 1950; Eysenck H.J., *A mish-mash of theories*, in «International Journal of Psychiatry», 1970, 9; Eysenck H.J., (1952). *The effects of psychotherapy: An evaluation*, in «Journal of Consulting Psychology», 1952, 16, 5; Frank J.D., *Persuasion and healing: A comparative study of psychotherapy*, 1961; Hubble M.A., Duncan B.L., Miller S.D., *The heart and soul of change*, in «American Psychological Association», 1999; Husband R.W., *Can an eclectic position be sound?*, in «Psychological Review», 1934, 41, 4; Ivey A.E., *Developmental strategies for helpers: Individual, family, and network interventions*, 1991; Iwakabe, S., *Psychotherapy integration in Japan*, in «Journal of Psychotherapy Integration», 2008, 18, 1; Klein, D.B., *Eclecticism versus system-making in psychology*, in «Psychological Review», 1930, 37, 6; Knobloch F., Knobloch J., *Integrated psychotherapy*, 1979; Lampropoulos G.K., *Bridging technical eclecticism and theoretical integration: Assimilative integration*, in «Journal of Psychotherapy Integration», 2001, 11, 1; Lazarus A.A., *In support of technical eclecticism*, in «Psychological Reports», 1967, 21, 2; Lazarus A.A., *Brief but comprehensive psychotherapy: The multimodal way*, 1997; Lazarus, A.A., *Multimodal therapy: Technical eclecticism with minimal integration,* in J.C. Norcross, M.R. Goldfried (eds.), *Handbook of psychotherapy integration*, 1992; Lazarus A.A., Beutler L.E., *On technical eclecticism*, in «Journal of Counseling & Development», 1993, 71, 4; Linehan M.M., *Cognitive-behavioural treatment of borderline personality disorder*, 1993; Mahoney M.J., *Power, politics, and psychotherapy: A constructive caution on unification*, in «Journal of Psychotherapy Integration», 2008, 18, 3; Messer, S.B., *A critical examination of belief structure in integrative and eclectic psychotherapy*, in J.C. Norcross, M.R. Goldfried (eds.), *Handbook of psychotherapy integration*, 1992; Messer S.B., *Unification in psychotherapy: A commentary* in «Journal of Psychotherapy Integration», 2008, 18, 3; Muller F.J., *Psychotherapy in Argentina: Theoretical orientation and clinical practice*, in «Journal of Psychotherapy Integration», 2008, 18, 4; Nichols W.C., *Integrative family therapy*, in «Journal of Psychotherapy Integration», 2001, 11, 3; Norcross J.C., Goldfried M.R., *The future of psychotherapy integration: A roundtable*, in «Journal of Psychotherapy Integration», 2005, 15, 4; Norcross J.C., Prochaska J.O., *A study of eclectic (and integrative) views revisited*, in «Professional Psychology: Research and Practice», 1988, 19, 2; Opazo R., *In the hurricane's eye: A supraparadigmatic integrative model*, in «Journal of Psychotherapy Integration», 1997, 7, 1; Prochaska J.O., DiClemente C.C., *The transtheoretical approach*, 2005; Shapiro F.S., *Eye movement desensitization and reprocessing (2nd ed.)*, 2002; Sommers-Flanagan J., Sommers-Flanagan R., *Counseling and psychotherapy theories in context and practice*, 2004; Thorne F.C., *Structuring eclectic psychotherapy for the client*, in «Journal of Clinical Psychology», 1959, 15; Vasco A.B., *Psychotherapy integration in Portugal*, in «Journal of Psychotherapy Integration», 2008, 18,1; Wachtel P.L., *Psychoanalysis, behaviour therapy, and the relational world*, in «American Psychological Association», 1997; Wampold B.E., *The great psychotherapy debate*, 2001.

THERAPEUTIC PARADIGMS AND THEIR MODELS

Table 0 Therapeutic paradigms and their models.

Psychodynamic paradigm	Analytic group psychotherapy
	Analytical psychology (C.G. Jung)
	Ego psychology (H. Hartman)
	Freudian psychoanalysis
	Group analysis
	Humanistic psychoanalysis (E. Fromm)
	Individual psychology (A. Adler)
	Interpersonal psychiatry (H.S. Sullivan)
	Psychoanalysis (Klein and Bion)
	Psychoanalysis (Independent or middle group of British analysts)
	Psychoanalysis (Lacan)
	Multiple code theory (W. Bucci)
	Mutative psychoanalytic process
	Psychodrama (J.L. Moreno)
	Relational psychoanalysis (S. Mitchell)
	Self psychology (H. Kout)
	Short-term psychodynamic psychotherapy
	Transactional analysis (E. Berne)
Behavioural paradigm	Acceptance and commitment therapy
	Behavioural model of classical conditioning
	Behavioural model of operant conditioning
	Compassion-focused therapy
	Functional analytic therapy
	Neo-behavioural therapy
	Third-generation behavioural therapies
Existential-humanistic paradigm	Client-centred therapy
	Existential psychoanalysis
	Logotherapy
	Psychosynthesis

Body-expression paradigm	Bioenergetics
	Expressive therapy
	Gestalt psychotherapy
	Gestalt psychotherapy (Spagnuolo Lobb)
Systemic-relational paradigm	Conversational therapy
	Functional family therapy
	Interactional focused therapy
	Milan school of family therapy
	Narrative therapy
	Strategic family therapy
	Symbolic-experiential family therapy (Whitaker)
	Three-generation model of psychotherapy
Cognitive paradigm	Cognitive model of operant conditioning
	Neuropsychological cognitive psychotherapy
	Cognitive-behavioural therapy (Aaron Beck)
	Cognitive-behavioural therapy with couples and families
	Cognitive-causal therapy
	Personal-constructs psychotherapy
	Post-rationalist cognitive development therapy
	Post-rationalist cognitive therapy
	Rational emotive behavioural therapy (REBT)
	Rational emotive therapy (RET)
	Well-being psychotherapy
Interactional-strategic paradigm	Brief solution-focused therapy
	Brief strategic therapy (Nardone's model)
	Brief therapy (MRI's model)
	Collaborative strengths-based brief therapy
	Creative therapy
	Strategic directive psychotherapy
	Ericksonian psychotherapy
	Explicit analogue interventions (EAI) brief therapy
	Hypno-systemic therapy
	Integrated strategic therapy
	Interactionist therapy
	Neuro-Linguistic Programming (NLP)
Eclectic paradigm	Eye movement desensitization and reprocessing (EMDR)
	Integrated psychotherapy
	Positive psychotherapy
	Reality therapy
	Self-relations psychotherapy
	Transtheoretical psychotherapy

DICTIONARY ENTRIES A–Z

A

ABC MODEL

In the context of cognitive-behavioural therapy, a pattern of interpretation of behaviours and beliefs and of their recurrence. In the behavioural version of ABC, A corresponds to the antecedent, B to the → behaviour and C to the consequences (and → reinforcements). Behaviour analysis (→ clinical behaviour analysis) consists of a detailed assessment of antecedents (A) and consequences (C) of a disturbing behaviour (B). In the cognitive version of ABC, A corresponds to the antecedent, B to the beliefs and C to the emotional and behavioural consequences. Cognitive ABC focuses on the cognitive component (→ cognition) that stands between an antecedent (event) and its emotional and behavioural consequences. *[G. Palmieri].*

REFERENCES. Beck A.T., *Cognitive therapy of depression*, 1979.

ABOUTISM

In Gestalt therapy, it is a defensive attitude aiming to "turn things around", especially those causing great anxiety, rather than address them directly. It can be noticed that most of the → defence mechanisms, also analyzed by Freud, are connected to an avoidance attitude (negation, repression, displacement, etc.). In the words of Perls: "avoidance is the main characteristic of neurosis and concentration it is obviously its corrective opposite [. . .] the function of psychotherapy is to help the patient to listen to those facts that he hides to himself". Beyond the perhaps excessive expectations given by the father of Gestalt to this attitude – as evidenced by expressions such as "Look at your thoughts, your emotions: whatever they are, they are yours, it is you; *through the close contact with a neurotic symptom* you will be in a position to dissolve it" – the process of change that is determined in an individual, through the exercise of awareness, is undeniable. The price is obviously connected with the emergence of unpleasant contents (Zerbetto writes: "it is often necessary *to go through* hell and not to go around it"). This indication evokes the paradigm of a process of self-knowledge, which is symbolically represented in the story of Oedipus – the hero who did not stop in front of the danger of "Know thyself", up to its final consequences – as well as in Dante's journey, which involves descent into the deepest hell and then leads to the prelude of "then we came forth to see again the stars". In fact, it is all about "stepping into the black holes of consciousness", from where we tend, instinctively, to run away. *[R. Zerbetto, R. Sciaky]*

REFERENCES. Perls F., *Ego, hunger, and aggression*, 1942; Zerbetto R., *Gestalt: la terapia della consapevolezza*, 1998.

ABREACTION

This concept, born with Freud's *Studies on Hysteria*, expresses the idea of an emotional discharge capable of releasing the → affect linked to the memory of a traumatic event, which, having the possibility to move freely, does not acquire the characteristics of a fossilized pathogenic nucleus. The → cathartic method, in which abreaction occupies a central position, expresses the possibility of transferring the affect that has remained unconscious in a narrative, "purifying" it, in this way, from its traumatic part. The excitation phenomena, produced during traumatic events, will find their resolution (abreaction) in the use of language that frees the patient from the reminiscences of what he experienced. "Man finds a substitute for this action in speech through which help the affect can well-nigh be abreacted" (Freud, *Studies on Hysteria*, 1895, p. 180). Freud adds that the persistence of traumatic memories, even after many years, is explained by observing that "the reason why the pathogenically formed presentations retain their freshness and affective force is because they are not subject to the normal waste through abreaction" (ibid., p. 182). *[M. Balsamo]*

REFERENCES. Breuer, J., Freud, S. (1895), *Studies on hysteria*, in *The Standard Edition*, II, 1953–1974.

ABSTINENCE

In psychotherapy, this term has different meanings depending on the paradigm of reference. For example, the psychodynamic perspective focuses on sexual abstinence, while abstinence from food is relevant in the treatment of eating disorders and abstinence from experiences considered as dangerous is highlighted in the treatment of phobias. Therefore, the term abstinence refers to a voluntary induced or forced conduct consisting in giving up something that would be desirable. Abstinence can be pathogenic but also desirable as an element of wellbeing or as escape from certain diseases. *[R.]*

ABUSE

A physical and/or psychological coercion aimed at influencing other people's freedom of action and thought, and exerted to obtain material, social, sexual or moral subjugation. The attempt to adopt and obtain control and power over other people can be expressed either directly or through conduct aimed implicitly at amplifying an already existing hierarchy. The phenomenon may concern different contexts and situations – such as family, school, workplace – and it can be repeated over time assuming the form of → mobbing, stalking, bullying. Several authors have pointed out that the harmful health effects may result both from direct and indirect experiences: an individual may be victim of a violent incident in person, or witness violent incidents or become aware of violent incidents, death or harm caused to another person. Such experiences may have important consequences for their health, leading to the development of disorders such as depression, anxiety and social withdrawal.

Abuse against children has been particularly studied. As evidenced by Hart and colleagues, it includes all the affective and cognitive aspects derived from the mistreatment of children such as negligence, omission of attention, aggression or verbal abuse; even emotional mistreatment, attitudes of isolation, denigration, lack of emotional responsiveness, neglect of psychological, medical and educational health, rejection and deprivation fall into this category.

The term abuse is also used in the literature on drug addiction and it defines a particular form of use of psychoactive substance characterized by an increased risk of somatic, affective and psychosocial harm, both for subjects themselves and for other people and society, even without a structured form of addiction, characterized by tolerance towards the psychoactive substance. *[R.]*

REFERENCES. Buka S.L., Stichick T.L., Birdthistle I., Earls F.J., *Youth exposure to violence: Prevalence, risks and consequences*, in «American Journal of Orthopsychiatry», 2001, III, 71; Di Blasio P., *Psicologia del bambino maltrattato*, 2000; Gulotta G., *Elementi di psicologia giuridica e di diritto psicologico-civile, penale, minorile*, 2000; Hart S.N., Brassard M.R., *A major threat to children's mental health*, in «American Psychologist», 1987, 42; Hart S.N., Brassard M.R., Karlson H.C., *Psychological maltreatment*, 1996; Parquet P.-J., Reynaud M., Lagrue G., *Les pratiques addictives. Usage, usage nocif et dépendances aux substances psycho-actives*, 1999.

ACCEPTANCE AND COMMITMENT THERAPY

Third-generation model of cognitive-behavioural therapy deriving from a linguistic and semantic theory called Relational Frame Theory (RFT) developed by S. Hayes and his collaborators. The principles of RFT are based on the relationship between thought and language, and on how the representation of things by human beings is deeply influenced by learning through symbolic processes that are no longer recognized as simple relationships derived from verbal stimuli. This causes the domain of language and thought to become so excessive that the body no longer adapts to the demands of the environment, but it is subjected to control through the symbolic representations of the environment itself. In acceptance and commitment therapy, this is referred to as "language hegemony".

RFT has shown that the human mind is capable of creating entirely arbitrary representations of the past, the present and the future, not based on direct experience. This means that human beings are capable of feeling pain, fear or any other emotion just through the memory of a past event or the imagination of a future event. For example, a person can develop an intense fear of highways without having ever experienced any negative episode or trauma on highways. If the mind is able to create authentic "virtual realities" that are perceived as real, it is not possible to control psychological distress by simply escaping from adverse situations. When facing a problem, the natural tendency of human beings is to check for the cause and to adopt strategies to eliminate it. On the contrary, according to this psychotherapy model, it is precisely the use of control and strategies for the elimination of the problem that, paradoxically, lead to increased suffering and to an apparent loss of control of symptoms that people would, instead, like to eliminate. In particular, the less people are willing to accept having a personal problematic experience, the more they end up producing it. Ironically, the strategies that have produced success in the evolution of the human species in relation to the outside world are the cause of suffering and psychopathology when applied to their inner world, because everything that is reasonably done to address the suffering ends up generating it.

This dysfunctional nucleus of responses has been described by acceptance and commitment therapy in the suffering pattern called FEAR: Fusion, Evaluation, Avoidance, Reason-giving. *Fusion*: the tendency of human beings to merge with the content of their personal experiences, which leads to the problem of "literality", that is, the loss of distinction between the symbolic activity and the event that acts as its referent. *Evaluation*: the tendency to categorize the qualities of referents, as if they were owned by the referents themselves (i.e. "right–wrong", "good–bad", "fair–unfair"); through the fusion process, evaluations become inseparable from the real events. *Avoidance*: human beings are prone to avoid unpleasant situations but, paradoxically, this type of experiential avoidance may stimulate and increase feared or unwanted inner experiences, such as thoughts, feelings, memories or body sensations. *Reason-giving*: it is the tendency to give reasons that explain the cause of particular forms of personal experience and/or behaviour; this is a growing problem in human dysfunctionality, mainly for two reasons: not only do people have extremely limited access to the multitude of influences that shape the history of their learning, but there is no convincing evidence that personal events are the "cause" of such behaviour.

The aim of this therapeutic model is to intervene on these dysfunctional tendencies by giving more attention to direct experience and reducing the tendency to take all the thoughts and inner catastrophic representations literally. The patient should be led to discover that control and elimination strategies are the causes of suffering, not their treatment; to realize that acceptance and will are viable alternatives to control and attempts at elimination; to understand that acceptance is possible if people learn how to separate themselves from the rules that compose language and thought.

The final result consists in realizing that the road to vitality, to the achievement of purposes and meanings, is a journey that consists in choosing the actions that need to be evaluated, which are executed in the service of the ultimate value of life. Therefore, "acceptance" means accepting one's own inner experiences without trying to control or explain them, otherwise an aggravation of suffering is produced; "commitment" refers to the ability to choose one's own behaviour according to one's own values, regardless of the discomfort caused by one's own feelings, thoughts and emotional states. In other words, the answer that this model of therapy gives to the limiting effects of FEAR is to: accept, choose, act (ACT, or Accept, Choose, Take action). *[R.]*

REFERENCES. Hayes S.C., Strosahl K.D., *A practical guide to acceptance and commitment therapy*, 2004; Hayes S.C., Strosahl K.D., Wilson K.G., *Acceptance and commitment therapy: An experiential approach to behaviour change*, 1999; Strosahl K.D., *Acceptance and commitment therapy*, in M. Hersen, W. Sledge (eds.), *Encyclopedia of psychotherapy*, 2002.

ACT

It is a specific product of action that can be identified as the simplest significant intentional behaviour unit performed by an individual to adjust adaptively their relationship with the cultural, relational and social → environment. In this light, the speech-act theory states that language and communication are expressive behaviours, with an actionable meaning that modifies interpersonal relationships. In particular, a speech act can be examined for what it is said (*locution*), for the purpose of enunciation (*illocution*) and for the effects that it determines on onlookers and in the surrounding world (*perlocution*). In this view, speech acts are linked to the pragmatic conception of human communication that values, in particular, the tangible effects of symbolic interaction. More generally, all the psychosocial literature on suggestion, persuasion and social influence, emphasizes the factual importance assumed by communication within the process of social construction of reality and, in parallel, the construction of social reality.

In the sphere of psychoanalysis, the theory of faulty actions (*parapraxes*) developed by Freud in the interpretative framework of the so-called psychopathology of everyday life, is also well known. These behaviours (*action slips*), are the result of a neurotic conflict between norms and social constraints and unconscious drives that free the latter to the detriment of those that the person performing the faulty action defines as their real intentions. Speech acts can also be seen as the pillar of the ritual events that characterize the different social cultures, with particular reference to expressions of religious beliefs and magical practices. In this sense, even obsessive-compulsive disorders can be defined as behavioural syndromes governed by repeated and encoded speech acts that assume a specific regulation role between the person, the significant others and the world. *[S. Smiraglia]*

ACTING-IN

A typical psychodrama technique consisting in the exploration of a person's inner world through the transformation of mental images in action on stage: the person (the protagonist) embodies their ghosts on the stage with the help of fellow group members (auxiliary-egos). The acting-in is a sequence of actions called for by the direction of the therapist and is designed to let subjects easily perceive ambiguous, obscure or denied aspects of themselves, in view of the enlargement of their own self-consciousness. This is a proper and productive act when it is appropriate to the representation that is taking place. It is called acting-in as opposed to the more well-known acting-out (→ defence-mechanisms), which indicates an inappropriate act taking place when the person comes out of their embodied role. In a therapeutic approach based primarily on verbal communication, this event occurs when the person uses expressive forms not considered by the setting. *[G. Boria]*

REFERENCES. G. Boria, *Psicoterapia psicodrammatica. Sviluppi del modello moreniano nel lavoro terapeutico con gruppi di adulti*, 2005; G. Boria, F. Muzzarelli, *Incontri sulla scena*, 2009; J.L. Moreno, *Psychodrama first volume*, 1946; J.L. Moreno, *Who shall survive?*, 1953.

ACTING-OUT → DEFENCE MECHANISMS

ACTIVATING EVENT

In rational emotive therapy, an activating event (or *activation*) represents one of the three main elements of the so-called → "ABC model" developed by A. Ellis, concerning the analysis of the thoughts that drive emotions and behaviours after an event. Ellis has proposed this model to improve clinical evaluations and to identify the therapeutic focus of the common emotional disorders; the model considers that every emotion or behaviour (C: *consequences*) experienced or enacted by an individual is not a product of the situation or the event itself (A: *activating event*), but rather of the interpretation of the thoughts that the event activates in the individual (B: *belief system*). Although at first sight this may seem a straightforward model, it is actually circular, as the elements influence and condition each other; an emotional state can trigger a mental process and vice versa. Activation consists in an external or internal (feelings or mental images) action that starts cognitive processes, which in turn are accompanied by an emotional reaction and by the activation of a behaviour. In individuals that are subject to panic attacks, *activating events* may be some typical situations in which there is no escape (for example: I am in an elevator, if I start to feel bad I cannot ask for help), or in which the feelings experienced by a person are capable of triggering catastrophic thoughts (for example: I feel pain in my chest, I might have a heart attack). In case of more serious disorders, such as psychosis, in the presence of delusions and hallucinations, the activating events can take many forms. In Chadwick and Birchwood's model, the activating events (A) are the auditory hallucinations (voices) heard by people and not their thoughts (B). If we consider voices as activating events (A) to which meanings (B) are given, it is possible to clarify that the emotional distress and behaviour expressed by the subject, are not a direct consequence of hallucinations but rather of beliefs, evaluations and explanations that the individual gives to them; beliefs are therefore treated as secondary delusions. *[M. Procacci, C. Petracca]*

REFERENCES. Chadwick P., Birchwood M., Trower P., *Cognitive therapy for delusions, voices and paranoia*, 1996; De Silvestri C., *Fondamenti teorici e clinici della terapia razionale-emotiva*, 1981; Semerari A., *I processi cognitivi della relazione terapeutica*, 1991.

ACTIVE AND DIRECTIVE PSYCHOTHERAPIST

Within cognitive behavioural psychotherapy, the style adopted by the psychotherapist in helping his patient. This means that the psychotherapist directs the therapy, keeping in mind, at every stage of the therapeutic process, where to direct his patient. In this context, being directive does not mean being authoritarian, so much so that the psychotherapist applies his or her own style in a manner that is decisively "Socratic". Additionally, although active and directive, the psychotherapist uses his style in a flexible manner, adapting it to the particular characteristics of the patient, with the objective of guaranteeing a functional relationship with the patient in order to help him attain his therapeutic goals. *[M. Di Pietro]*

REFERENCES. Ellis A., *Reason and emotion in psychotherapy*, 1962.

ACTIVE IMAGINATION

An introspective method invented by Jung and subsequently developed by Jungian analysts. This technique is focused on soliciting spontaneous images to enable the comparison with the unconscious experience. It aims at producing intentionally what happens naturally thanks to the transcendent → function, that is, by connecting consciousness and unconscious. Subjects are invited to turn their attention to the affections and fantasies that emerge in that moment, starting from a recent sensory perception. The meeting with these images, which demands a strict "ethics" position to avoid confusion between imagination and reality, allows the integration of consciousness with the multiple viewpoints of the unconscious, derived from personal experiences and by archetypal images. *[M. Tibaldi, A. De Coro]*

REFERENCES. Jung C.G., *Analytical psychology, its theory and practice: The Tavistock lectures*, 1968; Tibaldi M., *Pratica dell'immaginazione attiva*, 2011.

ACTIVE LISTENING

It is the core methodology in → client-centred therapy. Active listening is meant as a multisensorial, understanding, non-directive type of listening, that allows an empathic process (→ emphatic understanding) to take place. Its purpose is to facilitate a profound relationship with the other, enabling him to explore even those parts of himself that are unconscious, in order to find new resources for change. Active-emotional listening, which excludes judgement and advice, offers the person who is speaking the opportunity to express himself fully and unequivocally, to accept his limitations and to reveal himself with confidence. This kind of listening allows the therapist to tune in to him and assimilate his framework, while grasping those aspects of content and process that facilitate continuation of the dialogue. *[C. Montanari, F. Barbuto]*

REFERENCES. Rogers C.R., Stevens B., *Person to person: The problem of being human*, 1974; Gordon T., *Leader effectiveness training*, 1987; Rogers C.R., Russell D.E., *Carl Rogers: The quiet revolutionary*, 2002.

ACTIVE TECHNIQUE

Forms part of the model of psychoanalytic derivation developed by the great Hungarian psychoanalyst Ferenczi. This approach is based on a series of "cardinal" points that, in the period in which they were formulated, appeared as being revolutionary with respect to the theory of S. Freud; these are: 1) that → drive theory has its limitations: Ferenczi asserted that the disorder of the patient derives from traumatic relationships with a pathogenic environment; 2) the patient–analyst interaction should blossom into the development of new and healthier roles; 3) the analytic abstinence predicted by the → setting in reality can hide the hypocrisy and the indifference of the therapist and runs the risk of being a vehicle of emotional distancing or rejection that reminds the patient of situations of deprivation experienced in childhood; 4) the analyst that is able to achieve regression in the therapy session (→ defence mechanisms) produces the emergence of wounds that require → empathy and care; 5) verbal interpretation on its own is not enough: the patient is able to experience new emotional experiences only when he interacts with the therapist. Ferenczi, the *enfant terrible* of psychoanalysis, was the first to formulate concrete therapeutic interventions. With him, the analyst, the scientist of the soul seated behind the couch, was transformed into a therapeutic actor: he did not limit himself to simply listening and talking, but he would also use his body as an instrument of therapy. For example, in one of his more difficult cases, Ferenczi invited a patient who was struggling in therapy to move closer to him, and he stroked his head as a good mother would do. Today, many of these proposals have been adopted to a greater or lesser degree by psychotherapy, but in the 1920s Ferenczi's creative talent and human generosity sparked attacks from other, more conformist analysts, and the envy of Freud himself.

It is evident that active technique has some points in common with the action-method techniques of J.L. Moreno (→ psychodrama), but with an important difference: Ferenczi acted within the dual setting of psychoanalysis – that excludes the gaze and the participation of other people – whilst Moreno worked with auxiliary egos and in front of a group. Within the theatrical space, playful and symbolic, of psychodrama, the therapist that tries to achieve a profound contact cannot establish a relationship in the first person with the ghosts of the patient but can only help him to re-enact them. The director of psychodrama does not interpret the therapeutic roles as an actor, but he hands them over to the therapeutic assistants or to the other members of the group. In this way, the healing interaction, aimed at repairing the consequences of trauma or the deficits of the patient, takes place in a space and time different from that of reality. Defining the reparative action as psychodrama, the psychotherapist is encouraging regression and the active restructuring of trauma and deprivation, without falling into the trap and the ambiguity of an enactment that would short-circuit → transference. *[O. Rosati]*

REFERENCES. Ferenczi S., *The clinical diary of Sándor Ferenczi*, 1988; Haynal A., *The technique at issue: Controversies in psychoanalysis: from Freud and Ferenczi to Michael Balint*, 1988.

ADAPTATION

A concept used in psychotherapy to indicate the entirety of self-modelling changes on behaviour and thought, implemented by individuals during their life as an interactive response to the social and physical → environment and to their mental states in particular. This concept needs therefore to be distinguished from the concept of evolutionary adaptation, that is, the phenomenon concerning phylogenetic survival of living species, according to which only individuals with a genetic heritage "suitable" to respond to the constraints and the physical limits of the environment have the ability to reproduce. In psychotherapy, the general concept of psychological adaptation can be distinguished from the more specific concept of → social adaptation. Psychological adaptation corresponds to the autoplastic adjustment of behavioural, emotional and cognitive responses, depending on one's own perceptions of reality, motivations and needs, cognitions and beliefs, feelings and emotions and psychophysiological states. Adaptation can be spontaneous or deliberate: in the first case it is an automatic reaction learned on the basis of previous experience, and it is referred to as learned response; in the second case it is a voluntary response to a situation perceived as problematic or conflictual (*problem-solving*), and it is called creative adaptation. In psychopathology, an adaptation disorder is defined as a state of great distress and psychological pain produced by an unsuccessful management/resolution of the stressors. It is also possible to speak about a so-called pathological adaptation when there is a → chronicization of a disorder. In this case, pathological adaptation can be connected to the usefulness of the symptom – for example, the ability to draw attention or to feel protected, or even to be able to avoid addressing other problems – or it can be generated by temporary or structural situations, as for example in case of hospitalization and → psychiatrization, or in the absence of adequate therapies. *[R.]*

ADAPTIVE BEHAVIOUR

A term used to indicate a behaviour able to acquire or learn skills that are valued as "appropriate" by one's own culture and that are used by the person to effectively cope with daily life. The psychologist C. Hull tried to expand Pavlov's → behavioural model of classical conditioning by assuming that organisms act to reduce the tension that originates the *drive* to the behaviour itself. Therefore, any behaviour is initiated by an activation state of the organism, based on an internal state of necessity or stimulus, (hunger, thirst, sexual arousal, pain) or an external one (gratifications, rewards). If the behaviour is effective, the tension decreases: this represents a "reward" for the behaviour itself, and it fosters its repetition in similar contexts (learning by reinforcement). In addition, "intervening" variables can be identified between stimulus and behaviour. These variables are characteristics of the organism itself and able to mediate the relationship between stimuli and responses: for example, the tendency to respond in the same way, almost automatically, to the same stimulus, or the flexibility of behaviour repertoires; the motivation towards the extent of the reward; "high or low" excitatory potential, that is, the threshold above which a stimulus is capable of generating tension in the body. According to this model (known as SOR – Stimulus–Organism–Response) the environment (with its constraints and opportunities), the body (with its needs and its motivational components) and behaviours (with their reinforcing or punishing consequences) mutually interact: for example, when children seek the parent's proximity so that they can satisfy their needs, in order to ensure the attention of adults, they acquire a range of adaptive responses (learning) to please them (education, obedience, etc.). *[G. Lo Savio]*

REFERENCES. Amsel A., Rashotte M.E., *Mechanisms of adaptive behaviour*, in L. Clark, *Hull's theoretical papers*, 1984; Skinner F.B., *Science and human bevavior*, 1953; Tolman E.C., *Behaviour and psychological man: Essays in motivation and learning*, 1951.

ADHESIVE IDENTIFICATION → DEFENCE MECHANISMS

ADOLESCENCE

A phase of deep modification and reorganization of the psychic reality, corresponding to the maturation of the nervous system and the main biological systems, that accompanies the transition from childhood to adulthood. The most noticeable change is observed in cognitive abilities, which develop abstract reasoning skills, but it also involves the development of a personal sense of → identity, socialization and interpersonal affiliation processes, the complete development of sexual and gender identity, adult modulation of emotional and affective capabilities. The starting point of adolescence usually coincides with pubertal development, while it is more difficult to define the term chronologically, as it depends on the acquisition of a sociologically determined adult status and therefore varies according to the different socio-cultural contexts. Adolescence is one of the most important application fields of psychotherapy, both because in this period individuals are ductile and prone to change due to their inclination to personal development, and because, for the same reason, it is also the stage of life where the majority of mental and behavioural disorders are developed and expressed. Therefore, therapeutic work with adolescents shows some peculiar characteristics: on the one hand, the therapeutic change process benefits from dealing with a system that is already in transformation; on the other hand, particular attention should be given to the → therapeutic alliance, as the clinician is often called to manage the strong inner conflicts, transgression and shyness typical of this phase of transition to adulthood. *[R.]*

REFERENCES. G. Lutte, *Libérer l'adolescence: introduction à la psychologie des adolescents et des jeunes*, 1988.

ADULT

In transactional analysis, name given to one of the three → Ego-states described by Berne and defined as an independent set of feelings, thoughts, attitudes and behaviour suited to reality. It symbolizes the full capability of the neopsychic system (Adult) to work without the intrapsychic influence of the introjected contents of the → Parent and/or his non-integrated childhood experiences. The neopsyche integrates the qualities of the → archaeopsyche (→ Child) through *pathos* (emotions of passion, tenderness, spontaneity and empathy) and the universal moral qualities of the → exteropsyche (Parent) through *ethos* (moral values such as adult responsibilities, courage, loyalty and sincerity dependent on an ethical system of life) and processes the information gathered through *logos*, abstract thinking and *technos*, creative skills. Today we speak of the "Neopsyche/Integrating Adult", who has three types of tendencies: personal receptiveness and attractiveness, objective assessment of information and moral responsibility. These tendencies represent the exteropsychic, neopsychic and archeopsychic elements processed and "integrated" in the neopsyche. A person who has analyzed dysfunctional archaic experiences and integrated them in his or her Neopsyche/Integrating Adult is charming, brave, creative and empathetic from a phenomenological viewpoint. *[A. Liverano]*

REFERENCES. Berne E., *Transactional analysis in psychotherapy*, 1961; Id., *Intuitions and ego states*, 1977; Dryden W., *Dryden's handbook of individual therapy*, 1984; Liverano A., Piermartini B., *Il concetto di Adulto integrante e le sue implicazioni nella relazione terapeutica*, in «Psicologia, Psicoterapia e Salute», 2010, XVI, 1.

AESTHETICS OF CHANGE

The book, *Aesthetics of Change,* published in 1983, proposed a systemic-cybernetic (→ cybernetics) aesthetics for the practice and understanding of therapy. Following Gregory Bateson's idea that the complexity of systemic process should not be reduced to simplistic generalizations and reductionist formulas, aesthetics refers to the whole, irreducible, ecosystemic processes that hold human interaction and experience. Aesthetics of change, as understood in systemic therapy, is an extension of the classic philosophy of art and culture. Here it embodies a radical constructivist (→ constructivism) position that concerns itself with the ways we can construe and invent perceived worlds. Following cybernetician Heinz von Foerster, ethics and aesthetics become inseparable because how one acts brings forth what one senses, experiences and knows. Gregory Bateson proposed that aesthetics rather than pragmatics be the overarching context for the study of biological interaction, whether the subject is a redwood forest, the learning of a dolphin, or a family therapy session. Both in the study and the intervention, the focus is on interacting with the changing flux, the recursive nature of circular process that holds the ongoing creation of situational realities.

In 1983, Keeney published *Aesthetics of Change,* a return to the epistemological challenge Bateson had proposed. It resulted in an historic controversy in which members of the → Mental Research Institute, including Watzlawick, viciously attacked the perceived critique on pragmatics as irrelevant and unworthy of serious concern. Years later, Keeney sat on an Ericksonian conference panel in Orlando, Florida with Sophie Freud and Paul Watzlawick. Watzlawick personally communicated that Bateson's split with him had been a traumatic emotional crisis. He believed that he had tried to report Bateson's ideas in a respectful way, while acknowledging that Bateson felt he had been plagiarized.

Today it is instructive to see how the historic debate between pragmatics and aesthetic views of change mirror other ongoing debates in therapy between action and meaning, performance and narrative, rigour and imagination, art and technique, theory and practice. In the voicing of these differences, positions are easily taken that are framed as an either/or dichotomy. The challenge is to hold their necessary relations, without obscuring the benefits of their differences. *[B. Keeney]*

REFERENCES. Bateson G.,. *Steps to an ecology of mind: Collected essays in anthropology, psychiatry, evolution, and epistemology*, 1972; Harries-Jones P., *A recursive vision: Ecological understanding and Gregory Bateson*, 1995; Keeney B.P., *Aesthetics of change*, 1983; Keeney B. P., *Not pragmatics, not aesthetics*, in «Family Process», 21: 429–434, 1982; Morin, E., *On complexity*, 2008; Von Foerster H., *Observing systems*, 1981; Watzlawick P., Bavelas J. B., Jackson D. D., *Pragmatics of human communication: A study of interactional patterns, pathologies, and paradoxes*, 1967.

AETIOLOGY

The research and study of factors determining an illness or a → disorder. In psychology, when searching for a cause to explain why a behaviour happens or not, it is important to consider that both variables, internal and external to the individual, need to be taken into account simultaneously. In fact, the aetiology of the majority of disorders described in the *Diagnostic and Statistical Manual of Mental Disorders* (→ DSM) is unknown. Many theories and explanations have been indicated to clarify the origin of a psychological problem, but not always with convincing evidence. In all the disorders where it was possible to establish precisely and unambiguously a proper causal relationship, this has been included in the definition of the disorder. At the moment, as it is not possible to refer precisely to infectious agents or metabolic and/or physical alterations of medical competence, and as correlation or linear or circular causation (→ causalism) dynamics are not clear, the remaining pathologies are still waiting to be more carefully studied, relying on the progress of the methods of investigation and intervention. To this day, for example, in most cases it is not clear whether physiological processes influence emotional states or whether it is the psychic dimension that has an effect on metabolic, physiological and endocrinological aspects. In accordance with the principles of equifinality and multifinality enunciated by L. von Bertalanffy, it is a widely shared opinion that the origin of psychological problems can be traced back to a complex system of interrelationships between biological, social and psychological factors, not exclusively related to linear causation phenomena typical of medical investigation. *[R.]*

AFFECT

In Freudian theory, this term refers to emotions resulting from investments and drive discharge. According to Freud, if drives were not linked to representations or affective states, they would remain completely unknown. Freud clarifies that "representations are investments – basically of mnestic traces –, whilst affects and feelings correspond to discharge processes, whose final displays are perceived as [inner] feelings." Affective states are organized around the two basic polarities of pleasure and pain, but they differ in the whole complex range of painful or pleasant emotions (anxiety, guilt, euphoria, sadness, etc.). Affects play an essential role in regulating the psychic life, as defence mechanisms follow the pleasure principle and try to avoid painful affects. "We affirmed," Freud observes, "that in case of repression there is a separation between the affect and its representation, after which the one and the other meet their fate separately." Therefore, drive investments and corresponding affective states, can be connected to objects that change depending on the events that come in succession in the psychic life. Both "affective charge" and "representation" are "representatives" of drives. In other words, they are what, in psychic life, expresses the quantitative and energetic components of drives themselves. Therefore, holding or discharging a drive determines the production of an affect that accompanies, in turn, both the presentification of an image and the execution of some specific action, in relation to an object. Affects are, in essence, the determinants of emotional life.

With the development of the structural theory, the Ego becomes the location of affects and anguish in particular, and it becomes the specific structure responsible for the organization of the defensive processes. From a therapeutic perspective, affects are the essential elements involved in the manifestations of transference and the effective and efficient expression of transformation processes. The acquisition of a purely intellectual understanding of one's own mental state, unaccompanied by a full experience of its affective components, remains ineffective and does not involve any real possibility of maturation and change. *[P. Cruciani]*

REFERENCES. Ammaniti M., Dazzi N. (eds.), *Affetti. Natura e sviluppo delle relazioni interpersonali*, 1990; Freud, S., *On metapsychology*, 1991. Rapaport, D. *On the psycho-analytic theory of affects*, in «The International Journal of Psychoanalysis», 1953, 34, 177.

AGGRESSIVENESS

A number of different behaviours can be defined as aggressive (to a greater or lesser extent); they can range from physical violence to participating in a sporting event, from sarcastic comments to looking for a sexual partner, from the defence of one's own territory to the act of chewing food. The term (from the Latin *ad-gredior*, "I move forwards") designates a tendency to behave or to have hetero-/ self-destructive fantasies, or fantasies directed to self-affirmation. Concerning the first type of behaviour or fantasies, many authors tend to put particular emphasis on the intentionality of the act, thus limiting the definition to "conscious intent to cause harm". In contrast, theoretical models closer to the second type prefer to use the term "aggressiveness" just to designate behaviours directed to organisms' survival and reproduction of species, preferring instead the term "destructiveness" to indicate behaviours intended to damage or destroy. These two positions are united by the fact that a behaviour of self-assertion (for example, winning a sporting competition, getting the attention of a sexual partner, getting some food) can result in more or less intentional damage to other individuals, or at least have a value of predominance and subjugation. Psychotherapy often considers aggressive behaviour closely related to the emotion of → anger, and does not exclude doing cathartic work on it by encouraging patients to express freely, in a safe environment, emotions that have been repressed for a long time. However, there are different types of treatment for aggressive dysfunctional behaviours, consistent with the theoretical postulates of the different therapeutic models.

In literature, it is thus possible to find treatments that assert the importance of a cognitive management of aggressive reactions, and others that, on the contrary, are based on supportive-expressive techniques. But if we consider the most constructive sense of the term, that is, the one related to self-affirmation, psychotherapy allows patients to activate and express the resources that carry an aggressive value, in order to revitalize energy and constructive personal initiative. *[R.]*

AION

Jung chose this Greek word ("eon", "age"), to indicate both the era of Christianity and the new period that was about to start, and he used it as the title of one of his important works. In this work, he tries to provide an historical, mythological and psychological analysis of the division in the Western psyche (individually and collectively) between very high ethical standards and disastrous concrete behaviours. Jung points out the change of the psychic situation in the Christian era: the advent of Christ led to the split of the image that man had of himself (a projected image onto God, if we use the religious language of the time), between the opposites Christ and Satan (a mythological pair which today is moralized and psychologized in the pair good–bad). In other words, it can be said that consciousness came from the undetermined unconscious and it left darkness behind. It was a necessary step in human development, but this generated one-sidedness (the same of which consciousness consists), division and conflict (intra- and intersubjective: if man does not perceive his internal conflict, the conflicting counterpart reveals itself in the environment). In this division between light and shadow that marks the 2000 years of Christianity, the focus of consciousness has slipped from the initial religious spiritualism to today's scientific materialism, going through the whole spectrum of shades. As a result, the experience of the Self has materialistically slipped from the initial religious projection of Christ to the human psyche. Today it is possible to reunite the split parts of the Self into a work of awareness and culture: the bygone era of conflict, in which man was surrounded, and acted on, by the psyche, gives way to integration and awareness of the reality of psyche. *[G.M. Vadalà, A. Benvenuti]*

REFERENCES. Edinger E.F., *The Aion lectures*, 1996; Hannah B., von Franz M.L., *Lectures on Jung's Aion*, 2004; Jung C.G., *Aion: Researches into the phenomenology of the self* (1951), in *Collected Works*, IX/II, 1969.

ALCHEMY

Considered as a science until the eighteenth century in Europe – its origin is perhaps related to prehistoric metalworking (from the Arabic *al-kimiya*, "philosopher's stone") –, alchemy is a set of philosophical and esoteric knowledge and experimental procedures that aim to transform humble and imperfect matter into noble substance and to realize the elixir of life through a codified procedure. This consists of seven successive operations, using sciences (chemistry, physics, medicine, pharmacy, etc.), philosophical speculations and magical practices. In alchemy, philosophical speculations, symbolic aspects and experimental practices are mutually indistinguishable, as it is assumed that there is a mutual influence between the states of awareness of the alchemist and physical occurrences; he feels part of the transmutation and aspires to attain omnipotence and omniscience. The decline of alchemy began with the emergence of the scientific method. Jung sensed the correspondence between alchemical symbols and archetypes, hypothesized as active, in the collective unconscious. From the 1930s onwards, Jung's writings show his studies on alchemy; the alchemical process of transformation of matter becomes the footprint on which the process of individuation, that is, the realization of the true self of the subject, takes place in the knowledge of its different complexes and is realized in the psyche. The → transference and → countertransference, that play a central role in the therapeutic relationship, are exemplified in the analysis and depiction of an alchemical text of the thirteenth century by Arnold of Villanova, the *Rosarium filosoforum*. *[A. Cannavina]*

REFERENCES. Eliade M., *Arti del metallo e alchimia*, 1980; Jung C.G., *The psychology of the transference* (1946), in *Collected Works*, XVI, 1966; Id., *Mysterium coniunctionis* (1967), in *Collected Works*, XIV, 1970; Id., *Alchemical studies* (1967), in *Collected Works*, XIII, 1968.

ALIENATION

In the first phase of his teaching, Lacan sees alienation as an imaginary identification of the Ego with the narcissistic image that the Other reflects on it and hence a non-coincidence between the Ego and its ideal. At a later time, Lacan rethinks the theoretical foundations of alienation when clarifying the contrast between imaginary and symbolic, with a progressive attribution of importance to the latter on the establishment of subjective realities. Alienation finds a complete articulation in the way it relates to the big Other, a dimension that refers to a superindividual symbolic and linguistic order. Alienation is a constituting condition of each speaking human being as it is inscribed in a pre-existing symbolic order and it rises as a result of the dependency from the discourse of the Other *[S. Guido]*

REFERENCES. Lacan J., *Presentation on psychical causality*, in *Écrits: The first complete edition in English*, 1946; Id., *Aggressiveness in psychoanalysis*, in *Écrits: The first complete edition in English*, 1948.; Id., *The function and field of speech and language in psychoanalysis*, in *Écrits: The first complete edition in English*, 1953; Id. *The four fundamental concepts of psychoanalysis*, 1964, in *The seminars of Jacques Lacan XI*, 1977.

ALLIANCE

In the systemic-relational paradigm, alliance represents the interaction between the therapist and the family based on trust, respect and collaboration and it is aimed at addressing problems and difficulties. Psychotherapy is a generative act that occurs through the structural coupling between the therapist and the system they encounter. In order to create a fruitful agreement, the coupling needs a mutual courtship and accommodation; if the therapist assumes an attitude of availability, the customer (the family) easily put itself in a position of acceptance.

This process will allow going beyond blocking stereotyped repetitive formalities (homeostasis), and will generate a new relational reality at a higher level. Without alliance, the intervention of the therapist may take the form of a deliberate act and harden the family, stopping the → change and turning it into a relationship made of contrasts or sterile symmetry (→ complementarity). The therapist, as a change agent, makes themselves fully and professionally available to the other, facilitating a new situation, from which he/she will leave at the end of the intervention. The therapist can be considered as the mullah in the story told by von Foerster, who helps three brothers divide 17 camels bequeathed from their father: half of the herd is due to the eldest son, a third to the second son and a ninth to the third son. The mullah decides to add his own camel, and the herd becomes 18 camels. This makes the problem possible to be solved. At the end, the mullah takes the camel back and continues his journey. Therefore, alliance does not have a collusive nature, but it is a creation of a new system capable of new answers. *[F. Bruni, P.G. Defilippi]*

REFERENCES. Bandler R., Grinder J., *The structure of magic*, 1975; Maturana H., Varela F., *Autopoiesis and cognition*, 1980; Minuchin S., Fishman H.C., *Family therapy techniques*, 1981; von Foerster H., *Observing systems*, 1981.

AMBIGUITY

A feature of what is perceived by a person in a non-univocal way. In linguistics, a word, phrase or sentence has the property to have more than one possible meaning. In a broader sense, the term refers to behaviours, stimuli, situations, statements that can be interpreted in different ways and therefore do not appear so clear and unambiguous. In Gestalt psychology (→ Gestalt psychotherapy) ambiguous figures are popular. In these, the subject perceives two different things depending on how the relationship between figure and background is structured. In psychoanalysis, words or ambiguous phrases are often interpreted as signs of hidden feelings or unconscious desires. For this reason, in such approaches → projective tests are used. These instruments are deemed suitable for an evaluation of the subject's personality due to the ambiguous characteristics of the stimuli. *[R.]*

AMBIVALENCE

A term defined by non-ordinary logic to indicate a statement that cannot be defined either true or false, therefore violating the Aristotelian principle of the "excluded middle", according to which additional possibilities, other than the two proposed above, do not exist. The construct of ambivalence is particularly important in connection to the relationship that each individual has with themselves, the others and the world, because, within this complex network of interactions, the phenomena of ambivalence are not an exception but a rule. Some of the most relevant studies on ambivalence are those of the Palo Alto school concerning pragmatics (→ Mental Research Institute) which highlights the ambivalent aspects of human communication and its effects on people's actions. In psychotherapy, the construct of ambivalence is a transversal phenomenon since it is an essential feature of the therapeutic relationship, even when, as in some cognitive behavioural approaches, its influence wants to be restricted (if not eliminated). On the contrary, some forms of therapy, such as the strategic and systemic ones, use ambivalences as tools to develop and apply strategies for change, for example the prescription of a symptom. *[R.]*

AMNESIA

In Freudian psychoanalysis, it is the inability to recall traumatic childhood experiences, since these are eliminated from consciousness due to the interference of the defence mechanism of repression.

Traumatic amnesia distinguishes the contents of the "repressed" unconscious and should be discerned from occasional lapses of memory – that the consciousness of the subject can recover autonomously – from latent contents of dreamlike formations and from paramnesias (false memories). *[I. Sarno]*

AMPLIFICATION

A method of interpretation of unconscious productions added by Jung to Freud's method of → free association. Jung believed that each person encloses in their mental processes the etymons that humankind has universally lived and pass on with myths and fairy tales; amplification allows people to reach these archetypal and archaic contents that hide in the metaphors of dreams and fantasies, and that remain otherwise unknown to consciousness. *[A. Cannavina]*

REFERENCES. Jung C.G. (1934–1954), *Archetypes and the collective unconscious*, in *Collected Works*, IX, 1969; Carotenuto A. (eds.), *Trattato di Psicologia Analitica*, 1992.

ANACLITIC

In Freudian psychoanalysis, a basic concept of the first drive theory (anaclisis). It is defined as anaclitic (or "for support"), an object choice (directed towards an external love object), as opposed to a narcissistic choice (directed towards the Ego or the Self). In *Three Essays on the Theory of Sexuality*, Freud theorized the mother as an anaclitic object for libidinal drives, since the child relies on the memory of the first experiences of satisfaction of his/her vital conservation needs, loving the "object" mother who takes care of him. Freud's drive theory introduces a difference between *narcissistic* and *anaclitic* choice of the love object in adulthood: narcissistic is the choice of a person who has a real or imaginary resemblance with the subject itself, that chooses him/her precisely for that similarity; in particular, Kohut explained different types of narcissistic relationship and described also the related, specific types of → transference that develop during the analysis of narcissistic patients. Instead, the anaclitic object-choice is based on the need and desire to be symbolically nourished and protected, as was once done by mother and father.

The expression "anaclitic depression" was coined by Spitz and Wolf: this is a syndrome consisting of symptoms of anxiety, sadness, crying, refusal of food, isolation that affects some children around the age of nine months. Its appearance is caused by an absence of the mother figure for at least three consecutive months, after a good mother–child relationship during the first three months of life. If, before the end of a critical period, that is set between the end of the third month and the end of the fifth month, the mother is returned to the child, or an acceptable replacement can be found, disorders disappear with surprising quickness. Conversely, if the separation continues, the symptoms become more severe and can cause insomnia, apathy, weight loss, developmental delays and even death. *[S. Sagliaschi, M. Casonato]*

REFERENCES. Freud S. (1901–1905), *A case of hysteria, Three essays on sexuality*, and other works, in *The Standard Edition*, VII, 1953–1974; Id. *On narcissism: An introduction*, 1914; Kohut H.T., *The restoration of the self*, 1977; Id., *The two analyses of Mr. Z.*, in «International Journal of Psychoanalysis», 1979, 60; Spitz R.A., *The first year of life*, 1965; Spitz R.A., Wolf K., *The smiling response: A contribution of the ontogenesis of social relations*, in «Genetic Psychological Monographs», 1946, 34.

ANALYSAND

In Lacanian clinic, this term defines the subject during the course of their analytical path; whereas, one who has concluded their analysis is called "analysed". J. Lacan uses the term "analysand" to emphasize the active, rather than passive, position taken by the patient during the treatment. In fact, the analyst cannot know anything about what happens to the analysand other than through listening, learning in this way from the same analysand what led him to ask for an analysis. For their part, patients talk, although, ignoring the value of their own words, they are not able to gain access to the truth of what they say. The analyst is aware that the analysand "knows without knowing", because the unconscious dimension constitutes a knowledge not known, i.e. a knowledge that the subject does not know and does not recognize. *[S. Guido]*

REFERENCES. Miller J.A., *Delucidazioni su Lacan*, 2008.

ANALYTICAL EXISTENTIAL PSYCHOTHERAPY

A therapeutic practice that springs from the awareness that psychological hardship and existential discomfort cannot be addressed in isolation one from the other, as this would be a partial solution or even a failure. Born in Europe and in the United States of America as an evolution of Freudian thought, based on European existentialism, from L. Binswanger's speculations up to E. Fromm, in Italy it has been developed by A. Mercurio, in that anthropological and meta-psychological vein named "Sophianalisi".

Nowadays it is irrefutable how the vision of reality, and, even more, the vision of men, is based on the awareness of the essential interrelatedness and interdependence of all phenomena: physical, biological, psychological, social and cultural. It is from this holistic view of both life and man that existential analytical psychotherapy promotes the conscious implementation of the conceptual "framework" of a man capable of uniting harmoniously the multiple identities from which he is composed which define the Person. The analytically oriented psychotherapies, from both a theoretical and methodological standpoint, are derived from psychoanalysis, with which they share the therapeutic treatment process and its structure. Methodology in psychoanalysis is characterized by a → setting that establishes a particular relationship between the therapist and the patient as one that promotes the emotional investment on the latter with the transfer of affective and emotional experiences (what is defined as → transference).

Existential analytic psychotherapy also works through transference interpretation, but especially through the analysis of the wisdom and the projects held within each person. The theoretical foundations of clinical psychoanalysis derive from all S. Freud's, and his pupils', discoveries. The discovery of the unconscious, of emotional ambivalence, the existence of infantile sexuality, the universality of the elastically understood Oedipus complex, the interpretability of dream and delirium and the chance to use transference therapeutically (C. Brenner), all represent the base of the analytical work. On the other hand, existential analytical psychotherapy takes advantage of the European doctrine of existentialism and the way it takes mankind and its problems into consideration, especially regarding the subject–object dichotomy of Western thought. Therefore, it focuses its attention not only on the patient's disease, but it considers him as a person in all his potential for freedom, responsibility and quality of life. This point of view does not deny the validity of studying one's own dynamics and behavioural patterns, but it affirms that drives or dynamics, whatever they are called, can only be understood in the context of the structure of the existence of the particular person we are relating to.

The distinctiveness of existential analysis is to take care of the Being, of existence in particular, namely, the patient that sits in front of the therapist. It ascribes four fundamental instances to the human being: the Corporal Ego (it represents the body; it is the ability to feel with both internal and external senses and to issue vibrations); Ego (the instinctive and drive part, as described by Freud, which enables us to perceive the messages coming from the Corporal Ego; it acts and reacts in a deterministic way, it builds thoughts, words, symbols and reasonings, all this just by following the → pleasure principle logic); Cosmic Self (the heart of the person, which contains its project – at the same time unique and part of the others' project, as well as being part of the entire universe one, also known as Cosmic Self – and jointly the modalities that realize it; its fundamental feature is to transcend itself, namely to always aim to surpass itself, to evolve; it is the inner voice, sometimes awkward, but always wise and positive, ready to remind each what their thorough plan and the purpose of life is); the *Io Persona* (the spiritual instance that harmonizes and unifies together the Corporal Ego, the Ego and the Self, freely deciding whether to act in harmony or in opposition to the project that each individual has within its own Self; from the beginning of intrauterine life, it is responsible for choices of love or hatred, destructiveness or constructiveness).

GUILT COMPLEX AND ACTUAL GUILT. The feeling of guilt is a false guilt. It is the result of the adjustment process, by the child, to outright bans and patterns of behaviour imposed by parents, especially by their mother. According to existential analytical psychotherapy, the real fault is given by the judgment of the Self on the work of the *Io Persona*, that is, on the quality of its actions and decisions, especially if these are focused on destructive hatred. Our pride does not allow us to admit this guilt, which means we do not put into effect our potential and thus waste our lives. In other words, we constantly deviate from what is our profound project and purpose in life, feeling as if we are never fully realized. This is due to our desire to remain anchored to our childhood experience, with its burden of unmet needs and with the inevitable hatred for wrongs we have suffered; also, and above all, in order to remain anchored to self-pity and victimhood. Even if we are unaware or refuse to hear his voice, the Self continually signals us about this state of affairs. We could just change it by assuming responsibility and repairing the actual guilt with forgiveness (this kind of forgiveness has nothing in common with the religious one). Whenever one acts against life, including one's own, whether we realize it or not, one is always committing a real sin.

HATRED. Hatred is a form of defence from a sorrow caused by an ancient wound. All our childhood stories are filled by received humiliations and insults that generate indelible wounds which, most of the time, are removed and forgotten once we are adults. Those who have not been loved, approved of or recognized, or who were unwanted during their childhood, may not be able to make up for it as an adult, at least not in the same way a child would. Living, hoping, and trying in every possible way to bridge these shortcomings is the basis of a deep feeling of hatred. Bearing a grudge for not having received, induces the individual to hate for good the person who has not loved him, by anchoring himself in the past with the belief and the expectation that those who have not loved him will return to fill in his gaps. All this contributes to straying from the Self. Self-love is the only way that one can make oneself accept both one's past and one's hatred, so as to take them on as exclusively personal matters and forgive oneself. Contrary to what many think, hate is not an emotion, but it is an action and belongs to the spiritual dimension; namely it is subject to freedom of choice. If we weren't free, we could neither hate nor love. The only chance either to love or to hate is to be free.

THE SPIRITUAL DIMENSION. The term *Person* is the pivot around which both Antonio Mercurio's Existential Anthropology and Personalistic Metapsychology develops, which represents one of the modern guidelines of existential analytical psychotherapy. He founds an innovative ethics on the concept of *Person*, brilliant in its simplicity, but not so simple to achieve. The fundamental assumption is the existence in the human being of a spiritual dimension and its most important representative: the Self. By affirming that Man has a spiritual dimension we mean he is endowed with freedom, that is, he can choose whether to love or to hate.

The spiritual dimension exists, together with the psychic and body dimensions, from conception and presents itself as an elemental form gradually, becoming more and more complex. The modalities of the psychic and corporeal sphere are substantially reactive, whilst the spiritual dimension decides through the *Io Persona*: in other words, it selects the behavioural model in order to deal with the trauma that has hit it.

THE EXISTENTIAL UNCONSCIOUS. The first consequence of identifying the spiritual dimension is to introduce the concept of the psychic unconscious alongside the existential one, which is structured in factual, reactive and decision-making unconscious. All the pleasant and unpleasant events that have shaped the individual are recorded in the factual unconscious. All instinctive responses are contained in the reactive one, automatic to events that occur inside and outside the person, aiming to satisfy the principle of pleasure and self-preservation. Instead, in the decision-making we discover all decisions of love or hatred taken since conception. Repressed hatred lies in the decision-making unconscious and only by retracing decisions of hate we have taken in the past, and by assuming both its consciousness and responsibility, can we decide freely and anew whether to confirm or creatively transform them. It follows a new, complex and integrated modality of working with dreams and their interpretative mode that is extremely interesting within a clinical profile. *[D. Romagnoli]*

REFERENCES. Binswager L., *Wahn. Beitrage zu seiner phanomenologischen und daseinsanalytischen Erforschung*, 1965; Binswanger L., (1992), *Der Mensch in der Psychiatrie*, 1957; Binswanger L., *Ausgewählte Aufsätze und Vorträge, Bd. 1: Zur phänomenologischen Anthropologie*, 1947; Binswanger L., *Being in the world*, 1975; Boss, M., *Geist und Psyche. Psychoanlyse und Daseinsanalytik*, 1978; Foulkes S.H., Antony E.J., *Group psychotherapy: The psychoanalytic approach*, 1957; Freud, S., *The Standard Edition*, 1953–1974; Fromm E., *Psychoanalysis and religion*, 1950; Id., *The art of loving*, 1956; Id., *The sane society*, 1955; Id., *The art of listening*, 1994; Id., *To have or to be*, 1976; Mercurio A., *Amore e Persona*, 1978; Id., *Teoria della Persona*, 1978; Mercurio A., *Amore Libertà e colpa*, 1999; Mercurio A., *Antropologia esistenziale e meta psicologia personalistica*, 1991; Mercurio A., *La vita come opera d'arte*, 1995; Mercurio A., *Le leggi della vita*, 1995; Romagnoli D., *Per una concezione olistica dell'uomo*, in «A&P. Anthropology & Philosophy», 1997, 2, 1.

ANALYTICAL PSYCHOLOGY

Analytical Psychology is the self-designation of what was originally known as the "Zurich School" of psychoanalysis, which had its origins around the central figure of Carl Gustav Jung while he was member of the psychiatric staff at the Burghölzli Klinik in Zurich and then became the first president of the International Psychoanalytic Association (1910–1914). After meeting Freud at his home in Vienna in 1907, Jung quickly became the most important member of the early group of psychoanalysts and Freud's own "Crown Prince" designate. The term "analytical psychology" first occurs in the lecture "General aspects of psychoanalysis" delivered by Jung to the Psycho-Medical Society in London on 5 August 1913. It soon became the name of a separate and distinct school of psychoanalysis, officially after Jung's break with Freud and his resignation from the IPA in 1914.

In its practical application, which is known as Jungian psychoanalysis, Analytical Psychology is distinguished from Freudian psychoanalysis by its strong emphasis on the symbolic and by its understanding of the unconscious as potentially creative and forward-looking. In analysis, dreams are interpreted both reductively and prospectively, depending on the context and life situation of the patient. Psychological development is understood as a lifelong unfolding of innate psychological potentials and is referred to as "the → individuation process." With close colleagues in Zurich and especially within the context of The Psychological Club of Zurich, which was founded by Jung and some 40 followers in 1916, Jung worked out the main theoretical features of what was to become a general psychological theory and method for psychotherapeutic practice. Much of this early theorizing is included in Jung's massive work of 1921, *Psychological Types*, and in the first versions of what was to become the foundational text, *Two Essays on Analytical Psychology*. In both works, Jung presented a radically revized version of psychoanalytic theory, including a newly formulated theory of psychodynamic relations between conscious and unconscious that is rooted in symbols and shows an innate teleological movement towards growth of consciousness and personal meaning. In the first work, Jung also included his own definitions of psychological terms, which demonstrate not only his departure from Freudian views but also his deep intellectual roots in European and especially in German nineteenth-century philosophy and psychology. In *Two Essays,* he lays out his first version of the theory of the → archetypes of the collective unconscious and explains how they play an important role in the psychological life of the individual, especially in the → transference dynamics and unconscious contents that emerge during analytic treatment. After World War I, students began coming to Zurich from many parts of the world to study with Jung and his associates, and within a short period of time analysts began practicing in a Jungian mode in Europe and the United States. At first, training to become an analyst consisted in undergoing personal analysis with Jung himself or with one of his Zurich colleagues, attending seminars at The Psychological Club, and perhaps discussing ongoing cases with the Zurich Jungians, whereupon Jung might write a personal letter certifying that the individual was qualified to practice analysis according to his methods. Since those early days, Analytical Psychology has grown into a broad and diverse international field that currently numbers some 3,000 trained professional analysts on five continents. This body of analysts is organized globally through the International Association for Analytical Psychology (IAAP), which was founded in 1955 and since then has held triannual congresses whose proceedings have been regularly published. These collections show the astonishing level of development in the field as a whole since the inception of the IAAP. In addition, formal training institutes opened in several cities, importantly in Zurich, London, Rome, and New York, shortly after the end of World War II. These presently number more than 40 and are located throughout the world. Candidates for training come from a variety of academic disciplines, most typically from clinical psychology, psychiatry, clinical social work, and pastoral psychotherapy. In recent decades, many candidates have taken up training to become Jungian psychoanalysts as second careers, coming from many academic backgrounds and fields of endeavour other than clinical ones. This rich and diverse influx of talented people has contributed great breadth to the knowledge base of the field as a whole. For Analytical Psychology, Jung's own writings continue to form the bedrock of teaching and thinking. Most centrally these are the books and essays, which include works large and small on many clinical and cultural subjects, including mythology, religion, and (most importantly) alchemy, that have been assembled in *The Collected Works* (18 volumes). The Jung Archives, housed at the *Eidgenössische Technische Hochschule Zürich*, additionally contains many letters and documents not yet published in *The Collected Works*, in the several volumes of letters, and in the numerous publications of Jung's seminars. Jung's autobiography (written with Aniela Jaffé) titled *Memories, Dreams, Reflections* has been one of the most influential works in the Jungian canon. Recently, his monumental personal journal dating from the years 1913–1927 and called *The Red Book* has been published to great acclaim in the public domain. Among the key ideas that have characterized Analytical Psychology and Jungian psychoanalysis throughout their history are the following: a) the view that the individual's personality is characterized by an innate and lifelong striving towards growth and towards seeking the fullest possible expression of the self (individuation); b) the understanding of psychic energy (" → libido") that sees it as being organized by symbols that reflect a broad range of innate instincts and archetypal patterns as well as by personal complexes, including the Ego complex; c) the commitment to methods and techniques that work towards integrating the personality by bringing together conscious and unconscious components into an ever increasing but never completed state of wholeness. The frequency of analytic sessions varies from once to four times per week, depending on the local analytic culture and the specific training of the analyst, as well as according to the needs and means of patients. Dream interpretation plays a central role both for the analysis of transference and → countertransference as well as for use in the development of psychological integration and individuation. The field of Analytical Psychology has consistently and over its entire history displayed diversity and strong differences of opinion among its members, and the debates pertaining to clinical and theoretical matters have been frequent and vigorous, especially in the Jungian journals and at IAAP congresses. In the 1950s and 60s, a central division opened up between analysts who emphasized what Jung called reductive analysis (represented chiefly by the London members of the Society of Analytical Psychology and their followers, now often referred to as "the developmental school" in Analytical Psychology) and those who prefer to emphasize synthetic methods (the Zurich school, generally called "the classical school"). The former group tends to have affinities with neo-Freudian and → object relations ideas, while the latter have been somewhat linked with such movements as → psychosynthesis, Gestalt therapy and humanistic psychology. In the first generation after Jung, Michael Fordham of London was the chief proponent of the developmental school, while Marie-Louise von Franz of Zurich carried the banner for the classical school. While this tension still exists to some degree within Analytical Psychology, the dividing lines have softened with the passing years and more mutual understanding and cross-fertilization have occurred than was possible earlier. Today it is difficult to find pure types of either extreme in the wider field of Analytical Psychology. The diversity of perspectives and emphases among analysts and the strong debates that have taken place over the past 50 years have resulted in increased internal complexity and broader connections to many other schools of psychoanalysis and psychotherapy. In addition to numerous works with a clinical focus, members of the field of Analytical Psychology have over the last 50 years produced an impressive quantity of studies on cultural subjects of many kinds, ranging from myth, ritual and religion to the arts (literature, painting, sculpture, music) and most recently to popular culture (film, contemporary literature, television). Important in these areas have been works by Erich Neumann, Joseph Henderson and James Hillman. More recently, increasing attention has been given to a number of other disciplines that interface with Analytical Psychology, such as the cognitive sciences, the neurosciences and evolutionary psychology. After the massive shift in the world's political situation in the early 1990s, the interest in Jung's writings and in the theory and practice of Analytical Psychology and Jungian psychoanalysis has grown explosively in Eastern Europe, South America, Asia, and Africa. Journals of Analytical Psychology exist in Dutch, English, French, German, Italian, Japanese, Korean, Portuguese, Russian, Spanish and Swedish. Scientific studies testing the hypotheses of Analytical Psychology take place today in a wide variety of cultural contexts and in many universities and institutes throughout the world. *[M. Stein]*

REFERENCES. Bair D., *Jung: A biography*, 2003; Bishop P., *Analytical Psychology and German classical aesthetics: Goethe, Schiller, and Jung*, 2008–2009; Cambray J., Carter L. (eds.), *Analytical Psychology: Contemporary perspectives in Jungian analysis*, 2004; Hull R.F.C., Read H., Fordham M., Adler G. , McGuire Wm., *The collected works of C.G. Jung*, 1953–1979; Kirsch T., *The Jungians*; Jung C.G., *General aspects of psychoanalysis*, in *Collected Works*, IV, 1961; Jung C.G., *Psychological types*, in *Collected Works*, VI, 1971; Jung C.G., *Two essays in Analytical Psychology*, in *Collected Works*, VII, 1967; Samuels A., *Jung and the post-Jungians*, 1985; Shamdasani S., *Jung and the making of modern psychology*, 2003; Stein M. (ed.), *Jungian psychoanalysis*, 2010.

ANALYTIC GROUP PSYCHOTHERAPY

A form of psychotherapy of analytic orientation, carried out within a group setting made up of a therapist (or of two therapists) and of a small number of patients, directed towards the resolution of symptoms as well as towards the exploration of one's inner world, achieving a greater understanding and self-awareness.

For a long time, analytic group psychotherapy has been intended as a synonym of group psychotherapy. Even if the differences between the two therapeutic approaches seem to be greater today than in the past, it still remains a difficult task to define in a clear and univocal way what is to be intended for analytic group psychotherapy, because the boundary with group psychotherapy as well as with → group analysis is not clear-cut and delimited. In a certain sense, one may say that within the sphere of analytic group psychotherapy converge the contributions of all those scholars who have elaborated the construction of their clinical models in compliance with the psychoanalytic theory and later embraced other approaches and orientations, placing specific attention on the group as instrument and possibility of cure. In the light of such observations, it is difficult to classify the various contributions that have moved in such a direction, within a homogeneous and well-defined corpus. Even if the scholars of this branch have moved away from an initial stimulus deriving from Freudian thought, in their work with groups they have availed themselves of contributions from different theories, such as for example that of K. Lewis or from the Gestalt. The eclecticism characterizing such a branch has been well described by Tuttman who, in his "Theoretical and technical elements which characterize the American approaches to psychoanalytic group psychotherapy", has illustrated and offered a broad review of the American situation. With reference to Lewin's "theory of field", Pauletta D'Anna has produced interesting contributions – whose observations move from an analysis "of" the group to an analysis "in" the group – directed towards the identification of two different concepts of the object "group": the group as place of individual relationships and the group as specific psychological object. Analytic group psychotherapy is characterized by in-depth objectives that must not be limited to the "mere" remission of symptoms, but move towards a structural change of the personality and towards a more complex understanding of one's inner world. The concept of " symptomatic", in analytical terms, must be used and intended in a wider and more articulated sense, not limited to identifying only somatic dysfunctions (depression, insomnia, food disorders), but further stressing the psychic and interpersonal aspects connected to these. This means that the goal of an analytic group psychotherapy must be that of analyzing, first and foremost, the experiences of the patients which are making living difficult; their emotional/relational, communicative difficulties, the memory of unpleasant episodes, the anger, etc.

The duration of this kind of therapy is usually medium-term; the therapist must hold a solid, group-analytic training background, including a personal analysis, one or more observations in therapeutic groups and several supervisions. The many instruments used within the analytic group context are: the experience itself of the group → setting, as activated and coordinated by the analyst; the relational reciprocity; the relation between the inner relational world of the patients (internal group, psychic family field) and the unconscious dramatization of it within the group process; conscious and unconscious communication; the relationship mind–body. Following the development of the classical branches based on the works of Bion, Foulkes, J.L.Moreno and the French and German contributions, in Italy there has been a great production, mostly through Coirag (Confederation of Italian Organizations for the Analytic Research on Groups), thanks to the branch of research of group analysis – which is a type of analytic group work frequently used in both private and public contexts – of analytic psychodrama, of group analysis, etc. Among the many contributions that have emerged in recent years, the most relevant ones are those that have allowed a greater investigation of issues pertaining to the study of the group processes, the assessment of treatments, a greater knowledge of "self" and of psychopathology, the leading of groups and the various parameters of the setting. Today, the key issue has become that of avoiding thinking of the patient on the basis of the group, but, on the contrary, to think of the group on the basis of the patient – a simple reversal of perspective, which, however, gives back to the suffering individual the right to be cured and therefore the right to find a treatment setting suitable for him. This inevitably involves a competence of the therapist who must be able to renovate and modify (above all inside his own mind) the setting on the basis of the patient, without remaining prisoner to certain models that often become "fundamentalisms", which are probably reassuring but are certainly not very therapeutic. The aim is to express oneself not only in diagnostic terms. Common expressions, such as "a narcissistic patient", "a schizoid", "a borderline", are ways of intending clinical practice to be one that looks at an objectified patient and not at the individual, the tip of the iceberg and not the iceberg itself, the visible and not the invisible, the nosography and not the history, the pathology and not the sanity (those sane parts of the Ego belonging to all patients, even those in serious conditions), the statistics and not the single individual. Thinking in these terms reduces the patient to a single point of view, as de-contextualized, historicized and depersonalized. Even though it has been demonstrated that group psychotherapy works just as well as individual psychotherapy, there still remains a series of problematic issues regarding the difficulty of empirically assessing complex aspects such as subjective experience, the relation, analogical communicative processes, transference and countertransference dynamics. From the research work carried out by the Sicilian Laboratorio di Gruppoanalisi (Group Analysis Laboratory) there are two observations worthy of further investigation and reflection, which point out the importance that research work (if it is not strictly experimental or laboratory) can have for clinical practice: the first highlights the fact that dropouts from group psychotherapy seem to depend less on the patient's psychopathology and to a greater extent on the way in which the therapist relates with the patient (especially when he /she takes on an attitude that is either too close or too impersonal); the second shows how anorexia and bulimia, conceived for years as two sides of the same coin, seem to assume different implications within an analytic group therapy: in particular, this kind of approach seems to be more beneficial for patients suffering from anorexic disorders than for those suffering from bulimic ones. *[G.Lo Verso, I. Formica]*

REFERENCES. Foulkes S., Anthony E.J., *The psychoanalytic approach to group psychotherapy*, 1965; Pauletta D'Anna G.M.(ed.), *Modelli psicoanalitici del gruppo*, 1990; Tuttman S., *Theoretical and technical elements which characterize the American approaches to psichoanalytic group psychotherapy*, in «International Journal of Group Psychotherapy», 1986, XXXVI, 4; Vanni F. (ed.), *Saggi di psicoterapia di gruppo*, 1979.

ANAMNESIS

According to a medical-psychiatric model, anamnesis refers to the collection of information concerning the current problem, the medical history and the patient's biography in order to formulate a → diagnosis and define a therapeutic plan and prognostic hypotheses on the disease itself.

In psychological assessments, anamnesis tries to identify experiences and episodes that could be particularly meaningful and relevant to understanding the patient's problem, using different means and goals depending on the approach adopted. In some cases, anamnesis can include data-collection tools, designed to identify and select the most significant information in different areas of the patient's life (family, work, relationships, general health before the disorder, etc.). Even when using objective methods such as tests (→ psychological tests), a relationship driven by personal and subjective factors is established between the examiner and the examined subject.

The information and events reported by the subject are affected by distortions of memory and are collected in a relational context. For this reason, rather than trying, at all costs, to channel the information provided in a preordained pattern, it is important to pay attention to the global elements of the patient's situation, psychological relational aspects, nonverbal communication and to understand the disclosure of the patient situation in that "playing field" in the making, which is the clinical space. The collection of anamnestic information can also become an incentive and a means, available to the person, to reorganize their own story and possibly rewrite some basic points of it. *[R.]*

ANCHORING TECHNIQUE

In → neuro-linguistic programming, a technique that allows a person to "knowingly" reproduce particular moods that were previously determined, naturally generated and associated with a precise and unambiguous noise, smell, taste, gesture or word (sensory channels). The association process is that of an internal response to a random or controlled external stimulus. Whenever the signal is repeated, it is automatically reminiscent of the state of mind to which it was "anchored" (like listening to a song that evokes emotions). Anchors can be intentionally (artificially) created by associating a state of mind to one of the sensory channels mentioned above; they can be established with every representational system (kinaesthetic, visual, auditory), for example by tightening the fist while experiencing a feeling/emotion or by entering an imaginary space and drawing useful resources (spatial anchoring). In therapeutic neuro-linguistic programming, anchoring is an effective emotional switch, useful to overcome moments of panic, difficult situations, stimulate motivation and the achievement of objectives. Anchoring a state, a moment of unforgettable emotional involvement, is decisive in the presence of blocks and is very positive in life. *[F. Pilò]*

REFERENCES. Dilts R., Grinder J., Bandler R., Cameron Bandler L., De J. Lozier, *Neurolinguistic programming: The study of the structure of subjective experience*, 1980; Granata G., *Programming neurolinguistics*, 1999; Lankton S., *Magic practice: The basics of programming neuro-linguistics in language psychotherapy clinic*, 1980.

ANDROGYNOUS

That which contains within itself the nature of a man and a woman; the simultaneous presence of male and female behaviours and physical features, without any reference to sexual orientation or reproduction. In some texts, it is used as a synonym of hermaphrodite, which in science defines the reproductive organization of certain animal species. In Plato's *Symposium*, Aristophanes tells the myth of the androgyne, sons of the Moon, which, made arrogant by their independence and completeness, plotted for the conquest of Olympus. Zeus punished them by splitting each of them into male and female; but since the two halves were desperately looking for each other, he sent Eros to them, so that through the physical union, they could still feel like "one". Even in modern man, now far from the myths, the desire for completeness and entirety, linked to the psychological imaginary of androgyne, persists. It represents the archetype that alludes to concurrence of opposites and complete autonomy. Jung takes the concept of androgynous from alchemical philosophy and he emphasizes the spiritual sense of unification of opposites. *[A. Cannavina]*

REFERENCES. Jung C.G. (1917–1950), *Civilization in transition*, in *Collected Works*, X; Lacan J., Fink B., *Écrits*, 2006.

ANGUISH

An intense emotion of apprehension that involves a state of alarm accompanied by somatic reactions (tightness of the chest, dyspnœa, stomach contractions, alterations of the heart-rate, different types of pain). A state of great distress and fear, often accompanied by a feeling of catastrophe, is triggered when a person faces something perceived as painful or dangerous. Anguish does not refer to anything specific; it is about having a presentiment of an imminent danger, but without being able to give specific reasons and without knowing the source of it. This aspect differentiates anguish from → anxiety (although the two terms are often used interchangeably), since the latter is a normal physiological reaction, a process of adaptation when facing danger, useful in many cases to achieve a goal; while anguish is a situation of trauma determined by an excessive influx of stimuli to be managed in space and time. The philosopher S. Kierkegaard introduced anguish as the basic condition of man, which emerges whenever he stands in front of a choice. Anguish itself is not a pathological response, but it becomes pathological when it causes repetitive disproportionate behaviours or blocks compared to the situation that the person, according to their perspective, perceives as painful and/or dangerous and that immobilize him/her in a closed circle. *[R.]*

In Freudian thought, there are two models of anguish. In the first (1915–1917), anguish is the result of a frustrated or psychically non-elaborated sexual arousal, which ends up affecting the autonomic nervous system. It is therefore the result of operating defences that, preventing desires to access consciousness and motility, create an obstruction of libido which turns "chemically" into anguish. In the second model (1926), Freud suggests that anguish is the cause of operating defences: as a function of the Ego, anguish would signal the presence of a traumatic situation or danger. The fundamental economic characteristics of a traumatic situation is a sudden increase of stimuli that invade one's psyche, creating a situation of helplessness that leads to an "automatic anguish". According to Freud, birth is the prototype model of a traumatic and anxiety-inducing situation. When the Ego learns to anticipate a possible occurrence of a traumatic situation by means of thought, it can use the feeling of anguish as a signal to activate the necessary psychic countermeasures. The anguish connected to this type of purpose is called "signal-anxiety" and the situations in which it is triggered by the Ego are called "danger-situations". According to Freud, there are some universal danger-situations that can prevail in different moments of human development and that can cause psychic problems: the separation from the object, the loss of a loved object, castration, the loss of support of the Superego and the anguish of death. [*F. Gazzillo*]

REFERENCES. Brenner C., *The mind in conflict*, 1982; Freud S. (1925–1926), *An autobiographical study, Inhibitions, symptoms and anxiety, A question of lay analysis, and other works*, in *The Standard Edition*, XX, 1953–1974; Id. (1932–1936), *New introductory lectures on psycho-analysis and other works*, in *The Standard Edition*, XXII, 1953–1974.

ANIMA

In Jungian thought, the concept of anima is considered initially a synonym of psyche, meaning the totality of the psychic processes. Later on, Jung considered it mainly as an inner figure of the woman in man. He also identified four stages in this figure: purely biological, sexual (both at the aesthetic and romantic level), spiritual and *sophia*. Therefore, anima becomes for Jung the personification of the female figure in man's unconscious, his unconscious complementary part in respect to the attitude of consciousness. Anima is the part of the male psyche that man must integrate into his consciousness, to avoid being a victim of its negative side – an excessive and unregulated emotionality – or remain confined in a one-sided attitude of consciousness. Therefore, anima plays a role of connection between the unconscious, the consciousness of the → Id and the → persona, opening the latter to a real figurative thought in opposition to a conceptual thought, that is, linked to → feeling and → sensation, similar to poetic thought. The concept of anima was also the first to be taken to an archetypal dimension, starting precisely from the confrontation Jung undertook with his own unconscious after the break with Freud occurred in 1913. The break with Freud produced a powerful disorientation, to the point that, to recover from the crisis, he abandoned any reference to psychological theories and put his trust in his own fantasies and in the images generated by them. In this "confrontation with the unconscious" – as he called it – he discovered a vision of psyche as an autonomous reality, independent of consciousness; a reality expressed through the representation of figures that personify some typical themes that always appear in human history, in myths, in fairy tales, in dreams and fantasies. Later on, Jung called these themes → archetypes. Anima as an archetype – anima was the first theorized archetype – is therefore a concept that he found empirically through the images that were hidden behind the strong emotions that accompanied the visions of his "confrontation". *[F. Bellotti]*

REFERENCES. Hillman J., *Anima: An anatomy of a personified notion*, 1985; Jung C.G. (1921), *Psychological types*, in *Collected works*, VI, 1971; Id. (1912–1928), *Two essays on analytical psychology*, in *Collected Works*, VII, 1967.

ANIMIC FUNCTION

In Jungian psychology, a psychic function that expresses the deeper layers of the psyche, those related to both the personal → unconscious and the collective → unconscious. In particular, the activity of the animic function is emphasized in the oneiric expression of psychic life, that is, in the genesis of dreams. *[N. Fina]*

ANIMUS

In Jungian thought, animus is the corresponding figure of the opposite sex in the unconscious of women, who should perform a function similar to → anima in men, but not in an identical manner. In fact, Jung writes that while the figure of anima in men is singular and performs different functions, in women it would be more appropriate to talk about several male figures representing animus, but who all perform the same function: that of the spirit. This is an important distinction, as it introduces a profound difference between female and male psychology. In fact, the link function, both with the unconscious and with the world, that the figure of anima performs in men, is performed in women by consciousness. Therefore, animus essentially concerns women's attitude towards the spirit, which can, in fact, be interpreted in multiple ways. In synthesis, anima concerns a certain type of woman, while animus expresses different mental attitudes related to the different visions of the world. However, the same principles of anima apply also to the figure of animus: if animus is not integrated into feminine consciousness, the figure is projected, as on a screen, onto a real man, causing the woman to miss a bridge to her own unconscious. That is, when the Ego of a woman, unaware that everything that is unconscious is projected, identifies with the inner male figure, it becomes rigid and abstract, as it embraces attitudes that negatively affect femininity. However, it needs to be specified that the concept of animus, unlike anima, is an abstract concept, in the sense that Jung deduced it, as he was unable to have immediate knowledge of it. In the famous "definitions" that appear in the final chapter of *Psychological Types* (1921), the entry "animus" is not provided. Similarly, in the index of works, the bibliography related to the term anima is extremely limited. *[F. Bellotti]*

REFERENCES. Hillman J., *Suicide and the soul*, 1964; Jung C.G. (1925), *Development of personality*, in *Collected Works*, XVII, 1954; Id. (1936), *Archetypes and the collective unconscious*, in *Collected Works*, IX (part I), 1969.

ANTAGONISTIC RESPONSE

Within the behaviourist paradigm, a term introduced by Wolpe to describe the class of → responses that are the objective of the clinician in the procedure of → systemic desensitization. This technique is based on the principle of → counter-conditioning and aims at inducing the emergence of stimulus-conditions that evoke responses aimed at weakening such stimulus–response associations (→ stimulus–response relationships). The typical example is that of → relaxation (antagonistic response) in the presence of anxiety-provoking stimuli. If a stimulus-situation provokes anxiety, the therapist, according to Wolpe, should aim at inducing the emergence in its presence of relaxation-associated responses. This would take place by associating, in the individual's imagination (→ imaginal exposure) and/or in vivo (→ in-vivo exposure), the antagonistic response to the anxiety-provoking stimulus progressively according to a hierarchical structure, from the least anxiety-provoking to the most anxiety-provoking, until they are all counter-conditioned. *[G. Presti]*

REFERENCES. Kazdin A.E., Wilcoxon L.A., *Systematic desensitization and nonspecific treatment effects: A methodological evaluation*, in «Psychological Bulletin», 1976, 83, 5; Wolpe J., *The systematic desensitization treatment of neuroses*, in «Journal of Nervous and Mental Disease», 1961, 132.

ANTHROPOMORPHISM

The anthropomorphic model, systematized in the work of R. Harre and P.F. Secord, uses the term → personality to indicate a certain class of psychological processes (mental states, self-perception constructs, interactive schemes) produced by people that are in relation to each other and within interpersonal situations, social episodes, symbolic, regulatory and socio-cultural contexts. These processes, characterized by various degrees of self-awareness, are generated by actors involved in the construction of the reality that concerns them, while they suffer its effects as predefined by them or by others. Anthropomorphism is opposed to the mecanomorphic view previously adopted by clinical psychology. The assumptions of the mecanomorphic model can be found in theories, methods and techniques that consider personality as an objective entity, an identifiable psychic organism with its constituent elements (traits, symptoms, factors), with dynamics (intrapsychic instances, defence mechanisms, neurotic compensations), with certain biological requirements (temperament, genetic predispositions) or constraints (learned repertoires of behaviour, models of conduct, etc.). The mecanomorphic model assumes traits, dispositions, internal dynamics and external conditions that are imposed on the individual and determine their ways of thinking, perceiving and acting. Instead, the anthropomorphic model assumes that people use (through skills, rules and accessible meanings) those parts of themselves that can best support the directed action, the conscious or tacit action that pursues goals of adaptation or change in interactive situations.

In psychotherapy, the more traditional paradigms refer to one or the other perspective, while the more recent paradigms assert a position that goes beyond this antinomy and moves to constructivist perspectives (→ constructivism). *[R.]*

ANTICIPATION → DEFENCE MECHANISMS

ANTINOMY

In Jung's analytical psychology, the theory of neurosis has its foundation in the antinomian concept of psyche, which identifies the simultaneous existence of two opposing forces within the psyche.

Antinomies belong to human nature and can be endless: between the Self and the Other, subject and object, nature and culture, life and death, stasis and movement, collective and individual, spirit and body, conscious and unconscious. In Jungian thought, the antinomian concept is also at the base of the theory of → symbols.

The function of the symbol, which opens to further meanings comparing to the conflicting opposites, is based on the existence of contradictions, since there can be a symbol only if there is a need to recompose the → opposites. When this recomposition does not happen spontaneously, the antinomy can turn into a violent conflict within themselves and in a block of one's will, which leads to neurosis. The aim of therapy is to be able to grasp the signs that the symbol provides to facilitate the transition from laceration to recomposition that can create a new psychological situation. *[A. Benvenuti]*

REFERENCES. Aversa L., *Il problema dell'antinomia*, in Id. (ed.), *Fondamenti di icologia analitica*, 1995; Jung C.G. (1921), *Psychological types*, in *Collected Works*, VI, 1971.

ANTI-PSYCHIATRY

The term "*Antipsychiatrie*", coined in 1908 by the German psychiatrist Bernhard Beyer, came into being in response to two novel social phenomena: the growth of insane asylums during the nineteenth century and the mounting popular fear of "false commitment," that is, the imprisonment of sane persons in insane asylums. Beyer, like most psychiatrists, viewed criticism of psychiatry, regardless of its merits, as *lèse majesté*. He created the term "antipsychiatry" as a label with which to stigmatize and dismiss such criticism. This early use of the term "anti-psychiatry" gained no currency outside the German language and its use faded away during World War I.

In the late 1960s, a group of psychiatrists, led by David Cooper (1931–1986) and Ronald D. Laing (1927–1989), began to criticize conventional psychiatry, especially somatic treatments, and reinvented the term "anti-psychiatry" to distinguish its members from establishment psychiatrists and to identify themselves as morally superior and therapeutically more effective than their competitors. However, instead of advocating the abolition of the psychiatrist's legal power over the patient, epitomized by the paradigmatic psychiatric practices of involuntary mental hospitalization and the insanity defense, the anti-psychiatrists sought to replace traditional psychiatric power with their own power masquerading as anti-power. Recreating Beyer's nasty misnomer, the London anti-psychiatrists managed to attract attention to themselves and deflect attention from what they did. Imitating psychiatrists, the anti-psychiatrists constructed anti-theories of schizophrenia, which they called "existential-phenomenological accounts of madness"; established anti-hospitals, which they called "households" and defined as "ideal psychiatric communities"; and provided psychiatric treatments, which they called "trips," that often entailed the use of mind-altering (psychotropic) drugs, especially LSD . In short, the antipsychiatrists were a new breed of institutional psychiatrists, competing with conventional institutional psychiatrists. The upshot of all this sound and fury was that "anti-psychiatry" and "anti-psychiatrist" quickly became terms of abuse. Ironically, the anti-psychiatry movement is often said to be based on my contention that the phenomena psychiatrists call mental illnesses are behaviours or metaphorical illness, that is, not genuine medical problems. "A key understanding of 'anti-psychiatry'," explains Digby Tantam, Professor of Psychotherapy at the University of Sheffield, "is that mental illness is a myth" (Szasz, 1961). As I have shown, nothing could be further from the truth: "key understanding . . . that mental illness is a myth" forms no part of the anti-psychiatry movement. The psychiatrist qua health-care professional is a fraud, and so too is the anti-psychiatrist. In *Psychiatry* I show that psychiatry – an imitation of medicine – is a form of quackery. In *Antipsychiatry* I show that anti-psychiatry – a form of alternative psychiatry – is quackery squared. Once the term "anti-psychiatry" entered the language of psychiatry and everyday English, lexicographers and mental health experts offered a variety of definitions of it. According to the *Oxford Dictionary of Psychology* (2001): "Antipsychiatry [is] a radical critique of traditional (especially medical) approaches to mental disorders, influenced by existentialism and sociology, popularized by the Scottish psychiatrist Ronald D(avid) Laing and others during the 1960s and 1970s." The *Wikipedia* entry for "anti-psychiatry" reads, in part, as follows:

> Anti-psychiatry refers to a collection of alternative movements that challenge the fundamental theories and practices of (mainstream) psychiatry. . . . Coming to the fore in the 1960s, "anti-psychiatry" (a term first used by David Cooper in 1967) defined a movement that vocally challenged the fundamental claims and practices of mainstream psychiatry. Psychiatrists R.D. Laing, Theodore Lidz, Silvano Arieti and others argued that schizophrenia could be understood as an injury to the inner self inflicted by psychologically invasive "schizophrenogenic" parents, or as a healthy attempt to cope with a sick society. Psychiatrist Thomas Szasz argues that "mental illness" is an inherently incoherent combination of a medical and a psychological concept, but popular because it legitimizes the use of psychiatric force to control and limit deviance from societal norms. Adherents of this view referred to "the myth of mental illness" after Szasz's controversial book of that name.

Other authorities offer still different definitions, illustrating the uselessness of the category and the term. The *Oxford Dictionary of Sociology* identifies "anti-psychiatry" as follows:

> A term coined in the 1960s for writers who are highly critical of the ideas and practice of psychiatry. Precisely who is included within this group (which is always theoretically and politically heterogeneous) tends to vary. Frequently mentioned are the radical libertarian Thomas Szasz, the more left-wing, existentialist-inclined R.D. Laing and his colleague David Cooper, the Italian mental health reformer Franco Basaglia (all psychiatrists), and two sociologists – the symbolic interactionist Erving Goffman and labelling theorist Thomas Scheff. Sometimes Michel Foucault is also cited in this context. According to Australian journalist Alex Burns, anti-psychiatry "is generally associated with phenomenological philosophers like Thomas Szasz, Gregory Bateson and R. D. Laing . . . During the upheaval unleashed by May 1968, Anti-Psychiatry spread to Milan, Brussels, Paris and other major European cities. . . . As a political force, Anti-Psychiatry waned during the 1970s due to the demise of counter-culture (Marxist and Anarchist) politics, psychiatric care industry reform, and the popularity of Human Potential Movement therapies.

The authors of the encyclopaedic *Oxford Textbook of Philosophy and Psychiatry* correctly conclude: "The absorption of antipsychiatric themes into mental health practice has led some, especially in psychiatry, to believe that antipsychiatry is dead. That it is not, that antipsychiatry is alive and well, is evident." Indeed, the term "anti-psychiatry" is very much alive – as a powerful rhetorical weapon in the hands of psychiatrists and their supporters: it stigmatizes and invalidates critics of psychiatry, regardless of the content of the criticism. *[T. Szasz]*

REFERENCES. Beyer B., *Die Bestrebungen zur Reform des Irrenwesen*, 1912; Szasz T., *The myth of mental illness: Foundations of a theory of personal conduct*, 1961; Szasz, T., *Antipsychiatry: The paradigm of the plundered mind*, in «New Review», 1976, 3; Id., *Schizophrenia: The sacred symbol of psychiatry*, 1976; Id., *Knowing what ain't so: R.D. Lang and Thomas Szasz*, in «Psychoanalytic Review», 2004, 91; Id., *Debunking antipsychiatry: Laing, law and Largactil*, in «Current Psychology», 2008, 27; Id., *Psychiatry: The science of lies*, 2008; Id., *Antipsychiatry: Quackery squared*, 2009.

ANXIETY

A state of arousal of the body triggered by a situation regarded as being dangerous. Therefore, per se, it is neither a limit nor a disorder but both an important resource and a physiological condition which often protect us from harms and enables us to remain alert and improve performance. Anxiety can be broken into four main components: a *cognitive* component, which is characterized by one's ability or inability to understand the reasons behind one's own condition; a *somatic* component, which is characterized by an emergency reaction of the whole body and whose symptoms may include palpitations, increased sweating, feelings of vertigo, digestive disorders, breathing difficulties and panting, sudden hot flushes, etc.; an *emotional* component, which may result in peevishness, mood swings, feelings of dread or abject terror; a *behavioural* component, which is characterized by "flight or fight" responses, i.e. behaviour aimed at re-establishing one's psychological → homeostasis). A disproportionate or unjustified activation of the anxiety system, however, leads to anxiety disorders, which can greatly complicate life and hinder a person's ability to cope with even the most ordinary situations. According to Sullivan – the founder and main theorist of Interpersonal psychiatry – anxiety is not a unitary affective state but a set of emotions, with terror and panic being identified as its most severe forms. Euphoria, on the contrary, is envisioned as a state of wellbeing and ease in which anxiety is entirely absent. Anxiety occurs as the infant's apprehensive reaction to the fears and expectations of disapproval of his caregivers; it is transmitted within the affective relationship and becomes a pivotal feature in interpersonal relational processes. In order to avoid anxiety and preserve a sense of wellbeing and security, the infant's psychological functioning changes and generates the self-system. Through the self-system, he learns to use his anxiety as a compass in a way that allows the self-system to "choose" from many different stimuli, supposedly offering protection from anxiety, and, therefore, to guide the development of both the personality and the relational processes. The need for satisfaction is accompanied by the need for security, i.e. the need to bar from awareness every possible challenge to the operations of one's inner security. Although they might be experienced subjectively in the same way, fear and anxiety are different phenomena: the former represents one's response to an external danger, while the latter – once "acquired" – signals an inner peril. A successful treatment depends on the analyst's ability to monitor and manage both the patient's and his/her own anxiety– in order to enable new and previously precluded forms of relatedness. *[A. Cresti, S. Brizzi]*

REFERENCES. Crastnopol, M., *Anxiety*, edited by M.Lionells *et al.*, *Handbook of Interpersonal psychoanalysis*, 1995; Mitchell, S.A., Black, M.J., *Freud and beyond: A history of modern psychoanalytic thought*,1955; H.S., *The meaning of anxiety in psychiatry and in life*, in «Psychiatry», 1948, XI, 1–3; Sullivan, H.S., *The theory of anxiety and the nature in psychotherapy*, in «Psychiatry», 1949, XII, 3–12.

ANXIETY IMMUNIZATION

Psychological → anxiety immunization may take place on at least two levels. The first is purely behavioural and the second is cognitive. In the context of behavioural theories, the theory of "classical conditioning", which follows the theoretical scheme of stimulus–response reflex arc (→ stimulus–response relationship), suggests that anxiety is generated by associating a → neutral stimulus to an anxiety-inducing event. Therefore, behavioural immunization could take place by replacing the anxiety-inducing event with a pleasant stimulus. The most effective behavioural techniques to treat anxiety are: → relaxation, exposure (→ graduated exposure) and → systematic desensitization.

Relaxation techniques aim to replace the alert response with its opposite, relaxation. These include progressive muscle relaxation, → autogenic training, hypnosis (→ clinical hypnosis) and → meditation. All these techniques involve, on closer inspection, a more or less overt cognitive component. Subjects learn self-control and self-induction of perceptions (for example, the heaviness of the arm) through exercises of muscle tone to increase the degree of mastery of their emotional states. In this way, a person assumes a position of self-observation and psychological self-manipulation as opposed to the passive attitude towards emotions typical of anxious patients. Whilst relaxation focuses on the response, exposure techniques work on the stimulus. The idea is simple and it obeys the behavioural principle of → extinction: the subject is exposed to the stimuli related to the anxiety response and the extinction of the anxious response is induced. Also in this case, cognitive components combine with purely behavioural mechanisms such as the mechanical reduction of physiological reaction due to habituation. In fact, a prolonged exposure can facilitate the development of a critical attitude towards the pathological belief (→ irrational beliefs) that anxiety is unbearable and the search for responses different from avoidance. This behavioural factor precludes, by definition, the cognitive processing of anxiety and prevents the subject fully experiencing the anxiety-provoking situation and having a less catastrophic picture of it. Systematic desensitization combines learning alternative responses to anxiety with desensitization techniques and, above all, patients are trained to use scales to quantify their levels of anxiety in relation to stimuli. Also in the area of behavioural theory called "operant conditioning", some techniques developed by Skinner can be used for anxiety immunization. They may be used to obtain a decrease in anxious activation (→ activating event) and avoidance responses and an increase in alternative responses to avoidance. → Positive reinforcement can be useful to increase self-control responses; extinction can be useful against avoidance; the → shaping of an assertive attitude can be useful against social phobia; thought-stopping techniques are recommended against the overthinking states typical of anxiety. Cognitive therapies, amongst which the most common are the models of Ellis (→ rational emotive behavioural therapy) and Beck (→ cognitive-behavioural therapy), move the attention to the investigation, discussion and elaboration of explicit and conscious thoughts (→ disputing), which, according to cognitive theory, always underlie emotional states of distress. The basic principles of cognitive interventions are: encouraging the patient to reflect on their emotional states, considering emotions as questionable assumptions about reality and not as hard facts (for example, anxiety represents the hypothesis, not the certainty of an existing danger); ascertain the rationale and empirical foundations of emotional states (Why do I have anxiety? What do I fear exactly? How much is this anxiety justified?); and reconsidering one's own strategies of management of supposed dangers. Patients have only two weapons to manage feared risks: anxious avoidance and obsessive control. The therapist encourages the patient to develop more complex and less rigid strategies (→ therapeutic strategy), also by using behavioural techniques, such as assertive training, an intervention designed to help people to strengthen themselves, to self-define and structure themselves as individuals. In cognitive therapy, behavioural techniques are also used, but they primarily aim at reproducing the pathogenic behaviours that create suffering during and between sessions, in order to facilitate the identification of thoughts. The effectiveness of these techniques has long been documented. For example, in panic disorders, a prolonged in-vivo → exposure has a positive effect on emotional distress, but if a cognitive treatment is added, the catastrophic thoughts that accompany panic can also decrease. Even in the case of social phobia, some behavioural interventions, such as exposure in vivo and social-skills training are effective, as well as proper cognitive psychotherapy. In the case of generalized anxiety disorder, pure behavioural interventions, where subjects are trained to relax, are effective, but their effectiveness is increased when a cognitive treatment is added to them. *[S. Sassaroli]*

REFERENCES. Barlow D.H., *Anxiety and its disorders: The nature and treatment of anxiety and panic*, 1988; Beck A.T., *Thinking and depression II: Theory and therapy*, in «Archives of General Psychiatry», 1964, 10; Bernstein D.A., Borkovec T.D., *Progressive relaxation training: A manual for the helping professions*, 1973; Bouman T.K., Emmelkamp P.M.G., *Panic disorder and agoraphobia*, in V.B. Van Hasselt, M. Hersen (eds.), Sourcebook of psychological treatment manuals for adult disorders, 1996; Ellis A., *Reason and emotion in psychotherapy*, 1962; Emmelkamp P.M.G., *Self-observation versus flooding in the treatment of agoraphobia*, in «Behaviour Research and Therapy», 1974, 12; Galeazzi A., Franceschina E., *Il modus operandi della terapia cognitivo-comportamentale*, in A. Galeazzi P., Meazzini (eds.), *Mente e comportamento. Trattato italiano di psicoterapia cognitivo-comportamentale*, 2004; Marks I.M., *Fear, phobias, and rituals*, 1987; Mersh P.P.A., *The treatment of social phobia: The differential effectiveness of exposure in vivo and an integration of exposure in vivo, rational emotive therapy and social skills training*, in «Behaviour Research and Therapy», 1995, 33; Overholser J.C., Nasser E.H., *Cognitive-behavioural treatment of generalized anxiety disorder*, in «Journal of Contemporary Psychotherapy», 2000, 30; Skinner B.F., *Two types of conditioned reflex and a pseudo type*, in «Journal of General Psychology», 1935, 12; Smith J.C., *The factor structure and correlates of negative relaxation attitudes*, in Id. (ed.), *Advances in ABC relaxation: Application and inventories*, 2001; Wolpe J., *The practice of behavioural therapy*, 1969.

APPROACH

In a broad sense, it is a peculiar way of knowing and contacting what is other from themselves or the context. It is possible to talk about approaching other people, the environment, a problem or a situation in both a practical and a theoretical sense. In science, an approach is a specific perspective-method adopted to analyze and address a phenomenon (for example, by a discipline or by a particular school). In terms of method, we can speak about a quantitative or a qualitative approach when analyzing a phenomenon, about a behaviourist or a cognitive approach when considering a theoretical perspective, and in psychotherapy about a psychodynamic, a systemic relational or a brief strategic approach. The approach, as a perspective of analysis and contact, focuses on some descriptive aspects of the phenomenon and of the data that represent its evidence. Therefore, an approach is selective because it takes a specific observational perspective and limits the relevance of the data to the same perspective adopted.

Scientific approaches generate observational data and produce fact-finding effects that, in turn, lead to validating their heuristic value. In this view, each specific therapeutic approach leads the therapist to intervene on the patient's problems according to the epistemological premises (→ epistemology) of the theoretical perspective adopted. However, if this ensures an initial cognitive advantage (a theory is available), a dysfunctional effect can be to overlook what is not included in the theory or, taken to the extreme, to reject the conclusions that may pose a threat to the pragmatic and scientific validity of the theory itself. *[S. Smiraglia]*

ARCHAEOPSYCHE

In → transactional analysis, a complex system organizing the first forms of secure and insecure relational attachment to the mother. It is the engine of corporeal, emotional and cognitive experiences that are manifested regressively in adult age and characterized by creative thinking, fears and expectations organized on the basis of pre-logical thinking. From a phenomenological viewpoint, it is manifested through the Child Ego state. *[F. Guglielmotti, R. Leone Guglielmotti]*

REFERENCES. Berne E., *Ego states in psychotherapy*, in «American Journal of Psychotherapy», 1957, XI; Berne E., *Transactional Analysis in psychotherapy*, 1961; Id., *Intuitions and ego states*, 1977; Multari M., *Lo Stato dell'Io Bambino: un'analisi della letteratura dell'Analisi Transazionale*, in «Polarità », 1988, II, 1.

ARCHETYPE

In Jungian psychology, archetypes are the "centres" of the psychic dynamics that take place through an antinomian dialectic between consciousness and the collective unconscious. Archetypes were initially considered as primordial images and then as structuring forms of the human psyche. They would be able (with the same fascination as the experience of the sacred) to impose themselves on the Ego and to place it in a condition of passivity. Their many expressions are collectively traceable in myths, religious phenomena or folklore, and, subjectively, in certain dreams extraneous to individuals' conscious experiences and their personal unconscious. Archetypes can be perceived and delimited, but never fully described, as they are, by definition, dark parts of the psyche related to the *bios* and therefore not exhaustively attainable from consciousness. This view pertains to the naturalistic hypothesis of an objective, absolute and unconscious psyche, in opposition to the subjective and therefore limited nature of the Ego. Therefore, therapy would tend to amplify what emerges from the collective unconscious, in the belief that a "healing" correction of the one-sidedness of the conscious could arise from it. The individual nature of the egoic consciousness is particularly highlighted, as this is anchored on directional thought, logical language and on the distinction between subject and object. However, the archetypal theory asks the Ego to confront itself with an unclearly defined objectivity of the unconscious and of its archetypes who are seen as an objective dimension, opposed to consciousness and independent from it, and capable of limiting human interpretative possibilities. In short, it is true that Jung seems to favour a hermeneutic orientation and tries to emphasize the subjectivity of the interpreters of the psychic life; however, it is equally true that the archetypal theory outlines an "objective psychology", valid in every age and everywhere, in contrast to the relativistic option of existence of many psychologies. *[E. V. Trapanese, S. Fossi]*

AREA OF PREJUDICE

In transactional analysis, the area of prejudice – or illusion – is a pathological anomaly of the exteropsychic structure which contaminates (→ contamination) the functioning of the neopsyche. Contamination by the exteropsyche occurs when a person takes the introjected information, prejudices and slogans coming from the real parent as true. Contamination by the archeopsyche occurs when archaic aspects, not identified correctly, are experienced as the reality of the here-and-now. The result is phobias, superstitions and delusions. *[F. Guglielmotti, R. Leone Guglielmotti]*

REFERENCES. Berne E., *Transactional Analysis in psychotherapy*, 1961; Id., *Intuitions and ego states*, 1977; Stewart I., Joines V., T.*A. today: A new introduction to transactional analysis*, 1987.

ARGUMENTATIVE RHETORIC

Art of persuasion through the use of language. In psychotherapy it is used with the aim of producing a beneficial change in the situation of suffering of the patient. The psychological traditions that embrace the cybernetic-conceptual presupposition recognize in argumentative rhetoric a generative power of an alternative psychological reality. In this perspective, the therapist, therefore, can find in the *logos* the royal road towards → change, in that it indeed plays a fundamental role in order for change to take place. The efficient use of → language is configured, therefore, as an instrument that builds with the interlocuter the cognitive and emotional perspectives on which to trigger new experiences, which will help the patient to move from a pathological equilibrium to a functional one. Nardone observed that a rhetoric of the "explicative" type is used by the models of psychotherapy that are close to the classical cognitive tradition, that refer to a process of persuasion based on logical-rational categories, and that change is tied to the resolution of internal contradictions and to the errors in logical attributions. On the contrary, therapeutic models that refer to a process of persuasion that is based on the hypnotic or strategic traditions utilize, with the aim of achieving change, rhetoric strategies based on non-ordinary → logic; and, on the use of metaphoric and suggestive language that follows this kind of logic, change, in this case, is not the result of a logical-rational conviction, but of a → reframing of meaning that has a strong suggestive and emotional charge. *[R.]*

REFERENCES. Nardone G., Watzlawick P., *Brief strategic therapy*, 2005.

"AS IF" TECHNIQUE

A therapeutic prescription used in strategic approaches, consisting in asking the patient to behave, in small everyday things, "as if" the perception of their reality was different from the one they usually experience. The technique is based on the → logic of belief and it has the purpose of guiding the person to change, first, their behaviour and, as a result, their beliefs and their own perception of reality. The idea that different actions may lead to the construction of different perceptual-emotional realities has been theorized by many authors. In philosophy, the famous Pascal's wager can be recalled, where he suggested that non-believers who wished to find faith act "as if" they already believed, that is, putting in place all those typical believers' rituals until faith arrived. In psychology, Piaget has shown, on the basis of accurate observations, that children literally construct their own reality through exploratory actions rather than forming an image of the world through their perceptions and then acting accordingly. But it was for the German philosopher Vaihinger to give a clear and articulated formulation of this theory (1911) through countless examples of how humans operate always using unproven and non-provable assumptions (the "as if"), which, nevertheless, lead to concrete results. Born within strategic approaches, the first formulation of the "as if" technique in psychotherapy is due to P. Watzlawick. The technique consists in guiding the person to introduce a minimal change into what he/she does during the day to trigger a gradual snowball effect. By asking the person to change, once a day, the attitude that leads them to a dysfunctional construction of reality in a seemingly unimportant situation, the therapist generates a concrete → corrective emotional experience. This can easily be raised by increasing the patient's "as if" actions and attitudes, until a new functional reality, which will replace the previous one, has been constructed. By triggering a subtle process of strategic deception, the "as if" technique creates an invented reality. This allows the person to change their perception of reality, by exploiting the well-known phenomenon of → self-fulfilling prophecy for therapeutic purposes. *[R. Milanese, T. Garcia-Rivera]*

REFERENCES. Nardone G., Balbi E., *The logic of therapeutic change*, 2015; Piaget J., *The construction of reality in the child*, 1937; Vaihinger H., *The philosophy of "as if"*, 1924.

ASSERTIVENESS TRAINING

Articulated programme of cognitive-behavioural psychotherapy aimed at improving social skills and communication skills, with the aim of achieving an optimal equilibrium between one's own needs and the needs of others. Assertiveness training has applications in the clinical field as well as in the area of education and can be carried out individually or in a group. Through successive sessions the trainer deals with various components of verbal communication, nonverbal communication and paraverbal communication with the objective of acquiring behavioural models that are active and efficient in the different areas of relational situations. The activity of learning is supported by cognitive-behavioural techniques (learning through approximations otherwise known as → shaping, learning through imitation or → modelling, → cognitive reframing, etc.), video recording and practical exercises, (→ role-playing, group games, shame-attack exercises and risk-taking, etc). *[P. Orifiammi]*

REFERENCES. Anchisi R., Gambotto Dessy M., 1992, *Non solo comunicare. Teoria e pratica del comportamento assertivo*, 1992; Bauer B., Bagnato G., Ventura M., *Puoi anche dire "no!". L'assertività al femminile*, 2002.

ASSESSMENT

Historically, occupational psychology is one of the first fields in which assessment tools have been developed. These are used to make an evaluation of individual potential capabilities that can be oriented to the internal staff of business organizations or to the external staff in the case of selections. The purpose is to guarantee an acceptable congruence between people's individual characteristics and the demands of the assigned jobs. In clinical psychology, the term assessment refers in particular to psychodiagnostics, a discipline that is concerned with diagnosis (→ psychological diagnosis, → psychiatric diagnosis), through the use of inventories, questionnaires and personality scales, psychometric techniques, → psychological tests and → projective tests, clinical interviews, neuropsychological tests and observational assessments. Although the techniques used can differ, the assessment practice is mainly made up of two phases: the measurement and the hypothesis. In psychotherapy, assessment, which definition has been developed in the behaviourist field, adopts different evaluation tools according to the paradigm of reference. *[R.]*

ASTONISHMENT

In narrative therapy, the feeling, accompanied by a sense of bewilderment, that enables the disclosure of multiple points of view and perspectives; the therapist searches within himself for it and induces it in patients by means of irreverence, a state of mind which does not acknowledge given rules, or through rhetorically structured interventions (→ persuasion) that favour the development of alternative stories. *[G. Manfrida, E. Giachi]*

REFERENCES. Cecchin G., Lane G., Wendel A.R., *Irreverence: A strategy for therapists' survival*, 1992; Manfrida, G.M. (2011), *Plausible, convincing and appealing: Characteristics and development of therapeutic stories in a shared reality approach*, in «Journal of Systemic Therapies», 2011, 30; Sclavi M., *Arte di ascoltare e mondi possibili. Come si esce dalle cornici di cui siamo parte*, 2003.

ATTACHMENT PROCESSES

Relational processes involving the application of emotive-behavioural patterns of a genetic origin aiming at keeping children in close proximity to a protective figure in order to safeguard them. Attachment processes were introduced by Bowlby at the end of the 1950s and formed the basis for → attachment theory, which he developed and rendered empirical with the help of M. Ainsworth. Attachment processes are observable in the young of most mammals and, in some of them, remain for the entire lifetime. M. Ainsworth identified a standardized method of evaluation for patterns of attachment (→ attachment theory) in early infancy called the → strange situation. In its initial formulation, the patterns of attachment identified were: secure (B), insecure-avoidant (A) and insecure-ambivalent or insecure-resistant (C) *[D. Liccione]*.

REFERENCES. Ainsworth M.D.S., Blehar M.C., Waters E., Wall S., *Patterns of attachment: A psychological study of the strange situation*, 1978; Bowlby J., *Maternal care and mental health of the child*, 1951; Id., *Attachment and loss. Vol. 1 Attachment*, 1969; Id., *Attachment and loss. Vol. 2 Separation from the Mother*, 1973; Id., *Attachment and loss. Vol. 3*; Id., *The loss of the mother*, 1972; Id., *The making and breaking of affectional bonds*, 1979; Id., *A secure base: Clinical application of attachment theory*, 1988.

ATTACHMENT THEORY

According to Bowlby, attachment is a primary motivational system by which an individual establishes a sense of internal security. It constitutes itself over time as an organization that includes feelings, memories, desires, expectations and intentions that have particular relevance to the establishment and endurance of deep relationships. It is based on representational structures, → internal working models, which are built on the experience lived in early relationships. The attachment bond develops through predispositions to social interaction and to creating stable and lasting relationships that are present since birth. These predispositions are inscribed in the genetic code of individuals and they organize themselves with growth into complex behavioural systems that are expressions of a child's needs, such as the primary need for warmth, closeness and physical contact.

Like other behavioural systems, the attachment system is organized to ensure survival and to fulfil a particular biological function that Bowlby identifies as "protection from predators". The external goal of the attachment system is therefore to achieve and maintain a certain level of physical proximity with the caregiver (the one who takes care of the child) whenever conditions of vulnerability occur, while its internal goal is to motivate the child to achieve a sense of inner security.

In attachment relationships, children learn specific styles to regulate their emotional tension by referring to the emotional availability and the regulatory abilities of their attachment figures. For this reason, it was possible to identify and describe different patterns of attachment through the procedure of the → strange situation based on the quality of care received. The "secure attachment" style (B) is typical of those children who protest during separations from the attachment figure; they actively seek proximity and, equally easily, they are comforted by the same figure. The parent is in this case a → secure base from which the child can move away temporarily to explore. The child has a working model of the mother as an available figure and a working model of himself as worthy of care and effective in getting emotional support, in addition to having a functional affect regulation strategy. In contrast, the "insecure-avoidant" (A) attachment style is typical of those children who easily explore in the absence of the attachment figure, who separate easily without complaining and do not seek proximity on their return. Avoidance seems in these cases to work both as a mechanism to interrupt attachment behaviours – that is, functional in a relationship with a rejecting figure – and as a mechanism to exclude the pain linked to rejection. This allows the child to regulate harmful emotional states and their disorganizing influence. Instead, children with an "insecure-ambivalent" (C) attachment style, are very distressed by separations; they only explore a little because of the prevailing concern that they show towards the attachment figure and they exhibit an extreme passivity and inconsolability or anger and ambivalence.

In this case, children develop a working model of the negative self, characterized by strong confusion and lack of differentiation, towards which they can react passively or aggressively. Finally, some children's behaviour indicates the presence of a "disorganized/disoriented" (D) style, frequently related to issues of unresolved grief or trauma in their parents or to experiences of mistreatment and abuse. The disorganization of attachment is supposed to involve multiple contradictory and mutually dissociated representations of the self and the other, which will form the basis for a possible future psychopathological display. *[A.M. Speranza]*

REFERENCES. Ainsworth M.D.S., Blehar M.C., Waters E., Wall S., *Patterns of attachment: A psychological study of the strange situation*, 1978; *Attachment and loss, vol.1. Attachment*, 1969; Id., *Attachment and loss, vol.2. Separation – anxiety and anger*, 1969.

ATTEMPTED SOLUTIONS

An expression used to indicate the attempts made by clients and others (including partners, friends, former therapists, medical staff) to (unsuccessfully) solve the presented problems.

The → brief therapy MRI's model underlines the importance of investigating these attempts as their identification offers two kinds of useful information to the therapist. First, it tells the therapist "what not to do". All the ways that have been unsuccessful in solving the problem must not be prolonged or repeated in another similar variation. Second, in brief therapy MRI's model, the attempted solutions are considered as some of the main conditions underlying the persistence of a problem. One of the goals of the brief therapy MRI's model is the interception of these unsuccessful attempts. If clients are prevented from doing what has helped them to keep the problem alive, the problem will disappear. In many cases the attempted solutions follow a "main theme" (a common message). The identification of this theme can help to design the so-called "180 degree" manoeuvre also known as paradoxical intervention (→ symptom prescription). *[S. Geyerhofer]*

▷ Attempted solutions are a key construct also in the → brief strategic therapy Nardone's model; if the solutions that have been attempted do not have a good outcome, they end up complicating the situation and making it worse. The entire strategic tradition has evidenced how no logical connection exists between how a problem has developed and how it can be resolved. What is emerging instead in an increasingly clear manner is an understanding of the way in which a problem persists (→ persistence) and what people do, without success, in order to resolve it; in Watzlawick's words: "the attempted solutions *become* the problem". The construct of the attempted solution was introduced within the → Brief Therapy Project and presented for the first time in 1974 in *Change*. In this work, which signaled the birth of the first model of Strategic Therapy (→ brief therapy MRI's model), the construct of "difficulty" was distinguished from that of "problem". "Difficulty" is defined as an undesirable state of affairs that can be resolved with any actions dictated by → common sense, or else an undesirable situation for which no known solution exists and that, at least for the present, needs to be accepted. The "problem" represents, on the other hand, a specific situation that requires a solution and that can be considered as being the outcome of an erroneous treatment of the difficulty. There are three situations that have the power to transform a difficulty into a "problem": those in which one intervenes when one should not; not intervening when one should; and intervening in an erroneous way. In all three cases, generally, the tendency is that of repeating the same attempted solution notwithstanding its lack of success and the persistence of the difficulty. When a system is in this situation, it continues to pass through all the possible internal changes without, however, being able to induce an effective change in the system itself – something that would lead to the resolution of the problem. The interruption of this "pathological" equilibrium is obtained only by intervening on the dysfunctional solutions adopted by the patient (→ first- and second-order change). Consequently, the aim of the strategic intervention is that of interrupting the vicious circle that has been created between the attempted solution and the persistence of the problem through the use of specific therapeutic indications (→ prescription) that are able to subvert the pathological equilibrium of the system. The construct of the attempted solution represents, from this point of view, not only the principal vehicle for understanding the functioning of a problem, but also a privileged means of access to its resolution. In the work of Nardone and his group, the construct of the attempted solution appeared increasingly fecund as a "reducer of complexity" for therapeutic intervention and for the understanding of the functioning of the principal psychological disorders. By means of the different projects of → research intervention carried out at the Centro di Terapia Strategica in Arezzo, in particular by using this construct, it has been possible to create not only → treatment protocols that are particularly effective and efficient, but also a categorization of an operative nature of the different psychological disorders on the bases of a redundant class of attempted solutions (→ operative diagnosis). In the most evolved model of Strategic Therapy, therefore, the attempted solutions are configured not only as the principal means of access to the resolution of a problem, but also as a cognitive construct in that, once identified and blocked, it allows the therapist to understand how the problem functioned; in other words, a problem is understood by means of its solution. *[R. Milanese]*

REFERENCES. Nardone G., Watzlawick P., *The art of change*, 1993; Nardone G., *Brief strategic solution-oriented therapy of phobic and obsessive disorders*, 1996; Nardone G., Portelli C., *Knowing through changing*, 2005; Nardone G., Balbi E., *The logic of therapeutic change*, 2015; Watzlawick P., Weakland J.H., Fisch R., *Change: Principles of problem formation and problem resolution*, 1974.

ATTENTION

Process of focus and selection of one or more bodily or environmental stimuli, which makes their perception sharper and more defined and prepares the behavioural response according to these stimuli. The concentration of attention on specific information or stimuli is a complex process that involves the cognitive, emotional and motor sphere. In fact, the selective perception of certain stimuli is activated by a complex twist of needs and emotions, as well as expectations and memories. Individuals who suffer from a frustrated need tend to be selective in their perceptual field and to direct themselves primarily towards those stimuli that are deemed more suitable for the satisfaction of their needs. Similarly, individuals suffering from phobia tend to select and focus on information that may indicate the presence of the anxiety-arousing stimulus and to activate at the same time an increased muscle tension that elicits avoidance behaviour and escape. The concept of attention is important for all therapeutic models, albeit with different meanings and uses. Freud coined the term → free-floating attention, to indicate the attitude that the psychoanalyst should take in response to the patient's → free associations. In Gestalt therapy and body-oriented therapies, focused attention is crucial to introduce → awareness processes. Cognitive-constructivist approaches consider attention as a constructing process, as a synthesis and learning of important information available in the environment. In brief strategic therapy and hypnosis, working on distracting and shifting processes is often essential to treat various types of psychological problems: phobias, obsessions and compulsions in particular (→ stratagems). *[R.]*

ATTITUDE

Unlike → behaviour, attitude is expressed as a simple "predisposition to", but it does not imply a consequent behaviour. It is an inner impulse that can be consolidated in an action, but it can also stop at the level of the perception of the emotion in progress. Therefore, therapeutic change implies a substantial change in subjects' attitudes as well as in their behaviours. Some forms of therapy consider change of attitude as essential, in order to subsequently change behaviours, while others argue that in order to change attitudes, behaviours need to be changed first. More sophisticated approaches overcome this traditional dichotomy by intervening in parallel on both components. *[R.]*

▷ In Jungian analytical psychology, attitude is the disposition of the psyche to act or react in a certain direction and it always appears to be influenced by a conscious or unconscious "point of orientation". This is a vital distinction for a theory aiming to take into account unconscious mental processes and their interactions with conscious processes. However, a more or less stable hegemony of a habitual attitude of consciousness and Ego can be observed in each subject. In *Psychological Types* (1921), Jung outlines the profiles of habitual conscious attitudes and the unconscious psychic dispositions corresponding to them by "compensation". The habitual conscious attitude is an essential part of one's personal psychological equation, since without its contribution the idea of an individual psychology would be impossible. It also organizes itself as an individual response that affects the whole psychic process, and it shows itself with such a nature of "obviousness" that it needs to be considered not as a particular subjective factor, but as a general tendency. Habitual conscious attitudes are partly innate and partly acquired dispositions, capable of directing the activities that connect certain psychic contents to Ego and of excluding other contents theoretically connectable to Ego. Consequently, the habitual attitude of consciousness and Ego is the structuring factor of conscious personality and of the resulting repression in the unconscious of functional abilities that the hypothetical model of psychic life designed by Jung considered to be natural qualities of human psyche. *[E.V. Trapanese]*

REFERENCES. Jung C.G. (1921), *Psychological types*, in *Collected Works*, VI, 1971; Trapanese E.V., *Il problema dei tipi*, in L. Aversa (ed.), *Fondamenti di psicologia analitica*, 1995; Id., *Tipi psicologici e funzioni della psiche*, in A. Carotenuto (ed.), *Trattato di psicologia analitica*, 1992; Trevi M., *Adesione e distanza 2. Una lettura critica dei "tipi psicologici" di Jung*, 1993.

AUTHENTICITY

In Gestalt therapy, the concept of authenticity does not refer to the dichotomy between true and false, but to the difference between what is stereotyped and relevant to the situation, which, with its multiplicity of elements, calls diverse and contradictory reactions. The more the past life of a person finds its place and is represented in their behaviour, the more authentic is their answer: authenticity therefore refers to a sense of congruity rather than to an absolute truth. According to this point of view, the main goal of Gestalt work is to develop the necessary creativity to shape constructs that are large enough to give space to complex and interrelated elements when answering life stresses. *[P. Quattrini]*

▷Existential analytic therapy speaks about authenticity when existence reflects the true inner reality of individuals, characterized by singularity, by possibility, by anguished choice opposed to false security and to a bland superficial everyday life or a life reflecting hypocritically social behaviours. This approach speaks about human beings and about their authentic belonging to themselves by defining the individual as the place of their own truth. True identity springs from and coincides with one's self. Therefore, the truth of reality lies in its entirety: only the whole, not a part, can be born. The presence of various sources and forms of knowledge represents a guarantee of authenticity. To state that truth is something clear and accomplished would be like stating a subjectivity greater than objectivity. The Self is bigger than Ego; therefore, the perfect truth is incomplete and transcendent. Not only can objective truth be found in man, but it also continuously exceeds him and it should be understood as *sophia*, that is, wisdom, life, coexistence, transcendence, synthesis, opening. The *sophia*, unlike rational truth, requires the approval of mind, heart and soul: that is, man as a whole. Man remains the only source of confirmation and truthfulness. Therefore, objective truth needs to be considered as perspectival and, for this, reason objective. *[D. Romagnoli, S. Antonetti]*

REFERENCES. Mercurio A., *Teoria della persona*, 1978; Id., *Antropologia esistenziale e metapsicologia personalistica*, 1991; Id., *Teoria dell'inconscio esistenziale*, 1995

AUTOGENIC TRAINING

A self-relaxation technique invented in the first half of the twentieth century by Schultz, that has amongst its aims an increased control over one's → stress levels and levels of anxiety, a general reduction in the level of emotional tension and the recovery of energy and psychophysical wellbeing. It includes six basic exercises (the "heaviness" exercise, the heat exercise, the heart exercise, the breathing exercise, the solar plexus exercise, the "fresh forehead" exercise) that can be carried out both whilst seated and whilst lying down. *[G. Palmieri]*

REFERENCES. Schultz J. H., Luthe W., *Autogenic training: A psychophysiologic approach to psychotherapy*, 1959.

AUTOMATIC NEGATIVE THOUGHT

According to cognitive behaviour therapy, dysfunctional and systematic modes of interpreting and evaluating events and situations or specific classes of events and situations. Everything that happens is interpreted, by default, in a negative manner, and in a way in which the individual fails to give himself the time needed to evaluate a given situation in a more functional and constructive way for his own ends, for example, by taking into consideration alternative hypotheses and judgements. *[A. Meluzzi, R.S. Pecorara]*

REFERENCES. Beck A.T., Weishaar M.E., *Cognitive therapy*, in *Current psychotherapies* (9th Ed.), 2017.

AUTOPOIESIS

This term was introduced in the early 1970s by the Chilean biologist Maturana to indicate the distinctive characteristics of living systems, namely the process of continuous self-production and maintenance of their own components (from the Greek *autos*, "self" and *poiesis*, "creation", "production"). According to a circular logic, which is typical of Maturana's ontology, living organizations are understood as self-referential organizations (→ self-reference), which ensure the production and maintenance of their own components and whose functioning produces the organization itself. In other terms, the fundamental characteristics of an autopoietic system is that it maintains itself through its own means, and forms itself as a distinct unit from the environment through its own dynamic. An autopoietic system is, therefore, a homeostatic system (→ homeostasis) whose identity is defined by its specific → self-organization. The term not only had notable success in the area of biology, but also in the wider area of theory in → self-organized systems, second-order → cybernetics (H. Von Foerster) and in the study of complex systems. In psychology and psychotherapy, the concept of autopoiesis and self-organization has been used in the theory and practice of systemic approaches, cognitive-constructivists (e.g. M. Mahoney) and in V.F. Guidano's post-rationalist cognitivism (see the opening chapter, "The eight paradigms and models and their respective theoretical-applicative models"). *[D. Liccione]*

REFERENCES. Maturana H.R., *Ontology of observing: The biological foundations of self-consciousness and the physical domain of existence*, 1988; Maturana H.R., Varela F.J., *The tree of knowledge*, 1987.

AUXILIARY EGO

Within → psychodrama, each member of the group that is chosen by the protagonist to play a part in the psychodramatic representation. It is therefore an individual who is detached from the audience and is brought on stage to be an actor, giving concrete form to the characters of the "inner theatre" of the protagonist. Thanks to the auxiliary Ego, the protagonist can meet, outside of himself, the ghosts of his world, which are made distinct and tangible: this allows a clearer awareness of their characteristics and their emotional valence. The auxiliary Ego, as a real person, is the bearer of the ghost but does not coincide with it: he participates in the representation in a creative way and with an emotional charge that allows the protagonist to perceive the human spirit, which is the deciding factor in any therapeutic process. *[G. Boria]*

REFERENCES. Boria G., *Psicoterapia psicodrammatica. Sviluppi del modello moreniano nel lavoro terapeutico con gruppi di adulti*, 2005; Boria G., Muzzarelli F., *Incontri sulla scena*, 2009; Moreno J.L., *Psychodrama first volume*, 1946; Moreno J.L., (1953), *Who shall survive?*

AWARENESS

A state in which an individual realizes the meaning of an event or situation (personal, collective, past or present, internal or external). This term, generally used as a synonym for "consciousness", is, in fact, fundamentally different: while consciousness describes what it sees, awareness seeks to give it a meaning. Starting with this meaning, man gives a meaning to his → experience. The main discussions around the concept of consciousness originated in the seventeenth century with the French philosopher Descartes, who proposed the assumption of a separation between mind and body. Descartes gave consciousness the meaning of "subjective awareness", considering it to be the only form of knowledge that man cannot question. According to recent biology studies, man is not the only being with awareness: other animals have this perception, although less developed. Man would be able to achieve a higher degree of awareness (in some cultures, for instance the Buddhist, this is called "illumination") through personal-growth techniques, such as → meditation. In psychotherapy, the concept of awareness is used for different purposes and in different ways: in particular, the term self-awareness is used to indicate the ability to pay → attention to, encode and retrieve information concerning the Self, that is, to distance oneself from one's own feelings and realize what is happening. For example, Freudian psychoanalysis believes that people are unaware of how their unconscious moves (→ Id), whereas awareness is considered a typical characteristic of the → Ego (consciousness). Dreams represent meanings hidden in the Id that elude its control and rise to the consciousness of the individual. The therapist's task is to conduct an analysis of personal dynamic processes, especially the unconscious ones (defence mechanisms, drives, repressed traumas, etc.), to resolve conflicts and tensions (which, when not revealed and understood, generate pathologies) through → insight. *[R]*

▷ In Gestalt therapy, awareness is the ability to perceive one's own body (bodily-kinaesthetic component) and the outside world (sensory-perceptual component), the ability to be in contact with excitement, fear, awe, etc. (emotional component) and to perceive the creation and flow of thoughts, images, fantasies, etc. (imaginal and cognitive component). It is a continuous process, an underground flow, accessible to experience through the practice of the "awareness continuum", which consists in perceiving and sometimes verbalizing this flow of experiences in the moment when it is experienced; a practice – that needs some training – whose unique purpose is to become progressively aware of the uninterrupted flow of the perception of the self. Intentional activities, such as appraisal, interpretation or classification of what is happening, prevent the experience of awareness and are considered auto-manipulations. Perls coined five questions to facilitate this process: "What do you do?", "What do you feel?", "What do you want?", "What do you expect from life?" and "What are you avoiding?" The primary purpose is to help people to become aware of the "mode" in which they are working in the present moment, both as a social being and as an organism, to enable the identification with spontaneous experiences and to facilitate the process of repossession of denied parts of the self. The "continuum", which can evolve from a sporadic exercise in an attitude and a lifestyle, is close to Eastern meditation practices such as Vipassana and Zazen. *[R. Zerbetto, G. Carrera]*

▷ In transactional analysis, Berne defines awareness as a psychological state in which an individual is able to recognize which emotional states lead to a certain behaviour. Awareness, together with → spontaneity (the capacity to take adequate decisions in the → here and now) and → intimacy, form a triad of psychological elements that lead the individual to autonomy. This is described as a person's ability to use their own → Ego states to be functionally adaptive to their own environment. From a methodological point of view, the achievement of autonomy is considered by Berne as the ideal goal of a psychotherapy in transactional analysis. *[M. Novellino]*

REFERENCES. Berne E., *Games people play*, 1964; Moiso C., Novellino M., *Stati dell'Io*, 1982; Perls F., Hefferline R.F., Goodman P., *Gestalt therapy: Excitement and growth in the human personality*, 1951; Zerbetto R., *Gestalt: la terapia della consapevolezza*, 1998

AWFULIZING

In the field of Rational Emotive Therapy (RET), it is one of the four basic categories of → irrational thoughts identified by Albert Ellis. Awfulizing is a way of thinking that leads a person to evaluate as awful, terrible or catastrophic situations in which things do not go as they would wish. Furthermore, this way of thinking can lead to extremely negative or exaggerated evaluations of situations that may not in fact be "catastrophic", but are effectively disturbing (e.g. it would be awful if my boss didn't approve of me); alternatively, it can lead to beliefs that the outside world is full of terrible and catastrophic things. In general, awfulizing produces beliefs that do not follow the principles of logic and obstructs people from reaching their goals and objectives. *[S. Lenzi, L. Cambrini]*

B

BAD OBJECT

In psychoanalysis, an object of the drive that is qualified as frustrating, persecutory, painful, malevolent, deadly, hated, fearful. In Kleinian theory, it indicates the split object in the → paranoid–schizoid position, correlative of the → good object. The bad object may be partial (breast or penis) or total (mother, father), inner or external. In the phantasmic life of a child, the prototype of the bad object takes shape – Klein writes – following on from the experience of the removal or absence of the breast:

> the breast-fed ejects his love impulses and attributes them to a breast able to give satisfaction (good), as it ejects outside his disruptive impulses, attributing them to a frustrating breast (bad.) Meanwhile, by the introjection, a good and a bad breast take over into his interior.

The splitting of the object performs the defensive function of not destroying the good object, which is invested in an ambivalent way. *[G. Perfetto, A. Voltolin]*

REFERENCES. Klein M., *Some theoretical conclusions regarding the emotional life of the infant*, 1952

BAD ME → GOOD ME

BAD MOTHER → MOTHER

BASIC ANXIETY

According to Horney's interpersonal psychoanalytic approach, basic anxiety consists in a feeling of helplessness and loneliness in a hostile world. It develops when the caregivers do not accept the infant as he is – i.e. his needs, his feelings and his peculiarities – and they love him only in so far as he complies with their inner image of what an infant ought to be. If parents deepen love and protection for their child only when he obeys and abides by their wishes, they hinder all his movements towards autonomy and independence. As a result, at first the infant will tend to rebel against his parents but will subsequently submit to his parents' wishes in order to avoid not being loved. Occasionally he may still manifest oppositional behaviours but, ultimately, he will tend to conform to the behaviour pattern demanded by others in order not to experience loneliness. Thus, the conflictual process between one's dependency and one's autonomy results in basic anxiety, i.e. the neurotic phenomenon hidden behind the experience of feeling helpless and alone in a hostile world. Such experience arises from repressed hostility and from pre-emptively experiencing others as being hostile. In summary, as Horney maintains, basic anxiety is the response to a potential danger, whilst manifest anxiety is the response to a manifest danger. *[A.Cresti, S. Brizzi]*

REFERENCES. Horney K., *The neurotic personality of our time*, 1937; Id., *New ways in psychoanalysis*, 1939; Id., *Neurosis and human growth*, 1950 .

BASIC ASSUMPTIONS

In Bionian psychoanalysis, basic assumptions are possible contents of group mentality. They represent collective phantasies that are adopted to avoid the frustration of learning through usual procedures (which would imply suffering and stress). Such phantasies show themselves through three basic assumptions: the first one is "coupling", which relies on the fact that all the sufferings, problems and wishes of the group will be resolved by a future event or by a human being who is not yet born; hope is placed into a (omnipotent) couple, inside the group itself, from which a saving idea or a messianic leader will come. In order for this expectation to allow the survival of the group, it must never be accomplished. Within society, this basic assumption is represented by aristocracy. The second assumption is called "ight and flight" and is rooted in the phantasy that there may be a bad external object personified by an enemy. To preserve the group, the only defence is destroying it (fight), or avoiding it (flight); usually the group finds its leader in paranoid personalities. In therapeutic groups, the "enemy" may be one of its members, another group, a disease or even the therapist themself; within society it is represented by the army. Finally, "dependency" concerns the expectation of an external object (guide, leader, idea) to be able to provide security and grant the fulfilment of the wishes of every member of the group; in a therapeutic group, this role is easily attributed to the therapist (the expectation is that the job will be done entirely by the therapist, because he/she is the only person capable of finding a solution to all the problems). In the social environment, it is represented by the Church. *[G. Perfetto, A. Voltolin]*

REFERENCES. Bion W.R., *Experiences in groups*, 1961; Grinberg L., Sor D. E., Tabac de Bianchedi, *Introducciòn a las ideas de Bion*, 1972.

BEHAVIOUR

An individual's set of actions and reactions to external or internal stimuli (defined in the latter case as → motivations). Research on the genetic basis of behaviour has not led to locating which genes encode certain behaviours, but it could identify a variety of basic cognitive characteristics that predispose their implementation. Instead, from a neurophysiological perspective, it has been possible to establish that behaviours depend on nerve stimulations of sensory receptors that are transmitted to the brain. Of particular interest for psychology is the study of nerve reflexes, considered as innate behavioural adaptations that may give rise to → conditioned reflexes, which are considered to be the basis of learning. According to the "homeostatic model" (Cannon, *The wisdom of the body*, 1932), behaviour is guided by the motivation of restoring perfect balance in the physiological functions, with the consequent reduction of the tension produced by an unfulfilled need. Every psychological school (and therefore also psychotherapy) has its own interpretation of behaviour. The behaviourist approach is based on the assumption that behaviour is the only unit of analysis that psychology can scientifically study. The psychotherapy models related to behaviourism aim to build functional behaviours, to replace the dysfunctional ones, driving the patient to change gradually and consciously the behavioural reactions learned in the past. Psychodynamic models see behaviour from different perspectives: the strictest view affirms that, during the first five years of a person's life, the fundamental behavioural patterns of the individual are established. The more flexible views give the will of the individual a *chance* to promote therapeutic change and set their work on searching for the causes that have produced certain behavioural patterns in the past. Systemic, strategic, humanistic and expressive-bodily models assert that behaviour needs to be exclusively studied in the historical moment and in the interpersonal context in which it takes place. Their therapeutic work aims to change dysfunctional behaviour (which, according to these approaches, maintains the pathological situation) in order to perceive reality in different ways, but also to be able to study its organization. *[R.]*

Behavioural paradigm → Please refer to the opening chapter, "The eight paradigms and their respective theoretical-applicative models".

BEHAVIOURAL MODEL OF CLASSICAL CONDITIONING

The model of classical (or respondent) conditioning was developed by the Russian physiologist Pavlov. His famous experiment on dogs was inspired by the simple observation of an innate response of salivation typically produced in the presence of food. Pavlov noticed that dogs were reacting before having food in front of them. They were starting to salivate just by just seeing his approaching figure: the animals had associated the physiologist with the arrival of food. Pavlov decided to try to associate other stimuli with the food, like the sound of a doorbell or a light, to see if the phenomenon would happen again. The success of the experiment gave rise to the following assumption: if an unconditioned stimulus (food), which produces an unconditioned response – that is genetically defined – (salivation), is associated a number of times with a neutral stimulus, which is unable to produce that response itself (the sound of a bell), the neutral stimulus will gain the same power as the unconditional one, and, even in its absence it will be able to elicit the response (salivation). Later research highlighted another phenomenon that played an important role in the development of behavioural theories: stimulus generalization. The same conditioned response was also related to stimuli similar but not identical to the original one. Depending on the characteristics of similarity of the stimuli, it is possible to distinguish between primary generalization, where the stimuli are similar in terms of objective and measurable characteristics, and secondary generalization, where stimuli are similar in a subjective sense, depending on how they are perceived and experienced. Further studies also explored the possibility of dissociating the bond between conditioned response and conditioned stimulus, to verify whether or not the stimulus could return to being neutral. This process was called "extinction" and it was achieved by avoiding presenting, a number of times, the conditioned stimulus together with the unconditioned one. In the specific case of Pavlov's experiment, this consisted in presenting the food without the sound of the bell: in fact, the salivation response was no longer induced. Researchers found that, in order to recreate the bond, a smaller number of presentations were necessary for the "relearning", compared to the first learning. Therefore, they deduced that the response was not eliminated but only inhibited. This regained effectiveness of the conditioned stimulus was called "spontaneous recovery". The field was enriched by the studies of J.B. Watson, author of an article (1913) considered to be the manifesto of Behaviourism. Undoubtedly, the most famous experiment, where it is possible to observe the application of the pavlovian principles of classical conditioning, is the one called "Little Albert". Watson worked with Albert, a boy of about 11 months, with the goal of reproducing the model of learning experienced by Pavlov. Little Albert was playing quietly with a white mouse until it was presented to him in combination with a loud noise, which frightened him and brought him to tears. After a few repetitions, Albert began crying merely on seeing the mouse, long before the sound was produced. The fear of the little child was generalized onto white, furry objects, confirming the outcome of the studies already conducted by Pavlov. The theory of classical conditioning is crucial in the behavioural approach, since one can provide a more correct and objective description of the environment in which organisms move through the possibility of identifying defined stimulus–response units (→ stimulus–response relationship). Watson described emotions as the expression of a learning derived from environmental stimuli. The basic emotions (happiness, fear, anger) and other complex emotions can be linked to repeated conditionings. The model of classical conditioning, together with Skinner's operant conditioning (→ behavioural model of operant conditioning), was at the base of the theory of learning and maintenance of phobias theorized by Wolpe, which gave rise to the technique of → systematic desensitization. *[E. Rolla, S. Durando]*

REFERENCES. Galeazzi A., Meazzini P., *Mente e comportamento. Trattato italiano di psicoterapia cognitivo-comportamentale*, 2004; Meyer V., Chesser E.S., *Behaviour therapy in clinical psychiatry*, 1970; Rolla E., *Ricomincia da te*, 2003; Skinner F.B., *Science and human bevavior*, 1953; Wilson R., Branch R., *Cognitive behavioural therapy for dummies*, 2006; Wolpe J., *Behaviour therapy techniques*, 1966.

BEHAVIOURAL MODEL OF OPERANT CONDITIONING

The model of operant conditioning was formulated by Skinner in the 1930s. Skinner criticized the positions of the first behaviourism proposed by J. Watson and E. Guthrie and rediscovered the previous works of Thorndike. With them, he also rediscovered the American functionalist traditions. In fact, the work of classical behaviourists drew inspiration from Thorndike's studies but then they distanced themselves from them and embraced the reflexology currents of the Soviet school. Instead, Skinner was completely aligned with Thorndike's work. Thorndike was an important American scholar of the early 1920s, a rigorous experimentalist who analyzed the strategies implemented by various animals to obtain food. Through his studies, he was able to discover how the consequences of a behaviour are essential to its possible stabilization. His "trial and error" learning theory represents the scientific summary of these discoveries. In one of his classic laboratory experiments, Thorndike puts a hungry cat in a cage and some food, not directly reachable, outside the cage. To access the gratifying → reward, the animal needs to learn to press a lever, which activates the mechanical opening of a small door, allowing the cat to leave the cage. The result is a slow and gradual learning process, characterized by increasingly rapid and confident expressions of the fruitful behavioural response. Therefore, this is not an intelligent and intuitive resolution of the problem, but rather an automatic consolidation, over time, of the connection between the environmental stimulus and the most effective behavioural response. This form of learning is based on two main laws: the law of exercise, according to which learning improves by repeating the trial through continuous practice, and the → law of effect, by which learning occurs in relation to the effects of pleasure and satisfaction following the active behaviour of the animal. A rewarding consequence strengthens the connection between the stimuli of hunger and food and the response of pressing the lever, whereas an unpleasant consequence weakens it; an appetizing food satisfies the cat, an unpleasant one does not. Moreover, the experimental results also show that states of satisfaction are more important than unpleasant states; in fact, rewards reinforce (→ reinforcement) the connections between stimulus and response; instead → punishments do not weaken them directly, but make the behaviour more flexible, thus creating the possibility for any other response to be reinforced. In the wake of Thorndike's early work, Skinner supported the idea of a truly scientific and objective psychology. Skinner affirmed that to be a good scientist, it is essential to adopt a typical mindset characterized by order and a tendency towards progress. When behaviour is studied with this attitude, it reveals its harmonic laws, which can always be explained in terms of causes, or independent variables, and dependent variables, or effects. In this way, it is possible to realize that the main causes of behaviour are environmental, each of which must be understood in physical terms, because they are real objective factors. In his scientific production, Skinner always reiterated the superiority of conditioning as a form of learning. According to him, the merits of Pavlov's work, and of the subsequent work of Watson, were to provide a highly scientific and experimental paradigm that was simultaneously linear and complex: from the same stimuli, the same responses follow. The → behavioural model of classical conditioning can only explain how automatic reflexes work; therefore, it omits the complexity of freely emitted behaviours. Reflexes are innate and hereditary and always functional for survival, whereas conditioning is learned; it is sometimes irrational, not useful to the survival of the organism. In the set of causal laws, the mechanism of → reinforcement plays a central role. This follows a response deliberately emitted by a subject in reaction to specific stimulating environmental conditions. Skinner investigated the importance of the consequences of a behaviour, which retrospectively, affect the same behaviour by causing its reactivation. Skinner discovered how a behaviour tends to stabilize as it carries on obtaining the desired effect. This allowed him to verify the law of effect and to include it in his theoretical system. In every situation, a behaviour acts in the environment to obtain a specific consequence. Therefore, this behaviour is no longer simply "elicited" by stimuli, as required by Watson's theory, but is freely emitted with the clear aim of pursuing consequences. A reinforcement action follows, which by binding itself to the acted response, determines the stabilization of a behaviour. Therefore, environmental stimuli lose their rigidly determining value and take a more elastically discriminating one. In other words, a stimulus acts as an objective criterion, which can only predispose towards certain responses, but does not produce them. Through experimentation with animals in cages (→ Skinner box) seeking to solve difficulties in obtaining food, Skinner proposed an ABC-type pattern of conditioning. In this pattern, A (antecedent) is the state of the environment before the emission of the behaviour, B (behaviour) is the emitted behaviour and C (consequence) is the consequence obtained. Antecedents, or stimuli, are conditions that predispose to a specific response, for example the status of food deprivation of a rat. Instead, behaviours are responses spontaneously emitted by the animal to obtain food. Finally, consequences are food itself, which can be obtained or not. In the Skinner box experiment, a hungry animal in a cage, usually a rat, can accidentally press a lever that activates the delivery of food. In this case, the behavioural response of pressing the lever will be intentionally repeated in the future in a more direct and simplified way, under the same conditions. Instead, when no reinforcement follows a response, this tends to become less and less frequent, and eventually it disappears. In this case, the phenomenon is called operant → extinction and it is often accompanied by emotional effects of frustration or anger. Unlike extinction, oblivion occurs when a certain conditioning is lost over time because the predisposing conditions and the responses emitted, even successfully, no longer have the possibility of manifesting themselves. Consequences can be positively reinforcing, such as food; negatively reinforcing, such as the removal of an obstacle; or punitive, such as an electric shock. Reinforcement, either positive or negative, always increases the response; instead, punishment always extinguishes it. In fact, positive reinforcement adds rewarding stimuli and negative reinforcement eliminates adverse stimuli; instead, punishment consists in presenting adverse stimuli (positive punishment) or in removing positive stimuli (negative punishment). Like all behaviourists, Skinner stressed the ineffectiveness of punishment as a learning technique. This is totally inadequate and it is often associated with distorting behaviour whose nature is emotionally temporary and contextualized in its effect and therefore unpleasant and despicable. Reinforcement, which supports all learning, is not a reaction to pleasure or to a reduction of deprivation: these are just connected effects; reinforcement is a biological and evolutionary neutral component. Skinner proposed several applications of operant behaviourism: clinical, educational, social, educational and institutional. He also perfected a specific technique called shaping, which was later adopted in clinical psychology. In this case, a behaviour is shaped gradually towards the development of the desired one. This is a step-by-step learning, which is made possible by reinforcing only some specific responses emitted by an individual. Thus, the final desired behaviour, such as pressing the lever for a rat, can be built gradually, for example by reinforcing the animal's behaviour with a small amount of food whenever it moves close to the lever that it has to press. *[A. Tamburello, E. De Monte]*

REFERENCES. De Monte E., Tamburello A., *Storia del pensiero psicologico*, 2008; Skinner F.B., *Science and human bevavior*, 1953; Thorndike E.L., *Animal intelligence: Experimental studies*, 1911.

BEHAVIOURAL PATTERN

According to the Milan systemic family therapy (→ Milan school of family therapy) this term designs a specific behavioural model, an example or a sample. It indicates a sort of regularity that can be temporally and spatially observed in generating actions or behaviours; a repetitive and constant way to react to its underlying logic, reproducing structural characteristics of the considered behaviour. It differs from the concept of → personality because it pertains to behaviour and is not related to traits or intrapsychic aspects. Behavioural patterns can also become redundant, rigid and dysfunctional if structured and strengthened in the course of the time. *[G. Castelnuovo, G. Pietrabissa, E. Molinari]*

REFERENCES. Watzlawick P., Beavin J.H., Jackson Don D., *Pragmatics of human communication*, 1967.

Behaviourism → Please refer to the opening chapter, "The eight paradigms and their respective theoretical-applicative models".

BEING

A term introduced by Fromm as opposed to → having to express the more natural tendency of living. The "being" mode facilitates vital and dynamic relationships among people and accepts the normal and ongoing process of transformation of everything that lives, in obedience to individual skills and manners.

> The anxiety and insecurity engendered by the danger of losing what one has are absent in the being mode. If I am what I am and not what I have, nobody can deprive me of my security and my sense of identity [. . .]. The only threat to my security in being lies in myself: in lack of faith in life and my productive powers.

This existential mode represents the authentic being, an explorer of their own inner world, able to see their limitations and perceive the reality of their own Ego and of what surrounds them and free to express it. *[G. Rombolà Corsini, M. Zetti, E. Benelli]*

REFERENCES. Fromm E., *The art of loving*; Id., *To have or to be*, 1976.

BEING-IN-THE-WORLD

This term is quite commonly borrowed from the Heideggerian philosophy that existential psychoanalysis follows, in which there is no human existence without the world. The essence of human beings is existence, which represents the immediate truth, the fundamental nature of being-here and being-in-the-world. The world is not a thing, but the field of possibilities/opportunities of human transcending. Existence is possible only if based on the understanding of being and language would naturally be the unveiling of being. Man is his own history in a setting; each individual, from birth, finds himself cast in a world of common meanings. Opportunity is treasured in the ways of being of existence. Man, therefore, will be whom he has decided to be. His way of being is a can-be, a way to go out, an uncertainty and a risk. Existential psychoanalysis is the analysis of the most common or fundamental relationships and situations in which man finds himself, the possible ways of being of the being-here. The intentional behaviour of the being-here, the ways of dealing-with and the relating-to, are the ways in which a possible relationship with the world is created. The possibility of being is the spectrum of possibilities of the ways of being from which man must choose or, better yet, which he plans to be. Mental illness can be intended as "lack of being", as a limit to the possibility of being-in-the-world, as inability to use self-determination and self-planning. *[F. Ioppolo]*

REFERENCES. Binswanger L., *Zur phänomenologischen Anthropologie*, 1947; Heidegger M., *Being and time*, 1962.

BEING-THERE

A term borrowed from Heidegger's philosophy, from which existential analytic psychotherapy takes inspiration. In this model, "being" refers to the act of existing, a continuous movement that cannot be fully grasped: "being" as the flow of existence. "Being" is meant as experience of oneself, as being alive and vivid in everything one does and feels, as an active and not passive presence. "Being" is not a goal, a point of arrival, but a process; the truth of being is not the rationalistic one, but what emerges from the person in their entirety in the → here-and-now; being in constant motion and permanent transcendence of what has been already given. *[D. Romagnoli, S. Antonetti]*

"BE SPONTANEOUS" PARADOX

A particular type of paradox (→ logic of paradox), which was postulated by Paul Watzlawick. In an interpersonal situation, a person requires or presupposes a behaviour performed by another person, which, by its nature, can only occur spontaneously, and not when prompted: therefore, the request itself makes it impossible to fulfil what was required. In addition to "be spontaneous", other examples of this type of paradox are requests such as: "You should desire me", "You should want to study", "You should be happy". Anyone who receives these injunctions is in an untenable position. In fact, in order to comply with the request, a person should be spontaneous within a scheme of condescension and not of spontaneity, while the concept of "spontaneity" itself requires that an action is performed without being suggested or directly required. When facing this type of solicitation, a person has only two alternatives: refusing to comply (and therefore failing to satisfy the request) or trying to satisfy these paradoxical injunctions through willpower, and therefore doing the right thing but for the wrong reason (that is, failing also in this case). In the latter case, a consciously directed effort of will not only makes the occurrence of a normal spontaneous reaction impossible, but it often generates unintended, unwanted and unplanned spontaneous reactions. For example, this happens when people suffering from panic attacks try to control anxiety through an effort of will, with the result of increasing it to the point where they experience real panic. Another example is that of a person who tries voluntarily to fall asleep with the inevitable result of staying awake in bed in the grip of insomnia. Precisely due to its ability to inhibit spontaneity, the "be spontaneous" paradox is the logical criterion underlying the → symptom prescription. This is a technique frequently adopted in systemic and strategic approaches to unlock uncontrollable symptoms (→ worst fantasy technique; → hypochondriac check-up technique; → contradictory confirmation prescription). *[C. Hybarger, R. Milanese]*

REFERENCES. Nardone G., Portelli C., *Knowing through changing*, 2005; Watzlawick P., Beavin J.H., Jackson Don D., *Pragmatics of human communication*, 1967; *Change: Principles of problem formation and problem resolution*, 1974.

BETA-SCREEN

What Bion refers to as the beta-screen is produced by the psychotic part of the personality by reversal of alpha function, the means by which emotional experience is normally processed. This reversal interferes with the formation of the → contact-barrier, which is what promotes both a distinction and a communication between conscious and unconscious, and depends on alpha function. The beta-screen presents clinically as a confused state and seems to want to arouse emotional involvement on the part of the analyst, which restricts any intuitive response. Instead of interpretation the analyst finds himself wanting to make either accusatory or laudatory remarks about the patient, who is correspondingly deprived of mental nourishment, namely the truth. *[J. Symington]*

REFERENCES. Bion W.R., *Learning from experience*, 1962.

BIOENERGETIC ANALYSIS → BIOENERGETICS

BIOENERGETICS

A body therapy – also called bioenergetic analysis – based on depth- and body- analysis and on the analysis of relational processes. This approach looks at human personality mainly in energetic and bodily terms. Bioenergetic analysis was systematized in the early 1950s by Lowen, an American psychiatrist, a student and patient of W. Reich, who, along with J. Pierrakos, founded in 1956 the International Institute for Bioenergetic Analysis (IIBA). Fascinated by Reich's intelligence and personality, Lowen became his student and decided to be analyzed by him. After in-depth personal and theoretical research work Lowen decided to separate from Reich, as he did not agree with the Reichian hypotheses of Orgone energy (cosmic energy, hypothesized by Reich and used by him for therapeutic purposes) and the excesses of character of the master. However, he remained always consistent with the Reichian vision of the somatic approach to neurosis, which constitutes the key assumption of bioenergetic analysis. Lowen's work is based on two Reichian principles: the concept of functional identity between somatic and psychological aspects and the fundamental correlation between emotional and psychological inhibition and insufficiency of respiratory functions. The fundamental thesis on which Reichian therapy was based, taken from bioenergetic analysis, is that of a functional identity between "muscular armour" and "behaviour armour", that is, the physical attitude of a person and the structure of their Ego. Lowen resumes the Reichian theory according to which tensions and contractions of any part of the body affect breathing and cause a lack of integrity in the individual, both on a physical and psychological level. Bioenergetic analysis aims to dissolve chronic muscular tensions in the body and to restore the natural expressiveness of the organism: in fact, any chronic muscle tension – a physical counterpart of a psychological inhibition – represents an inhibition and expresses specific feelings. Starting from these concepts, Lowen developed bioenergetic analysis as a therapeutic, analytical, somatic-relational, systemic method. Being in contact with one's own body is a guiding principle of bioenergetic analysis, which is based on the assumption that the more a person is emotionally disturbed, the more is far from the contact with their body. The goal of bioenergetic analysis is therefore to bring the patient into contact with the fundamental relationships of their lives: the one with the environment in which they live and the one with the "ground", considered as a physical and psychological space on which the person stands. The key themes are the functional identity between psyche and body, the unity of the person as an organism, the connection between energy and chronic muscle tension, the denial of the death instinct and of the central role of "genital"» sexuality as an expression of mental health (orgasm reflex). However, unlike his master, Lowen does not believe that the reactivation of the orgasm reflex corresponds linearly to the restoration of emotional health. On the contrary, he claims that this concerns the larger ability of a person to experience pleasure in life and the feeling of rootedness in one's bodily and emotional reality (*grounding*). Therefore, there is a broader view of the concept of pleasure, intended as a constant dynamic between relational processes and self-regulation. According to Lowen, pleasure is expressed in the ability to feel and to express ourselves with absolute self-mastery. The fundamental process of any bioenergetic therapeutic movement can be summarized in the Lowenian diagram: self-perception, self-expression and self-possession.

The ultimate goal is self-mastery, intended as the ability of the individual to manage their vital processes, their emotions and the perception of their personal power, a concept that anticipates all the theories of → empowerment in clinical psychology. Being in contact with one's own body is the principle that guides bioenergetic analysis: people in contact with their own body have no illusions about themselves and about life, they accept their feelings as expressions of their personality and have no difficulty in expressing them; this is the first and fundamental stage of any bioenergetic process. Self-expression is perhaps the most innovative and characteristic aspect of bioenergetic analysis: the energetic process is not activated by just verbalizing one's own feelings, but by returning to the individual the freedom and the opportunity to be in contact with their entire range of emotions (even the most awkward) through targeted exercises, so that these emotions can repossess their own expression. Hitting a mattress, screaming one's own anger or "shouting" one's own pain are bioenergetic techniques that, if supported by adequate integration of the analytical moment, are useful in order to retrieve, in a healthy way, suppressed emotions that can be very destructive for one's personality. Expressing them, also with the body, can allow for the reorganization of a balance altered by previous traumatic experiences that have created chronic muscular and psychological tension. Through the study of developmental experiences and the observation of physical and mental characteristics of patients, Lowen identified five main characters that are seen and quantified especially in energetic terms. Character structures, which correspond to the developmental phases of an individual, are interpreted in terms of "energetic charge". Starting from the less charged to the most energetically charged structure, Lowen identifies the schizoid character, the oral character, the psychopath character, the masochist character and the rigid character. These characters correspond to different developmental stages of the individual and their expressive blocks. According to Lowen, each individual is born with a positive self-regulating core characterized by energetic expansion and contraction. The environmental influence, including especially the parental couple, frustrates the attempts of individuals to realize their full potential. The problems encountered in the character types correspond to the blockage of a respective stage where individuals do not receive adequate support to the development of their Self. In the study of personality, Lowen outlines five basic rights-needs that characterize human existence: the right to exist (in the schizoid disorder); the right to have needs (in the oral disorder); the right to receive support (in the psychopathic disorder); the right to be free (in the masochist disorder); the right to be sexual (in the rigid disorder). The exterior denial of these rights-needs will determine defensive stratifications in the individual. At a somatic level, the inhibition of these rights is expressed by muscle tension and contraction, while at a psychological level the individual constructs and lives the illusion of an ideal Self in which the same issues are denied. Lowen's innovative approach is the systematization of an interpretation key where messages of individual parts of the body reveal their psychological correlates. It is precisely through "reading" the bodies of his patients that Lowen transformed psychological issues into five basic characters, detectable not only through psychological adaptation but also through energetic and bodily characteristics. Many years after the definition of the five basic characters, Lowen provided an innovative reading of the concept of narcissism – studied for the first time in its bioenergetic and bodily aspects –and outlined it not only as a character itself but also as a trait crossing over all other characters. His book *Narcissism* pays particular attention to body language that, in the narcissist person, transcends verbal expression and represents itself only in the role or through images. Moreover, the book resumes a social vision, typical of Reich, not limited merely to clinical aspects but underlining how a society obsessed by perfect bodies, facilitates and takes to extremes the mind–body and the emotion–image scission, typical of narcissistic pathology. The goal of bioenergetic therapy and character analysis is to bring people to consciousness, to loosen their character armour and regain a sufficient degree of flexibility to allow them to rely on their internal resources and to be truly in contact with the environment. This is how Lowen defines *grounding*. This concept represents one of Lowen's most important innovations, along with the necessity to work with patients by keeping them in an erect posture rather than lying or sitting down. He believed that a supine posture, with which Reich used to work, had a regressive characterization, opposite to the *grounding* position, which represents the contact with the present, with reality, with adult aspects. Therefore, *grounding* is both a psychological and a strictly physiological concept. According to Lowen, neurotic personality is determined by a sense of insecurity corresponding to poor contact of the feet with the ground. Therefore, starting by working on legs and feet means working with the sense of insecurity and reducing the need for dependence on external approval. Over the past 40 years, many therapies have changed: bioenergetic analysis, from a directive approach, has become a model that pays attention to the wide range of relational aspects and to the "meeting" between therapist and patient, completely deserving the definition of "somatic-relational psychotherapy", given to it by R. Hilton – one of the leading figures of bioenergetic analysis. *[P. Moselli]*

REFERENCES. Lowen A., *The language of the body*, 1958; Id., *Bioenergetics*, 1975; Id., *Narcissism*, 1983.

BIOFEEDBACK TECHNIQUE

In the behavioural paradigm, a self-regulation methodology through which it is possible to learn how to modulate, on a voluntary basis, some biological variables that usually are beyond conscious control, in accordance with the principles of → operant conditioning. Self-regulation occurs through an equipment that, via electrodes connected to the patient in a non-invasive way, converts biological signals in an acoustic or visual stimulus (*feedback*) in real time. The return signal acts as a → reinforcement for the individual's response that works in the desired direction (for example the reduction of muscle tension). The most used psychophysiological variables are: heart rate (HR), average variability of this frequency (HRV), muscle tone (EMG), peripheral temperature (THE), electrothermal response (GSR) and the electrical activity of the brain *(neuro feedback)*. The biofeedback technique has proven to be effective in treating muscle-tension headache, insomnia, generalized anxiety and attention deficit hyperactivity disorder. *[D. Coradeschi]*

REFERENCES. Anchisi R., Gambotto Dessi M., *Manuale del biofeedback: psicologia e medicina comportamentale*, 1996; Basmajian J.V., Biofeedback: *Principles and practice for clinicians*, 1979.

BIOPHILIA

A tendency to focus attention on life forms and on everything that reminds one of life and to assume a life-preservation mode, fighting death. From an ethical point of view, it recalls respect for life.

According to Fromm, the concept of biophilia is related to → necrophilia. As reported by Fromm, biophilia, as the primary disposition of individuals, should be found in the "productive" orientation of a person who

> fully loves life, is attracted by the process of life and growth in all spheres. He prefers to construct rather than to retain. He is capable of wondering, and he prefers to see something new to the security of finding confirmation of the old.

Considered as a primary potentiality, it develops only if there is a contagious love for life that prevents the appearance of love for death (necrophilia). It emerges in a society that guarantees

> safety, in the sense that the basic material conditions for a dignified life are not threatened; Justice, in the sense that no one can be an end for the purposes of another; freedom in the sense that every person has the opportunity to be an active and responsible member of society.

[E. Benelli, I. Battaglini]

REFERENCES. Fromm E., *Man for himself: An inquiry into the psychology of ethics*, 1947; Id., *The heart of Man: Its genius for good and evil*, 1964; Id., *Anatomy of human destructiveness*, 1973.

BIRTH TRAUMA

The trauma of birth is the ultimate, biological data of psychic life, the one beyond which it is impossible to go and starting from which, psychic life itself, in its totality, has to be explained. The Rankian construct gives title to his eponymous book, dedicated to S. Freud, whose publication marks Rank's detachment from the psychoanalytic mainstream, making him closer to later perspectives of psychology (humanistic, transpersonal). The central thesis is that anguish, with all of its consequences, is a derivative of birth. The → Oedipus complex, upon the paternal equation of which the coeval theorization of psychoanalysis is based, is by these means brought back to the pre-oedipal phases and → castration equalled the separation from the mother. The transference → libido, as Rank subsequently affirms, is libido towards the mother. It is in relationship to the birth trauma that constructs of "will" and "analytical situation" have to be understood. The first is given through the act of being (re)born and the second as a device by which "repetition" of the trauma is possible, that is, therapeutic use of reality, that is (re)birth. Freud's criticism of Rank's construct is that it intended to accelerate, wrongly, the analytic process. On his side, Rank would have conceived it following the systematic practice of scheduling the end of analysis. Such a technical device allowed him to discover, through patients' reactions, the existence of the repetition of birth during the analytic treatment. *[G. Antonelli]*

REFERENCES. Rank O., *The trauma of birth*, 1924.

BIZARRE OBJECT

The concept was formulated by Bion in 1967, to indicate an object composed by a nucleus – the proper object – and by a "halo" generated by the projection around it of fragments of the psychic apparatus. The constitution of bizarre objects is the consequence of the action of the mechanism of projective identification (→ defence mechanisms) on real objects. In its pathological expression such a mechanism is used by the psychotic part of the personality. Parts of the Ego, or Superego, fragments of psychic functions, once they are ejected, are perceived by the patient as though they are encysted in real objects and are not distinguished from them. For example: if the patient projects his own sightseeing function into a television set, he will perceive a "television that observes me". Such a dissociation can be so massive as to provoke the collapse of the symbolic function and the consequence would be the transformation of words and thoughts into things and, finally, in the setting up of a delirious dimension. *[A. Voltolin]*

REFERENCES. Bion W.R., *Second thoughts*, 1967; Lopez Corvo R., *Diccionario de la obra de Wilfred R. Bion*, 2002

BLACK BOX

In the behavioural paradigm (see the opening chapter, "The eight paradigms and their respective theoretical-applicative models"), a metaphor of the concepts of mind–brain indicates an "unknowable virtual space" inside the body. Here, neurobiological and cognitive-affective processes take place, which are not possible to observe directly and which interconnect the environmental input and the output behaviour. The black box was proposed by behavioural psychologists, within the stimulus–response model (→ stimulus–response relationship); it highlights the scientific unknowability and the irrelevance of behaviour, and emphasizes the role of stimuli and environmental contingencies.

Currently, studies and research in the cognitive field (cognitive function, memory, thought, etc.), neurosciences and mind modelling (on the brain, neural networks, units–neurons, synapses–connections, network algorithms, etc.) are contributing to the unveiling of the "contents" of the black box. *[A. Attianese]*

REFERENCES. Neisser U., *Cognitive psychology*, 1967; Skinner B.F., *About behaviourism*, 1974.

BLOCKAGE

In character analysis (→ bioenergetics), it is the somatic equivalent of a defensive formation used as a "solution" to a situation of → conflict. Reich identified in the blockage of vital energy the mechanism of formation of the "character armour" (→ character). Reich believed that the entire psychic dimension has a somatic correlation in the individual, assuming the theory of functional identity between psyche and soma, which underlines the close connection between emotional and muscular blockages and describes seven types of blockages in the human body: ocular, oral, cervical, thoracic, diaphragmatic, abdominal and pelvic. These blockages not only indicate the rigidity of the body in the individual, but denote lack of flexibility, affecting, in this way, mental health. *[M.L. Manca, P. Moselli]*

REFERENCES. Lowen A., *Bioenergetics*, 1975; Reich W., *The function of the orgasm*, 1968; Id., *On character analysis*, 1933.

BLOCKING ANSWERS TO INHIBIT QUESTIONS

Clinical-empirical research carried out at the Centro di Terapia Strategica in Arezzo, has revealed a paradoxical non-ordinary logic that seems to maintain and enrage obsessions. Patients often describe their obsessions or pathological doubting as a sort of a continuous siege from an ever-growing enemy.

The more they attempt to fight the intrusive thought, the more it fights back, entrapping them in a never-ending battle of the mind. Their usual attempted solution of fighting the too-forceful enemy is the best way to fall victim to it. By following and exploiting its logic, it was possible to design the technique of "blocking giving answers to inhibit the question". This prescription leads the patient to shift his attention from his failed → attempted solution of fighting the question onto blocking giving answers. Avoiding giving answers to the intrusive thought saps its strength, whereas fighting the original question only forces it to come back even stronger. Therefore, during the → strategic dialogue, the person is invited to reframe (→ strategic reframing technique) the logical attempt to fight the original thought, yet avoid giving answers that further feed the original question. This technique follows the stratagem, "to leave afterwards so as to arrive beforehand". While accepting and acknowledging that the question is too strong to battle, the person is invited to avoid pursuing finding answers. Obsessive patients recognize that, at this point, no answer is a good-enough answer, and, moreover, by answering the question they are caught in a never-ending vicious circle that further amplifies their anxiety, distress and doubts. This therapeutic indication follows Kant's maxim that "there are no correct answers to incorrect premises". This seemingly simple technique is very effective with the majority of patients caught in pathological doubting, yet when the thought is too strong or the patient is too vulnerable and tumbles easily into giving answers, another → stratagem is applied to the prescription: an → illusion of alternatives. The patient is instructed to either block giving an answer to inhibit the question or, if it is too strong, to get hold of pen and paper and transcribe, in detail, question and answer, question and answer, to the point of exasperation. By writing down questions and answers, the thought is inflated to such a point as to bring it to its self-annulment. Paradoxically (→ logic of paradox), the exhausted mind finally shuts out the intrusive thought. With this illusion of an alternative, the patient is caught in a win–win situation, i.e. in one way or another, either by blocking giving answers, or by exasperating the thought, he will gain control by blocking the usual vicious circle that enrages the obsession, and finally defeat it. *[C. Portelli]*

REFERENCES. Nardone G., *Psicosoluzioni*, 1998; Nardone G., Portelli C., *Knowing through changing*, 2005.

BODY

Of physical and material nature, as well as being an evolving organism, the body contains and allows the expression of individual potential and ability in the most general sense. In humans, in terms of its specific biological predisposition, the body is the first means of interaction with the external → environment. Many of the reflections on the body are affected by the ancient philosophical concept by which it is the antithesis of the soul. The psychological perspectives inspired by realism believe that the "psychological body" can be fixable to the physical entity that substantiates it; in terms of phenomenology, on the other hand, the body is the set of representations that are produced in us, and has no objective reality independent of the one who perceives it; for the idealists, the body is real, not in itself but to the thinking subject, as a synthesis of forms of intellect and feelings; for the socio-constructionist and from the interactionist perspective. No bodily experience is posible without a particular collective consciousness of the body and of its different meanings from a historical-cultural perspective. Two key concepts express the different connections to the objective dimension of the real body and the subjective one of the body as built and perceived: they are those of the "scheme" and the "images" of the body. The term "body scheme" refers to the conceptual construct of a neuro-cognitive nature that governs the direct perception of one's physical self by integrating and comparing past sensory experiences with present perceptions at the cortical level and vice versa; the expression "body image" refers to the way in which the body appears to oneself. The images of the body include emotional, cognitive and affective aspects that are closely linked to relationships with significant figures and to personal history; they also shift over time and over situations. Some important diseases, such as eating disorders and somatoform disorders, arise from the difference between the perceived body and the ideal body. The body for some forms of psychotherapy such as → bioenergetics is the fundamental vehicle for intervention. *[R.]*

Body-expression paradigm → Please refer to the first chapter, "The eight paradigms and their respective theoretical-applicative models".

BOND

In psychology, an emotionally significant connection between two or more subjects. Each person experiences daily different kinds of bond: bonds of kinship, social and work bonds and affective relationships. Often, these bonds can become entwined or even overlap. Each bond in which a person takes part can be defined based on its intensity, that is, on the force that keeps the relationship strong. In fact, psychologists use the terms "strong" and "weak" to describe bonds. An example of a strong bond is → attachment (→ attachment theory), namely, the intimate → relationship that children develop from birth with their mother and with the most significant figures who take care of them. A specific quality of a bond is reciprocity: the characteristics of the → interaction are determined by the conscious or unconscious contribution of all the subjects involved. A bond can become pathogenic or pathologic when it is too stiff or when the reciprocity between the individuals is heavily unbalanced, or when it contains expressed or hidden conflicts. The term therapeutic bond is used to indicate a particular type of relationship that is established between therapist and patient (or patients) and which aims to induce change, thus becoming an important therapeutic factor. *[R.]*

BORDERLINE

Starting in the 1930s and the 1940s, this term has been used to indicate people considered borderline between → neurosis and → psychosis. Psychiatric nosology refers to "*borderline* personality disorder" to indicate people that, starting from adolescence, are characterized by a pervasive difficulty to get into positive relationship with themselves and with others, both in the affective and the work sphere. In particular, in interpersonal relationships – where intense conflicts are frequent – people tend to overestimate or underestimate what is happening and build personal experiences characterized by continuous interpersonal failures. These people are frightened by social rejection but they trigger it continuously, due to their impulsive relational modalities. Unable to set limits, they can fall into numerous destructive excesses (substance abuse, suicide attempts, self-destructive behaviours, promiscuous sexuality) because of the constant emotional, intense and highly unstable peaks in the perception of themselves. The perspective of psychiatric nosology is, however, an oversimplification, claiming to measure in a mechanomorphic (→ mechanomorphism) way the possible expressions of psychological distress. In fact, the term "*borderline*" simply defines the concept of "border-line". Between "who" and "what" this boundary is set is determined by the theory of reference. If one takes a different perspective, the *borderline* construct can represent the boundary between many different realities. *[R.]*

BRIEF SOLUTION-FOCUSED THERAPY

A future- and goal-oriented approach to brief therapy was developed in the early 1980s by I.K. Berg, S. de Shazer and their colleagues at the Milwaukee Brief Family Therapy Centre. This is a highly disciplined approach, strongly pragmatic rather than theoretical, and developed in an inductive way. The roots of this therapy can be found in the early works of the → Mental Research Institute (MRI) in Palo Alto, in the work of M.H. Erickson and in the philosophy of L. Wittgenstein, as well as in Buddhist thought. The approach can be described through the eight guiding principles that follow: 1) *If it is not broken, don't fix it*: this can be considered as the general principle of this psychotherapy. It means that if the client has already solved their problem, nothing else needs to be done, no theory, model or philosophy of intervention is needed. It may seem obvious, but some schools of psychotherapy advocate the importance of therapeutic interventions oriented to "growth" or to go more "in depth". Brief solution-focused therapy puts itself antithetically against these concepts; therefore if there is not a problem that the person lives as such, there should be no therapy; 2) *If it works, insist*: if the client has already started to solve a problem, the therapist must encourage him to "do more" of what he is already doing with good outcomes. This psychotherapy does not judge the quality of a client's solution, if this is effective. The therapist has the simple role of helping the client to persevere in what he has done and what has worked; that is, to replicate their own "positive" exceptions (→ search for exceptions technique); to do so, the therapist must investigate in detail those exceptions, obtaining a detailed description of how the client acted and of their reactions. Identifying what has worked, can guide them to repeat the success and their situation will further evolve in a positive direction; 3) *If this does not work, do not insist*: complementary to the second principle, the third suggests that, however good a solution may seem, if it does not work, it is not a good solution. A rather bizarre characteristic of human nature is the tendency to try to solve a problem by repeating the same solutions that have already failed (→ attempted solutions). This does not just apply to the client. Many theories suggest that, if the client does not improve, or does not solve the problem, the fault is in the client (and not in the therapist or in the theory); in brief solution-focused psychotherapy, if the client does not overcome the problem, then the "tasks" that have been assigned to them to overcome it need to be changed so that they can experiment with different behaviours; 4) *Small steps can lead to big changes*: this type of therapy may be understood as a minimalistic approach, in which the construction of the solution is accomplished by a series of small steps that are therefore better managed: one small step will produce changes, which in turn will produce more of them, which will result in a much larger systemic change. It follows that helping clients to take small steps to improve their own situation, helps them to move forwards gradually, introducing the desired changes step by step in their daily lives. The process ends when clients describe their situation as improved "enough" to put an end to the therapy; 5) *The solution is not necessarily directly related to the problem*: almost all other approaches to change require a clear definition of the problem to be solved in order to develop a solution strategy; on the contrary, brief solution-focused psychotherapy develops solutions through the description provided by the patient of what will be different once the problem is solved. To do this, it uses a key technique called the → miracle question. Once a detailed description of the "miraculous" scenario has been obtained, therapist and client proceed with the analysis of what has already been done and what worked in the past, that is, the → search for exceptions technique. This path leads to a therapy that spends very little time on investigating the originating causes, the nature of the problem, the pathology of the client or on the analysis of dysfunctional interactions. It focuses instead almost exclusively on the present and future: a real leap of paradigm compared to those models of psychotherapy that focus primarily on the past; 6) *The language to develop the solution is different from that required to describe the problem*: to use the words of L. Wittgenstein: "the world of the happy is quite different from that of the unhappy". Usually the language of the problem is negative, focused on the past (to describe the origins of the problem), and it often feeds the maintenance of the problem itself. On the other hand, the language of the solution is usually more positive, hopeful, focused on the future, and emphasizes the transitory nature of the problems; 7) *Not all the problems occur "all the time"; there are always exceptions that can be used*: this principle, following the concept of the transience of the problem, reflects most of the interventions used in brief solution-focused therapy and suggests that people are always able to see exceptions to their problems, even the smallest ones, and these exceptions can be used to make small changes; 8) *Future is both created and negotiated*: this principle provides a powerful basis for practicing this therapy; people are not considered to be determined by their past history, their social background or by a psychological diagnosis. Based on a constructivist approach (→ constructivism), this principle suggests that the future is a place full of hope where people are the architects of their own destiny. The role of the therapist in this psychotherapy is different from that performed in many other therapeutic approaches: the hierarchy within the therapeutic relationship tends to be more egalitarian and democratic than authoritarian, the style of conducting the session is gentle, never directive. I.K. Berg and S. Dolan argue that therapists of brief solution-focused therapy should avoid expressing judgements of their clients or giving any kind of interpretation about the meanings behind their wishes, needs and behaviours. They must expand their chances rather than limit them and take only the role of one who "stimulates", without pushing the client to do anything in particular. Within the psychotherapy sphere, this model – as it is based on the concept of → resilience and as it uses solutions and exceptions that the customer has already experienced in the past to fix their own problems – is one of the most popular and is used worldwide. Not only has it been applied to a wide range of clinical issues – including family and couple problems, sexual abuse and schizophrenia – but also in interventions within social services, educational, school and business settings. *[R.]*

REFERENCES. De Shazer S., Dolan Y., Korman H., Trepper T., McCollum E., Berg I.K., *More than miracles: The state of the art of solution-focused brief therapy*, 2007.

BRIEF STRATEGIC THERAPY – NARDONE'S MODEL

The advanced brief strategic therapy model, developed by Giorgio Nardone and his collaborators at the Centro di Terapia Strategica in Arezzo, embraces a whole array of specific protocols for the treatment of various psychological disorders, i.e. phobic-obsessive disorders, eating disorders, depression, couple problems, dependencies, child-related problems and so forth. Since its foundation in 1987, initially under the supervision of Weakland and Watzlawick, the centre has carried out ongoing empirical-experimental research involving thousands of patients in the treatment of various psychological problems. The key idea of this work was to develop from general models of therapy, specific protocols of treatment for particular pathologies holding rigorous sequences of therapeutic manoeuvers with → heuristic and predictive (→ predictability) power. The most important and renowned results were achieved mainly with phobic-obsessive and eating disorders with high efficacy and efficiency outcomes, which were scientifically recognized to be actually the highest in the psychotherapy field (87 per cent of solved cases in a median duration of seven sessions).

During these 30y years, this systematic process of → intervention-research, has become an important instrument of knowledge, applicable to the resolution of most human problems encountered in clinical, educational and organizational settings. In a sort of spiral evolution, nourished by the interaction between empirical interventions and epistemological reflections, this study has led to the detectection of a series of specific rigid models of interaction between the subject and his reality, which we coined "→ perceptive-reactive systems" that seem to maintain and often aggravate the problematic situation. This evolved model of the strategic approach goes beyond the nosographic classifications of psychiatry and clinical psychology, which provide a static description of the phenomena, to adopt a more operative means of categorization of human problems, which guides the operator to understand how a system works, to make it work better. By operative knowledge, we mean a cybernetic-constructivist (→ cybernetics, → constructivism) type of description of the modalities of persistence of the problem, i.e. *how* the problem feeds itself through a complex network of perceptive and reactive retroactions between the subject and his or her personal and interpersonal reality. Without any claim to *a priori* knowledge of the phenomena at hand, the strategic therapist seeks, in the complexity of the presented situation, to be a "reducer of complexity", which will allow him to start working on the reality that needs to be modified and which will gradually reveal its functioning. From this standpoint, it is trivial to know how a problem was formed in the past, but it is interesting to know what actually protracts it in the present so as to understand what can be done. In order to change a situation, one should be able to stop its persistence, by identifying and blocking the "circular causality" between how a problem persists and the ineffective ways people try to solve the problem. Therefore, to induce change, it is important to concentrate on the dysfunctional solutions that are being attempted. If we manage to block or change the recursive dysfunctional solutions, we interrupt the vicious circle that nourishes the persistence of the problem, opening the way to inevitable change. Based on the studies of the Palo Alto school, such a reducer of complexity has been found in the construct of → attempted solutions. When a problem emerges within a certain context (individual, couple or family, organization) there is a tendency to reapply interventions that have been successful in solving similar problems in the past. Even when strategies strongly fail, rather than applying alternative solutions, there is a tendency to apply the same strategy more vigorously, based on the illusion that doing "more than before" will be more effective. Such attempts to reiterate the same ineffective solution eventually give life to a complex process of retroactions in which the efforts to achieve change actually keep the problematic situation unchanged. As Watzlawick maintained, the attempted solution actually becomes the problem. The strategic therapist is a sort of action researcher; the only epistemological variable of knowledge that he can control is his own strategy, i.e. our "attempted solution". If the strategy works, it enables the researcher to understand the functioning of the reality that is being studied. This is in line with Lewin's concepts of change and stasis, which denote that in order to understand how a process works, one needs to introduce a change and observe its variable effects, i.e. knowing through changing. We come to know a reality by operating on it, gradually adjusting our interventions, adapting them to the new elements of knowledge that emerged step by step. The Advanced Therapy Model is the final result of such an empirical-experimental process, guided by models of mathematical logic, which can be continuously checked and verified, and which furthermore, owing to its formalization, can be replicated (→ replicability) and didactically transferred (→ transferability). This approach to therapy and research renders this model not only highly effective and efficient but even highly predictive. This enabled us to evolve brief strategic therapy from an artistic-creative practice into a sort of rigorous advanced technology. This *saltus* in the model was achieved without losing its characteristic inventive aspect, which is necessary for its ongoing innovation process, while respecting rigorously scientific criteria. Therapy became an ongoing investigative–intervening process, where every intervention is tailored to every single case and individual patient. As Milton Erickson affirmed, every person owns unique and unrepeatable features, such as his interaction with himself, the others and the world. Thus, even though there are common features and redundancies, each case always represents something original. Every human interaction, including the therapeutic relations, results in being unique and unrepeatable. Only if the therapist manages to understand and tune in (→ tuning technique) with the underlying logic and the "language of the patient", can he proceed to "successfully" and thoroughly investigate the problem presented and eventually chose the most adequate manoeuvers to arrive at its solution. In this way, the therapeutic intervention can truly maintain its capacity to adapt itself to every new person's peculiarity and situation, while remaining rigorously adapted to the structure of the intervention. The strategic therapist avails himself of a series of flexible tactics and tools that can be adjusted to the different patients and problems under treatment. His interventions are not developed from scratch, but, following the logic of the type of problem and its → resistance to change, he chooses the most appropriate strategies, tailoring them to the specific case. Moreover, the strategic therapist, who we like to define as a problem-solver, gradually corrects and adjusts the model of intervention based on the effects observed during the problem-solving process (→ self-correctiveness). While this model is rigorous and systematic, it also has the important characteristic of being flexible and self-correcting. It can be modified and adapted throughout its interaction with the reality to which it is applied. In line with Popper's work, this saves it from rigid, "self-immunizing" positions. The possibility of correcting the intervention based on its observed effects exists at every single phase of the problem-solving process. That means that effectiveness is not measured only between the beginning and the end of the therapy, but is gradually evaluated for each single move and manoeuver, so that the model of intervention constantly confirms or corrects itself during its application. The Advanced Brief Strategic Model is based on the premise that it is impossible and even misleading, to pretend to know *a priori* the right route to reach an objective; the only way is to start travelling along that route, overcoming, step by step, the obstacles encounted and "riding the good waves" and the resources of the person or system. Developed from a constructivist approach, this model privileges the idea that humans construct their behaviour based on their perceptions of lived or imagined experience. An intervention aimed at changing a situation must provide a different experience in the perception of the reality to be changed – as Alexander would say, a → corrective emotional experience. This opens the way to different reactions, which, if consolidated, bring the person to second-order change (→ first- and second-order change), i.e. it changes a person's perception of reality, producing consequently a change even at the emotional, cognitive and behavioural levels. Such → corrective emotional experiences are triggered by means of strategic interventions based on non-ordinary → logic, such as the → logic of paradox, the → logic of contradiction and the → logic of belief. Since Gödel demolished the possibility of a rigorously rational logic in his treatise on "Undecidable propositions", mathematical logic has evolved towards the development of models that consider contradiction, self-deception and paradox to be rigorous and predictive procedures in the construction of human beliefs and behaviour.

Based on these new types of logic, we can systematically apply non-ordinary logical procedures to construct → stratagems capable of leading to objectives or solutions of problems that would seem unreachable and unsolvable if approached through ordinary logic. Most human problems are nonlinear phenomena, which are often treated using ordinary logic, bringing them to point of exasperation. Most human psychological problems such as phobias, obsessive-compulsive disorders, depression, eating disorders and also presumed psychosis are not irrational or illogical, but follow a non-ordinary logic. So the strategic therapist follows and utilizes the underlying non-ordinary logic of the problem to bring it to its self-annulment. By revealing and exploiting the non-ordinary logic the strategic therapist is enriched by alternative → stratagems that put into question and eventually change rigid perceptions and actions. This enables the individual to rediscover his resources, which have been imprisoned in the "vicious circle" of interaction between attempts to solve the problem and the persistence of the problem.

Thanks to its rigorous yet self-corrective properties, the Advanced Brief Strategic Model has been successfully applied in various contexts, from the clinical to the educational, from interpersonal relationships to the organizational world, with astonishing results. In spite of this, our constant mission remains that of finding always more effective and efficient means – in our strategies, communication and therapeutic relationship – that take us beyond what has been achieved so far. In accordance with Abrahamson, we are constantly engaged in continuous action research, giving equal weight to scientific rigour (i.e. treatment efficacy) and clinical utility (i.e. treatment effectiveness). *[C. Portelli, G. Nardone]*

REFERENCES. Milanese R., Mordazzi P., *Strategic choaching*, 2015; Nardone G., *Brief strategic solution-oriented therapy of phobic and obsessive disorders*, 1996; Id., *Oltre i limiti della paura*, 2000; Id., *Non c'è notte che non veda il giorno*, 2003; Id., *Cavalcare la propria tigre*, 2003; Id., *Problem solving strategico da tasca*, 2009; Nardone G., Balbi E., *The logic of therapeutic change*, 2015; Nardone G., Milanese R., *Il cambiamento strategico*, 2018; Nardone G., Portelli C., *Knowing through changing*, 2005; Nardone G., Verbitz T., Milanese R., *Prison of food*, 2005; Nardone G., Watzlawick P., *The art of change*, 1993.

BRIEF THERAPY – MRI'S MODEL

In 1965, Richard Fisch proposed a "brief therapy clinic and evaluation project" to Don D. Jackson, founder and director of the → Mental Research Institute (MRI) in Palo Alto, California. It led to the establishment of the Brief Therapy Center (BTC), which became MRI's most widely recognized project. The BTC first opened its doors to clients in early 1967, at a time when Jay Haley (who left MRI in 1967) and Jackson (who died in 1968) also participated, and where Richard Fisch, its director, John Weakland and Paul Watzlawick teamed up and developed what is known as MRI's Brief Therapy. MRI's Brief Therapy, which continued to be worked on and refined for years after initial publication of the model and its tactics, could be said to encapsulate ideas that came to prominence in the years after World War II, such as → cybernetics (when the problem presented by the client in therapy is seen as being maintained by feedback loops in the → here-and-now); systemic thinking (when problems are deemed to be created and to exist in interactions, and therefore intrasystemically rather than intrapsychically); and → constructivism (when the only valid "reality" to be worked with is the client's), ideas that changed our way of thinking about human behaviour, communication and human interactions. They made way for a new approach in centreing psychotherapy both strategically (with a → problem-solving step-wise model that is goal-oriented) and tactically (with new considerations for shaping client–therapist interactions), thus forging a kind of therapy that was quite novel at the time, both conceptually and in its therapeutic practice. Grounded in the work of the Bateson Research Project, influenced by Milton H. Erickson's hypnosis (→ Ericksonian hypnotherapy), and having adopted many of the premises of the family therapy developed and practiced by Don D. Jackson, the research endeavour at → MRI's BTC, with an interest in reducing sessions to a minimum and a focus on how problems were formed and how they could be resolved, culminated in the creation of a minimalist, bare-bones approach that gets to the essence of what needs to be done to induce change quickly and effectively. MRI's Brief Therapy is both problem-focused and interactional, and is conducted following three basic steps: the *first step* consists of closely identifying and narrowing down the spectrum of problems (presented and defined by the client) to the one problem chosen by the client to be worked on "first", requiring the client to prioritize his or her concerns. The therapist then asks for the interactive context in which the problem selected to be worked on manifests itself, and helps identify the behavioural sequences in that interaction that best elucidate the problem. In this way the problem is made specific and concrete. So, if a client comes to therapy complaining about his relationship with his spouse, the therapist will have the client list the different aspects of his relationship that are problematic for him; then the client will be asked to state which aspect he would like to work on or "fix" first, since this therapy involves working on one narrowly defined problem at a time. The therapist will invite the client to relate a typical interaction where the problem is present, and will inquire into the most specific details of the behavioural sequences that pinpoint the workings of the problem in question. The *second step* involves the Brief Therapy team's most original contribution – the need for inquiring about the client's → attempted solutions. The team had discovered that no matter how a problem began, the very solutions that clients implemented in their best effort to fix it not only *did not* work, but tended to increase its magnitude. Therefore, after identifying and delimiting the problem to be worked on, and because problems are considered to be maintained by ineffective solution attempts, the therapist inquires about all those "attempted" solutions (the ways the client has tried to solve the problem, including the advice received from others) that have not worked (or not well enough, for if they had, there would no longer be a problem). As a *third step*, once the problem-maintaining, ineffective behaviours, i.e. attempted solutions, are pinpointed, the therapist has to identify the common message contained in them, and help the client find a message-altering solution, one that constitutes a 180-degree reversal from the ineffective solutions that have kept the client "stuck" in the problem. (The metaphor of a "180-degree reversal" is used to indicate the radical change of behaviour the new solution requires to allow for the problem to no longer exist.) Clients are often assigned homework containing the alternative message. The expectation is that changing words and actions create different interactions, which in turn will change perceptions, opening the way for a different experience.

Just as the client must engage in communications (i.e. behaviours) that constitute a 180-degree shift from the problem-maintaining attempted solutions, so too the therapist must be on the alert so as *not* to repeat what others have advised or tried (that obviously failed to achieve a meaningful resolution for the client). It often means acting in a manner counter to what "common sense" would perhaps dictate. So if a previous therapist, or a friend, encouraged the client to keep trying (to lose weight, to support or put limits on her partner, etc.), in Brief Therapy the therapist must then "discourage" the client from doing so. Furthermore, the therapist will often point to the "disadvantages" of change, or prescribe the very symptom (→ symptom prescription) the client is complaining about, in keeping with the notion that only a 180-degree reversal from what has not worked has a chance of helping the client get "unstuck".

Brief Therapy *à la* MRI fully implements the paradigmatic change from viewing problems as located within the individual's psyche to seeing problems as located within systemic processes in the here-and-now. It incorporates an anthropological understanding of human phenomena, where the meaning of behaviour is searched for in its "cultural" context, with "culture" varying from family to family. Behaviours as such are seen as neither right nor wrong, nor as sick or healthy, but are likely to be looked at from the point of view of whether they work for the client, or not, in the particular interaction under discussion. It is thus that Brief Therapy is said to operate with a non-normative (and therefore non-pathologizing), ahistorical approach. When a client comes to therapy with a problem, it is important to look at *how* the problem is a problem for the client and *how* it manifests itself interactively in the present, rather than to search for an origin to the problem in the past or through an assessment of pathology. It works with the notion that people construct their own realities based on their accumulated experience, and that we must always consider the client's "position" (how the client constructs the situation in question) vis-à-vis the problem. A mother may complain about her child's laziness and refusal to put sufficient effort into his homework, while the father may think that the teachers are too demanding and that the child is faltering as a result of his inability to keep up. The mother's *position* here is that the child is "lazy" or "bad", while the father's *position* is that the child is "not able" to do his work. It is this position that the therapist interacts with while aiming for the client to alter his or her construction of the problem. In keeping with this goal, one of the important ways of intervening in Brief Therapy is by offering the client a "reframe" (→ reframing), an alternative view of what the client considers to be symptomatic of the problem, yet keeping the reframe within plausible limits of the client's position.

At the BTC, the idea of a systemic therapy was expanded to include work with individual members of the system, for it is understood that a significant change in one member of the system will have repercussions in its other member(s). So when a family's or a couple's problems are dealt with in Brief Therapy, the therapist can opt to work with only one member of that system (couple, family, or organization) and still achieve changes in the system as a whole. It gives the therapist a choice as to whom to work with, allowing him or her to pick the more motivated member(s), or the one(s) most available or willing, without compromising the systemic change sought. So when a wife wants "couple's therapy", but states that her husband is not willing, the Brief Therapist can work with her alone on the couple's problem. While not precluding work with several members of the system jointly, the added option of working with them separately can simplify interacting with their respective positions. All of the foregoing accounts for a great reduction in the number of sessions needed to fix the problem, and for making this approach not only befitting cross-cultural treatment conditions, but well-suited to most populations throughout the world. *[K. Anger, B. Anger-Diaz]*

REFERENCES. Watzlawick, P., *Change: Principles of problem formation and problem resolution*, 1974; Fisch R., Weakland J.H., Segal, L., *The tactics of change: Doing therapy briefly*, 1982.

BRIEF THERAPY PROJECT

The Brief Therapy Project came to life in 1967 at the → Mental Research Institute (MRI) in Palo Alto, California, becoming its most acclaimed research endeavour. In 1965, Richard Fisch approached Don D. Jackson, founder and director of the MRI, with the idea of setting up a "brief therapy clinic and evaluation project", funding for which Jackson was able to secure. It led to the establishment of the Brief Therapy Center (BTC), where Richard Fisch, John Weakland and Paul Watzlawick collaborated in the development of a step-wise, problem-focused, strategic therapy model that did away with most of the theoretical underpinnings of what was then conventional practice (long-term, intrapsychic, pathology-based psychotherapy, with a historically linear perspective). With an interactional, circular view of problem formation and resolution, focused on the → here-and-now, therapy at the BTC evolved within a systemic framework and a constructivist (→ constructivism) epistemology. It pioneered practices that while common today, broke with tradition, such as the recording of sessions, the use of the one-way mirror to observe and intervene in ongoing sessions, working as a team – all within a time-limited context. *[B. Anger-Díaz, K. Anger]*

REFERENCES. Fisch R., Weakland J.H., Segal L., *The tactics of change: Doing therapy briefly*, 1982; Watzlawick P., Weakland J.H., Fisch R., *Change: Principles of problem formation and problem resolution*, 1974.

BT-STEPS

It is a form of computer-aided self-help by cognitive behaviour therapy for obsessive-compulsive disorder. With guidance from BT-Steps, patients identify the triggers for their compulsive rituals and obsessive thoughts, work out personalized goals to overcome these, and learn to do self-exposure and cognitive homework exercises to reduce their obsessive-compulsive problem. BT-Steps users also had minimal brief human support by phone and/or email. Improvement guided by BT-Steps and an associated manual has been as great as that from face-to-face cognitive behaviour therapy. NICE (the National Institute for Health and Care Excellence in England and Wales) recognizes the clinical efficacy of BT-Steps for the management of obsessive-compulsive disorder. Access to BT-Steps has been by interactive voice response on the phone plus a self-help manual, and is planned in future to be used on the internet at home. *[I. Marks]*

REFERENCES. Marks I., *Living with fear: Understanding and coping with anxiety*, 1978; Marks I., Cavanagh K., Gega L., *Hands-on help: Computer-aided psychotherapy*, 2007.

C

CAPACITY TO THINK

According to Bion, a mental faculty "which is rudimentary in all of us", especially when it concerns the phenomenon of life itself. It requires an inner space free from the invasion of stimuli, both external and internal. This is achieved by focusing the attention on the present moment. It is necessary to have the strength to tolerate frustrations, rather than avoiding them through an indiscriminate evacuation of unsatisfactory experiences. An attitude of tolerated doubt "without any irritable reaching after facts and reason" facilitates the coming together of fragmentary facts in a new understanding, that is, thinking. Also, it facilitates their subsequent spreading, which is a precondition for a new coherence to emerge. *[J. Symington]*

REFERENCES. Bion W.R., *Learning from experience*, 1962; Keats J., *Letters to George and Thomas Keats*, 21 December 1817 quoted in Bion, W.R., *Attention and interpretation*, 1970.

CASE RECORD

An empirical sample of patients belonging to specific psychodiagnostic categories, subject to statistical control of the efficacy and duration of treatment. The typically studied variables in clinical case records are: socio-cultural indicators, incidence of disorder in population, clinical progress, familiarity of disorder, → efficacy and → efficiency of psychotherapy. In medicine, case records determine the most appropriate type of intervention protocol for the observed symptomatology. Similarly, in psychotherapy, they guide the psychologist in determining and choosing the most effective intervention for the problem reported by the patient. *[R.]*

CASTRATION

In Freudian psychoanalysis, a concept used to explain the overcoming of the → Oedipus complex (the father threatens the son with castration). Since the child has, in the unconscious, the necessary sexual fantasy and energy to activate it, this creates the conditions for the emergence of a neurosis that concerns all humanity. The term is used for the removal of a real penis and takes different forms in males and females. The first experience the threat of castration as punishment for their sexual desires towards the mother. Conversely, the female perceives the lack of penis as a serious injustice and she tries to deny this condition or to fix it for her entire life. In response to objections to the fact that these anxieties had a solid foundation, Freud said that castration was an event that occurred in the "primitive horde" and that, therefore, each male was born with the predisposition to have fantasies that might be related to that experience. Instead, the female would not address adequately the Oedipus complex, due to the absence of a castration anxiety. *[G. Fossi]*

▷Lacanian psychoanalysis adopted the Freudian concept of castration, interpreting it as the totality of the consequences of the threat (of the ghost) of castration in the male child and the absence of a penis in the female child. This approach considers castration to be the outcome of a symbolic function that does not concern a real organ – the penis – but the signifier that represents it, namely the phallus in its imaginary dimension. The function of castration is closely related to the → Oedipus complex, which Lacan organizes in three logical (and not chronological) phases. That is, they do not correspond to the so-called child development "stages": in the first stage, the child, male or female, wants to be the phallus that attracts the desire of the mother; in the second stage, the father, in his symbolic function, implements a double interdiction: towards the child, to whom he interdicts the mother, and towards the mother, to whom he forbids making the child her own object and completion. This interdiction, if effective, marks for the child the end of the omnipotence of the mother, who must bow to the paternal interdiction and separate herself from her child. In the third stage, the actual father shows himself to the child as the one who, having imposed his law, has the phallus and for this reason is the mother's favourite. At the end of three logical phases the Oedipus complex closes, ideally, with the renunciation of the desire to be the mother's imaginary phallus and with the acceptance of their shortcoming, and thus of the mother's castration in addition to their own. In fact, the acceptance of the shortcoming is what characterizes the accomplished castration and what allows a sexed position to be taken: for the male child through the identification with the father and for the female child through accepting herself as the object of desire of men. *[M. Fiumanò]*

REFERENCES. Freud S. (1900–1901), *The interpretation of dreams*, in *The Standard Edition*, IV–V, 1953–1974; Lacan J. (1966), *The signification of the phallus*, in *Écrits: A selection*, 1972; Id., *The seminar of Jaques Lacan IV: The object relation*, 1956–1957.

CATHARSIS

A tension decrease resulting from verbal or emotional expression of life experiences that deeply involve the patient. The term is traditionally used by hypnotherapists (→ hypnosis) to define the phenomenon of "mental liberation" that, in a state of hypnotic trance, leads the person to express repressed or traumatic emotions. *[R.]*

▷ In *Poetics*, Aristotle describes catharsis as the purifying effect of a dramatic work on the audience. On the contrary, according to J.L. Moreno, father of psychodrama, catharsis consists in the action of anyone who performs their life, becoming actor–author of self. So, he introduces into the world of the theatre and of psychotherapy a new professional role, that of therapeutic directors halfway between doctors and priests who, instead of expressing their work, devote themselves to a kind of theatre that treats people. Moreno, holistic doctor of the soul, is not an inventor but a discoverer: the psycho-catharsis is always related to spontaneity, while the professional actor could suffer from a "histrionic neurosis" that prevents them from finding the true meaning of their life. It should be noted that catharsis in psychodrama is not limited to the outburst of suffering and goes beyond → abreaction of repressed feelings, culminating in the creation of new images and new encounters, which release the existence of the patient. The main character of the game, with the help of the group, leaves the old context that imprisons them and enters a world more free and wider in which he/she takes new roles and learns to transform their network of relationships. In summary, the catharsis begins when the patient stages "their" characters in search of an author and culminates when the crucial turning point (*peripeteia*) of their destiny takes place. *[O. Rosati]*

REFERENCES. Moreno J.L., *Psychodrama first volume*, 1946; Rosati O., *Da storia nasce storia*, 1993.

CATHARTIC METHOD

According to Freud, catharsis is a psychotherapeutic method that allows a person, after having remembered or relived a traumatic event, to discharge an excess of pathogenic energy caused by the trauma itself. The cathartic method was utilized between 1890 and 1895 by Breuer and Freud. This method was directly connected with hypnosis, during which the subject could recover the memory of the event. At a later time, Freud abandoned hypnosis and tried to persuade patients to remember the event. This allowed them to release the affect caused by the traumatic experience, stored up in body innervations and provoking hysterical symptoms. The entire theory expresses, on the one hand the drama of the hysterical crises at that time, which were illustrated by Charcot; on the other hand, it shows the energetic paradigm of nineteenth-century neurology. Our brain is activated by an energy different from the energy of metabolic processes; it is a nervous energy with qualitative characteristics; in the Freudian theory, its origin is first traumatic and then sexual. The accumulation of this energy is painful or pathogenic; the discharge is pleasant or therapeutic. Nowadays, this concept has become less important. With the formulation of the structural theory (→ Id, → Ego, → Superego) and the development of Ego theory, psychoanalysis has progressively left the cathartic method behind. *[G. Fossi]*

REFERENCES. Breuer J., Freud S. (1895), *Studies on hysteria*, in *The Standard Edition*, II, 1953–1974.

CAUSALISM

Epistemological perspective (→ epistemology) that presumes the possibility of identifying a linear cause–effect relation amongst different factors inside a psychological phenomenon. The most ingenuous version of causalism applied to psychology is represented by the idea that what is lived in the present is the effect of what was lived in the past (linear causalism), or also by the idea that the temporal concomitance (or the strict nearness) of events implies necessarily their causal link (temporal causalism). Though this positivist perspective of causalism has been widely acceptedc in the physical and mathematical sciences since last century – just thinking about Godel's, Einstein's and Heisenberg's contributions, that is, principles of indecisiveness, relativity and indetermination –, causalism survives in psychotherapy because of an ingenuous perspective of observation of psychopathological phenomena. There are two models of causalism still disseminated in the psychological sciences. The first is mechanic causalism (or empiric), directly imported from physical sciences, according to which a precise relation between psychological qualities and behavioural reactions exists. The second is teleological causalism (or rational), which considers human behaviour as directed by purposes instead of by causes. Some psychotherapeutic models, in particular within the psychodynamic paradigm, still refer to causalistic principles and consider the solution to the discomfort of their disturbed patients to lie in the uncovering of past causes. *[R.]*

CAUSALITY

The causal perspective brings every aspect of psychic life to a set of general normative forces and tends to give to these aspects "legal" explanations or explanations that refer to other previously mentioned elements. The use of a discrete set of heuristic categories is encouraged by the likelihood that the general similarity of mental processes in individuals should have, as a basis, similarly general laws. The "reductive analytic" method (according to Jung, typical of psychoanalysis but it can also be used by analytical psychology) aims to know how the individual psyche has come into being. Therefore, not only does it aim to explain this individuality in the present, but also traces future developments with reference to the causes that determined its current configuration. Within this definition of causality, psychotherapy descends into the problem of the potential finalistic sense (→ finalism) of psychic processes. *[E. V. Trapanese]*

CENSORSHIP

In Freudian psychoanalysis, a permanent function of the mental apparatus that is destined to build a barrier between unconscious contents, which push to become conscious and to realize themselves in behaviour or fantasies, and the conscious/preconscious system. An analogous, but less potent, barrier exists between conscious and preconscious contents. Particularly important is the censorship working during dreams against the fantasies wanting to become conscious. These fantasies could, however, appear masked by the oneiric work (→ condensation, → displacement, → symbolism) and obtain, in this way, partial satisfaction. In fact, as the satisfaction of fantasies is impossible while asleep, censorship is less rigid compared to wakefulness: for this reason, dreams have become the "royal" road to the unconscious. *[G. Fossi]*

REFERENCES. Freud S., (1900–1901), *The interpretation of dreams*, in *The Standard Edition*, IV–V, 1953–1974;

CENTROVERSION

Within Jung's analytic psychology, a term that refers to the movement of the psyche from the periphery towards the centre, a tendency that becomes evident in the individuation process. The movement is not linear, but follows a spiral formation around a hypothetical centre; it is also called *circumambulation*, as a dance rotating around a centre. In the first half of one's life, centroversion manifests itself in the compensation between consciousness and unconscious, that remains unaware, as the Ego ignores its dependence on the wholeness. In the second half of one's life, centroversion becomes evident to the consciousness in the constellation of the Self as the consciously experienced psychic centre of the wholeness. This psychic process, aiming towards a goal, is expressed in a sequence of images, which appear finalized, without being induced by any external suggestion. *[M. Gay]*

REFERENCES. Jung C.G. (1916–1952), *The structure and dynamics of the psyche*, in *Collected Works*, VIII, 1969; Id., (1944), *Pychology and alchemy*, in *Collected Works*, VIII, 1968; Neumann E., *The origins and history of consciousness*, 1954.

CHANGE

In the philosophical-religious sphere, a term closely connected to the concept of becoming. In fact, it relates to the concepts of birth and death, identity and diversity, eternity and finiteness. Heraclitus, the Greek philosopher of eternal becoming, argued that *pólemos* ("conflict") governs all things and that perennial change derives from this play of forces permeating nature: nothing is forever, nothing remains the same, everything changes, turns, flows (*panta rei*). From an evolutionary perspective, it is argued that species evolved and survived thanks to their capability – each different from the other – to adapt to change. Regarding human behaviour, as change, communication and interaction are inevitable, it follows that human behaviour is a source of constant changes both within the same person and in its relationship with the outside world. Obviously change can go towards both an ameliorative and pejorative (or pathological) modification of the system. When it comes to therapeutic change, we talk about a change that is not fortuitous, but focused on a definite direction, which should be defined *a priori* as a therapeutic goal. This work involves – as a relational system – the "disturbance" of a homeostatic (→ homeostasis) or autopoietic (→ autopoiesis) system, that always adapts to the new achieved state. Hence the importance of knowing in advance the direction towards which change can be induced. According to this non-linear logic of change, there are three different types of change: catastrophic, when it is quick and immediate, caused by an "experience" on the basis of which the subject can only change their previous mental and behavioural scripts; gradual, generated step by step by introducing many small changes until a goal is reached; exponential geometrical, caused by a chain reaction where the first change will lead to an inevitable sequence of changes up to an almost "explosive" scenario. *[R.]*

CHARACTER

Within character analysis (→ bioenergetics), a defensive structure investigated by Reich used to define psychological resistances and chronic muscle contractions that jointly oppose the success of therapy. Reich realized that many patients expressed hostility and → resistance to change using a nonverbal language. He noticed that patients tended to resort to psychoanalytic treatment to become free from symptoms, but wanting to preserve their own vision of themselves and the world. Although symptoms were perceived as disturbing, this vision was uncritically accepted, as it was usually the result of the morality of the times (Reich worked in the early decades of the twentieth century, when there was a restrictive morality that, by preventing free expression of sexuality, was a cause of neurotic suffering, like, for example, hysteria). Psychological resistances and chronic muscle contractions determine a psycho-corporeal organization, that is, the character of a person, whose bodily aspects, the "muscle armour", are functionally identical to the psychological defensive organization. The character, or "character armour", represents the acquisition, within personality, of what Reich calls "imposed anti-emotional and anti-libidinal morality". Reich distinguishes between people with a healthy genital character, with an energy free from fixations, whose body is capable of self-regulation and of fully surrendering to orgasm, and neurotic characters, whose bodily and psychological organization prevents the emergence of repressed impulses and defends itself against pleasure. Lowen, the most important follower of Reichian thought, takes up the theme of character and reorganizes its etiology, starting from the personal history of each person in the encounter with the environment. According to Reich, there are five fundamental rights/needs that, during the development phase of each human being, seek satisfaction in succession: being accepted by the world, needing, being independent, being supported, being sexed. If the environment frustrates these needs/rights, chronic muscular contractions and psychological defences emerge and make up the character. *[R. Filoni, P. Moselli]*

REFERENCES. Lowen A., *The language of the body*, 1958; Id., *Joy: The surrender to the body and to life*, 1995; Reich W., *On character analysis*, 1933.

CHARACTER ANALYSIS

A therapeutic and diagnostic method. Precondition for intervention in every Reichian therapy and in bioenergetic analysis (→ bioenergetics). *[P. Moselli]*

CHARACTER ARMOUR

An expression coined by W. Reich to define the character organization (→ character) of individuals. A character armour represents a person's chronic mental mobility limitation against the pleasure–displeasure principle. This protection mechanism finds its expression, both qualitative and quantitative, in the denial of libidinal impulses; also on the somatic side, through some sort of energy retention rings that are placed throughout the body and limit its expressiveness, starting from the bodily blocks identified by Reich: from the ocular to the pelvis block. *[P. Moselli, L. Parmeggiani]*

REFERENCES. Mercurio A., *Antropologia esistenziale e metapsicologia personalistica*, 1991.

CHARACTER TYPES

According to Fromm, as in other modern characterological classifications, character types do not constitute fixed taxonomies and standardized categories, but are more likely to represent the tendencies present, to a greater or lesser degree in every individual. Fromm articulated his theory of characteriology within the context of his wider range of studies of the theory of personality. He departed from the basic assumption that there is a reciprocal conditioning that takes place between an individual and society, and based his theory on the concept of "productivity". The characters clarified by Fromm constitute a typology empirically validated with statistically based research, and using → projective tests, operating within the doctrine expressed in all his works. In his theory of personality, he describes it as being that combination of personal and subjective inclinations with which each individual, in all his humanity and in his total uniqueness, describes and informs, in a concrete manner, his relationship with himself, the world, the Other.

Within personality theory, Fromm distinguishes the character from temperament, and he considers this pair as being the foundation of the individual personality. The temperament is the total of the inherited psychological characteristics and is made up of the constitutional factors that find expression in the reaction of the individual to the stimuli coming from his environment; the character is that combination of qualities acquired by the individual, of his characteristics, of the traits with which he relates to the Other and to society, and is conditioned by the filters to the stimuli coming from both the inside and the outside. Fromm also refers to Hippocrates, who distinguished four different kinds of temperaments – choleric, sanguine, melancholic, phlegmatic –, in this way underlining the relationship between temperament and biology.

According to Fromm, the character forms as a result of experience and is also a combination of competencies that are able to modulate the temperament in the functioning of personality; the character influences behaviour by leaving its imprint on the actions of the individual. Fromm defines the family as being "the psychological agency of society". Within the family, Fromm observes that both the process of assimilation as well as that of socialization contribute to the formation of the character, which is determined by the incessant energy of human nature channelled in these continuously developing processes. The character develops into the psychological structure of man, within the context of the family and of society, on the basis of "passions"; the concept of character for Fromm substitutes the concept of → instinct, used by

S. Freud in the theory of the → libido. The passions give "consistency, direction and movement according to the reactions to the fundamental conflicts of existence. Love, tenderness, the need for justice, for independence, for the truth, hate, sadism, masochism, narcissism are all human passions".

The orientation towards the world that derives from this process is characterized in two ways: productive and non-productive. The first can be found in those individuals that tend to fulfil their potentialities by participating, in a productive and constructive manner, in life in society; whilst the second are those that are not able to fulfil their Ego to its full potential. The productive character is the result of a lifetime of development to the full; the individual with a productive character is not alienated, he is mature and full of love, a love that takes place through respect towards the Other, awareness, a sense of responsibility, knowledge, sociability. Fromm discusses and distinguishes five types of love in his book *The Art of Loving*: fraternal, between parents and children, erotic, towards oneself and towards God. The productive character is a point of reference, for Fromm, in the scrutiny of the negative aspects of a non-productive orientation, where he evidences various character types: *receptive*, characterized by a lack of sense of initiative, dependent on the external world, with a tendency towards optimism, and towards confidence; *exploitative*, dominated by dependence on the external world, whose attitude is aimed towards obtaining things through the use of cunning and strength (with a tendency towards being suspicious and cynical); *hoarding*, characterized by lack of faith in the external world, focused on himself, setting up a wall between himself and the world; his sense of justice is expressed through the use of the phrase "What is mine is mine, what is yours is yours". The *hoarder* is an example of a character type that has an unchangeable attitude; *marketing* expresses a condition typical of contemporary man; it is the most flexible and open to change, in that he bases his success on his ability to change: "I am as you would like me to be".

The character types do not constitute a fixed taxonomy and have standardized categories; instead, more accurately, as in all the other modern characterological systems, they represent tendencies that are present to a certain degree in every personality. There are men and women in whom a particular tendency appears to be more accentuated than others, but also cases in which a tendency manifests itself with hints that are less apparent. Productivity does not necessarily exclude the belonging to a non-productive type, in that productivity itself is not a variable but a mode of orientation of the character, and can be attained through different methods by each human being. In *Anatomy of Human Destructiveness*, Fromm described a negative character type, defined as being "necrophiliac" (→ necrophilia): attracted to death, alienated from life; this orientation can be contrasted to the tendency towards → biophilia, and represents the extreme, defined by Fromm himself as being pathologically distanced from the value of the character with a productive orientation. As in the other typologies, the necrophiliac will rarely be found in a "pure form"; whilst it is more likely that there are, in man, elements of the character traits associated with this specific classification, in its full force it deserves to be the object of close clinical examination. *[I. Battaglini, E. Benelli]*

REFERENCES. Biancoli R., *Erich Fromm therapeutische Annäherung oder die Kunst der Psychotherapie*, in *Der unbekannte Fromm. Biographische Studien*, 1987; Id., *L'approccio psicoterapeutico di Erich Fromm*, 1987; Fromm E., Man for himself: An inquiry into the psychology of ethics, 1947; *The art of loving*, 1956; Id., *Anatomy of human destructiveness*, 1973; Id., *To have or to be*, 1976.

CHARISMATIC THERAPIST

The psychotherapist is an essential instrument of psychotherapy, whether it is individual therapy, couples therapy or family therapy. The term charismatic, in reference to the psychotherapist, can however be ambiguous in its meaning, particularly when by charismatic one means the capacity to create uncritical subjection and not a predisposition towards → change and new → redefinitions validated by an authoritative attitude. The more this sense of authoritativeness is present in the relationship, without rituals and drama, the more the therapist will be able to contribute positively to change. The relationship is, by definition, one of change: the more this takes place with the active participation of the individual involved, the more effective it will be. On the other hand, the more the therapist puts the patient into a passive role, and is overactive and unwilling to delegate, in this way manipulating the patient, the higher the risk of the change being fictitious and limited. The charisma of the therapist becomes positive only when it enables the family system to start the process of self-determination and not of hetero-determination. A therapist who has good charisma will help the system he is treating achieve the ultimate goal of becoming autonomous and no longer dependent on him. In the field of systemic therapy these themes have been discussed by Miller. *[F. Bruni, P.G. Defilippi]*

REFERENCES. Miller J.G., *Living systems*, 1978.

CHILD

In the area of transactional analysis, it is the name given to one of the three → Ego states described by Berne. The Child Ego state corresponds to the egoic fixation of significant infantile experiences during an individual's development. This fixation remains in the Ego and it can reactivate itself and provoke an experience of ways of thinking and feeling in the "here and now", with appropriate behavioural styles, such as to produce an adaptation to the environment analogous to that experienced in the "there and then" of childhood. Phenomenologically, individuals of an adult age respond to a stimulus as if they were still the child of that period of development. Berne hypothesized an underlying biological structure at the stage of the Ego Child, which he defined as archaeopsychic (→ archaeopsyche), a depository for the experiences tied to primary needs. He distinguished an archaeopsychic Ego state free from the inhibitory influences given by environmental pressures – defined as Free Child – and another, on the other hand, controlled by the same pressures – defined as Adaptive Child. In transactional analysis, the Child is considered as an elective place of expression of the phenomenon of transference (in the patient) and countertransference (in the psychotherapist). Mistakenly, the Child was considered a primary origin of pathological communication, and as such, an area of personality in itself pathological. From a psychodynamic point of view, this became the main source of the recovery of the emotional and intuitive potential of the patient. *[M. Novellino]*

REFERENCES. Berne E., *Games people play*, 1964; Id., *Transactional analysis in psychotherapy*, 1961; M. Novellino, *Psicoanalisi transazionale*, 2005.

CHRONICIZATION

A gradual process through which a psychological disorder becomes a structural characteristic and a constant in the psychic organization of an individual. Chronicization typically occurs as a result of the repeated absence or inadequacy of effective treatments in solving an increasing psychological difficulty, which may initially not be recognized as such (for example due to diagnostic or family negligence); or it has been recognized but improperly treated (for example as a result of "institutionalization"); or, finally, it can be addressed belatedly, although functionally (in these cases, there could be a partial recovery from symptoms but without a substantial change in the dynamics of the disorder). There is no agreement among scholars about when to consider a disorder to be chronic, whether years or a few months after the onset of the first → symptoms. Instead, there is greater agreement about the empirical rule according to which it is not correct to speak of chronic disorders before the attainment of adulthood (meaning the post-pubertal age), where there is a progressive stabilization of hormonal and psychological functions. *[R.]*

CHTHONIC

In Jungian analytical psychology, a quality of the "earthly" and "dark" sphere. "All archetypes, in addition to a positive, favourable, clear, facing upwards character, have also a facing downwards, partially negative and unfavourable and partly simply chthonic character". It compensates for an excess of its opposite, although its irruption to consciousness can be negatively experienced. *[A. Benvenuti]*

REFERENCES. Jung C.G. (1934–1954), *Archetypes and the collective unconscious*, in *Collected Works*, IX, 1969.

CIRCULAR CAUSALITY

In systemic interactional psychotherapy, a principle according to which, within a system, a component can influence another component which in turn can influence the first one, generating a recursive ring. This principle is opposed to linear causality (→ causalism), according to which a cause produces an effect and this effect is not able to modify the antecedent: A causes B and B does not change A. With the concept of circularity, instead, this unidirectionality fails: A and B are cause and effect of each other. When describing or explaining the causal components of a systemic change, a single factor cannot be identified as a unique cause of a subsequent behaviour. In cybernetic systems (→ cybernetics), all is connected to everything, and this holistic and complex connection is expressed through actions and feedback characterized by a circular causality. In a system such as the → family, a member's behaviour simultaneously influences and represents a response of the other's conduct, in a relationship of reciprocal causality. *[E. Molinari, F. Pagnini, G Pietrabissa, G. Castelnuovo]*

REFERENCES. Bateson G., *A systems approach*, 1971; Selvini M. P., Boscolo L., Cecchin G., and Prata G., *Hypothesizing-circularity-neutrality: Three guidelines for the conductor of the session*, in «Family process»,1980, 19(1); Watzlawick P., Beavin J.H., Jackson Don D., *Pragmatics of human communication*, 1967.

CIRCULAR QUESTIONS

Within the approach of the Milan school (→ Milan school of family therapy) a technique aiming to collect, and at the same time introduce, information in the "family system". Collecting information helps to formulate and validate hypotheses regarding the dynamic structure of a family (generation of hypotheses). The transmission of information aims to change people's individual and family → epistemology. According to Bateson, "information is a difference which makes a difference". In this way, each family member contributes at a meta-level (meta-communication) to the development of an image of the structure of the family and to an understanding of the circular nature of relationships in the family. *[R.]*

REFERENCES. Bateson G., *Mind and nature: A necessary unity*, 1979.

CLASSICAL CONDITIONING

Within the behavioural paradigm, classical conditioning – also called respondent or Pavlovian conditioning – investigates the process of learning a new relationship (→ conditioned response) between a response already available in the repertoire of an organism (→ unconditioned response) and a new environmental event (→ stimulus). This can be conceptualized as a transfer of function, by which what was previously a neutral stimulus becomes capable of producing the response that originally was elicited by an → unconditioned stimulus. An unconditioned response is a permanent correlation between an external agent and a response of an organism; a conditioned response is the formation of a new temporary bond between one of the countless environmental factors perceived by the organism and a certain reaction available in the repertoire of an organism. *[P. Orifiammi, P. Moderato]*

REFERENCES. Moderato P., *Interazioni umane*, 2005; Skinner F.B., *Science and human bevavior*, 1953.

CLIENT

This term appeared in clinical psychology with the advent of humanistic approaches, born in opposition to psychoanalytic theories and therapies. It was introduced by C.R. Rogers with his client-centred therapy model, as he considered it more suitable to his idea of subject: active, responsible and participating in the process of change. This is in opposition to the term → patient used at that time to depict a passive subject who entrusted themselves to an expert, who, from the height of their knowledge, chose the direction of the therapy. According to the humanistic and existential approach, the therapist should not play the role of an expert who judges what is "healthy" or "sick", but rather facilitate clients in expressing their innate ability of → self-regulation and → self-realization. Irrespective of the therapeutic orientation, this term is now preferred, by many psychotherapists, to the more classic term "patient", both to emphasize the non-medical nature of their intervention and to avoid pathologizing the subject. The widest meaning of the term "client", compared with "patient", underlines the possibility that even someone with difficulties not necessarily characterized by outright psychopathology, may turn to a therapist, as emphasized by interventions such as consultation (→ consultancy) → counselling or → coaching in many non-clinical fields such as schools or other contexts. *[R.]*

CLIENT-CENTRED THERAPY

Pragmatism, empiricism, phenomenology and existentialism form the main philosophical background of the client-centred therapy founded in the 1940s by Rogers, who subsequently extended the application of his paradigm to all helping relationships under the name of the person-centred approach. Rogers founded, with Ch. Devonshire and Zucconi, the Person-Centered Approach Institute, active in Italy and in other European countries in the fields of education, research and consulting, which today also collaborates with some United Nations agencies.

When the field of psychotherapy was still marked by mechanistic-reductionist views, Rogers was the first psychologist to formulate a holistic-systemic paradigm founded on a concept of human nature characterized by an innate tendency towards self-awareness, self-regulation and health; a paradigm based on empirically verifiable and verified hypotheses. In fact, Rogers introduced the use of tape recorders and, for the first time, conducted research by recording entire psychotherapy sessions and by publishing transcripts, making boldly transparent in this way what happens in clinical → settings.

According to Rogers, human nature is positive, trustworthy and rational. Every human being has, within themselves, an actualizing tendency, that is, a force, a source of energy directed towards the development of all the abilities that are useful to maintain, self-regulate and develop the innate potential of an organism. Rogers always speaks about the human being as an organism: it is a holistic view that considers the individual as an inseparable unity of psyche and soma. Rogers has democratized the relationship between professional and user and has promoted, in psychotherapy, the necessary awareness of uses and abuses of power, of the ubiquitous relational policies generated consciously or unconsciously by professionals in designing and managing clinical setting. His contribution is of great significance: it has been and still is essential to thoroughly understand the implications of the fact that any therapeutic approach is necessarily based on a specific view of human nature, which is, in turn, based on values that then determine the policies of the helping relationship and influence its processes and results. Not only does Rogers define the quality of a relationship as a crucial aspect to determine the effectiveness of psychotherapeutic treatments in each approach, but he anticipates hypotheses, later confirmed by neuroscience and research on mirror neurons, on the importance of empathy as an adaptive ability. An effective therapist is able to establish with their client a "facilitating" relationship marked by the ability to make contact, with deep respect, acceptance, understanding, authenticity/congruency. This type of relationship promotes self-awareness, self-regulation and positive change. That is, it determines a process that gradually leads individuals to be more in touch with their organism and their experience, increasingly free from moral constraints imposed from the outside, and at the same time it will lead individuals to express a "natural morality", to be constructive towards themselves and others by becoming an increasingly fully functioning person. In fact, in "client-centred therapy", the ability of human beings to be in touch with their own nature is considered essential. According to Rogers, being fully in touch with oneself, others and the world is a synonym of mental health and of optimal development of one's own potential. When organisms are no longer in touch with themselves, individuals lose the ability to make choices using their internal *locus* of evaluation, a sort of compass necessary to navigate and effectively manage one's life.

In the personality theory formulated by Rogers, the structure of the Self is formed based on the quality of environmental relationships, in particular as a result of evaluations expressed by others. The ability of parents and significant persons to establish a relationship characterized by acceptance and respect with the child will allow them to develop a Self consistent with their own organism (also called organismic Self) – a depositary of their needs and the ability to realize them. In Roger's holistic view, mind and body are inseparable and the ability to be in touch with one's own needs is a prerequisite to being able to meet them and a synonym of mental health. However, if the relationship with the parents is perceived by the child to be a source of judgement, threat and insecurity, the structure of their personality may develop as dysfunctional and neurotic; the innate ability of children to understand themselves and to self regulate may be blocked and distorted as they lose contact with their own organism. In this case the child introjects the values and constructs of parents and significant persons, that is, other people's ways of evaluating experiences, though they are perceived as their own. This process of introjection is, for the child, a real form of reification, a detachment from their organism, which hitherto has formed the evaluation centre of experiences.

The Self that takes shape, formed on the basis of distorted sensory and visceral experiences, becomes a "false Self", which the individual, once adult, will try to preserve with their behaviour at all costs. The experiences considered inconsistent with the structure of this Self are perceived as a threat; the greater the number of threatening perceptions, the more rigid and defensive the structure of the Self will become. The Self will be committed to defend, suppress and distort everything perceived as a threat. This state of internal discrepancy between the organism, its experience and the representation of the Self that regulates behaviour, prevents and/or misrepresents important aspects of the symbolization process (that is, representing an experience made available to consciousness) and generates anxiety, tension and uncertainty in the individual. Neurosis and psychosis are obvious examples of this process. With the recurrence of perceived threats and resulting defensive actions, as in a vicious circle, the distorted or denied experiential area widens increasingly. The less a person is in contact with their organismic Self, the more incongruous and dysfunctional they are and the less able to accept themselves and others. Rogers hypothesized, and then confirmed with extensive research, his theory of therapy: through a non-judgemental, empathetic and authentic relationship, people change the way they construct their own experience becoming able to relate in a more respectful, empathetic and authentic way, and they improve their relationship with themselves, others and the world. This has significant implications, not only for the promotion of change in psychotherapy and in helping relationships, but in the overall field of interpersonal relations. *[A. Zucconi]*

REFERENCES. Rogers C.R., *Counselling and psychotherapy*, 1942; Id., *Client-centered therapy*, 1951; Id., *A theory of therapy, personality and interpersonal relationships, as developed in the client-centered framework*, in S. Koch (eds.), *Psychology: A study of science*, 1959; Rogers C.R., Gendlin E.T., Kiesler D.J., Truax C.B., *The therapeutic relationship and its impact: A study of psychotherapy with schizophrenics*, 1967; Rogers C.R., Kinget M.G., *Psychotherapy and human relations*, 1962; Zucconi A., *Denominatori comuni nelle varie forme di psicoterapia, Atti IV, Congresso di Psicologia Umanistica*, 1982; Id., *La Bussola del Professionista. Da Persona a Persona*, in «Rivista di Studi Rogersiani», 2006; Id., *Effective helping relationships: Focus on illness or on health and well being?*, in B. Lewitt (eds.), *Reflections of human potential: The person centered approach as a positive psychology*, 2008; Zucconi A., Dattola G., *La relazione terapeutica nella terapia centrata sul cliente*, in P. Petrini, A. Zucconi (eds.), *La relazione che cura*, 2007; Zucconi A., Faini E., Sulprizio G., *L'uso del potere in psicoterapia: la posizione della Psicoterapia Centrata sul Cliente di Carl Rogers*, in «Idee in Psicoterapia», 2009, 2, 1; Zucconi A., Howell P., *Promuovere la salute con un approccio centrato sulla persona*, 2003; Zucconi A., Silani G., *Le conferme delle neuroscienze alle ipotesi della Psicoterapia Centrata sul Cliente di Carl Rogers ed alla teoria dei fattori comuni delle psicoterapie*, in «Idee in Psicoterapia», 2008, 1, 3.

CLIMBING TECHNIQUE

In → brief strategic therapy, Nardone's model, a technique used in order to break down the goals of therapy into smaller steps, inspired by what the alpine guides do before climbing a mountain. Instead of departing from the base of the mountain, they study the path to be followed, starting from the top of the mountain, and proceeding backwards, tracing the route to be taken and its steps up to the point of departure. Working backwards, from the summit to the point of departure, it becomes much easier to predict the best route to take and therefore to build it up according to its different stages, predicting intermediate stages and the possibility of changing the route to be taken if unexpected difficulties are encountered. Analogously, when dealing with a complex objective that is posited as the ultimate goal of the intervention, it is fundamental to guide the persons involved into breaking down the path to be taken into at least ten small steps, each of which must correspond to the achievement of a specific sub-goal. In order to be able to do this, the client is asked first of all what would be the point of arrival (the number 10), and then, working backwards, what would be steps 9, 8,7 and so forth, until one is able to identify the smallest objective, in other words, the step number 1. In this way, the individual is guided to defining in extremely concrete terms every single step in the process of the resolution of the problem, departing from the final objective and working backwards to the point of departure. All of this takes place in such a way as to subdivide the process of the resolution of the problem into stages, which correspond to equal micro-objectives. Thanks to the subdivision of the objective, the person who is entrusted with resolving the problem (whether he is a consultant or a psychotherapist) can utilize specific strategies (→ stratagem) and intervention techniques at every single stage, thereby significantly increasing his operational capability. The underlying logic of the climbing technique is that of disassembling something that is complicated in order to make it simpler and more manageable, in such a way that it becomes possible to verify the → efficacy of the intervention at every single stage of the process and that it becomes possible to eventually correct it if it does not achieve the desired outcome. In this way, if the intervention does not yield results, the problem-solver is able to change the technique employed without compromising the final result. Additionally, the subdivision of the objective represents an excellent way of circumventing the → resistance to change. This will allow the person taking part in the process of change to achieve the final objective without needing to engage in particularly extraordinary behaviour and without feeling overwhelmed by an excessive sense of responsibility, as a result of the fact that they will succeed in doing a "big" thing as the simple result of the addition of many small things. This mental strategy, which may appear to be counter-intuitive, allows the easy building up of the sequence of actions to be undertaken in order to resolve a problem departing from the smallest, but concrete, possible change. For this reason, the mountain climber technique is successfully employed in clinical as well as in organizational contexts. *[G. Nardone, R. Milanese]*

REFERENCES. Nardone G., *Problem solving strategico da tasca*, 2010; Nardone G., Mariotti R., Milanese R., Fiorenza A., *La terapia dell'azienda malata*, 2000.

CLINICAL

Originally, clinic was the practical teaching of the doctor at the patient's bed. In psychology, the term was used by L. Witmer in 1896 for the evaluation of children with mental and physical disabilities. Today, the term designates a research method or a practical application of medical and psychological knowledge. The main object of study of clinical psychology is the individual or small groups of individuals. In psychology and psychotherapy, clinic, meant as a method, aims to gain knowledge through consulting sessions and the relationship between individuals or between individuals and small groups. Clinical investigation happens primarily through the use of free or structured interviews and tests (→ projective tests, → psychological tests). A fundamental postulate of this method is that individuals are studied in their natural environment and not under laboratory conditions. For this reason, the → clinical method is usually opposed to the → scientific method, which favours the study of the individual or individuals in laboratories where experimentalists claim to have better control of variables. This theoretical position is strongly criticized by clinicians who consider laboratory conditions as artificial, and therefore prevent the possibility of studying the individual authentically and globally in their natural → environment. The practical-applicative discipline refers to the use of psychological knowledge to perform → psychological diagnosis, intervention and rehabilitation, education, prevention and management of health care organizations. The clinical psychologist is an expert in normal and pathological processes of mental functioning, knows how to design and conduct research and interventions and knows and can use the main diagnostic methods and psychological treatment of individuals and groups. *[R.]*

CLINICAL BEHAVIOUR ANALYSIS

In cognitive behavioural therapy, it represents the extension of behaviour analysis to the fields and to the themes of interest of → clinical psychology. In 2000 Dougher and Hayes defined clinical behaviour analysis as that part of behaviour analysis that: a) applies hypotheses, principles and methods of contextual and functional behaviour analysis to problems, → settings and topics that clinical psychologists deal with when working with patients in outpatient settings; b) includes the identification of variables and processes that play a role in the development, maintenance and treatment of clinical disorders; c) pays specific attention to the role and use of verbal events in psychological disorders and their treatment, in a modern scientific interpretation of the processes and principle involved in language and cognition. Clinical behaviour analysis is an active approach to behavioural change in which patient and therapist work together considering past and present → patterns of interaction with the world, and planning steps towards a richer and more meaningful life. It is an evidence-based therapy (see → third-generation behavioural therapy). *[P. Moderato, G. Miselli]*

REFERENCES. Dougher M.J. (eds.), *Clinical behaviour analysis*, 2000; Hayes S.C., Bissett R.T., *Behavioural psychotherapy and the rise of clinical behaviour analysis*, in J.A. Austin, J.E. Carr (eds.), *Handbook of applied behaviour analysis*, 2000; Hayes S.C., Strosahl K., Wilson K.G., *Acceptance and commitment therapy: An experiential approach to behaviour change*, 1999; Moderato P., Presti G., Miselli G., *La terapia cognitivo-comportamentale entra nel terzo millennio*, in S. Di Nuovo, G. Falgares (eds.), *Per una psicologia psicologica*, 2008.

CLINICAL HYPNOSIS

Riding a wave of substantial empirical support for its effectiveness in the domains of psychotherapy and behavioural medicine, clinical → hypnosis has emerged as a viable treatment for a variety of medical and psychological conditions. Hypnosis is a global term, however. In fact, hypnosis is comprised of many different components easily applied in a variety of goal-oriented psychotherapies, including cognitive-behavioural and psychodynamic approaches. Since hypnosis can take many different forms and be applied in a variety of ways, there are many different theoretical viewpoints attempting to explain hypnotic phenomena as well as widely divergent practical applications across treatment models. Hypnosis involves the mechanism of selective attention, a narrowing of focus and an increased absorption in suggested experiences. Hypnosis is not generally regarded as a therapy in and of itself. Rather, it is considered a therapeutic tool for creating a more relaxed, focused and attentive context for delivering the therapy. Thus, the salient question to ask is *not*, "How does hypnosis compare to cognitive-behavioural therapy (CBT) (or some other specific form of therapy) in treatment success rates?" Rather, the appropriate question is, "If CBT is performed *without* hypnosis and CBT is performed *with* hypnosis, does the addition of hypnosis enhance the efficacy of the treatment?" The evidence is substantial that the answer is yes. Of course, no treatment is successful with all clients, but the ability of hypnosis to enhance treatment results in most individuals is quite impressive. How a clinician structures an intervention employing hypnosis will necessarily differ according to each individual client's unique profile and goals. Generally, hypnosis sessions are about 20 to 30 minutes in length, embedded within the larger therapy session. Hypnotic procedures typically, but not always, involve directing the client to close his or her eyes, relax, focus intently on the clinician's words, and actively engage in the internal process of adapting the ideas and perspectives (i.e. suggestions) the clinician offers into a meaningful approach to the specific problems or symptoms under consideration.

In hypnosis, responses occur at levels outside of the client's awareness that further intensify the hypnotic experience. People are able to manifest a variety of talents that are collectively termed "hypnotic phenomena." These include: 1) *age regression* (defined as the intense and experiential absorption in memory such that memories can be recalled in vivid detail and perhaps even relived as if occurring in the now, allowing for the reframing of memories, for example); 2) *age progression* (defined as the intense and experiential absorption in expectations, a vehicle for establishing positive → self-fulfilling prophecies, for example); 3) *analgesia and anaesthesia* (the ability to reduce or even eliminate sensation, exceptionally valuable in the treatment of all kinds of pain); and, 4) *dissociation* (the ability to break global experiences into component parts and selectively amplify or de-amplify a part depending on therapeutic objective, such as encouraging a controlled detachment from overwhelming emotions). There are many other hypnotic phenomena that become accessible in hypnosis that are also beneficial to employ in the course of psychotherapy, and the interested reader may choose to learn more than this brief article can address. Suffice it to say that as one considers what is possible in hypnosis (and the limits of what can be achieved have not yet been defined), wherever one can influence mental or physical processes it quickly becomes apparent thathypnosis will be valuable.

WAYS TO USE HYPNOSIS IN PSYCHOTHERAPY. Hypnosis essentially amplifies experience. So, if one wants to focus the client on the cognitive dimension of experience, perhaps to teach a client to recognize and correct so-called → cognitive distortions (i.e. errors in information processing), one might use hypnosis to help make such identification and correction a more natural and even more reflexive process.

Hypnosis can be used to help *manage symptoms*. This is a more superficial, yet meaningful, application of hypnosis. For example, using hypnosis to reduce anxiety or rumination so that an anxious or depressed client can enhance his or her sleep may not be a particularly "deep" intervention. Clinically, however, it is an enormously valuable one since sleep disturbance is a key issue in depression. As another example, teaching someone to manage pain with hypnosis to reduce subjective distress and depression is not psychologically "deep," but can literally save peoples' lives. Hypnosis can be used to *foster skill acquisition*. Teaching clients specific skills (e.g. social skills or → problem-solving skills) is a standard part of almost any therapy. Hypnosis is a vehicle of experiential learning, which involves teaching practical skills to be absorbed on many different levels. Thus, it is a proactive and empowering approach, and a vital element of effective treatments.

Hypnosis can be used to *establish associations and dissociations*. To which aspect(s) of experience do we want the client to be more connected (or associated)? To which aspect(s) of experience do we want the patient to be more detached (or dissociated)? For example, someone who is lacking emotional awareness can benefit from an emotionally focused (associative) intervention (e.g. "You can learn to be more aware of your feelings and use them a source of information in making decisions"); while someone who is hyperemotional might benefit from a more cognitively based (emotionally dissociative) intervention (e.g. "You can learn to think logically about the best way to make decisions regarding these issues"). The ability of hypnosis to build strong links between challenging situations and helpful responses is the primary reason why hypnosis can be so easily integrated into virtually any model of treatment.

There are many other ways to use hypnosis in treatment, including building positive expectations to counter hopelessness, reframing emotion-laden memories, enhancing perceptual flexibility, instilling better coping skills, and increasing self-efficacy. Hypnosis as a subject of serious study, both in clinical and neuroscientific domains, is already reaping great dividends, and, as new applications emerge, hypnosis has great potential to become a part of every clinicians' treatment repertoire. *[M.D. Yapko]*

REFERENCES. Moore M., Tasso A., *Clinical hypnosis: The empirical evidence*, in M. Nash, A. Barnier (eds.), *The Oxford handbook of hypnosis*, 2008; Yapko M., *Hypnosis and the treatment of depressions: Strategies for change*, 1992; Yapko M., *Treating depression with hypnosis: Integrating cognitive-behavioural and strategic approaches*, 2001; Yapko M., *Trancework: An introduction to the practice of clinical hypnosis*, 1990; Yapko M., (ed.) *Hypnosis and treating depression: Applications in clinical practice*, 2006.

CLINICAL METHOD → SCIENTIFIC METHOD IN PSYCHOLOGY AND PSYCHOTHERAPY

CLINICAL PSYCHOLOGY

Discipline based on a practice that is essentially psychological, that differentiates itself from a predominantly medical one. The therapeutic interventions are configured as methods aimed at changing mental states, behavioural patterns and relational systems. Denominated in different ways, the methods of clinical psychology have the aim of obtaining the best functional and adaptive conditions, whether this be composed of one or more individuals, in group situations and and/or institutions. The psychotherapies themselves occupy a central position in these activities. The working context of clinical psychology involves a large variety of problematic situations, relative to the personal and/or social level, in which psychopathology constitutes one – but not exclusively so – indication, together with other situations that involve themes of maladjustment, in whatever way these are evidenced and related to personal and social aspirations for → change. *[R.]*

CLINICAL SCHEMES OF PERSONALITY TYPIZATION

Organizational modalities of interpersonal knowledge based on category abstractions generated for the purpose of evaluation, diagnosis and prognosis. These abstractions allow the attribution of a set of psychological features to individuals that can be grouped on the basis of a distinctive aspect. This attribution process is employed not only by experts but also by lay people for pragmatic purposes in order to predict and explain the actions of others; this process employes the criteria of "normality and pathology" (→ norm; → pathology) as a category construction and, consequently, attributes behaviour and actions to specific features (genetic, psycho-biographical, environmental, educational, psycho-affective, etc.).

The clinical schemes of → personality typization provide inferential shortcuts that allow the observer/diagnostician to deduct a lot of information from a few elements, by adopting different criteria (categorical, deterministic, structural). Since the clinical schemes of typization are based on prototypical and stereotypical (→ stereotype) constructions, they represent the procedure chosen for psychopathological typologies. These schemes often make the mistake of transforming hypothetical, conventional constructions – semantically connoted by value judgments – into a matter of fact. The clinical schemes of personality typization can be conventionally useful, but not necessarily true. *[A. Salvini]*

REFERENCES. Salvini A., *Gli schemi di tipizzazione della personalità in psicologia clinica e psicoterapia*, in G. Pagliaro, M. Cesa-Bianchi (eds.), *Nuove prospettive in psicoterapia e modelli interattivo-cognitivi*, 1995.

COACHING

A consultancy service to individuals or groups. It is characterized by a set of techniques and directives, training, motivational methodologies and aims that enable and support the customer in the process of acquisition of goals and/or in the development of specific skills and expertise. Specifically, the key elements of the coaching relationship include: identifying specific objectives regarding improvements of performance parameters in the professional and/or social behaviour of the customer; defining and evaluating specific strengths and weaknesses of the person who asks for the coaching intervention; building an interpersonal relationship aimed at acquiring defined and pragmatically recognizable objective results at an individual level (quality and quantity of new knowledge and behavioural changes), at a group level (changes in operational efficiency and effectiveness) and at an organizational level (improvements in management activities). The coaching intervention, although on the boundary line between organizational disciplines and interpersonal helping practices, differs both from the typical forms of business → consultancies (counselling, training, mentoring, tutoring) and from psychotherapeutic activities. In fact, its scope, in its proper application, is not psychopathology, with its search for causal connections and diagnosis; moreover, its methodology does not use rigid theoretical models when reading and interpreting the individual or organizational realities on which action is taken. The coaching intervention is especially a "process intervention" focused on producing quick significant changes in a customer's present and future behaviour. The expression "process intervention" aims to emphasize that the ultimate goal of coaching is not to provide predefined solutions to customers but rather to help customers acquire the necessary cognitive and behavioural techniques to produce the desired solutions autonomously and independently. It is a process where clients do not receive existential "truths", but conceptual tools that can be used to define their own aspirations, focus on the objectives that are necessary for their fulfilment, motivate themselves to make efforts, develop professional and interpersonal skills and, finally, enhance their awareness of those skills. Therefore, coaching cannot in any way be considered a form of psychotherapeutic intervention and, indeed, no specific qualification in this area is necessary to practice it. *[P. Mordazzi]*

REFERENCES. Milanese R., Mordazzi P. *Strategic coaching*, 2015.

COGNITION

In psychology, a set of functions that allow a person to gather information (*input* phase), process them and use them in the surrounding world (*output* phase). These include → memory, → attention, recognition and understanding of the information coming from the outside world, the ability to give adequate responses and to make oneself understood with words and actions and orientation in space and time. The ultimate goal of these functions is to allow behaviours to adapt to the needs of the → environment or to change the environment according to one's own needs. The term "cognitive development" refers to the development of intellectual activities. J. Piaget divided this process into four different stages: sensorimotor (0 to 18 months), based essentially on reflexes and then on dynamic relationships between objects; preoperational (18 months to 6 years), which precedes the child's ability to start utilizing proper logical "operations" to solve problems and where the child is not able to take a different point of view than their own (egocentrism); concrete operational (ages 6 to 11) where the child learns the reversibility of processes and learns spatial and temporal relationships; formal operational (ages 11 to 13) where inductive and deductive reasoning and the ability to reflect on one's own thought emerge (→ development stages (Piaget's)). Instead, the beginning of problematic cognitive situations is the basis for the development and acquisition of specialized knowledge, which is a constant process in an individual's life. According to L. Festinger's theory of "cognitive dissonance" (i.e. inconsistency between thoughts, emotions and behaviours), man attempts to minimize contradictions between what he thinks and what he lives. This can be done in three different ways: by producing a change in the environment; modifying one's behaviour; modifying one's cognitive world. Creating → experiences that can change how reality is perceived (through cognitive structures) becomes, in fact, a goal in all those psychotherapies based on the assumption that cognitive change can be achieved only through concrete experiences;

however, most therapeutic interventions utilize the mere awareness of how change should happen at every stage as an instrument to obtain such a change only as last resort. For example, according to the cognitive approach, as the human mind works like a data processor that continuously checks for congruence between its own " behavioural project" and existing objective conditions, every single change must go through awareness and rational consciousness to be acted upon. *[R.]*

COGNITIVE-BEHAVIOURAL THERAPY (AARON BECK'S MODEL)

Aaron T. Beck, M.D., developed Cognitive Therapy (CT) in the early 1960s. CT is often used synonymously with Cognitive Behaviour Therapy. Beginning in the late 1950s, Dr. Beck, a psychiatrist and psychoanalyst at the University of Pennsylvania, conducted several studies, which he predicted would validate the psychoanalytic theory of depression. But his research produced opposite findings. He then started to investigate other explanations for depression.

Beck found that a characteristic common to all depressed patients was negative, unrealistic thinking, especially a negative view of the self, one's world and the future (the → "cognitive triad" of depression). He also found that helping patients evaluate their depressed thinking more realistically led to an improvement in their mood and behaviour. Borrowing elements from behaviour therapy, he measured patients' moods (having created the Beck Depression Inventory in 1961), structured therapy sessions and assessed the impact of interventions. He engaged in straightforward problem-solving with patients, collaboratively assigned → "homework", taught them cognitive and behavioural skills and elicited their feedback. From the beginning, Beck made clinical observations that helped him formulate theories that have since been validated in hundreds of studies. He and his residents and trainees also performed one of the first randomized controlled psychotherapy outcome studies, published in 1977, comparing the efficacy of CT for depression to an antidepressant; both were found to be equally effective. (Later studies demonstrated that CT is effective for mild, moderate, and severe depression and is about twice as effective as medication in preventing relapse). In the following decades, Beck and colleagues, worldwide, studied a wide range of psychiatric disorders, psychological problems and medical conditions with psychological components. They have identified the key cognitions and → behavioural patterns for each, developed specific interventions and established the efficacy of CT treatment in several hundred research trials. Regardless of the disorder being studied, the underlying theory of CT, the "cognitive model", remains constant. It is not the triggering situation itself that directly leads to patients' reactions. It is their *perception* of the situation, the specific "automatic" thoughts they have about a situation, that lead to their emotional, behavioural and physiological response. Automatic thoughts are the most superficial level of cognition. They are the actual words and/or images that seem to spontaneously arise in patients' minds. Automatic thoughts (→ automatic negative thought) contain consistent themes for an individual. These themes, also referred to as underlying "beliefs", are related to the basic way patients see themselves, their world and other people. Patients' beliefs shape their perception of reality. Patients experience symptomatic relief when they respond adaptively to their automatic thoughts. They experience enduring changes in their mood, behaviour and physiology when they change their maladaptive, basic beliefs.

CT has certain underlying principles, regardless of patients' disorders: CT treatment is based on the cognitive formulation of patients' disorders and an individual cognitive conceptualization of the specific patient. Therapists begin to collect data about patients at their first encounter and continue to collect data until termination. Important data include (1) historical information that may shed light on the development and maintenance of patients' basic beliefs, (2) factors that precipitated patients' disorders, and (3) current information about patients' typical automatic thoughts, behavioural patterns and emotional and physiological responses. The conceptualization is data-driven and therapists continue to share and refine their understanding of patients at every session. CT treatment necessitates a strong therapeutic relationship. Therapists need good → counselling skills: genuine warmth, → empathy, caring, regard, and accurate understanding. They collaboratively make therapeutic decisions with patients and seek feedback. They are alert to changes in patients' mood and verbal and nonverbal behaviour during sessions. When they notice a change, they may gently interrupt the session, ask patients what is going through their minds and solve the problem if patients are having negative thoughts about them. Therapists also elicit feedback at the end of sessions to make sure the alliance (→ therapeutic alliance) is strong and to ascertain whether patients feel treatment should be altered in any way.

CT treatment involves active therapists and patients. Cognitive therapists tell patients that they would like to work as a team to help overcome their disorder. Both therapists and patients take an active role in specifying problems, devising solutions, identifying, evaluating and responding to dysfunctional cognitions, and setting self-help assignments. Initially therapists may take more of a lead in these activities, but patients gradually take more responsibility as they become socialized to treatment and learn important cognitive and behavioural skills. CT treatment is goal-oriented. From the first session, therapists help patients recognize problems and turn them into concrete behavioural goals. They ask, "What are your goals for treatment? How would you like to be different as a result of treatment? How would you like your life to be different?" Patients' goals then help guide treatment. CT focuses primarily, though not necessarily exclusively, on the present. To alleviate patients' suffering as soon as possible, cognitive therapists discuss their current difficulties. Most patients recover from their disorder with this primary focus on the present. Some, particularly those with longstanding difficulties in relationships, work or general functioning, benefit from some discussion of past events, usually towards the middle of treatment. It is useful for them to understand how they came to develop negative beliefs about themselves, their worlds and other people, how these beliefs solidified as time went on, and how these beliefs are affecting them today. Imagery (→ imaginal exposure) and other experiential (→ in-vivo exposure) techniques can help them change their beliefs at both the "intellectual" and "emotional" levels. CT treatment emphasizes relapse prevention. From the first session, therapists not only help patients solve problems and change their thinking and behaviour, but they also teach them how to do so themselves (→ self-therapy). In this way, patients become their own therapists and know what to do if they start to experience symptoms after their disorder has remitted. CT treatment is generally time-limited. Cognitive therapists seek to produce remission as soon as possible. Many patients with straightforward depression or anxiety are treated for 6 to 20 sessions. Patients with more complex disorders or personality disorders may require up to a year of treatment, or even more. Patients with chronic severe mental illness, such as bipolar disorder and schizophrenia, also benefit from a longer course of treatment, followed by periodic booster sessions. CT sessions are structured. At the beginning of sessions, cognitive therapists check on patients' moods and experiences from the past week, and help them set an agenda, that is, specify the problems they want help in solving. In the middle part of sessions, therapists review patients' homework and, in the context of helping them solve a specific problem, teach them relevant cognitive, behavioural and problem-solving tools. At the end of sessions, therapists and patients summarize the most important points of the session, review the self-help assignments (usually involving both cognitive and behavioural change) patients have agreed to, and therapists elicit feedback. CT sessions emphasize → cognitive reframing. A strong focus in most sessions is the identification of dysfunctional cognitions the patient has been experiencing or is likely to experience in the coming week. Therapists use guided discovery, often through a process of Socratic questioning, to help patients evaluate and respond to their inaccurate and/or maladaptive thoughts (→ irrational thoughts) and beliefs. They engage in collaborative empiricism, that is, they jointly investigate the accuracy of patients' thinking. When patients make negative predictions (e.g. I won't be able to understand anything I read" or "If I get really anxious, my heart will start beating fast and I'll have a heart attack,"), they may also use "behavioural experiments" to test these ideas, in session or between sessions. Therapists do not use exclusively cognitive and behavioural strategies. They may borrow techniques from other treatment modalities (e.g. Gestalt therapy or psychodynamic psychotherapy) within the cognitive model. To summarize, CT is generally a time-limited, educative, problem-solving psychotherapy that is based on the cognitive model. Its theory and treatment have been demonstrated to be valid and efficacious in hundreds of research trials. *[J.S. Beck]*

REFERENCES. Beck A.T., *Cognitive therapy of depression*, 1979; Beck A.T., Alford B.A., *Depression: Causes and treatment*, 2009; Beck J.S., *Cognitive therapy: Basics and beyond*, 1995.

COGNITIVE-BEHAVIOURAL THERAPY WITH COUPLES AND FAMILIES

At the end of the 1950s, A. Ellis was already using rational emotive therapy to work with couples. Since then, and until the 1980s, little was published in scientific literature on cognitive-oriented therapy. In parallel, the principles of behaviour modification were applied first to interaction patterns among family members, and later to their successful application with couples experiencing difficulty. This type of work with couples was followed by many case studies that involved the use of family interventions when treating child behaviour. Behaviourists recognized the very powerful effect of family members on children's natural environments and began to integrate them into the treatment process. Later, a refined and more complete style of intervention with family units was described in detail in *Reprogramming the social environment* (Patterson *et al.*). The professional literature has continued to apply behavioural therapy to family systems, with a strong emphasis on bargaining skills, negotiation strategies and environmental reprogramming; the implementations here reported are directed towards families with children with behavioural problems.

The cognitive approach, or, as it should be described, the cognitive component of behavioural therapy has since obtained more attention, as it has provided an addition to behaviour-oriented family and couple therapy. In addition to the work of Ellis, an important study by Margolin and Weiss suggested the effectiveness of the cognitive component of behavioural psychotherapy with couples, prompting further investigation into the use of cognitive techniques with dysfunctional couples. Actually, only a few studies have examined the impact of additional → cognitive reframing interventions on behavioural protocols, typically replacing some cognitive-oriented with behaviour-oriented sessions, in order to maintain equality between the compared treatments. The results suggested that the combination of cognitive and behavioural interventions was just as effective as purely behavioural interventions; however, the interventions focused on cognitive aspects tended to produce a more cognitive change, while behaviour-oriented interventions modified behavioural interactions.

DEVELOPMENT OF THE THEORY. Consistent and compatible with → system theory, cognitive-behavioural therapy applied to couples and families has, as its premise, the fact that the members of a family influence each other; as a result, the behaviour of a family member produces specific behaviours, thoughts and emotions in the other members of the system, who, in turn, provoke certain thoughts, behaviours and emotions in the other member. As this cycle repeats itself, the volatility of family dynamics increases, making family members vulnerable to a negative spiral of conflict. When the number of family members involved increases, obviously, the complexity of the dynamics increases as well. Cognitive psychotherapy places a strong emphasis on → mental schemes of individuals, that is, on what was also defined as "core beliefs". Since this construct of a mental scheme has been applied to the treatment of families, therapeutic intervention has been based on the assumption that family members interpret and evaluate each other and also evaluate emotions and behaviours that are generated in response to their own evaluations. Although the cognitive-behavioural theory does not claim that cognitive processes cause every family behaviour, it emphasizes that cognitive appraisal plays a significant role in the existing interrelations between events, thoughts, emotions and behaviours. Together with the cognitive component of cognitive-behavioural psychotherapy, the cognitive reframing of → irrational thoughts has a fundamental impact on the change of dysfunctional behaviours and vice versa.

EMPIRICAL FOUNDATIONS OF COGNITIVE-BEHAVIOURAL PSYCHOTHERAPY WITH COUPLES AND FAMILIES. The first studies on behavioural therapy with couples and families paved the way for the most recent research. In fact, pragmatic application of the social exchange theory and learning strategies, used to facilitate a more satisfactory interaction between couples experiencing difficulty, have later appeared in professional literature. In the aforementioned *Reprogramming the social environment* the authors applied the procedures of → operant conditioning and contingent negotiation (strategy aimed to improve cooperation by requiring an *a priori* implementation of specific behaviours followed by a reward or the suspension of a punishment) to develop in parents the ability to control children's regressive behaviour. Subsequently, behaviour-oriented therapists added communication and → problem-solving skills as additional tools to use when working with couples and families. Research confirms the premise of social-exchange theory (whose central element is to consider exchanges as the basis of any action, institutional and cultural entity, beyond the differences that exist between institutions and between cultures), indicating that the members of couples experiencing difficulty exchange more unpleasant behaviours than those with functional relationships and those who have followed a behavioural therapeutic intervention. In the late 1970s, cognitive elements were introduced as an auxiliary component of the behaviour-oriented treatment in therapies with couples and families. In the 1980s and 1990s, cognitive factors became an increasingly important focus in research and in the literature on couple therapy, and cognitive aspects were addressed more directly and systematically compared with other theoretical approaches to family therapy.

Similarly, behavioural approaches to family therapy were expanded to include the "cognitions" that family members have towards each other. Ellis was one of the first to introduce a cognitive approach in family therapy. Cognitive-behavioural orientation is now considered one of the main approaches to family therapy. Epstein produced an excellent report on the empirical situation of cognitive-behavioural psychotherapy with couples; a more recent overview, both on family and couples therapy, with further emphasis on familiar schemes, is provided by Dattilo and Epstein. Unfortunately, the domain of cognitive-behavioural psychotherapy with couples has more quantitative studies (studies that follow a research method structured in different phases according to a deductive approach where theory precedes research) compared to family therapy. The most recent studies on families include the treatment of schizophrenia in the early 1980s, in addition to studies conducted by C. Barrowclough and N. Tarrier.

FUTURE DIRECTIONS. The future of cognitive-behavioural therapy with couples and families looks promising, especially if implemented in the context of a systemic approach. Its integration with other methods of couples and family therapy is increasing and growing exponentially worldwide. This aspect is highlighted in a text by Dattilo, who shows a great integration potential with many of the 16 different types of couple and family therapy described. The techniques and strategies of cognitive-behavioural therapy are very versatile in dealing with the contemporary issues of couples and families. Theoretically, since the vast majority of therapeutic approaches to couples and families involve thought and perception, the majority of therapies can be defined as "cognitive", or at least with a cognitive component. For similar reasons, many therapies can be considered as behavioural, in part because international communication and exchange are often behavioural, and all behaviours are a communicative act. Since the human condition also includes emotions, many psychotherapies are oriented, to a significant extent, towards emotions. As a result, any therapy can be viewed through a variety of lenses: cognitive, behavioural, emotional and so on. Cognitive-behavioural therapies have moved a step further and suggested that behaviours, thoughts, emotions, physiological and interpersonal components are integrated, so that, if any of the elements change during the course of therapy, it causes a chain reaction in the others. It seems that most of the psychotherapy approaches are moving towards a perspective of integration; this clearly includes cognitive-behavioural approaches, in particular with couples and families. In addition, the application of cognitive-behavioural psychotherapy with couples and families from different cultures is essential to better understand strengths and cultural boundaries in this field. *[F.M. Dattilio]*

REFERENCES. Beck A.T., *Love is never enough: How couples can overcome misunderstandings, resolve conflicts, and solve relationship problems through cognitive therapy*, 1989; Bitter J.M., *Theory and practice of family therapy and counselling*, 2008; Dattilio F.M., *Case studies in couple and family therapy: Systemic and cognitive perspectives*, 1998; Id., *Cognitive-behavioural family therapy: Contemporary myths and misconceptions*, in «Contemporary Family Therapy», 2001, 23(1); Id., *Comprehensive cognitive-behaviour therapy with couples and families*, 2009; Dattilio F.M., Epstein N.B., *Cognitive-behavioural couple and family therapy*, in G. Weeks, T. Sexton, M. Robbins (eds.), *Handbook of family therapy: Theory research and practice*, 2003; Dattilio F.M., Padesky C.A., *Terapia cognitiva della coppia*, 1990; Epstein N.B., *Cognitive-behavioural therapy with couples: Empirical status*, in «Journal of Cognitive Psychotherapy», 2001, 15(2); Epstein N.B., Baucom D.H., *Enhanced cognitive therapy for couples: A contextual approach*, 2002; Margolin C., Weiss R.L., *Comparative evaluation of therapeutic components associated with behavioural marital treatments*, in «Journal of Consulting and Clinical Psychology», 1978, 46.

COGNITIVE-CAUSAL THERAPY

Founded in Italy, in the early twenty-first century by Tamburello and his research team, as a review and synthesis of the thirty-year clinical and therapeutic experience gained by the Skinner Institute in Rome, it operates a conceptual revolution of the theoretical foundations of cognitivism, framing it in a logical and ontological reference. Psychic life is re-evaluated in its basic aspects thanks to a fine and wise, rational elaboration. These concepts are operationally connected to diagnostic procedures attentive to the principles causing discomfort and to a therapeutic practice tending to a → cognitive reframing that could activate the good and balancing unexpressed potential of the person.

The essence and principles of this perspective suggest what the primary senses of the person are and the origin of their possible suffering: a subjective nucleus, which is always a source of harmony and adaptation, although several possible and accidental contingencies of imbalance and mental suffering can torment the person. Individual essence is a unique and inimitable potential capital of talents and harmonizing and balancing forces: each person possesses, in their intimacy, a range of capabilities and potentialities that, if expressed freely, would lead to perfect harmony with the world. Unfortunately, the existential contingencies are often a source of imbalance and suffering: these "accidents" imprison the essence by limiting its expressiveness and freedom of action. Individuals, driven by their ephemeral needs, move away from their intrinsic and natural perfectibility. In fact, the gap between health and mental pathology lies between essence and accident. In the subjective core, nothing is disorganized: everything has the qualities of a balanced and orderly array; pathology is a malevolent masking of this essence in favour of excessive and misleading existential aims that are sources of disharmony. If harmony and order are necessary and inviolable traits of all human beings, dysfunctionality and suffering are contingent and unnecessary effects of subjective life experiences.

With a careful assessment, it can be identified that the origin of discomfort lies in a series of destabilizing causes, which, although acting in proximity to the individual essence – that is always inviolable – cannot contaminate perfection, but may seem essential, precisely because of their proximity. The task of psychotherapy, then ,is the clinical investigation of the causes of individual distress. In this complex investigation work, the role played by logic, in all its historical and theoretical branches, becomes essential. Deductive and inductive logic becomes an irreplaceable interest for the clinician and an opportunity for wisdom and procedural growth for psychology and psychotherapy in general. The logical investigation of pathogenic causes leads to highlight the mutual connection between two complex space-temporal dimensions. In fact, every person lives their present contingency alternating cognitive, emotional and behavioural states. These are generally linked to a few primary interests and several secondary goals; that is, some motives drive their conduct by determining the degree of adaptation to reality and subjective wellbeing. If these motives are misleading, because interested in unreachable and unrealistic excesses, the result will be a clearly disorderly conduct, with conflicting thoughts, emotions and behaviours, resulting from undeniable suffering. This is the synchronic dimension of every person, dominated by contingencies and illusions. In addition to living their present contingency, people also live their own existential unspecific continuity, which transcends experiential immediacies and is projected into the future.

Therefore, psychic life is, much more than it appears, an unstoppable progress of experiences and interiorities that follow one another, some getting lost in time, others stabilizing in the perpetuation of the Self, all ultimately gathering in what lives in every present contingency. Any motive, as well as any thought, emotion, behaviour or aim, lies on a layering of other motives and experiences that are lost in time, regardless of their pathogenic or adaptive value. Thus, a pathology is, as well as a good harmony, the product of the temporal continuity of one's life. This is the diachronic dimension of each person, the one that rises from contingencies and then descends upon it with all its weight. The therapist can use a logical investigation tool, schematized for practical purposes in a table with seven sequential columns (hence the name "seven-column analysis"), capable of disclosing the knowledge of synchronic and diachronic dimensions of who is suffering and asking for help. First, this tool sheds light on the synchronic dimension of the patient, revealing regular and fluid causal interconnections. The primary interest of the moment, representing the patient's pathogenic motive, activates, based on its criteria and on environmental conditions, the cognitive, emotional and behavioural conduct expressing pathological suffering and pursuing, assiduously, those multiple secondary goals, which, as sources of pleasure and satisfaction, reinforce discomfort. When the columns in the table are read following a causal sequence, each of them represents a psychic aspect that can be: cause of another psychic aspect that follows; effect of a previous one; first cause or final cause of the sequence. The first column regards the primary interest, which, with its focus on needs, moves the psychic forces. The second column contains operational and normative criteria that translate the basic need into a mental active tendency, focused on its immediate implementation in the environment. The third column shows the environmental antecedents that stimulate the conduct. The next three columns include, respectively: thoughts, emotions and behaviours that provide a lived and sincere expression of these criterial tendencies and underlying motives. Finally, the seventh column shows specific and secondary goals that represent the stimuli and reinforcing conditions of each conduct.

By imagining a series of seven-column tables placed on top of each other, it is then possible to clarify the diachronic dimension of suffering, up to its existential causes. Each synchronic dimension becomes stratified over time, creating an additional similar dimension that overlaps it. In the same way that geological layers are structured one upon one another, so that the current layer lies on the previous ones and owes them its subsistence, so psychological layers are stratified on multiple underlying and overlying layers. Like geological structures, which have a primal layer underlying all others, so, too, do psychic structures have a primal layer, a causing principle on which the subjective essence, that is, the uncaused and potential human intimacy, is based. This essence can remain completely buried or, if free to express itself, can emerge to the surface, making its way through each layer and demolishing any structural impediment: as lava explodes from the bowels of the Earth, it overwhelms everything with its power. This is the end of every existential path and also of each clinical path of growth. Eventually, the subjective essence is always a source of harmony and wellbeing. Negative contingencies of life can, however, suppress its expressiveness. In this case, it can be said that many are the unexpressed potentialities and few those disclosed. However, although unspoken, the essence itself remains inviolable. The positive contingencies of life can, instead, facilitate the expressiveness of the subjective essence. Also in this case, the essence remains inviolable, because, as a source, it comes before any of its expressions. However, the unexpressed potentialities are just a few, and instead those disclosed are many. Starting from these ideas, a new additional tool can be created that acts as a beacon on the clinical path guiding its evolution. This is the "order matrix", that is, a model of subjective perfection, which, adapting to the essence of each person, reveals their possible expressions. Therefore, it follows a psychotherapy aimed at comparing the contingent state of disorder and suffering to the potential state of harmony and wellbeing towards which the person should be directed. Any form of cognitive reframing marks a transition from a painful present to a possible world of serenity, which, once materialized, would shape and activate at least part of the regenerating and creative potential remaining unexpressed. The investigation of talents and personal capabilities should be a must in every therapy, an area of positivity that, ultimately, has to impose its presence on everything that is pathological and limiting. Finally, cognitive causal therapy utilizes the main clinical techniques of the cognitive behavioural approach but these are aimed at a reduction of individual suffering, which can only come from the individual itself, once free to express its innermost potential. *[A. Tamburello, E. De Monte].*

REFERENCES. De Monte E., Tamburello A., *Storia del pensiero psicologico*, 2008; Id., *Una logica integrata per la psicologia clinica*, 2010; Tamburello A., *La nuova psicoterapia cognitiva. Dalla diagnosi di profondità alla terapia causale*, 2007; Id., *Psicoterapia cognitiva e profondità causale*, 2008; Id., *Nuove procedure di psicodiagnosi e psicoterapia cognitiva*, 2008.

COGNITIVE CONCEPTUALIZATION

In standard cognitive psychotherapy, cognitive conceptualization is an individualized understanding of a client's psychological problems. The therapist begins to construct a cognitive conceptualization during the first contact with the client and continues to refine the conceptualization until the final session. An accurate cognitive conceptualization helps the therapist and client achieve two main goals of effective cognitive psychotherapy: 1) alleviating the client's distress and 2) building the client's → resilience. Cognitive conceptualization helps the therapist to: 1) synthesize client problems based on cognitive-behavioural theory and research; 2) describe problems using language aimed towards normalizing the client's experiences; 3) promote the client's interest and foster engagement in therapy; 4) make challenging problems more manageable; 5) guide the selection and sequence of cognitive behavioural techniques; 6) identify the client's strengths; 7) select the most cost-efficient interventions tailored to the client's needs; 8) anticipate difficulties and obstacles that might arise in therapy; 9) understand therapeutic roadblocks and formulate alternative strategies to achieve treatment goals; and 10) provide high-quality supervision *[A. Montano]*

REFERENCES. Beck J. S., *Cognitive therapy: Basics and beyond*, 1995; Kuyken W., Padesky C. A., Dudley R., *Collaborative case conceptualization: Working effectively with clients in cognitive-behavioural therapy*, 2009; Neenan M., Dryden W., *Cognitive therapy: 100 key points and techniques*, 2004.

COGNITIVE DISTORTIONS

Within the cognitive behavioural model of psychotherapy, cognitive distortions are viewed as the product of faulty or biased information processing that leads to consistent and systematic errors in thinking. Cognitive distortions are hypothesized to play an important role in the maintenance of a range of emotional disorders. Originally formulated by A.T. Beck, six different types of thinking errors were identified and later extended by his daughter, J.S. Beck. Cognitive distortions, although not mutually exclusive, can now be listed in the following 12 categories: all-or-nothing thinking; catastrophizing; disqualifying or discounting the positives; emotional reasoning; labeling; magnification/minimization; mental filter; mind reading; overgeneralization; personalization; "should" or "must" statements; and tunnel vision. One of the initial goals of cognitive-behavioural psychotherapy is to enable clients to identify or label the different types of thinking errors linked to their dysfunctional thoughts in order to help them explore and question the validity of their thoughts *[A. Montano]*.

REFERENCES. Beck A.T., *Cognitive therapy and the emotional disorders*, 1976; Beck J.S., *Cognitive therapy: Basics and beyond*, 1995.

COGNITIVE MODEL OF OPERANT CONDITIONING

Operant conditioning is a theoretic learning paradigm discovered and systematized by B. Skinner in the 1930s, during the neo-behavioural period. It establishes a strong relational bond between behaviours adopted by a human or animal organism and its stabilization over time due to the environmental reinforcements that follow it. In the first cognitive therapy, called rationalist or cognitive-behavioural, the close link with behaviourism, of which this is both a review and a direct expansion, is particularly visible in the use of operant conditioning as a therapeutic technique adapted to new theoretical and methodological needs. However, over time, cognitive therapy, especially in its recent constructivist leanings, focused on other cognitive paradigms to overcome old behaviourist paradigms, although adapted and reinterpreted. At the beginning of the first cognitive psychotherapy, particularly significant are the studies of Bandura and R. Walters on a form of learning called "social imitation", where some importance is given to → operant conditioning as well. Bandura and Walters highlighted the complexity of social imitation that is not reducible, as argued before them by Miller and J. Dollard, to a simple reproduction of behaviours observed in others. They turned their interest to the complexity involved in the emulation process, where the other person acts as a model and where the reproduction of his/her behaviour requires the involvement of multiple factors (→ social imitation or modelling). In fact, in addition to simple imitation, identification and assimilation processes to the imitated model are involved. This could be a real character, if alive, or virtual, if no longer alive as a historical figure, or never existed and is purely imaginative as a literary or a movie character. Social imitation processes depend, at least in part, on the consequences of emulated behaviours: we tend to copy rewarded patterns (→ reinforcement) more than those punished (→ punishment): in this case, they are called indirect or vicarious reinforcement or punishment. The results of this type of learning can be of three types. First, some new behaviours, acquired by imitating others, could remain unexpressed and unacted. These behaviours become "acted" only in the presence of a conscious desire to do it;

in both cases, reinforcement plays only a secondary role. Different is its impact in response inhibition or disinhibition: inhibition refers to the block and loss of a habitual response because the emulated model, in similar situations, does not put it in place. A vicarious punishment pushes the emulator to abandon a usual behaviour to avoid the risk of suffering the same consequences. In contrast, disinhibition consists in recovering a lost response because, in similar situations, the emulated model acts as the imitator was acting previously, before losing the answer. In the latter case, the desire for a particular behaviour is always active, despite no longer being acted, and just observing a model that puts it in places pushes the emulator to recover it immediately. A vicarious reinforcement pushes the individual to reactivate an abandoned but always desired behaviour. Finally, the third outcome of social learning, called induction, can be to act an already learned behaviour that was abandoned because unwanted. In this case, the model raises in the observer a desire that was absent before, giving a new and positive value to the abandoned behaviour. The following developments of the first cognitive psychotherapy, or cognitive-behavioural therapy, broadened the perspectives of investigation and application of the operant conditioning paradigm. A. Ellis and Beck, considered the true fathers of this psychotherapy school, resumed and revized Skinner's ABC model, which acquired the features of a proper cognitive diagnostic functionality. In fact, the symbol A indicates a set of environmental conditions, from a behavioural perspective, that predispose to a particular answer B, which, however, is no longer only behavioural, but also, and above all, emotional and cognitive. Finally, according to the theoretical parameters of operant conditioning, the "C" consequences allow the stabilization of all responses, that take shape as reinforcing or punitive conditions, which can be both environmental, or external and cognitive, or internal. The idea of internal cognitive reinforcements and punishments represents the main innovation introduced by Ellis, Beck and all the emerging cognitive psychotherapy in the operant conditioning paradigm. In this respect, the works of L.E. Homme and J.R. Caution in the 1970s, for example, should be read. Homme introduces the concept of *coverant*, that is, a hidden operant behaviour, not so different from overt behaviour. According to Homme, the *coverant* could consist of images, thoughts, memories and more that are subject, as overt behaviours, to the same operant rules based on reinforcements and punishments. However, Cautela goes further. Inspired by Homme's concept of *coverant*, he developed a series of psychotherapy techniques where the paradigm of operant conditioning plays a central role, although in the cognitive non-visible dimension, and, for that reason, defined as covert. For example, in covert positive reinforcement, Cautela asks patients to reinforce themselves through imagination, after having performed or simply imagined a desired behaviour. Differently, in covert negative reinforcement, he asks patients to imagine an unpleasant situation and then to avoid it by implementing the desirable response. In contrast, in covert modelling, Cautela first invites subjects to imagine a situation where the model performs the desired behaviour, then a situation where the person himself performs the behaviour and, finally, to perform the same behaviour in a real situation. In addition, in covert sensitization, Cautela requires patients to imagine themselves while performing an unwanted behaviour and then repeatedly link it to a strongly unpleasant situation. Finally, during covert response, Cautela invites patients to imagine themselves while performing an undesirable behaviour and to consider a possible cost, as a punishment or a loss of positive reinforcement, in order to avoid it in real life. In conclusion, the operant conditioning paradigm acquires, in the first cognitive psychotherapy, a revolutionary significance, by tying itself to an internal and hidden cognitive dimension where it assumes imaginative and mnestic traits that the former behaviourism avoided and neglected. *[A. Tamburello, E. De Monte]*

REFERENCES. Bandura A., *Social learning theory*, 1977; Beck A.T., *Cognitive therapy and the emotional disorders*, 1975; De Monte E., Tamburello A., *Storia del pensiero psicologico*, 2008; Schuyler D., *A practical guide to cognitive therapy*, 1991.

Cognitive paradigm → Please refer to the first chapter, "The eight paradigms and their respective theoretical-applicative models".

COGNITIVE REFRAMING

Cognitive reframing is a process of questioning or reattributing dysfunctional ways of thinking and formulating new, more adaptive thoughts. In all forms of cognitive reframing, the key role of the therapist is to actively help the client become clearly aware of his/her dysfunctional thinking in terms of the self, the world and the future, and then challenge the validity of its content. The basic principles of cognitive reframing, which is a key feature of psychotherapies belonging to the cognitive paradigm, originate from the early ideas of Greek and Latin philosophers; according to which, individuals had some degree of choice between an adaptive and a dysfunctional reaction when confronted with adverse circumstances. For example, Epictetus claimed that individuals were not disturbed by events themselves but by the way they interpreted these events. According to the cognitive model, core negative beliefs influence intermediate dysfunctional beliefs that, in turn, give rise to automatic thoughts associated with situations, hence resulting in emotional, behavioural and physiological consequences. Cognitive reframing works across the three layers of this model, starting from the one on the surface, which is represented by automatic thoughts. By using relevant negative automatic-thought diaries and forms, the therapist helps the client elicit and modify his/her own dysfunctional thoughts and errors of logic (known as "cognitive distortions"). An example of this form is the Thought Record Form, which is intended to assist the client in effectively recognizing and responding to negative automatic thoughts, hence reducing negative emotions. A previous version was known as the Daily Record of Dysfunctional Thoughts. This form requires that clients enter details of triggers of emotional disturbance, specifying situations that are negatively appraised with resulting negative emotions and unhelpful behaviours. There are also specific questions aimed at challenging associated cognitive distortions.

After this step, the therapist identifies intermediate beliefs by using the downward arrow technique. Here, the cognitive therapist explores the central meaning of the client's cognitions by searching for common themes that may be embedded within his/her dysfunctional thinking, and then elicits a specific unhelpful rule, attitude or assumption, which is later modified using other strategies such as Socratic questioning and behavioural experiments. Finally, the therapist works collaboratively with the client to identify core beliefs, which are likely to have developed during his/her childhood. An effective and systematic modification of core beliefs, through historical tests, restructuring early memories, or core belief worksheet, is thought to make clients less likely to relapse in the future. *[A. Montano]*

REFERENCES. Beck J.S., *Cognitive therapy: Basics and beyond*, 1995.

COGNITIVE TRIAD

In cognitive-behavioural therapy, a concept introduced by Aaron Beck in relation to the state of depression (→ depressive scheme). He noted that depressed patients suffer from faulty information processing (→ functional balance). They do not perceive reality clearly and see three aspects of their experience in an unrealistically negative light: themselves, their worlds and their future. Depressed patients may view themselves as helpless, inadequate, defective, weak, inferior, unlovable or bad. Their self-image (→ self-concept) influences their perception of current experiences. They may assume they will fail whatever they try or that they are not strong enough to get along on their own. As a result of these beliefs and assumptions, they may avoid situations that could produce counter-evidence and may be deprived of experiences that could provide a sense of pleasure or mastery. When they do engage with the world, they are often highly self-critical, undervalue their efforts and discount their achievements. A → negative view of their world also characterizes depressed patients. They may believe that the world poses obstacles to their wellbeing, that other people are superior and likely to evaluate them negatively. Small reversals are over-generalized and interpreted in a maladaptive way. Neutral experiences may be construed as negative. Positive experiences are often discounted or disregarded. Depressed patients view their future as hopeless. They believe that they will never be able to solve their problems and that their lives will never improve. They anticipate only hardships and negative experiences. They predict failure and suffering. As a result of unremitting, negative thinking, patients experience low mood, apathy, lack of motivation, avoidance and a sense of helplessness. Their hopeless ideas can lead to suicidal thoughts. [*J.S. Beck*]

REFERENCES. Beck A.T., *Cognitive therapy of depression*, 1979. Clark D.A., Beck A.T., Alford B.A., *Scientific foundations of cognitive theory and therapy of depression*, 1999.

COLLABORATIVE STRENGTHS-BASED BRIEF THERAPY

The collaborative strengths-based brief therapy model has been evolving since 1985. It is a flexible, integrative and eco-systemic approach that is theoretically informed by the best elements of solution-focused brief therapy, positive psychology, MRI brief strategic therapy, client-directed, outcome-informed therapy, narrative therapy, collaborative language systems therapy, expressive therapy art and writing methods, Buddhist → mindfulness meditations and practices, Navajo Native American rituals and healing and the Stages of Change model. The integration of these practices led to the development of a model capable of combining different elements into specific and systemic intervention protocols for various classes of problems. The "collaborative strengths-based" model, besides being an effective and efficient method for brief therapy, provides a perspective through which human problems can be interpreted. From a theoretical point of view, it is based on a number of key assumptions, highly pragmatic ideas that influence the thoughts and actions of the therapist. Change is inevitable and there is always a time when clients' problems do not show themselves: this is an assumption derived from the brief solutions-focused psychotherapy of de Shatzer and Berg; in this model, the solution of a problem is built by progressively extending the positive exceptions (→ search for exceptions technique) brought by clients and by directing them to the vision of a future in which everything will be solved. All clients have the necessary resources to solve their problems; they are the "experts" of their lives: the therapist enables them to guide the intervention and uses resources and solutions that already exist within the client and/or family; these resources are amplified through the use of specific communicative manoeuvres and "therapeutic" experiments that they need to complete between sessions. Problems are seen as ineffective attempts to solve difficulties: in line with the strategic approach, → attempted solutions are identified in order to change the persistent patterns of behaviours that retain the problems. Problems develop when the lives of clients lack balance, purpose and meanings: it gives specific attention to the social, cultural and even spiritual aspects of the people asking for help; moreover, the traditional psychiatric diagnoses are challenged as they are considered stigmatizing and an obstacle to change. All clients desire to overcome their overwhelming problems: the traditional concepts of resistance and opposition are seen as counterproductive and useless; within a collaborative perspective, the therapist tries to find and create specific ways of working with every client. Interventions are successful when they are built starting from the objectives of the clients, their theories of change and their preferences:

this reduces dropouts and increases the efficiency of the intervention. Reality is "negotiable" and there are many different ways to see clients' issues: therapists are inspired by a constructivist epistemology (→ constructivism), they assume a position of "not-knowing" and they try to introduce a modification in the belief systems of the clients in relation to the problematic situation. By changing beliefs and the language used, it is possible to change the problematic behaviour. Starting from these theoretical assumptions, the "collaborative strengths-based brief therapy" can be used with any kind of problem, any age and any treatment setting.

The client is put in the position of the expert. Regardless of how clients come to the therapist and the type of issues presented, they are encouraged to decide the goals they want to achieve, and the treatment modalities: the agenda of the sessions, who takes part in them and their frequency. In addition, at the end of each session, they can choose the prescriptions and the therapeutic rituals they want to practice in the interval between the sessions by selecting them from a list submitted by the therapist. In accordance with the client, the therapist works closely, both in and out of the session, with all members of the client's social network who are involved in and concerned about their problems. Whether they be professionals, friends or relatives, all those who are willing to help are encouraged to create an "intervention" team to resolve issues in the most effective and efficient way. This ecological-batesonian approach to family therapy makes it possible to offer interventions at an individual, family, peer group, social network level, up to the involvement of extended social systems and the community in which the patient belongs. The main focus of the treatment is the identification of, and focus on, clients' strengths, competencies, aspects of → resilience and past successes, even in areas different from that of the problem. The goal is to use all the resources, experiences and capabilities of the client in the area of the problem to help them solve their difficulties. The therapist pays much attention to gender issues, cultural aspects, broader social factors and elements of social injustice that often play a role in the development and persistence of human problems. Another important aspect of this therapy is the fact that, at the end of each session, the therapist considers, with the client, the quality of the therapeutic relationship and the client's level of satisfaction in the process of change. By taking care of the therapeutic relationship and by making the necessary adjustments to ensure clients' satisfaction, it is possible to increase their motivation, reduce the chances of abandonment of the therapy and to increase the chances of success in achieving objectives. The ecological, flexible and integrated approach that underlies the collaborative strengths-based brief therapy, provides the therapist with a multiplicity of perspectives on the difficulties of clients and offers them different types of intervention to strengthen, in a collaborative way, their abilities to achieve the desired goals. The combination of versatility and precision makes this model suitable not only for therapeutic intervention, but also as a frame of reference for supervision and → coaching. It is also used for groups of parents and adolescents. The approach of this therapy has proved to be very effective and capable of producing very rapid changes in patients, even in a single session. Therefore, it can be especially useful for operators of public amenities and it is recommended in all the contexts where therapists work with a large number of clients and where the duration of treatments is limited. *[M. Selekman]*

REFERENCES. Anderson H., *Conversation, language, and possibilities: A post-modern approach to therapy*, 1997; Anderson H., Gehart D.R., *Collaborative therapy: Relationships and conversations that make a difference*, 2007; de Shazer S., *Clues: Investigating solutions in brief therapy*, 1988; Id., *Putting difference to work*, 1991; de Shazer S., Dolan Y., Korman H., Trepper T., McCollum E., Berg I.K., *More than miracles: The state of the art of solution-focused brief therapy*, 2007; Hubble M.A., Duncan B.L., Miller S.D., *The heart and soul of change: What works in therapy*, 1999; Norcross J.C., *Psychotherapy relationships that work: Tailoring the relationship to the individual client*, 2002; Selekman M.D., *Pathways to change: Brief therapy with difficult adolescents*, 1993; Id., *Working with selfharming adolescents: A collaborative, strengths-based therapy approach*, 2006; Id., *The adolescent and young adult selfharming treatment manual*, 2009; Id., *Collaborative brief therapy with children*, 2010.

COLLECTIVE

In Jungian analytical psychology, all the psychic contents that do not belong to a single individual, but rather to a society, a population, or to humanity as a whole, are defined as "collective". Not only concepts, opinions and ways of thinking belong to these collective contents but also feelings, sensations and insights shared by a large number of individuals. According to this definition given by Jung, the concept of "collective" refers to the extra-personal dimension of the unconscious (→ collective unconscious), and consciousness (or "collective consciousness"). According to the antinomic concept of psyche proposed by Jung, everything that is collective (general) stands opposite to what is individual, but such opposition does not concern two entities, but two different interpretations of the same phenomenon or phenomena. *[E. V. Trapanese]*

COLLECTIVE UNCONSCIOUS

In Jungian thought, an original and uniform germinal disposition of the human psyche that underlies the conscious psyche and one's personal → unconscious. It would include all the contents that are not the result of personal acquisitions, but of functional capabilities inherited by the psyche, that is, the inherited brain structure. This would represent what gives meaning even to conscious mental processes. At least two interpretative hypotheses stem from this radical conception of the unconscious. According to the first hypothesis, the collective unconscious and its → archetypes would represent the prime foundation of the biopsychological human being and the shaping forces of the whole psychic life. According to the second, the collective unconscious should be considered a heuristic category, useful to define: the set of contents removed for adaptive reasons, the functional abilities inhibited by the development of the conscious personality and finally the elements that form the "opaque background" of the psyche. Nowadays, the concept of collective unconscious is controversial since it seems impossible to attribute a unique meaning to it and since it can be conceived as a naturalistic psychologization of the symbolic forms of culture. In fact, every idea and every expressive human activity finds its imaginary foundation in an archetype, so that man is called upon only to draw from the enormous treasure of primordial images kept in the collective unconscious. Therefore, this view proposes an image of the psyche flattened by the early development of human history. *[E. V. Trapanese]*

COMMON SENSE

Common sense is a system of knowledge in which individuals or groups attribute reality and truth, and in which they have confidence. This system is founded on shared beliefs about the physical, human and social world, providing explanations to events, rarely questioned, and interpretations of their own and others' behaviour, which may be useful to master the environment and to keep it under some level of control. Heider outlined a model of "common sense psychology", or naive psychology that leads individuals' behaviour, interpersonal relationships and opinions in social situations. Although these opinions are not always explicit, they often work suitably as a scientific theory that makes inference possible. According to Bem, such beliefs would be characterized by a conceptual structure based on syllogistic reasoning, and centrality, considered as the effect of one belief on another. A belief is deep-rooted if it is trustworthy, if it has centrality and significance, if it is accessible cognitively, and if the whole belief system (→ logic of belief) is recognized as coherent and organized. This is related to psychotherapy because the last is evaluated by individuals on the grounds of their belief system, and because the psychotherapeutic work arises from the theory of common sense used by individuals in structuring the image of themselves and their malaise, in order to elaborate different perspectives for examining the reality and intervening on it. *[P. Meringolo]*

REFERENCES. Bem D.J., *Beliefs, attitudes, and human affairs*, 1970; Gulotta G. *Psicologia, senso comune e buon senso*, in M. Cesa-Bianchi, A. Antonietti (eds.), *Dentro la psicologia. Contesti, teorie, ricerche, personaggi*, 2002; Heider F., *Psicologia delle relazioni interpersonali*, 1958.

COMMUNICATION

In its most general sense, a transmission or conveyance of information, from one entity to another, by various kinds of means (as described in the mathematical theory of information) or, even more generally, an exchange of messages whose forms can be studied by different disciplines (such as linguistics, sociology, cybernetics, etc.). According to linguistics, there are three areas of study of communication: structure (that investigates the transmission of a message), semantics (that investigates meanings) and pragmatics (that investigates the effects of communication on behaviour).

According to the Russian linguist Jakobson, in every communicative exchange there is a sender (the one who sends the message), a receiver (the one receiving the message) and a context (the totality of the general situation and of particular circumstances in which communication occurs). To ensure that communication is possible, a code (common to both sender and receiver) and a contact (physical or mediated by another channel between sender and receiver), able to establish and maintain communication, are also needed. Watzlawick analyzed the pragmatic and relational aspects of communication (→ pragmatics of human communication) and formulated five axioms that have revolutionized the approach to the study of psychopathology. Therefore, according to this interactional logic, able to produce changes on human behaviour, communication consists in a twofold activity: to inform and persuade. Every type of → therapeutic talk, aimed at producing change, utilizes its own rhetoric, usually consistent with its own theoretical principles. Consequently, it is possible to identify rationalistic and demonstrative therapies (such as psychoanalytic, behaviourist and cognitive therapy) and injunctive and suggestive therapies (such as hypnotic and strategic therapy). Since communication is the main vehicle of therapy, each approach has formalized different communication techniques to guide patients to overcome their problems/disorders. *[R.]*

REFERENCES. Jakobson R., *Linguistics and poetics*, 1960; Watzlawick P., Beavin J.H., Jackson Don D., *Pragmatics of human communication*, 1967.

COMPARATIVE METHOD

In analytical psychology, it configures the possibility of retrieving analogue and comparable psychic expressions in cultures or contexts different from each other. Its assumption is the hypothesis formulated by Jung about the existence of a → collective unconscious and of its primordial images (→ archetypes); examples are universality of the image of → mandalas, mythic-psychopathological parallels (the → Oedipus complex). The hypothesis has been developed in a diachronic sense by Neumann, for whom the coordinates of the evolution of collective consciousness as described in myths – the Ouroboros (the snake that bites its own tail, a symbol of original undifferentiation), the Great Mother, the Hero, the murder of the mother and of the father, the Ego's consolidation – repeat themselves during each individual's development. From a clinical point of view, the comparative method coincides with the "hermeneutic" possibility of amplifying the material brought by the patient into the session. *[G. Antonelli, A. Dorella]*

REFERENCES. Jung C.G. (1934–1954), *The archetypes and the collective unconscious*, in *Collected Works* IX/I, 1969; Neumann E., *The origins and history of consciousness*, 1949–1954.

COMPASSION-FOCUSED THERAPY

"Compassion-focused Therapy" (CFT) is derived from and based on so-called "compassionate mind training", originally developed by Paul Gilbert to treat people with high levels of shame and self-criticism. According to this view, such people find it particularly difficult to be supportive and reassuring to themselves, in part because they never learned to be so, as a consequence of their frequent traumatic, critical and shaming environment. A greater ability to reassure oneself and show compassionate feelings for oneself has proven beneficial for many chronic problems. CFT is one of several new forms of therapy that Hayes has defined as the so-called "third generation" of cognitive-behavioural therapy (CBT). These innovative therapies, originated in the first half of the 1990s, also include Acceptance and Commitment Therapy (ACT), Dialectical Behavioural Therapy (DBT), Functional Analytic Psychotherapy (FAP), Integrative Behavioural Couple Therapy (IBCT) and Mindfulness Based Cognitive Therapy (MBCT). These approaches are based on the tradition of Cognitive-Behavioural Therapy (CBT), although they differ in some respects. In fact, while not abandoning the strategy of direct change, they place the emphasis on contextual and experiential change strategies that modify the function of problematic psychological events, without intervening directly in changing their shape or frequency. So they widen the focus of the intervention from the reduction of symptoms to the development of skills aimed at significantly improving the quality of life. Even with severely disturbed patients, such new therapies emphasize → empowerment and increased behavioural repertoire, not only the mere reduction of problem behaviours. This emphasis on building skills in a non-pathologizing way, on normalization and acceptance can also be found in the assumption that therapists, being as human as their patients, are struggling with many of the same difficulties. The theory behind CFT stems from recent developments in neuroscience on positive emotions, and these have suggested the existence of two basic systems able to regulate positive affect. The first one (which we call "motivating") aims to achieve and act, while the second one (so-called "soothing") is focused on achieving happiness and satisfaction, as well as peace and "safeness" in social relations. In this sense, when we are satisfied, we don't strive to achieve something more. Furthermore, the "soothing" system would have evolved as a regulator of the "threat recognizer", a system that tends to seek "safety" from dangers: for example, in mammals with a system of attachment, parent closeness and care can make a puppy, for example, feel calm and secure. In a normal course of events, repeated experiences of safety by parents stimulate and integrate the soothing system as a natural regulator of threats recognized; on the contrary, negative early experiences can alter this process, making difficult the access to the soothing system as an affect regulator. Thus, in some people, for example those with paranoid aspects, the system is particularly responsive to threat and the soothing one, for various reasons, is inactivated; consequently they feel that in order to be safe they must be highly vigilant with respect to the environment; if the paranoid ideas become delusional, with the appearance of hallucinated hostile voices, then, along with the external world, the internal one becomes a source of threats, further activating the system precisely specialized in responding to them. The therapeutic approach of CFT, most exhaustively exposed in a recent handbook, helps people to interpret their problems, such as excessive safety behaviours, bringing them to be more understanding and compassionate towards such behaviours, diminishing the shame arising from them and depathologizing and normalizing them. The therapist supports the person to empathize (→ empathy) with the fear and distress (→ stress) underlying the safety behaviours, developing tolerance for some of these fears. He/she also discusses the function and value of compassion towards oneself. Compassion is made up of the following important components: sensitivity to one's own and others' discomfort and needs; concern for one's own and others' welfare; a non-judgmental attitude; sympathy, the ability to be moved by one's own and others' distress; empathy, an understanding of one's own and others' minds, having a theory of mind, decentralizing; distress tolerance; the ability to not avoid and of "staying" with one's emotions and memories, with an attitude of → mindfulness. These goals are pursued through the use of various procedures. The person (or persons, as the CFT can be carried out usefully in a group) is taught how to generate feelings of warmth and self-acceptance in response to their thoughts of self-criticism. These feelings are then used in the process of examining threat-centred thoughts, in order to practice attention, thinking and behaviour focused on compassion towards oneself. When people begin to feel "safer", they may be able to recognize their own interior style, critical and hostile to themselves. According to CFT, self-criticism is a safety behaviour, which, at least initially, may be useful, because, according to the prudent so-called "better safe than sorry" strategy, having a critical attitude towards oneself can induce one to take precautions and to improve. If this strategy, however, is used too often, it can induce "external" shame (towards others) and "internal" shame (towards themselves), thereby maintaining the activated threat system, preventing one from feeling safe. Trying to create warm and compassionate feelings towards themselves, people can gradually develop new ways of thinking and feeling, rather than considering their thoughts (→ cognition) and → emotions as wrong and pathological. Just as, if we are hungry and see a sandwich, the production of saliva and stomach acid can be stimulated, a similar effect can be induced by the simple mental image of a sandwich. Consequently, both external and internal stimuli can create effects; people are gradually rendered able to understand the relationship between imagination, thought and physiology. This process is also valid for external and internal criticisms, which are both able to stimulate the threat systems; this equally applies to all sources of calm, reassurance and acceptance, both external and internal ones, which can activate the soothing system. If people understand this, they may come to consider CFT as a kind of "physical therapy for the brain". The self-critical thoughts of people are considered in the context of their history, so they come to consider them understandable and to develop empathy for their distress. Through progressive muscle relaxation they are helped, by guided imagination, to visualize a compassionate picture or to bring back emotionally connoted memories in which they were sympathetic to someone or others were so to them. The process of imagination is based on the "here-and-now" and people are asked to focus on compassionate modes as the unconditional acceptance (→ positive and unconditional acceptance) and to generate a feeling of warm affection with this image. Once able to view the more compassionate side of themselves and the associated feelings of warmth, people are invited to reassess their self-critical thoughts, and, in the meantime, they are brought to consider how they can relate and behave in a more compassionate manner in relation to themselves.

These procedures can be usefully inserted in the processes of classical CBT and have been used so far in addressing, individually and in groups, subjects characterized by severe self-criticism, shame towards themselves (also due to significant physical and aesthetic problems,, with auditory hallucinations and even malicious voices. CFT is an interesting new development in CBT, which combines elements from evolutionary psychology and Eastern disciplines in a creative synthesis, and has relevant therapeutic potential, but must still be evaluated by randomized and controlled clinical trials. *[D. Dèttore]*

REFERENCES. Carter C.S., *Neuroendocrine perspectives on social attachment and love*, in «Psychoneuroendocrinology», 1998, 23, 779–818; Depue R.A., Morrone-Strupinsky J.V., *A neurobehavioural model of affiliative bonding*, in «Behavioural and Brain Sciences», 2005, 28, 313–395; Gilbert P., *Social mentalities: Internal "social" conflicts and the role of inner warmth and compassion in cognitive therapy*, 2000, in Gilbert P., K.G. Bailey (Eds), *Genes on the couch: Explorations in evolutionary psychotherapy* (pp. 118–150).; Gilbert P., *Compassion: Conceptualisations, research and use in psychotherapy*, 2005; Gilbert P., *Compassion-focused therapy: Distinctive features*, 2009; Gilbert P., Irons C., (2005). *Focused therapies and compassionate mind training for shame and selfattacking*, in P. Gilbert (ed.), *Compassion: Conceptualisations, research and use in psychotherapy* (pp. 263–325).; Gilbert P., Procter S., (2006), *Compassionate mind training for people with high shame and selfcriticism: Overview and pilot study of a group therapy approach*, in «Clinical Psychology & Psychotherapy», 2006, 13(6); Hayes S. C., *Acceptance and commitment therapy, relational frame theory, and the third wave of behavioural and cognitive therapies*, in «Behaviour Therapy», 2004, 35, 639–665; Hayes S. C., Strosahl K., Wilson K. G., *Acceptance and commitment therapy: An experiential approach to behaviour change*, 1999; Jacobson N.S., Christensen A., *Integrative couple therapy: Promoting acceptance and change*, 1995; Kohlenberg R. J., Tsai M., *Functional analytic psychotherapy: Creating intense and curative therapeutic relationships*, 1991; Linehan M.M., *Cognitive behavioural treatment for borderline personality disorder*, 1993; Linehan M.M., *Skills training manual for treating borderline personality disorder*, 1993; Mayhew S.L., Gilbert P., *Compassionate mind training with people who hear malevolent voices: A case series* repor, in «Clinical Psychology and Psychotherapy», 2008, 15, 113–138; Schore A.N., *Affect regulation and the origin of the self: The neurobiology of emotional development*, 1994; Segal Z.V., Williams, J.M., Teasdale J.D., *Mindfulness-based cognitive therapy for depression: A new approach to preventing relapse*, 2002.

COMPENSATION

A necessity arising from the essential → need of balance and fairness that characterizes human actions in the context of their social life. Unlike the term "reward", which indicates a value that reflects motivation and behaviour (conjunction), the term compensation underlines a contribution that balances a loss and that is not closely related to an action (disjunction). The money obtained for a job is a reward, but the money found on the ground after losing a job is a compensation. Compensation re-establishes improperly and indirectly a condition of balance without cancelling the relevance of the unsatisfied element or request. Although unsatisfactory as regards the desired object, compensation has a profound psychological meaning as it contributes to the illusion that justice is a law governing the universe ("just-world" hypothesis by M. Lerner), meaning that some form of justice "should" exist and that therefore bad luck or chance are not prevalent in the world (theories of attribution; *locus* of control). *[S. Smiraglia]*

▷ In Jungian analytical psychology, it is a natural self-regulating function of the psyche that operates keeping a continuous dialectic relationship and exchange between the conscious and the unconscious. When consciousness excludes unpleasant contents, these contents settle in the unconscious where they work as a natural counterweight to conscious attitudes and continue to be expressed in actions, thoughts and feelings, or dreams. The compensation acted by the unconscious establishes the psychic balance. An excessive one-sidedness of consciousness creates a barrier between the conscious and the unconscious, which can stiffen and lead to a conflict (neurosis), or even to a dissociation (psychosis). Therapy aims to restore this function with a work of awareness and integration of repressed contents. *[A. Benvenuti]*

REFERENCES. Jung C.G. (1921), *Psychological types*, in *Collected Works*, VI, 1971; Id. (1951), *Fundamental questions of psychotherapy*, in *Collected Works*, XVI, 1966; Id. (1957), *Schizoprenia*, in *Collected Works*, III, 1960.

COMPENSATORY STRATEGIES

An important concept, particularly in the understanding and treatment of patients with personality disorders, is that of "compensatory strategies". These are largely dysfunctional patterns (→ dysfunctional balance) of behaviour that Axis II patients display across situations and across time. They represent an attempt by patients to cope with their highly negative beliefs about themselves, their worlds and other people. These behavioural strategies are idiosyncratic to the patient. One patient, for example, believes at heart that he is incompetent. He therefore displays behaviour such as avoiding challenges. Another patient, with the same belief, copes with this painful idea by hiding any sign of weakness, unduly preparing and checking her work, and pushing herself to achieve highly. Conditional assumptions help explain why patients use certain compensatory strategies. They believe, "If I [use my compensatory strategy], I'll be okay but if I don't, my core belief will come true". *[J. S. Beck]*

REFERENCES. Beck A.T., Freeman A., Davis D.D., Associates, (2004), *Cognitive therapy of personality disorders* (2nd ed.); Beck J.S., *Cognitive therapy for challenging problems: What to do when the basics don't work*, 2005.

COMPLEMENTARITY

According to the analytic psychology of Jung, this term suggests a reciprocal relationship between two entities, which only together will constitute a totality or make sense. An example can be the mutual complementarity between conscious and unconscious: it is not possible to mention one of them without referring to the other, or even the mention the individual without referring to the general. *[A. Benvenuti]*

▷ In the systemic-relational paradigm the complementarity describes a pattern of relationships where individual or group behaviours and inspirations reciprocally differ, completing each other. This kind of relationship, if harmonic, allows the establishment of a dynamic and → functional balance. During the course of the years, Bateson, studying the Naven ritual of Iatmul natives in New Guinea, was the first to talk about complementarity (as well as symmetry).

According to Bateson, every culture progressively establishes its own behavioural pattern, to which individuals must conform. Therefore, the common proprieties result from the relationships between groups and individuals within the community. These relationships, because of the dichotomous nature of Occidental or Western thought, possess bipolar features, of which typical examples can be authority–submission, admiration–exhibitionism, care–dependency and, even if expressing mainly one of these two terms, individuals also present the other end of the relationship. Therefore, the cumulative interaction between individuals, groups and cultures brings about a process of differentiation in rules of individual behaviour, defined by Bateson as "schismogenesis", that can be expressed in a complementary (for example, in the structuring of social strata, classes, cast) or symmetric manner (for example, in the creation of factions, clans, villages, nations).

Watzlawick, Beavin and Jackson have applied these assumptions to couple and family therapy and, in particular, J. Haley has argued that complementary behaviour is characterized by two different positions: one-up (typical of the person who controls and defines the relationship, dominant position) and one-down (peculiar to the individual in a secondary and inferior position). Differences in partners in the couple or families' behaviours reflect and reinforce each other, creating an interdependent relationship in which respective roles are accepted by the various actors involved (for example, the mother–child relationship, doctor–patient, teacher–student).

In other words, the complementary schismogenesis occurs when one of the protagonists of the interaction behaves in an opposite way to the other one. Therefore, it is not a dysfunctional relational scheme in itself. It becomes problematic if a person, permanently and pervasively, recruits and retains a one-up or, on the contrary, a one-down position, determining a relational hardening. For instance, problems related to complementary relationships can occur if one member of the communication, asking for self-confirmation, receives in return a disconfirmation, subsequently developing a sense of frustration and despair, which can also move to the other interlocutor. In addition, certain individuals show their pathology only if observed along with their "complementary", appearing well-adapted in any other communication context. The theory of *folie à deux*, ideated by two French psychiatrists, C. Lasègue and J.P. Falret in 1877, perfectly fits this find. Complementary conflicts are usually less explicit and more subtle than those that are symmetrical, characterized by a high level of intrinsic relational competitiveness. *[G. Castelnuovo, G. Pietrabissa]*

REFERENCES. Bateson G., *Steps to an ecology of mind: Collected essays in anthropology, psychiatry, evolution, and epistemology*, 1972; Jung C.G. (1935), *Principles of practical psychotherapy*, in *Collected Works*, XVI, 1966; Trevi M., *Per uno junghismo critico*, 2000; Watzlawick P., Beavin J.H., Jackson Don D., *Pragmatics of human communication*, 1967.

COMPLIANCE

An explicit or implicit positive response of a subject to suggestions, prescriptions, treatments and indications. In medicine, psychiatry and clinical psychology, adherence to treatment and therapeutic indications are a crucial factor for the success of a treatment; an excellent prescription or indication, in fact, may not work if it is not followed by the patient. Patients may not follow the given directions for several reasons: because they do not understand them, they do not agree with them, they are frightened by them; because they do not feel understood, they are overwhelmed by dominant feelings and emotions (fear, → pain, → pleasure, anger); because the proposed suggestions and changes are too big and/or they drastically alter the patient's lifestyle; because the → secondary gain consequent to the pathologic condition surpasses the disadvantages; because of the fear of recovering and much more. *[R.]*

CONCEPTUAL REALISM

Level of reality attributed to a certain class of events configured as being psychological, social and cultural, which, on the basis of conventions and their effects, transform themselves from being conceptual entities into objects that exist in reality. This property, identified by Salvini as being the "ingenious realism" of → common sense, in the positivist psychologies and in → psychiatric diagnosis, is based on the presupposition of reification, or rather, the coincidence between the word and the nominated object, that transforms constructs of meaning into empirical entities, making them manifestly independent from dialogues and intentions. From this point of view, a wide range of events are considered by the observor as existing in reality, also in light of the effects that they produce: whether these are social artefacts, beliefs, objects, emotional states, acts and actions, implying in certain cases also the presence of corresponding physiological states. For example, a certain event, construed and perceived as being threatening can become real in its physiological effects by activating a sympathetic-mimetic response (perspiration, increase in heartbeat or in the rate of breathing, etc.). Realities that are invented, imagined, attributed or narrated can find confirmation in the subjective experience of the individual and fulfil an adaptive or maladaptive function in symbolic or relational contexts, acquiring the cognitive and emotional properties of entities that are conceptually real and perceived as such. *[R.]*

REFERENCES. Salvini A., *Pluralismo teorico e pragmatismo conoscitivo: assunti metateorici in psicologia della personalità*, in E. Fiora, L. Pedrabissi, A. Salvini, *Pluralismo teorico e pragmatismo conoscitivo in psicologia della personalità*, 1988.

CONDENSATION → DREAM

CONDITIONED REFLEX → CONDITIONED RESPONSE

CONDITIONED RESPONSE

Also known as a conditioned reflex, it was "discovered" at the beginning of last century by Pavlov, a Russian scientist (→ behavioural model of classical conditioning) from his studies in physiology. This was the first scientific research into the study of learning processes and it provided a model that could be tested and verified. This is how a conditioned response is generated: an → unconditioned stimulus (US) is presented that is able to elicit an → unconditioned response (UR), that is, a response that is genetically programmed and not learnt, for example, if we show a dog some meat, it will start to salivate. Then, this stimulus is paired with a → neutral stimulus (NS), (for example ringing a bell) that is not able to elicit an unconditioned response (salivation). By showing the meat (US) and ringing the bell at the same time (NS), salivation of the dog is elicited. After repeated presentations of the association US + UR, the NS will be able to elicit the UR on its own. From this moment the NS can no longer be described as being "neutral" and will be described as being a → conditioned stumulus (CS), and the response elicited will be called a conditioned response or conditioned reflex: the sound of a bell ringing (CS) will elicit salivation in the dog (CR). *[E. Rolla, S. Durando]*

REFERENCES. Pavlov I.P., *Conditioned reflexes*, 1903.

CONDITIONED STIMULUS

Within the behaviourist paradigm a conditioned stimulus is defined as being a → neutral stimulus that, as a result of repeated presentations in association with an → unconditioned stimulus, becomes able, by itself, to induce an → unconditioned response that from that moment onwards will be denominated as being a → conditioned response. Renowned are the experiments of I.P. Pavlov in which, following repeated associations with the unconditioned stimulus "meat", (that is, the presentation of food), the sound of a bell ringing or a light had acquired the power of inducing salivation in dogs. *[E. Rolla, S. Durando]*

CONDITIONING

In the behavioural paradigm, a type of → learning consisting of a shaping effect elicited by the environment on an individual's behaviour. In the behavioural therapy based on classical or respondent conditioning, first investigated by J. Watson, conditioning assumes the trait of an instinct-based mechanism. A response, elicited automatically by an environmental stimulus, is learned and stabilized over time so that in the future, the same behaviour will follow the reappearance of the same stimulus. In the behavioural psychotherapy based on operant conditioning, investigated especially by B. Skinner, conditioning refers to a response emitted spontaneously by an individual. According to this model there are two possibilities: in conditioning by → reinforcement, people experience an environmental condition that is a source of pleasant stimuli. Therefore, they tend to stabilize their behaviour over time as they aspire to re-experience the same pleasant condition in the future. In conditioning by → punishment, people experience an environmental condition that is source of unpleasant or adverse stimuli, and they tend to extinguish (→ extinction) their behaviour because their desire is to avoid re-experiencing the same unpleasant condition in the future. However, in both cases, a behaviour undergoes a process of learning that can stabilize or limit it over time. *[A. Tamburello, E. De Monte]*

REFERENCES. De Monte E., Tamburello A., *Storia del pensiero psicologico*, 2008; Hill W.F., *Learning: A survey of psychological interpretations*, 1963; Reber A.S., *Dictionary of psychology*, 1985.

CONFLICT

A state of tension that appears at the intrapsychic level (within an individual), interpersonal level (between individuals) or intergroup or global level due to a perceived incompatibility of aims or scarce resources. A conflict, as an expression of opposing forces, generates instances of change in the situation and in the relationship between the elements in tension, which can show themselves also in the form of → aggressiveness and violence. Unresolved conflicts may also underlie personal withdrawals such as avoidance and depression. In that regard, there is a close interdependence between intrapsychic conflict and interpersonal conflict and one can refer to overt or latent conflicts, realistic or unrealistic conflicts, and other- or self-directed aggressiveness. In the psychodynamic perspective, the → drive resulting from a conflict reveals itself in feelings, ideas and behaviours that reflect the specific → defence mechanisms that are activated. If, because of this instance of change, a conflict can lead to aggressive and destructive behaviours, it may also provide the basis for creative and ameliorative expressions compared to the status quo. A conflict can lead to overcoming situations characterized by personal discomfort and relational impasse and it can push individuals and groups to look for more advanced and advantageous solutions (divergent thinking). Game theory assumes particular relevance when investigating conflicts with the classic distinction between zero–sum games (I win–you lose) and variable sum games (we both win or lose). With reference to this last point, a conflict can make differences of interest explicit, which, rather than degenerate, can translate into opportunities for negotiation and promote the development of cooperative behaviours. *[S. Smiraglia]*

▷ In psychoanalytic theory the concept has assumed a growing importance because it had to replace a real → trauma, also if assuming a growing metapsychological nature moving away from clinical experience. At the beginning conflict was shaped by the conscious activity of the mind and a mental representation incompatible with consciousness (for example the memory of an incest) and social norms of the subject. After the development of speculation concerning unconscious activity (metapsychology) the conflict takes place between sexual and Ego instinct . After the introduction of structural theory, the conflict occurs among Ego, Id and Superego. With the last theoretical period we have a conflict between life and death instincts. This conflict was cautiously explored by Freud but became fundamental for Melanie Klein as the cause of neonatal schizophrenia (→ paranoid–schizoid position). *[G. Fossi]*

REFERENCES. Eiser R., *Cognitive social psychology: A guidebook to therapy and research*, 1980; Festinger L., A theory of cognitive dissonance, 1962; Fossi G., *La psicologia dinamica: un'eredità del XX secolo*, 1983; Freud S. (1938), *An outline of psycho-analysis*, in *The Standard Edition*, XXIII, 1953–1974.

CONFLICT NEGOTIATION TECHNIQUE

In the field of systemic-relational mediation, intervention technique used by a mediator in order to facilitate the resolution of → conflict between two or more parties. First phase: the mediator helps the parties to admit to both the existence of a conflict as well as to the necessity of resolving it; second phase: encourages the involved parties to suggest possible options for the resolution of the conflict; third phase: helps the parties to choose the best solution for the resolution of the conflict. The conflict can be at the level of the "content" and/or at the level of the "relationship": the resolution of the conflict at one of these levels does not automatically lead to the resolution of the conflict at the other. *[M. Menafro]*

REFERENCES. Busso P., *Lotta e cooperazione. Percorsi per un'evoluzione ecologica del conflitto*, 2004; Canevelli F., Lucardi M., *La mediazione familiare*, 2000.

CONFLUENCE

In Gestalt therapy, a condition of scarce differentiation between individual and environment, with a basically undifferentiated hyper-osmosis in the flow of information between the internal and external world. This function expresses itself positively in the early stages of one's growth, amorous intimacy, empathic sharing and mystical experiences of transcendence of the Ego. On the other hand, it expresses itself negatively in the inability to differentiate the individual from the environment in an elective and discriminative way. *[R. Zerbetto, A. Poletto]*

REFERENCES. Perls F., Hefferline R.F., Goodman P., *Gestalt therapy: Excitement and growth in the human personality*, 1951; Zerbetto., *Il Sé come membrana: modello, metafora, episteme*, in Id. (ed.), *Psicoterapia della Gestalt: per una scienza dell'esperienza*, 1994.

CONFUSION OF TONGUES

A concept introduced by Ferenczi in a disputed paper, published in 1933. The confusion is intended between the child's "language of tenderness" and the adult's "language of passion". The adult may mistake (the language of) tenderness for (the language of) passion, therefore projecting his/her own sexual desire onto the child. The reaction of the adult, denying the reality of the seduction, results, for the child, in an experience of abandonment, guilt and an impaired perception of reality. Such experience causes a form of inner division, compromising the Ego functions, particularly in the area of object relations. In this specific case Ferenczi introduces the concept of "traumatic confusion". In 1908 he had already mentioned "masked sexual acts", perpetrated by adult relatives, to which children fall victim; he had subsequently spoken about a "sort of pitfall" set up by parents for the child, so envisaging later "mystification" and → "double-bind" constructs. The confusion of tongues applies not only to the adult–child, but also to the analyst–patient relationship: the analyst's failure in communicating empathically with the patient reactivates the ancient trauma, reinstating the traumatic confusion of tongues. The analyst hides such inability behind a mask of professionalism, an attitude branded by Ferenczi as "professional hypocrisy". *[G. Antonelli]*

REFERENCES. Ferenczi S., (1908), *The analytic interpretation and treatment of psychical impotence*; Id., *Confusion of tongues between child and adults*, 1933.

CONFUTATION → RATIONAL ANALYSIS

CONGRUENCE

In the context of client-centred therapy, a state of agreement between experience and its representation at a conscious level, that is, the ability to symbolize experience without defensively distorting it. According to Rogers, congruence is synonymous with mental health. It is the ability to be deeply in touch with oneself, others and the world. A good level of congruence characterizes self-aware people, it allows people to be authentic, to communicate and to be what one really is without erecting barriers or facades. A good level of congruence makes a person capable of transparency, which Rogers considers to be synonymous with authenticity. Incongruence is synonymous with dysfunction and lack of contact. The goal of client-centred therapy is to help the organism of the client improve its contact/congruence ability. This helps to restore the innate tendency towards self-congruence and → self-regulation of the human organism. The level of congruence of the therapist, that is, good contact with their own process, with the construction of their own experience in an unbiased manner, allows them to have good contact with the client's process. This is considered by Rogers to be a more reliable instrument of knowledge of the other person than diagnostic tests. *[A. Zucconi]*

REFERENCES. Rogers C.R., *Client-centered therapy*, 1951; Rogers C.R., Kinget M.G., *Psychotherapy and human relations*, 1962; Zucconi A., *La bussola del professionista*, 2006; Id., *Odissea nello spazio relazionale: la psicoterapia centrata sul cliente e l'approccio centrato sulla persona dal 1942 ad oggi*, 2007.

CONSCIENCE

In psychoanalytic theory, the meaning of this term is ambiguous. According to Freud, on one hand it represents a part of the moral functions; therefore, it appears as the result of parental criticisms introjected by individuals. At a later time, Freud conceptualized it as a function of the Superego. In this case, it was meant as a sense organ, suitable for perceiving psychic qualities, which identifies states of instinctual tension and of the discharge of excitement in the qualitative form of pleasure and displeasure. From a functional point of view, the perception–conscience system of mnemonic traces is opposite to the preconscious–unconscious system. From an economic perspective, it is characterized by having free energy available, which is used to perform the attention process. *[G. Fossi]*

CONSCIOUS → UNCONSCIOUS

CONSTRUCTIVITSM

An epistemological perspective according to which reality is the product of the cognitive actions of the subject. This approach contrasts the idea of an existing objective, *a priori* and ontologically determined reality that can be "discovered". Constructivism asserts that the only possible reality is the one that depends on the mental operations of the observer, and, as such, it is created by the act of knowing itself. In Glasersferld's opinion, "reality" can be measured only on the basis of the concepts of pragmatism, practical efficacy and usefulness, or, to use his own expression, on the concept of "viability", that is, on the basis of what is functionally "viable". According to the well-chosen expression used by Watzlawick, any knowledge would always be an "invented reality".

Starting from this epistemological premise, some important applications follow in the field of psychotherapy. First, it is the attention given to "psychological relativism", meant as a subjective construction, different from individual to individual, of every mental phenomenon. This enables the interpretation of psychic suffering in the light of personal experiences and individual perceptions, avoiding the normative and organicist perspectives of psychopathology (→ psychiatrization → labelling → psychiatric diagnosis). Second, by replacing the concept of "truth" of knowledge with "adaptation" of knowledge, constructivism opens the way for interventions focused on the functional/dysfunctional (→ dysfunctional balance) adaptation processes of individuals to their own perceived reality. These can go from learning new meanings to developing alternative behaviours by introducing the theoretical construct of "operational awareness" as the methodological foundation of every therapeutic intervention.

Many theoretical approaches in psychotherapy have adopted constructivist ideas (interactive-strategic, relational-systemic and cognitive paradigms in particular). Currently, three main approaches can be identified: radical constructivism (which takes inspiration from the work of H. von Foerster, von Glasersfeld and Watzlawick); critical constructivism (Mahoney and Guidano); and Kelly's "personal construct theory". Radical constructivism denies the possibility of an existing reality independent from the presence of an observer. Consequently, it asserts the impossibility of a purely objective knowledge. Differently, critical constructivism keeps the "realistic" idea of a reality that is independent from the mental processes of the observer. Therefore, this approach does not deny the existence of a "real" physical world, although it emphasizes the subjective aspects of knowledge. Finally, personal construct theory focuses on the possible alternative dimensions of meaning that guide the act of knowing and consequently the development of perceptions, concepts and "worldviews".

The constructivist perspective is linked to an ancient philosophical tradition that can be traced back to some Greek philosophers such as Protagoras. His aphorism "man is the measure of all things" can be considered as the first formulation of a view that emphasizes the creative nature of experience.

In the late Middle Ages, the first manifesto of constructivist thought can be identified in the philosophical ideas of G.B. Vico, according to which, man is "the creator of his own ideas" and "truth lies in what is done".

In the modern age, this term was mentioned for the first time in psychology by J. Piaget to describe children's cognitive and conceptual development as a consequence of an active construction of reality.

The first proper constructivist theorization can be attributed to Kelly's work on personal constructs. The consequent development and dissemination of constructivist ideas was driven forwards by various authors. Among them it is important to mention Watzlawick, H. von Foerster, U. Maturana and F. Varela. The most complete systematic theorization of constructivism was provided by the German philosopher and cybernetic von Glasersfeld. *[A. Bartoletti]*

REFERENCES. Bridgman P.W., *Reflections of a physicist*, 1955; Ceruti M., Bocchi G., *La sfida della complessità*, 1985; Diels H., Kranz W., *Die Fragmente der Vorsokratiker*, 1952; Kelly G., *The psychology of personal constructs: Theory and personality*, 1955; Guidano V.F., Liotti G., *A constructivistic foundation for cognitive therapy*, in Mahoney M.J., Freeman A., *Cognition and psychotherapy*, 1985; von Glasersfeld E., *Radical constructivism: A way of knowing and learning*, 1995; Watzlawick P., *How real is real? Communication, disinformation, confusion*, 1976; Id., *The invented reality*, 1981.

CONSULTANCY

A professional service required by whoever seeks advice or help to solve a contingent problem, to set a goal and plan the most suitable ways of achieving it. Consultancy concerns the most diverse areas: family, education, sport and vocational guidance. Consultants perform an evaluation of their object of study and guide clients to achieve their goal by relying on experience and by using the most suitable tools in relation to the situation (questionnaires, tests, interviews). Generally, consultancies, which last for a limited period of time and concern a specific problem/goal, are part of the various intervention procedures in psychology. An effective consultancy allows applicants to gain clarity on the mechanism underlying the problem that led them to ask for it or on how to reach their goals more effectively: discovering the effects of their own actions on themselves and others; increasing their ability to make autonomous and focused choices by introducing new perspectives on the critical situation, which facilitate the possibility of identifying more functional actions and ways of thinking; being accompanied in pursuing new ways identified by applicants themselves, in order to achieve the established objectives within agreed timelines. Various types of consultancies can be distinguished: when it is directly oriented towards the individual who has a problem, the consultant is the person who directs the client towards the best ways to address the situation. From this point of view, consultancy can be distinguished from psychotherapy, as it is not aimed at solving clinical problems but rather at helping the person to face "non-pathological" difficulties that may be met in different areas of their lives. Consultancy can also concern organizational situations, in both private and public settings, where consultants make their knowledge available to individuals, groups or companies to reach a more effective management of organizational structure dynamics. Finally, consultancy can be a relationship between two colleagues, in which one asks the other for aid, opinions or supervision in relation to a professional situation that is difficult to manage. The consultant works indirectly, guiding the colleague to address effectively the difficulty with their patient/client. In such cases, the advice often achieves a double result: contributing to the resolution of the specific issue and allowing the colleague to learn something that could be used later in their career. *[R.]*

CONTACT-BARRIER

According to Bion, the contact barrier marks the splitting between unconscious and conscious, functioning as a permeable membrane. Thus, it regulates the passage of the elements between the two instances. The contact barrier will condition memory according to the form by which the passage of elements between conscious and unconscious is controlled. It derives from the work of the "alpha function" (the process transforming rough psychic elements into thoughts). It is formed by the continuous proliferation of "alpha elements" (psychic elements, the features of which can be used both as thoughts of the dream, or as thoughts of wakefulness). In their generation, alpha elements tend to cohesion: they unite, aggregate and order in sequence, to form a narration. In subjects who show some disturbances in their capacity of thinking, or have a worn-out or badly developed "alpha function", as happens with some psychotic subjects, the barrier of contact can be damaged, so that the conscious becomes overexposed to sensory impressions that come from external reality (phantasies and projections by the unconscious). If the contact barrier loses its ability to discriminate the intrapsychic from reality, "alpha elements" (thoughts) turn themselves into "beta elements" (sensory impressions are transformed into "beta elements" – sensory impressions of emotional experiences, rough psychic elements, which are not intelligible): these are → bizarre objects. The capacity to dream and remember dreams depends on the integrity of the contact barrier. A deficiency at this level is observable in psychotic subjects who present what they believe to be dreams, but are probably not oneiric thoughts (formed by alpha elements) but hallucinatory phenomena (what Bion properly defines as "transformations into hallucinosis"), characterized by the anguishing presence of beta elements. *[G. Perfetto, A. Voltolin]*

REFERENCES. Bion W. R., *Learning from experience* 1962; Grinberg L., Sor D. Tabak de Bianchedi E., *Introducciòn a las ideas de Bion*, 1972; Meltzer D., *A Kleinian development, 3*, 1978.

CONTACT BOUNDARY

In Gestalt therapy, a metaphor indicating the area where the parts involved make any kind of exchange. → Contact is a metaphor used to indicate a specific quality of relationship that transforms the people involved: a relationship where "electricity" passes between the parts involved, and that implies an effect of one on the other. Of course, the meeting between the two elements can only be partial, otherwise it would be an overlap, not a contact. However, contact boundary does not exist as a structure, as such, nor does it exist on the border of the Ego. This is a concept directly related to contact boundary and it simply refers to the extension of the psychic world that the person is able to manage. The consequences that can be drawn are metaphorical and, obviously, they cannot be confused with deductions. The term "contact boundary" refers to the parts of themselves that people bring into play when encountering the other, and to the place, always in a metaphorical sense, where they meet. The image of touching borders evokes the details of the event without interpretations, and, from a phenomenological-existential perspective, it facilitates the view of the → defence mechanisms in place. Concerning the distance between people, the difference between being and not being in touch refers to the difference between inhabited and uninhabited space. Metaphorically speaking, being in touch implies that this space, large or small, is inhabited by relational movements and vital processes that take place between the parts involved. In synthesis, this expression is a metaphor for all the emotional, cognitive and practical operations in which people are willing to get involved. *[P. Quattrini]*

REFERENCES. Brentano F., *Psychology from an empirical standpoint*, 1874; Perls F., Hefferline R.F., Goodman P., *Gestalt therapy: Excitement and growth in the human personality*, 1951; Polster E., Polster M., *Gestalt therapy integrated: Contours of theory and practice*, 1973.

CONTACT FUNCTIONS AND DYSFUNCTIONS

In Gestalt therapy, a biopsychosocial dimension of the relationship with ourselves and with others. The term refers to something different from the term communication, which is more abstract, as it implies a transfer of symbolic information. The focus shifts from the primacy of thought (which reaches its peak in the Cartesian "cogito ergo sum") to a Heideggerian "dasein" (being-there in the world), preceding the very possibility of thinking-about-it, and from here to the "being-with", in full awareness of a body that "we are" and not that "we have". From this perspective, Gestalt therapy focuses its attention on those borderline phenomena in which the particular relational style of each person is expressed – and that passes through the "theory of the Self" – which was defined by F. Perls as "function of creative adjustment" between an organism (or an individual, if endowed with self-reflection) and environment. This view is echoed by D. Anzieu who, in his "skin-ego", highlights that "experience occurs at the boundary between the organism and the environment, primarily the skin surface and the other organs of sensory and motor response". He linked this to what was claimed by Freud when describing the "contact-boundary" function in reference to the "paradoxical" feature of a boundary that both hinders and allows the transfer of information. In this perspective, relational processes depend on how effectively osmotic the "membrane Self" can be, therefore enabling and selecting the passage of information in the twofold direction – internal-world–external-world, and vice versa. Hence the different possibilities of individual–environment interaction, defined as: → confluence, egotism, introjection, projection, → retroflection → proflection and → deflection. *[R. Zerbetto]*

REFERENCES. Freud S. (1851), *Project for a scientific psychology*, in *The Standard Edition*, I, 1953–1974; Perls F., Hefferline R.F., Goodman P., *Gestalt therapy: Excitement and growth in the human personality*, 1951; Zerbetto R., *Il Sé come membrana: modello, metafora, episteme*, in Id., (ed.), *Atti del IV congresso internazionale di psicoterapia della Gestalt. Per una scienza dell'esperienza*, 1994.

CONTAINED → CONTAINER

CONTAINER

A term used by Bion closely linked to the term "contained" to designate two complementary functions (which may be carried out by different elements of psychic life) such as relationships between objects, meanings of words, ideas (as analyst and analysand). In different moments, the elements involved in the relationship can reverse their roles: the container can act as the contained and vice versa. The relationship that links the container and the contained always determines a mutual transformation. Bion developed this concept by reflecting (as is typically done in British psychoanalysis) on specific relational modalities (mother–child in particular) that play the role of "containment" – protection, emotional stimulation and support – and facilitate development and maturation: "a patient," says Bion, "will describe various objects as *containers*, such as his mind, the unconscious, the nation; others as *contained* such as his money, his ideas. The objects are many, but the relationships are not." The relationship between the container and the contained keeps its essential characteristics in very different contexts. Bion analyzes this relationship hypothesizing three fundamental categories:

> by "commensal" I mean a relationship in which two objects share a third to the advantage of all three. By "symbiotic" I understand a relationship in which one depends on another to mutual advantage. By "parasitic" I mean to represent a relationship in which one depends on another, to produce a third which is destructive of all three.

These concepts have broad application in relation to processes of transformation promoted by psychotherapy. Therefore, the relationship between the container and the contained can be used to understand the relationship between analyst and patient, the events that occur during its evolution and the transformations that it can produce; it is therefore an element of great importance in the Bionian conception of the therapeutic process. *[P. Cruciani]*

REFERENCES. Bion W.R., *Learning from experience*, 1962; Id., *Attention and interpretation: A scientific approach to insights in psychoanalysis and groups*, 1970.

CONTAMINATION

In Berne's psychopathological theory of transactional analysis, which also includes the condition of → exclusion, contamination is a phenomenologically dysfunctional state in which the individual perceives as objective reality the → here-and-now feelings and beliefs coming from their unresolved infantile experiences and from parental models that are not re-elaborated. In terms of → Ego states, people perceive themselves in their → Adult states, but they react according to patterns belonging to their → Child and/or → Parent states. According to Berne, contamination is at the basis of all the intrapsychic and relational disorders; therefore, it becomes the focus of the therapeutic work. A classic example of contamination by the Parent of the Adult are prejudices, that is, opinions about themselves and others, learned from parental figures and never critically re-elaborated. An example of contamination of the Child by the Adult is of lasting infantile phobias, such as a school phobia, which becomes performance anxiety in adult individuals. *[M. Novellino]*

REFERENCES. Berne E., *Transactional analysis in psychotherapy*, 1961; Novellino M., *Psicoanalisi transazionale*, 2004; Id., *Seminari clinici. La cassetta degli attrezzi dell'analista transazionale*, 2010.

CONTEXT

A set of elements related to each other, which within a text or a situation provide a meaning to both the whole and the individual parts. Therefore, context is responsible for attributions of meaning. Depending on the discipline, the word "context" may indicate different realities: for example, in chemistry, the term physical context indicates the characteristics of the environment within which certain reactions occur; in architecture, ergonomics and workplace safety, physical context indicates the set of elements of a room or a place that affect the psychological state of the occupants (including size and arrangement of living spaces and furniture, light, ventilation, temperature, noise, etc.). In all these cases the term "context" can be synonymous with "situation". In linguistics, a portion of text or a text in its entirety is defined as linguistic context. L. Wittgenstein supported the idea that context is essential to understanding the meaning of a word and that the meaning of a word or a concept depends on its context. In psychology, the communicative (or extratextual) context is particularly important. It represents the general circumstances of the communicative act that allow a message to acquire one particular meaning rather than another. Indeed, the same message, placed in different contexts, can have different meanings. As most of → communication takes place in conditions of semantic → ambiguity, the reference to the context is essential to attribute correct meanings. In this regard, it is useful to recall the phenomenon of the "exploitation of the context" whereby, within a communication, participants take full advantage of the characteristics of the context to shorten the communication or express themselves concisely. In psychotherapy, the context within which the therapeutic relationship takes place is often defined as → setting. Two elements can be identified in it: the set (the totality of the spatial-temporal characteristics within which the relationship takes place) and the "relational rules" that modulate the therapist–patient relationship. If the therapeutic context determines the meaning of that particular communication, it is important to remember that it is influenced by the reference theory adopted: therefore, the characteristics of the setting vary from theory to theory (in psychoanalysis, for instance, taking care of the analytical setting is of great importance). *[R.]*

CONTRACT

It is the supporting pillar of all the operative applications of transactional analysis. The contract expresses both a philosophical principle – as every professional relationship between a transactional analyst and a client is based on an explicit sharing of responsibility on the aims of the intervention and on the modality of its procedure, through a clarification about the respective roles – and the initial phase of the methodology of the intervention. In this phase, the transactional analyst aims to energize the → Adult Ego state of the client, in order to prevent the possible start of → psychological games that would undermine the possibility of an effective work. The contract includes an "administrative" aspect, which corresponds to the construction of a work → setting, and a therapeutic aspect, linked to the definition of the objectives of change. Regarding the level of depth of the therapeutic work, one distinguishes between: "focal therapy" contracts (brief psychotherapy with transactional analysis), aimed at a symptomatic cure; "restructuring therapy" contracts, aimed at curing the patient's → script, with consequent intrapsychic and general relational changes; and "analysis" contracts, aimed at the understanding of one's dynamic unconscious, which are used in particular in didactic analysis by transactional analysts in training. *[M. Novellino]*

REFERENCES. Berne E., *Principles of group therapy*, 1966; Novellino M., *Seminari clinici. La cassetta degli attrezzi dell'analista transazionale*, 2010.

CONTRADICTORY CONFIRMATION PRESCRIPTION

In → brief strategic therapy Nardone's model, is the key → prescription with patients who feel constantly refused by others, thus reverting to avoiding human contact in order to protect themselves (→ attempted solution). In line with this operative hypothesis, the strategic therapist invites these patients to act like an anthropologist, that is, to go around gathering all clues of refusal, while systemically categorizing "the sensed refusal" onto a scale from 0 to 10; 0 being total refusal and 10 full acceptance. This prescription works on various levels. First, without disqualifying the patients' belief (→ logic of belief), it inexplicitly conveys that not all "the others" will act in the same way and thus refuse them outright. By looking for different shades of refusal, patients will challenge the prophecy (→ logic of belief), that is, "everyone refuses me unconditionally", which leads them to either avoid or, if forced, to proceed to fulfil the negative prophecy (→ self-fulfilling prophecy), establishing antagonistic rapports. Second, shifting the patient's attention from their fear of refusal onto carrying out the task, brings them to do something that they would have had great difficulty doing if asked explicitly, i.e. avoid avoiding. "By sailing the sea unknown to the sky" (→ stratagem), the therapist surmounts the patient's → resistance to change, allowing them to undergo a → corrective emotional experience that will challenge their rigid perception and consequent reactions. By getting closer to others, looking for refusal, more often than not individuals find consent and acceptance, thus putting into question their perceptions and their relationship with others. By making them study "others" and categorize them in different ranks, they are led to discover and perceive their enemy as a more manageable entity. Others are no longer perceived as a scary massive battalion but rather as a number of approachable small troops with their respective weak points which can be "barraged" more easily. Moreover, in line with the Contact Hypothesis, getting closer to the feared object renders it familiar and thus the "feared enemy" can more easily become a friendly companion. *[C. Portelli]*

REFERENCES. Nardone G., Balbi E., *The logic of therapeutic change*, 2015.

CONTRAPOSITION

Cognitive, emotional, relational and social situation. Contraposition implies an opposition, usually antinomically polarized, and an activation of hostile and aggressive feelings and actions that can be acted on, denied or elaborated. The scheme is dualistic and works by exclusion, conversion or persuasion, as in the case of a semantic or ideological contraposition. In cognitive psychology, there is cognitive dissonance when two constructs, intentions or actions come into competition or in opposition: one example is the so-called "akrasia" where people act in opposition to their own choices. In psychoanalysis, a contraposition between instances may activate → defence mechanisms, which have the purpose of hiding the → neurotic conflict, which shows itself as a compromise through the symptom. In relationships between → groups, contraposition is typically processed through self-defensive cohesiveness, hierarchical and authoritarian dynamisms and through socially accepted forms, like competitiveness and competition, in which hostility and aggression are contextually regulated. In psychotherapy, contraposition can be used by the therapist (for example, mediation in couple therapy) to elicit resources and awareness in order to change the problem. *[R.]*

CONTROL-MASTERY THEORY

In the psychodynamic paradigm, according to the theory formulated by Weiss, Sampson and colleagues at Mount Zion Hospital in San Francisco, the activity of the human being is not aimed uniquely at the discharge of psychic → energy in order to achieve goals related to the satisfaction of drives. They asserted that the psyche is not driven only by the compulsion to repeat (→ repetition compulsion) past experiences; in his behaviour man also aims to improve, to adapt better to his environment, to look for new situations that will allow him to discredit his pathological beliefs that make him suffer and that put him in difficulty. According to this theory, the patient unconsciously searches, according to what is called an "unconscious plan" – a fundamental concept of this approach –, new experiences and persons that are able to pass the "tests" that he himself "fabricates" with the aim of discrediting pathological beliefs arising from childhood experiences.

The task of the therapist is therefore that of passing the tests of the patient (→ testing by the patient) and going along with the "unconscious plan" by making interpretations that are consonant with it. The Plan Formulation Method was proposed in order to help the therapist diagnose this "plan" in a credible manner and in a short period of time with the aim of "passing" the tests given to him by the patient. Psychotherapy is seen as being a situation of safety in which the patient can remember and re-experiment the painful situations of the past, integrating them into his global personality. *[S. Sagliaschi]*

REFERENCES. Weiss J., *How psychotherapy works: Process and technique*, 1993; Weiss J., *The role of pathogenic beliefs in psychic reality*, 1997; Weiss J., Sampson H., Mount Zion Psychotherapy Research Group, *The psychoanalytic process: Theory, clinical observation, and empirical research*, 1986.

CONVERSATIONAL THERAPY

Within the systemic-relational paradigm, this term indicates a therapy – also called dialogical therapy – that is collaborative, discursive, relational and open to dialogue, made by a set of principles that come from postmodern theories and hermeneutics. These principles represent a possible divergence from the classical conception of psychotherapy, in which the theories formulated to understand humans, their lives and their behaviours are based on inherited, taken-for-granted and ultimately static categorical knowledge. Conversational psychotherapy offers an alternative vision in understanding human systems (simple and complex), their lives and behaviours. Human beings are considered as unique and active participants who are involved in the construction of knowledge. This psychotherapy proposes a different mode of understanding "language" (and words), and emphasizes the connection between language and change. "Understanding" is meant as a dialogical and participatory process (which does not mean agreement, and is fraught with uncertainty). It highlights the role of perception in understanding and relating to the worlds in which we live and the fact that we always wear multiple interpretive lenses. It focuses on the inconspicuous (more often invisible) power of discrepancies that are part of our language, our words, our relations and our societies. These assumptions include: observing a critical and questioning attitude on knowledge; privileging a circumscribed knowledge (e.g. expertise, truth, wisdom, values, conventions, narrative etc.) created under a community of people (family, organization, class, etc.), who have direct knowledge of themselves and of their situation; seeing the construction of knowledge as an interactive-interpretative process in which each part contributes to its creation, fluidity, sustainability and change (therefore, this process is not elementary, definitive, fixed or identified); considering language and knowledge as dynamic and creative (for example, words do not "reveal" meanings, but become meaningful in their use and in how they are used); considering both language and knowledge as relational and generative and therefore intrinsically capable of creating change. Therefore, transformation or change are intrinsic to therapy. These assumptions represent the attitude or the "philosophical" position of the therapist. It refers to how the therapist thinks, acts and responds together with the client. This attitude has some distinct and interconnected features that guide the therapist's ideas, give information about how they think about the relationship and the conversation with the client and help the therapist to create and build a metaphorical "space" for them. This philosophical position is used as a practical philosophy, a conceptual guide and not as a formula; it is not a set of techniques. The characteristics of this type of therapy can be summarized in six points: 1) *Conversational relationship of mutual inquiry*. Attracting and engaging the other person in a collaborative relationship and in a dialogical conversation means inviting them through the therapist's way of being. This way says that the client and their situation have a special significance for the therapist, that there is respect for their views and that what clients have to say is taken into consideration without being judged. This gives rise to a relationship and a process characterized by a combined activity called "shared inquiry" or "mutual inquiry". All feedback, comments, questions of the therapist are provided by the conversation and are consistent with it. 2) *Relational competence*. Therapist and client bring their competencies to the session. Clients are expert in themselves and their world; the therapist is expert in a process and a space concerning collaborative relationships and dialogical conversations. Considering the importance of the client's competence does not mean disregarding the therapist's skills. Focusing on the client's knowledge of their life warns against assessing, favouring and venerating the therapist as the one who knows more and better than clients themselves. This does not suggest to pretend a lack of experience. Rather, the competence of the therapist is to create and maintain a basis of collaborative relationship and dialogic conversation. 3) *Not knowing*. It refers to how a therapist reflects on construction of knowledge and on the purpose and manner in which this is introduced into the therapy. It is a humble attitude concerning what therapists think they should know and the belief that therapists do not have access to inside information; they can never fully comprehend another person and they always need to learn more about what was or was not said. A collaborative therapist keeps the emphasis on understanding "with" another person, rather than knowing the person, the circumstances or the results obtained, better than the person themselves or even in advance. Collaborative therapists are aware of the risk that such *a priori* knowledge may cause them to place subjects in certain categories of problems. This interferes with the willingness to care about that person and to learn something about their uniqueness and the originality of their life. However, assuming the perspective of not-knowing does not mean being ignorant or abandoning and not using what a therapist knows (for example, theoretical knowledge, clinical experience, life experience). 4) *Being public*. Therapists have private thoughts, both in the form of professional, personal, theoretical evaluations, and in the form of experiential understanding (e.g. diagnosis, judgments or hypotheses). These thoughts affect the ways in which therapists hear and listen, and this affects their reaction. Thus, therapists should not entrench themselves behind their invisible thoughts, but have to make themselves visible, "public". Being public offers food for thought and dialogue and provides a wide range of topics to talk about or ways to do it. This is a way that the therapist can adopt to contribute to the conversation. 5) *Living with uncertainty*. Therapeutic conversations are more like natural conversations, where the reaction of each person influences and encourages the response of the other. These are not guided by structured "maps" or preconceived questions. Instead, they are spontaneous activities in which the client and the therapist create together the journey and determine its destination. What is built is different from, and is much more than, what one would have created by themself, without the other. When the client and the therapist meld in this type of spontaneous attempt, there is always uncertainty about where they are headed and how they will reach it. 6) *Transforming each other*. In this type of relational process, of "united testimony", each party involved is influenced by the other (or others) and is exposed to the risk of change (including the therapist). This is not a unilateral process guided by the therapist, nor must the therapist be passive or receptive. The therapist is actively involved in a complex interactive process of continuous response not only with the client but also internally with their own experience. As conversational partners, they constantly coordinate their actions with those of the other and they are constantly influenced by the other. Consistently, with their philosophical and therapeutic assumptions and their philosophical attitude, therapists are not instruments of change, they do not solve or "fix" the client's problem, they cannot determine the meanings that the client gives to the therapist's actions nor how the client is influenced by them. The transformation, or change, is rather a natural consequence of the collaborative relationship and of the dialogic conversation. Ultimately, the task of the therapist is to enable a process in which these things an happen and can be maintained. *[H. Anderson]*

REFERENCES. Andersen T., *The reflecting team: Dialogues and dialogues about the dialogues*, 1991; Anderson H., *Conversation, Language and possibilities: A postmodern approach to therapy*, 1997; Anderson H., Gehart D.R., (eds.), *Collaborative therapy: Relationships and conversations that make a difference*, 2007; Bateson G., *Mind and nature: A necessary unity*, 1979; Deleuze G., Guitarri F., *A thousand plateaus: Capitalism and schizophrenia*, 1987; Foucault M., *The archeology of knowledge*, 1969; Heidegger M., *Being and time*, 1962; Hoffman L., *Family therapy: An intimate history*, 2002; Merleau-Ponty M., *Il visibile e l'invisibile*, 1968; Seikkula J., Alakare B., Aaltonen J., *Open dialogue in first-episode psychosis ii: A comparison of good and poor outcome cases*, in «Journal of Constructive Psychology», 2001, 14; Shotter J., Katz A., *Living moments in dialogical exchanges*, in «Human Systems», 1996, 9(2); Strong T., Paré D. (eds.), *Furthering talk: Advances in the discursive therapies*, 2004; Vygotskij L., *Thought and language*, 1934; Id., *Philosophical investigations*, 1953.

COPING

Mentioned for the first time by Lazarus, the term can be used as a synonym of "effective answer" or "problem-solving ability". In the context of cognitive-behavioural therapy, it indicates the set of mental and behavioural strategies put in place to deal with a given situation. It also refers to the management of one's own emotions and stress derived from being in contact with a problematic situation. *[G. Palmieri]*

REFERENCES. Lazarus R., Folkman S., *Stress, appraisal and coping*, 1984; Snyder C.R., *Coping*, 1999.

CORE-SCHEMATA

In cognitive-behavioural therapy, a set of beliefs about the self (→ self-concept) and the world that are central to one's basic sense of identity (→ personal identity). Core-schemata are the basis of the processes used to interpret experiences and tend to be manifested consistently across a broad range of situations. They help people develop expectations about the way the world is and understand what is going on. They are fundamental in clinical settings as, when activated, they tend to generate a high level of affect which may, under certain conditions, involve or be associated with suffering. Since they involve knowledge about oneself and oneself in the world, core-schemata are fundamentally linked to experiences of attachment (→ attachment processes) and the concept of internal working model described by J. Bowlby. *[R.B. Ardito]*

REFERENCES. Bowlby J., *A secure base: Clinical applications of attachment theory*, 1988.

CORRECTIVE EMOTIONAL EXPERIENCE

An expression introduced by Alexander in 1946 to indicate those specific emotional experiences that allow the patient to «correct» the traumatic influence of previous negative experiences. According to Alexander, the most significant and long-lasting therapeutic changes would not take place by virtue of a mere evocation of repressed past memories, but by virtue of real experiences - lived by the patient in the present, in the relationship with the therapist or in their daily life - able to reverse the effect of the past ones. The concept of corrective emotional experience was revived and extended in the brief strategic approach (→ brief strategic therapy Nardone's model), which has made it one of the main cornerstones of their therapeutic process. As highlighted by Watzlawick and Nardone, any change, in order to be quick and efficient, must first produce a concrete experience of perceptual-emotional change in the person and only subsequently undergo a cognitive reflection. To minimize a patient's → resistance to change, therapeutic change must then start with the phase of experience and only later be translated into cognitive awareness. Corrective emotional experience in strategic therapy is achieved through random "planned" events, that is, situations that appear as fortuitous to the patient, but that are carefully prepared by the therapist to produce the desired corrective effect. This experience can be caused both within the therapeutic session, for example using → strategic dialogue, and between sessions thanks to the use of behaviour → prescriptions that patients must introduce in their daily life. *[R.]*

REFERENCES. Alexander F., French T.M., *Psychoanalytic therapy*, 1946; Nardone G., Milanese R., *Il cambiamento strategico*, 2018; Nardone G., Watzlawick P., *The art of change*, 1993.

COUNSELLING

In client-centred therapay, *counselling* is an active dialogical process between a counsellor and a client (or more clients in the case of counselling for couples, families or groups), characterized by an interpersonal exchange based on principles of empathy, authenticity, congruence, love for the truth and the integration of many psychological models and communication skills. In various fields of application (supportive relationship, training, company and community areas), it aims at helping the client (or clients) to examine and analyze reality, to clarify systems of thought that are dysfunctional for the realization of their projects, to resolve crisis situations or suffering states or forms of discomfort in life and in relationships, to make decisions and to process conflicts and to deal with specific problems. The practice of counselling is specifically based on the achievement, in an agreed amount of time, of responsibly negotiated targets that meet the deep intentions of the subject. These targets promote routes of awareness and self-knowledge, personal wellbeing, improve the connection with others and implement functional resources to increase self-esteem and feelings of self-efficacy, to find their own inner harmony and to regain the deepest meaning of one's own life and death. *[F. Nanetti]*

▷ To avoid creating confusion, it is necessary to underline that the term *counsellor* is also used in English-speaking countries within humanistic methods, but in those cases it identifies a figure that cannot replace a psychologist or psychotherapist: in fact, Italian legislation does not recognize counselling as a profession and does not contemplate a specific training procedure, while as far as professional psychology and psychotherapy are concerned, it requires the achievement of a degree in psychology or medicine and four years specialization in psychotherapy. *[R.]*

COUNSELLOR

A counsellor is a professional operator who facilitates a supportive relationship aimed at helping clients to make more independent choices in their lives in order to increase their self-awareness. He focuses on health as well as mental and physical wellbeing, he helps to orientate the person and he supports them in the development of their resources. The basic skills of the counsellor are concerned with *knowing how to be* an empathic, congruent, authentic person, conscious of his own values, feelings and thoughts and willing to offer unconditional acceptance. The counsellor uses many techniques: active listening, which avoids judgment and interpretation; exploration, using open and closed questions; clarification to encourage elaboration; paraphrase to help clients focus on the content of their message and to emphasize this message when expression of feelings at this point would be premature; reformulation to encourage awareness and expression of emotions, while testing out their intensity in order to learn how best to handle them; and clarification to connect multiple elements, to identify a recurrent theme and to summarize for further goal-setting. In this way, the relationship is built on recognition, respect and congruence, promoting self-understanding and self-exploration. *[C. Montanari]*

REFERENCES. Giusti E., *Dizionario di counseling*, 1995; Hough M., *Counselling skills and theory*, 1999; Rogers C.R., *Counselling and psychotherapy*, 1942.

COUNTER-CONDITIONING

Within cognitive-behavioural psychotherapy, it is a procedure borrowed from classic (or respondent) conditioning on which → systematic desensitization is based. It consists of the repeated association between the anxiogenic stimulus and an antagonistic response to anxiety, usually relaxation, in order to produce a progressive "reciprocal inhibition" between the stimulus and the associated response until the extinction of the anxiogenic response occurs. In clinical practice, after the start of relaxation, the visualization of the anxiogenic item (→ imaginal exposure) is elicited until the subject begins to feel anxiety. Relaxation is induced again and the patient evaluates the degree of anxiety he/she experienced according to the "SUD" scale. Even in the presence of mild anxiety, counter-conditioning must be repeated until total extinction, before moving on to the next item. *[E. Luisetti]*

REFERENCES. Galeazzi A., Meazzini P., *Mente e comportamento*, 2004; Meazzini P., *Trattato teorico-pratico di terapia e modificazione del comportamento*, 1984; Wolpe J., *The practice of behaviour therapy*, 1969.

COUNTER-PARADOX

A term coined by a group of therapists belonging to the → Milan school that indicates an intervention aimed at counteracting the paradoxical communication of psychotic families. They gained interest in the pragmatic effects of communicative paradox from the studies of G. Bateson's group, who had worked on the emergence of psychosis in paradoxical communicative contexts. The Milan school therapists claimed that the therapeutic context proposes the typical challenge of families with schizophrenic communication: the therapist's attempt to change a family is mirrored by the presumption of the family members to control the relationships unilaterally. Therefore, the counter-paradoxical technique of the group avoids challenging the family to make a change, and thus to negatively characterize the problem and the relationships. Instead, the therapists communicate their appreciation to the member carrying the symptom; the latter is defined as useful for the family unit, even as an act of love and loyalty as he/she avoids worse problems (for example, the disintegration of the system). In this way, by allying with the homeostatic tendency of the system (→ homeostasis), they introduce the idea that the sufferer is the "designated patient" to support the family homeostasis. *[M. Giuliani]*

REFERENCES. Selvini Palazzoli M., Boscolo L., Cecchin G., Prata G., *Paradox and counter-paradox*, 1978.

COUNTER-RITUAL TECHNIQUE

A key instrument of → brief strategic therapy Nardone's model in the treatment of obsessive-compulsive disorders (OCD). This is a condition that shows itself in various forms, with repetitive behaviours or thoughts through which the person tries to neutralize an obsession. The counter-ritual consists of a set of ritualized actions or thoughts that the therapist prescribes to the patient using the same non-ordinary → logic underlying compulsive rituals, in order to redirect them and bring them to their self-annihilation.

This technique stems from the recognition that any attempt to persuade patients to block their compulsions through a rational explanation, feeds the problem instead of solving it. In fact, OCD patients are highly resistant to change and able to follow the directions of the therapist only if these seem to direct them towards "a seemingly more efficient" behaviour to achieve the same purpose of their rituals. The patient will be more inclined to cooperate if the suggested counter-ritual follows the same logic, dynamics and conditions of his/her ritual. For example, if the compulsion is to check or wash something multiple times, using the same logic, the patient is prescribed the following counter-ritual:

> between now and the next time we meet, every time you will implement one of your rituals, you will have to do it five times, neither more nor less. You can avoid doing that, but if you do it once, you will have to do it five times, neither more nor less. You can avoid doing it, but if you do one, you do five.

This apparently simple prescription follows an ancient Chinese stratagem: "Lead the enemy up the attic and then remove the ladder". In fact, by proposing an → illusion of alternatives, the prescription will lead to an inevitable change, both in case the patient does not perform the ritual, and in case they decide to repeat it five times. In the latter case, prescribing the ritual, which is spontaneous, as something voluntarily acted on, depriving it of its spontaneity turns it into a real torture (→ be spontaneous paradox; → symptom prescription). The prescription implies the acknowledgment by the therapist of the necessity of the compulsive ritual, but at the same time the therapist takes full control of it, deciding how many times this has to be repeated. In most cases, patients report that their counter-rituals had become really tedious and confess that, unexpectedly, after a while they preferred to avoid performing them. This unblocking usually leads patients to question the real usefulness of their compulsions and, in parallel, to a clear and progressive decrease of the anxiety and fear that the ritual was supposed to control. An important aspect of this strategic → prescription is the fact that it is transmitted to the patient with a particularly injunctive communicative style: the wording is based on a hypnotic linguistic assonance and it is redundantly repeated, with a post-hypnotic message expressed with a stronger voice ("You can avoid doing it"). If the patient's compulsions have a more elaborate structure, a simple prescription is not appropriate and it is necessary to build an ad hoc counter-ritual, always following the same logic, dynamics and methods of the compulsive ritual. In order to tune this (→ tuning technique), the therapist, using → strategic dialogue, must investigate all the features of the ritual: if it is based on fear or pleasure, whether or not it has a specific sequence, if it is rational or magical, if it is precautionary-propitiatory or reparatory, if it includes actions or it is just mental and so on. Only through this investigation will the therapist be able to build a proper and effective counter-ritual and unblock more resistant disorders. *[C. Portelli]*

REFERENCES. Nardone G., *Brief strategic solution-oriented therapy of phobic and obsessive disorders*, 1996; Id., *Oltre i limiti della paura*, 2000; Id., *Cavalcare la propria tigre*, 2003; Nardone G., Watzlawick P., *The art of change*, 1993.

COUNTER-SCRIPT

In the area of transactional analysis, defensive sub-modality of the → script. The latter derives from defensive reactions of the child to parental → injunctions, while the counter-script is constructed by the child in reaction to parental counter-injunctions, which consist of verbal messages that transmit the known expectations of the parents regarding the child. If the injunctions have an inhibitive nature ("Do not . . ."), the counter-injunctions are transmitted by "You should" – be perfect, be strong, hurry up, be helpful, try. Both the injunctions and the counter-injunctions are internalized in the → Parent Ego state, and produce an internal dialogue that reproduces the relational dynamics that the child experienced with the parental figures. This internal dialogue recreates an adaptation of the → Child Ego state, with consequent states of impasse, which become the object of intervention on the part of the psychotherapist. *[M. Novellino]*

REFERENCES. Berne E., *"Hello!" . . . and then what?*, 1972; Novellino M., *Psicoanalisi transazionale*, 2004; Id., *Seminari clinici. La cassetta degli attrezzi dell'analista transazionale*, 2010.

COUNTERTRANSFERENCE

A complex of experiences and fantasies of the analyst, generated in the analytical relationship with the patient and especially as a reaction to → transference. Although some elements of countertransference can be found in Freud's body of work, it is a concept developed by later authors. Freud used this term in 1909, in a letter to C.G. Jung; he talked about it at the Nuremberg Congress in 1910, and he also used it the same year in a letter to S. Ferenczi. In 1926, H. Deutsch cites this term as a seemingly "paranormal phenomenon" happening during psychoanalytic sessions.

Initially, the countertransference is treated as a potentially damaging distortion of the analyst's experience that, originating from unanalysed issues or the therapist's blind spots (each unresolved repression in the clinic setting coincides, according to W. Stekel, with a "blind spot" in the therapist's analytical perception), affect negatively his analytical ability. In 1929, Jung considers countertransference as an essential instrument in analytical work. As well as transference, countertransference became more considered and, from being regarded as a damaging distortion, became an opportunity to unconsciously seize the dynamics of the patient or to resonate with their world. D.W. Winnicott (1965) describes the "countertransference hate" that the analyst can experience against specific patients and that poses delicate problems of progressive revelation. P. Heimann (1950) believes that the analysis of countertransference helps the analyst to better understand the patient and the reactions that the patient himself activates in people that are in contact with him. In this way, countertransference becomes a "depersonalized" phenomenon, facilitating knowledge. The author, by claiming that countertransference is an expression of a part of patients' personality, opens the way to the attention paid by Klein and Bion to the role of projective identification and counter-projective identification in transference and countertransference phenomena. Racker distinguishes between *complementary* and *concordant* countertransference. He connects the first to a projective identification mechanism and to a replica of a premature objectual relationship with the analyst. The second highlights the analyst's empathic abilities towards the patient. According to F. Fornari (1979), the analyst would experience within himself parts of the patient's personality and he/she would be able to return them, "cleared". According to G. Atwood and R. Stolorow (1984), there is only an interchange between two subjectivities within a bipersonal interactive (intersubjective) field that creates a specific dimension in psychoanalytic treatment. According to J. Weiss (1993), countertransferal feelings of confusion or discomfort may indicate a passive-into-active testing put in place by the patient (the patient assumes towards the therapist the same traumagenic conducts that one of their caregivers had put in place against them, hoping that the therapist will not be subjugated, but that he will face it constructively) using the analyst to carry out an exchange of roles compared to the current situation that allows the analyst to understand them better. *[M. Casonato, S. Sagliaschi]*

REFERENCES. Bion W.R., *Elements of psychoanalysis*, 1963; Fonagy P., *Attachment theory and psychoanalysis*, 2001; Klein M., *The writings of Melanie Klein, I–IV*, 1975; Racker H., *Transference and countertransference*, 1968.

CREATIVE ILLNESS

According to C.G. Jung, a condition from which the sick person emerges with a new vision of the world, a new *Einstellung* (attitude) or a new philosophical insight. Frequently observed among shamans, mystics, philosophers and artists, the creative illness was called "sublime hypochondria" by Novalis. H.F. Ellenberger refers to it with particular regard to S. Freud and Jung. It may be associated with neurotic and psychotic phenomena: depression, somatization, auditory and visual hallucinations. The attention is constantly directed towards the inside, focused on a dominant thought. Even when the relational, family and social life remains untouched, the experience is marked by total isolation (→ introversion). The conclusion leaves the subjects vested with exhilaration and with a new energy, so as to make them feel they have been through an experience of universal value. *[G. Antonelli, E. Santori]*

CREATIVE POTENTIALITY

In individual psychology, the ability to express personal creativity through action. To biological and instinctual determinism, A. Adler opposed personal, creative strength as a variable interposing between the environment and the subject. The creative way of building one's own personal attitudes towards life is characterized by the way a person's skills and environmental influences are utilized and finalized. Such a constant work of invention and and re-creation of oneself was named "creative self". "The human being has a unitary personality shaped (by) himself. He's, so to say, both the author and the work". The aim of psychological-individual therapy – played out in the empathic sharing of the "creative couple" analyst–patient – is to gradually free a patient's creative Self from neurotic and compensatory mechanisms in which he has entrapped himself. *[L. Cerioli]*

REFERENCES. Ansbacher H.L, Ansbacher R.R., *The individual psychology of Alfred Adler*, 1956.

CREATIVE SELF

In individual psychology, the harmonious and consistent creative self is simultaneously an autopoietic (→ autopoiesis) function of the psyche and a structure that fosters one's own → lifestyle towards creative adaptation to environmental demands. It is responsible for the uniqueness of the individual: it is the substance of subjective intentionality; it governs the structure of the personality; and it interprets experiences and makes them meaningful. For individual psychology, creativity is a universal attitude, an optimal outcome of the conflict/comparison between the feeling of impotence/omnipotence and the internalization of social demands. On an intrapsychic and relational level, the creative self orientates and encourages one's own lifestyle according to a perspective created by the individual: man is simultaneously a project of himself, an author and a work of art. Thanks to this, the individual transcends the ordinary stimulus/response pattern. In psychotherapy, the activation of the creative self is an agent of change and the aim of → change itself. *[A. Bianconi, B. Simonelli]*

REFERENCES. Adler A., *The fundamental views of individual psychology*, in «International Journal of Individual Psychology», 1935, 1,1, 5–8; Fassino S., Abbate Daga G., Leombruni P., *Manuale di psichiatria biopsicosociale*, 2007.

CREATIVE THERAPY

This non-schooled orientation to therapeutic practice, developed by Bradford Keeney (2009), proposes that therapy must be creatively alive for it to be engaging and effective. Like theatre and other transformative arts, if a clinical session feels boring or dead, it probably is. Furthermore, if it isn't alive, it isn't going anywhere. "Creativity" – rather than theory, method or technique – is what awakens meaningful and transformative therapy. Creative therapy encourages inspired presence rather than stale imitation. It embraces the process of developing something new, uncommon, and unique. Not simply "new for new's sake", but tailor-made both to fit and help liberate the immediate circumstances. Rather than replicating or reproducing a template to be hammered onto every clinical session, creative therapy custom builds a therapeutic encounter as the occasion requires. Respecting the authenticity of each moment, it brings about original clinical work on the stage of therapeutic transformation. If we believe each human being is unique, along with all the social interactions and contexts that contain the performance of everyday living, it follows that every clinical session should hold the possibility of conceiving a uniquely invented therapy. With this outlook, the creative therapist is ready to create, compose, construct, form, parent, give rise to, grow, bring forth, bring about and bring into being an authentic, made-in-the-moment, one-of-a-kind session.

While recognizing the value and importance of diverse models, schools and paradigms of psychotherapy, we must learn how to move creatively with our clients, or our sessions will go nowhere.

We must learn to go beyond the guidance initiated by previous clinical trainings. An emphasis upon creativity provides a revitalized reframing of therapeutic conduct that is applicable to all systems of practice. No matter what therapeutic orientation one practices, it must breathe and circulate creativity in order for sessions to come alive. Creative performance calls for the transformative presence of a therapist's (and client's) unique personal resources and talents, imagination, unpredictability, spontaneity and improvisation. Creative therapy is always changing and evolving, ready to utilize what both client and therapist bring to the table. We need to become architects of a new stage that directs its spotlight on the resources, gifts and transformative lessons delivered by any particular experience, whether it voices suffering or joy. Most importantly, we need to get on this stage and emphasize the performance rather than the interpretation of transformation. Another way of saying this is that the art of awakening a session requires moving outside of all the contexts that perpetuate the therapy game. With our clients, we must walk into an alternative theatre of creative transformation, where we play with, rather than brood over, whatever is presented. Here all experience is grist to the alchemical processes that utilize rather than cannibalize whatever life and death bring to the table. Creative therapy serves to liberate counsellors and therapists to be more creative and transformative. Our aim is nothing less than the re-contextualization of therapy as a creative improvisational art that emphasizes resourceful utilization rather than adding more rhetoric; that highlights, underscores, gives more detail or invents explanations and understandings of impoverishing experiences. You are invited to participate in the world of therapy as a performing art. Build your own stage and bring your own improvisational style. Have the courage to be part of the newborn hope that is possible when we pack up our therapeutic belongings and move towards becoming a more transformative art. *[B. Keeney]*

REFERENCES. Erickson, B.A., Keeney, B. (eds.). *Milton H. Erickson, M.D.: An American healer*, 2006; Keeney, B., *The creative therapist: The art of awakening a clinical session*, 2009.

CREATIVITY

The ability to produce ideas or new things, to find new relationships between ideas and things and find new ways to express them. Its distinctive features include novelty and moving away from traditional patterns and models and using, at times, seemingly illogical and paradoxical strategies (→ logic of paradox). The concept of creativity started being considered by psychology in the early 1900s. There have been many authors who have worked directly or indirectly with the concept of creativity; amongst them E. de Bono, with the construct of "lateral thinking". This way of thinking looks for solutions to complex problems through unorthodox methods, or with elements that would normally be ignored by logical thinking. In the field of psychotherapy, referring to Von Neumann's → game theory, some authors use the metaphor of a chess game to explain what is meant by the creativity of the therapist. He must modify the system of predictable moves to find new, unexpected and seemingly illogical winning strategic solutions within the infinite range of possible combinations in a communicative interaction between two or more people; in this way, the complexity of the game, and the range of possibilities to "play" it, are enormously amplified. *[M. Soriani Bellavista]*

CRISIS

A transient state of particular difficulty or confusion, which can be experienced at individual or social level. A person experiences a change from a state of equilibrium, that existed before the event, to a state of indecision and difficulty in managing a situation experienced as problematic. Change can be sudden and short-lived (as during a panic attack) or long-lasting, due to an imbalance created over time and not properly managed (as during a couple crisis). Aside from the duration, there is a shift from an initial discomfort to a situation that may induce, if badly managed, dysfunctional effects but, if properly addressed, a new and functional balance. Sometimes a state of crisis is inevitable, as during → adolescence, when physical, psychological and social factors are involved in the change that brings the individual from childhood to adulthood. Also, the death of a loved one results in a particularly difficult moment. The way a person addresses these situations is therefore preparatory to change: if handled efficiently they can increase feelings of capability and growth in the individual, facilitating the emergence of new ideas, new thoughts, new behaviours. A therapeutic intervention during an acute crisis has the function and the goal of helping the patient overcome the phase of intense emotional distress in a short time and leading them towards building a new emotional stability. *[R.]*

CULTURE

A broad concept used by different disciplines with different meanings. In the humanities, it is defined as the process of personal development that an individual undertakes to "cultivate" their own spirit. In anthropology and sociology, it indicates the set of customs, beliefs, attitudes, values, ideals and habits of a population or society. Generally, the existence of a culture is assumed in any significant social or ethnic group; the notion of "cultural identity" would depend on this. The characteristics of culture are: transferability (that is, it undergoes processes of → learning that take place through cross-generational communication); operativeness (it allows the individual to approach the world thanks to preselected models); selectivity (it makes selections of functional models according to the environment and the historic period); dynamism (even if it lasts over time, it is not stable, since it interacts with other cultures, creating mutual influences); layering (phenomenon whereby, within the same society, there are cultural differences based on age, gender, income, education, etc., which differentiate people's behaviours). In psychotherapy, the patient's cultural affiliation must be carefully considered by the therapist to establish a good → therapeutic alliance and a good intervention, in any theoretical context. Since culture is one of the contexts within which meanings are shared, the therapist must know how to "build" their intervention considering the cultural aspects of the person in front of them. *[R.]*

CURE

In common usage, the term is often synonymous with "therapy" and refers to the set of remedies, more or less complex depending on the case, with which an illness or a pathological condition is trying to be defeated. In this sense, the term has been used since ancient times (for example by Hippocrates) and it is closely connected to the concept of → healing. However, in 1900, M. Heidegger, began to talk about cure in philosophical terms, by defining man as the only entity able to take care of "being": according to the philosopher, existence, in its essence, is "existence cure". According to anthropologists, cure is a universal aspect of human life, as it is a condition experienced by everyone, both passively (the need of cure) and actively (the need to cure others in order to build meaningful relationships). From this perspective, the act of "curing" highlights the existence of relationships that man establishes with himself, with others and with the world, and curing actions depend on how man is considered in a particular → culture. For example, in Western medicine, cure is represented by the set of prescriptions (pharmacological or not), treatments and advice provided by a doctor, in order to eliminate or contain a pathological condition, especially physical. However, in some Eastern cultures, the concept of cure is often wider: a → symptom is tackled on a physical, a psychological and a spiritual level simultaneously. In most Western psychotherapies the concept of cure is linked to interventions aimed at overcoming a → blockage or a → crisis, or to producing a → change that the individual cannot achieve alone. The theoretical orientation of a psychotherapy defines time, means and objectives upon which to build an intervention. *[R.]*

CYBERNETICS

"Cybernetics" comes from Norbert Wiener's use of a Greek word meaning "the art of steering". In its simplest form, cybernetics is about the action that is taken and re-taken to move towards achieving a goal. More formally, cybernetics is the science of recursive patterns of organization, the study of how dynamic circular interactions constitute a whole coherence. *Simple (first-order) cybernetics:* the study of stability and change in simple circularly organized patterns of interaction, originally depicted in terms of input, output, information and control. In therapy, first-order cybernetics is illustrated by "interactional diagnosis" (→ diagnosis-intervention), where a therapist utilizes how a system responds to an effort to change it in order to redesign subsequent interventions for transformation. For a problem-and-attempted-solutions context, the relevant first-order cybernetic system involves the circular relationship of solutions that maintain problems (→ attempted solutions). Such a problem–solution interaction is stable and maintains its ongoing pattern through negative (self-correcting) feedback. *Complex (second-order) cybernetics:* the higher-order recursion of cybernetics, applied to itself – the cybernetics of cybernetics –, studies the diverse stabilities and changes of circularities embedded within other circularities. Here we discern different orders of circularity, recursion and organizational participation, the most important of which is the inclusion of the observer and therapist. The emphasis on the constructivist action (→ contructivism) of an observing therapist shifts us from discovery to invention and engaged participation. The latter underscores the steersmanship of the distinguisher, the one who makes distinctions that bring forth a particular experience. In therapy, the contribution of the therapist in constructing a reality is emphasized over the observable assessments of the presumed other, the client. Rather than regarding a therapist as distinct from a client, we move to more circular ways of underscoring the therapist–client interactional system. A second-order change is a change in the pattern of problem–solution interaction that may be delivered by a different order of solution or a different order of therapy. Gregory Bateson built a view of complex cybernetics based on a hierarchy of orders of cybernetic circuits. Heinz von Foerster created a complex cybernetics based on the formalism of recursion and eigenvalue (stability achieved through recursion). Finally, Humberto Maturana and Francisco Varela established a complex cybernetics by abandoning cybernetic metaphor and introducing the idea of autopoetic (self-produced) systems (→ autopoiesis).

In summary, simple first-order cybernetics is the science of *observed* systems, whereas complex second-order cybernetics is the science of *observing* systems. These are not opposed views, but different orders of perspective regarding cybernetics, the science of making descriptions. A cybernetic orientation to therapy is also recursively embedded, with both first-order and second-order ways of defining and prescribing our co-participation and co-constructions with clients. *[B. Keeney]*

REFERENCES. Bateson, G., *Steps to an ecology of mind*, 1972; Keeney, B., *Aesthetics of change*, 1983; Maturana, H., Varela, F., *Autopoiesis and cognition: The realization of the living*, in R.S. Cohen, M.W. Wartofsky (eds.), «Boston Studies in the Philosophy of Science», 42, 1973; von Foerster, H., *Understanding understanding: Essays on cybernetics and cognition*, 2002; Wiener, N., *Cybernetics: Or the control and communication in the animal and the machine*, 1948.

D

DASEIN → BEING-THERE

DAY'S RESIDUE

In psychoanalysis, perceptions, emotions and thoughts of the day immediately preceding a dream, that protract the activity of thought during sleep. These escape the narcissism of the dream, that shifts the libidinal investment from the representations of objects to the Ego, because they are associated (already in the state of semi-awakening during sleep itself) to repressed wishes. They can be considered as being the instigators of the dream, but only as a result of their role as the vehicle of an unconscious desire that tries to make its way to consciousness. During sleep, the day's residue converges towards the preconscious dream desire, that does not necessarily exist during waking life, and which, when configured, tends to be irrational in nature. *[S. Thanopulos]*

REFERENCES. Freud S. (1900–1901), *The interpretation of dreams*, in *The Standard Edition*, IV–V, 1953–1974.

DECONFUSION

Third phase of the methodological process of → transactional analysis described by C. Moiso and M. Novellino. After having contemplated the strategic phases of therapeutic alliance and of decontamination (→ transactional analysis) of the → Ego states, the psychotherapist helps the patient to elaborate, on a deep emotional level, the intrapsychic conflict that emerged cognitively during the work that has already taken place. What was understood by the → Adult Ego state is re-experienced through the contact with the → Child Ego state, and in this way, the Adult can reintegrate a corrective experience which will lead him to find new decisional and relational (relearning) options. The historical premise for deconfusion goes back to the work of Berne on "regressive analysis" in 1961, in which the founder of transactional analysis proposed a technique of a hypnotic-regressive type, to favour the emotional re-emergence of disturbing childhood experiences: it is to be noted that this technique was carried out using the analytic couch. This point is essential to correctly understand how the development of the deconfusion phase has taken two paths, in some ways antithetical: one is that of the "re-decision technique" of B. and M. Goulding, of a cathartic type, the expression of an integration between transactional analysis and Gestalt therapy: the liberation in the → here and now of ancient emotions as the premise of a change of the → script decision. The second is that of the psychodynamic transactional analysis of Moiso and Novellino, with the successive application of the transactional psychoanalysis of Novellino to the → setting of the individual psychotherapy, based on an interpretive elaboration of the dynamics of transference, and which recovers that prior individual work on the analytic couch of Berne. The use of the couch, therefore, characterizes a psychodynamic method with an interpretive base, aimed at the unconscious dynamics of the therapist–patient relationship, compared to a cathartic method, oriented at the conscious level of the relationship. *[M. Novellino]*

REFERENCES. Berne E., *Transactional analysis in psychotherapy*, 1961; Novellino M., *Psicoanalisi transazionale*, 2004.

DEEP STRUCTURE

In the first works of Chomsky, one of the fathers of theoretical linguistics, the deep structure of a phrase corresponds to its meaning, whilst the superficial structure refers to the different syntactical and grammatical ways of presenting this meaning. The concept of "deep structure" has been variably utilized in various psychological theories in order to indicate the totality of "fundamental" psychological processes, in contrast to psychological processes that are "superficial", the former being more structured and stable with respect to the latter. From this point of view, a change in the Self (→ self-concept) can be "deep" when it deals with the central nuclei of behaviour and "superficial" when it affects superficial aspects of the psyche of the individual. *[D. Liccione]*

REFERENCES. Chomsky N., *Syntactic structures*, 1957; Id., *Aspects of the theory of syntax*, 1965.

DEFENCE MECHANISMS

Inferred psychic processes (sometimes associated to observable behaviours) acted by a person in order to eliminate or relieve negative sensations (distress, insecurity, danger) and related to conflictual or stressful situations recurring in external reality and/or internal world. Defences work mainly in an automatic and unconscious way; only the recourse to mature defences (e.g. humour, self-observation, self-affirmation) is combined with consciousness and intentionality. Since ancient times, for example in Aesop's fable of "the fox and the grapes", the mind's ability to shape illusions in order to protect itself from pain and frustration has been demonstrated. In a scientific context, the notion of psychic defence was first introduced by Freud at the end of the nineteenth century. Despite the several interpretations proposed by psychodynamic traditions, today it is a concept that exists in a greater variety of theoretical and disciplinary approaches: from psychiatry (→ DSM) to cognitive psychology, from attachment theory to developmental psychopathology. Even if in the original Freudian concept defences were used to avoid consciousness, unacceptable thoughts, impulses or desires, recent psychoanalytic contributions have emphasized their role in maintaining self-esteem and self-cohesion. Research translated each single defence mechanism into empirical terms and organized them in "hierarchical" levels (from high to less adaptive); nowadays, the rigorous study of this construct has been permitted by the use of some clinical instruments, with regard to age and context of use. Evaluating the defensive style (on a quality or quantity level) has promoted the development of various issues such as: research on the relationship between defensive style and psychopathological pattern; on diagnostic organizations; on a mental or physical health index; on adjustment skills and psychotherapy processes. *[V. Lingiardi, F. De Bei]*

REFERENCES. Bick E., *The experience of the skin in early object-relations*, 1968; Bion W.R., *The Italian seminars*, 1985; Freud A., *The ego and the mechanisms of defense*, 1936; Freud S. (1921), *Group psychology and the analysis of the ego*, in *The Standard Edition*, VIII, 1953–1974; Klein M., *Envy and gratitude*, 1957; Meltzer D., *The Kleinian development: The clinical significance of the work of Bion*, 1978; Id., *Adhesive identification*, in Id., *The apprehension of beauty*, 1981; Meltzer D., Bremner J., Hoxter S., Weddell D., Wittenberg I., *Explorations in autism: A psycho-analytical study*, 1977.

BRIEF GLOSSARY OF DEFENCE MECHANISMS

Acting-out

Dealing with emotional conflicts and stressors by acting without thinking or worrying about the possible negative consequences. This term originates from the psychoanalytic field, where it was used to refer to feelings or transference wishes which are "acted" rather than thought. Over time, the meaning of this term has expanded to include behaviours originating outside the clinical setting. Therefore, acting-out has become an "impulsive act", which can take different forms of expression: from excessive anger, uncontrolled behaviour, up to real self-destructive acts (such as overdose, suicide attempts, dangerous driving). This allows the subject to "release" impulses or painful feelings, instead of enduring them and reflecting on the causal events. *[F. De Bei]*

Adhesive identification

In Kleinian and Bionian psychoanalysis, Klein, Bion, Meltzer and Bick give much importance to the setting-in of premature defences and of a sensory adaptation to external reality and define it as a process of "adhesive identification". Such an occurrence is due to the absence of a motherly container, valid enough to face the primary anguish of separation. In the Freudian equation between stranger and enemy, which Klein interprets in terms of absence/persecution, indifference is lived as hate. The lack of a motherly container puts the newborn baby in a state of disintegration (primary autism). The phenomenon is observed even in adults, when, all of a sudden, they are no longer capable of performing anything, as they have been assaulted by anguish and confusion. According to Meltzer, it is a form of identification based on imitation and not on introjection: "it produces a dependence similar to a sort of "clutching", where the existence, separated from the object, is not recognized". *[M. Cirlà, A. Voltolin]*

REFERENCES. Meltzer D., Harris M., *The apprehension of beauty: The role of aesthetic conflict in development, art and violence*, 2008

Anticipation

A way to mitigate or cope with emotional conflict or stressors by taking into account realistic alternatives, anticipating emotional reactions to future problems and actually experiencing the anguish in the future. Through this mechanism (for example, "How will I feel when this happens?") it is possible to plan a better adaptive response and mitigate the effects of stressful tensions or conflicts occurring in the future (for example: "I knew that talking to my parents about the decision to leave school would be stressful so, before I met them, I tried to imagine their answers and how I should deal with them"). *[F. De Bei]*

Denial

Not recognizing an aspect of internal or external reality that is, on the other hand, obvious to others. Denial allows a potentially negative feeling (such as shame, guilt, or other painful affects) to avoid reaching consciousness. For example, a person can say that she or he has been abused, denying at the same time any negative reaction, or avoiding the subject, or answering questions with an angry response ("You must be sad", "Sad? No, absolutely, I can't understand how you could think that"). A psychotic denial may appear when it is linked to an impairment of reality testing: in this case the subject refuses to recognize a physical object or a concrete event that is part of their present experience. *[F. De Bei]*

Devaluation

A behaviour aimed at dealing with conflicts and stressors by attributing exaggerated negative characteristics to oneself or to others. The use of derogatory, sarcastic or negative statements to oneself or others is used to increase self-esteem and to reject the consciousness of feelings such as shame, vulnerability or inferiority. Through the use of devaluation, an individual makes a comment on an object, a behaviour or action, in a negative way, in order to eliminate the painful affects associated with it. In this sense, devaluation may be considered the opposite of omnipotence. *[F. De Bei]*

Displacement

A behaviour in which a feeling originally directed at a person or an object is guided to a different person or object usually less feared or considered less threatening. In this way, an affection or action is recognized and expressed, although to a different "target". For example: "It's been a terrible day at work . . . I yelled at my wife at the slightest excuse when I got back home." In the psychoanalytic model, displacement is considered to be the underlying mechanism of phobic phenomena, where the feared situation may represent the conflict, both directly (sexual phobias) and indirectly (for example, knives or scissors phobia). *[F. De Bei]*

Dissociation

A transitional alteration of some integrated functions such as consciousness, memory and identity. This term can refer both to a specific defence mechanism and to broader phenomena related to normal and pathological mental functioning: amnesia, absorption, feelings of depersonalization, derealization, multiple concurrent streams of consciousness. As a defence mechanism, dissociation allows a specific affection or impulse (experienced as too dangerous or anxious to be fully recognized) to act outside consciousness. Depending on its intensity and pervasiveness, dissociation may affect the life of the subject to a greater (major dissociation) or lesser (minor dissociation) degree. The latter leads to a partial alteration of the integrative functions of consciousness: a short-term and reversible condition with localized episodes that do not involve personal life, work or social life. In the case of a major dissociation, this occurs as a discontinuity of consciousness leading to loss of coherence in self-image and in the emotional, cognitive and behavioural organization. In this case, there may be a significant impact, not only on the private sphere, but also at a relational, social and working level. The term has acquired a semantic extent due to the fact that, in recent years, the mechanism has crossed the boundaries of the psychiatric nosology; it entered into the vocabulary of different theoretical models and found a place both in the world of relational theories of psychoanalysis (increasingly based on a vision of the self as a decentralized, multiple and fluid entity) and in attachment theory, as a defensive response to an unpredictable and traumatic care-giving environment. *[F. De Bei]*

(continued)

(continued)

Humour

Ability to understand the irony of fun aspects occurring in conflictual and/or stressful situations. Humour has to be clearly connected with conflicts and stressors, and has the effect of dissolving tension by making it more bearable. In addition, unlike devaluation, which uses derisive comments at someone's expense, humour tends to relieve tensions in an acceptable way. An example of this mechanism is illustrated by Freud in his *Jokes and their relation to the unconscious*: it is Monday, and a man condemned to death, going to the gallows, exclaims: "What a great beginning to my week." *[F. De Bei]*

Hypochondriasis

Dealing with conflicts or stressors through the repeated use of complaints or requests for help that hide feelings of hostility or reproach towards others; hostility is then expressed by rejecting suggestions, advice or help offered. Requests and complaints, which may relate to somatic concerns or general problems of life are, therefore, used as a form of indirect reproach: help is rejected because ineffective, impossible to follow, "not good advice", thus impeding any step towards resolution. *[F. De Bei]*

Idealization

An overestimation of the characteristics and qualities of a person who is perceived as superior or better than he or she is. Therefore, idealization is a process concerning the object, since the object is "amplified" and "psychically elevated". In addition to the relationships with the Other, idealization can take place even within the libido of the Ego. For example, with reference to the first case, during falling in love, the love object is typically perceived as beautiful and amazing beyond its real characteristics. Even a chance encounter can lead to overestimating the happiness that we would have shared with that person, especially when there is no possibility of giving substance to the relationship. In the case of idealization as an expression of the libido of the Ego, it is a part of the Self to be idealized, almost always in correlation with the dynamics of infantile narcissism. One's own characteristics are overestimated; however, these cannot be expressed or can be neurotically unsatisfactory, also due to the excess of qualities by which the Ego represents itself (ideal Self). In this respect, the reference to the libidinal infantile process is essential. According to Freud, the development of the Ego requires a removal from primary narcissism and the transfer of libido on an ideal of the Ego, which takes into account (reality principle) the conditions imposed from the outside. The persistence of the narcissist dynamic can only debase the ability of individuals to be personally satisfied, and their capability of making real investments. This increases the perceived distance between reality and ideality, up to extreme forms of social fall-back and neurotic frustration. *[S. Smiraglia]*

Identification with the aggressor

It is the act of assuming an aggressive attitude towards others by an individual who has suffered a traumatic relational experience, in the same way as the person experienced it when he or she was dominated by the aggressor. This mechanism is used to avoid succumbing to feelings of humiliation, annihilation, impotence. The discovery of this type of bizarre and tremendous defence is usually attributed to Anna Freud (1936). As a matter of fact, if not the term, at least the dynamic that this mechanism refers to, needs to be backdated and attributed to S. Ferenczi. The context in which this defence manifests itself is relational and traumatic. *[S. Panizza]*

Intellectualization

A way to dealing with emotional conflicts and stressors through an excessive use of abstract thinking or generalizations, so as to control or minimize disturbing feelings. By changing the focus, intellectualization helps people to distance themselves from their own feelings: personal issues give way to generalizations, general principles, etc. Instead of referring to their own experience, individuals speak in general terms ("Am I glad? True happiness is hard to reach"), or talk about themselves, but in the second or third person ("Certainly, my sadness arises from exaggerated parental expectations and other experiences lived during my growth") *[V. Lingiardi, F. De Bei]*

Isolation of affect

A behaviour aimed at dealing with emotional conflicts or stressors by separating ideas from their originally associated feelings. Through this mechanism, the memory of a traumatic or painful experience is separated from emotions. Therefore, an individual can speak about an experience as if it did not concern them or did not cause any emotional response (for example: "After the car accident I was not distressed at all, I simply got up and went back to work"). *[F. De Bei]*

Omnipotence

An attitude aiming at facing conflicts or stressful events by acting as someone who is superior to others or with special powers or abilities. This mechanism is used to protect one's self-esteem, which is implicated whenever sources of stress induce feelings of disappointment, helplessness, worthlessness. Omnipotence subjectively minimizes these experiences through statements or fantasies of unlimited success, power, beauty, intelligence, etc, or by using particular substances (e.g. cocaine) or activities (e.g. jogging) as an artificial mean to increase self-esteem and feelings of success or competence in other areas of life. *[F. De Bei]*

Passive aggression

An indirect and silent expression of aggression, hostility or resentment towards others. Passive aggression often occurs in response to requests for independent acts or services or for the lack of gratification of dependent wishes. An accommodating front is used, consciously, to mask deep resentment and hostility transmitted by: failures, procrastination, silly or provocative behaviour intended to attract attention, etc. This behaviour can arrive at the point of obtaining an unconscious failure or being over-heedless (for example, failing to take necessary drugs such as insulin, antihypertensive drugs, lithium, etc.) in order to have a "pay-back". *[F. De Bei]*

(continued)

(continued)

Projection

A mechanism by which wishes, feelings and thoughts, which are the cause of stress or conflict, are attributed to other people. Unlike projective identification, projection does not influence the behaviour and affections of the people to which it refers. This mechanism preserves the subject from the conflicts and stress associated with the awareness of the presence within themselves of the projected elements. However, this leads to the development of a hostile attitude of suspicion (paranoia) towards the people to which these elements have been attributed. When the use of this mechanism is associated with severe impairment of reality-testing, the term used is delusional projection. *[F. De Bei]*

Projective identification

A way of dealing with conflicts and stressors by attributing one's own unacceptable feelings or thoughts to someone else. Unlike simple projection, however, the subject does not totally ignore what is projected, but he misinterprets it as a justified response towards the other. In fact, the subject frequently provokes in others the same feelings that, incorrectly, he first attributed to himself. Therefore, it is difficult to assess "who has started first". On a theoretical level, projective identification is perhaps the most complex defence mechanism. First introduced by Melanie Klein, this concept was developed by many post-Kleinian authors, such as H. Rosenfeld, Bion, Meltzer, T. Ogden, O.F. Kernberg, J. Sandler. Today, it is studied not as a "simple" defence mechanism, but as a special interactive form of emotional communication. G.O. Gabbard has divided the "progress" of this mechanism into three phases: the patient disclaims and projects into the therapist parts of the Self and/or bad internal objects; the therapist begins unconsciously to feel and/or act as the projected bad object in response to the interpersonal pressure exerted by the patient ("counter-projective identification"); the therapist contains and changes the projected object, which is then re-introjected and assimilated by the patient ("introjective identification"). Projective identification involves an interactive factor of particular prominence: unconsciously, through verbal and nonverbal channels, the subject pushes the other to feel, think and behave in accordance with the images of the Self or with the objects that he has projected into them. For this reason, from their feelings of countertransference, a therapist may infer the characteristics of the parts of themselves or of the internal objects that the patient placed in them through projective identification. The therapist's ability to contain and reflect upon these representations projectively identified in him, without acting on these feelings, is essential for the therapeutic work. Close to the concept of projective identification are the "intersubjective interpersonal shifts" developed by P. Fonagy and M. Target: this notion explains how borderline patients induce their therapists to behave and feel like the "alien selves" inside their Self. *[V. Lingiardi]*

Rationalization

A conduct aiming at providing socially acceptable and apparently logical explanations, even if incorrect, about one's own behaviour. Rationalization is used to justify to others or oneself a behaviour, motivation or feeling that causes discomfort or conflict, through factitious, though plausible, reasons. The subject is usually unaware of the true underlying motivation and perceives only factitious grounds, a socially acceptable reason. Perhaps the most famous example of this mechanism lies in Aesop's fable of the fox and the grapes: "I don't eat the grapes because they are not yet ripe, not because I cannot reach them." *[F. De Bei]*

Reaction formation

Unacceptable behaviours, thoughts or feelings are replaced with diametrically opposite equivalents, in order to avoid intolerable feelings of guilt. Reaction formation may have a highly "specific" quality, as in the case of individuals who show excessive deference to someone who they actually hate, or in the case of individuals who take care of someone with whom they are actually very angry; it can also have a "generalized" quality, in the presence of a real character trait, such as in individuals who seem to never get angry, never speak ill of anybody, are always too "sympathetic." *[F. De Bei]*

Regression

The act of returning to an older system (topographical regression), way of expression (formal regression) or time (temporal regression). Since the "primitive psychism" is undying and desire is indestructible, the future is always susceptible to being modelled on the past; this condition may apply to the most varied fields: to dreams, psychopathology, biology, development of civilization. In *The Interpretation of Dreams* S. Freud connotes regression as a path that leads thoughts "away from motility" and "back to perception". The result of this inversion is the dreaming hallucination. With regard to the phases of psychosexual development, regression concerns the return of the libido to former modalities of organization and satisfaction. With regard to the functioning of the psychic apparatus, regression is about the reversal from the "secondary process" to the "primary process" and, in parallel, from the reality principle to the pleasure principle. In connection with the analytic treatment, regression, even induced by the setting, may be therapeutic. On this question, S. Ferenczi may have fallen into an impasse: on the one hand, regression – even in the form of repetitions of trauma – must be induced; on the other, it can enter a vicious circle in which repetitions of the trauma turn out to be therapeutically unproductive and the patient's requests harder and harder to satisfy. M. Balint, a disciple of Ferenczi, has defined this regression as "malignant" (irreversible, aimed at gratification) as opposed to "benign" regression (reversible, aimed at acknowledgment). In the latter, the patient who has relived the trauma is able to achieve a "new beginning", that is, to love free from anguish. *[G. Antonelli]*

Repression

The first Freudian works considered repression as the mechanism responsible for the formation of hysterical symptoms and defined it as a specific mechanism activated by an "effort of will". This effort would remove from consciousness all the ideas and images that are incompatible with the predominant representations of the Ego, which would also be excluded from further associative elaboration. Repression is considered the "cornerstone on which rests the whole edifice of psychoanalysis". In its narrow sense, it indicates the process that allows a person to reject and/or maintain thoughts, images, memories connected to the drives in the unconscious. This process is

(continued)

(continued)

triggered when the fulfilment of a drive is likely to produce sorrow against other needs. In 1915, Freud formulated a general theory of repression by distinguishing *primal repression* from *repression proper* or secondary repression and from the return of the repressed. Primal repression is applied to the representatives of the drive that do not access the consciousness. This drive remains fixed and creates a first unconscious core, which constitutes a pole of attraction towards the items to be repressed. Differently, repression proper – or secondary repression– is a process that actively rejects unacceptable contents from consciousness and confines them to the unconscious, where they are subjected to the attraction of primary repressed contents. The third step in the repression process is the return of the repressed, which was considered responsible for the appearance of symptoms. *[N. Dazzi]*

Retroactive annulment

Also known as "undoing", it is the use of behaviours or thoughts symbolically aiming at denying or erasing thoughts, feelings or past actions. More generally, it is an attempt to "fix" an affection, impulse or action that induces guilt or anxiety, by minimizing it. This attempt can be retrospective, when a statement is followed by an immediate clarification with an opposite meaning, or anticipatory, when an observation begins with phrases such as: "Probably I'm wrong but . . .", as if the speaking person wants to nullify the meaning of what they are about to say. Or again, it may consist of real acts of reparation for actions deemed evil (for example: "After I lost money at the racecourse, I bought some flowers for my wife"). [*F. De Bei*]

Reversal

Freud used this expression to indicate those cases where the aim of the drive is transformed into its opposite, thus changing the activity into inactivity. It is one of the mechanisms that Freud hypothesized to underlie phenomena of sadism–masochism and voyeurism–exhibitionism. Anna Freud has included the reversal among the more primitive defence mechanisms such as passive aggression, complaint and refusal for help. *[V. Lingiardi]*

Splitting

A way of dealing with emotional conflicts or stressors by separating opposite affective states without the capacity of integrating positive and negative qualities into a unified image. Given the impossibility of experiencing ambivalent affects at the same time, the splitting does not allow a person to have more balanced views and expectations of oneself and others; these views tend to alternate between opposite polarities: totally good, strong and loving, or totally bad, weak and rejecting. M. Klein and O.F. Kernberg are two psychoanalytic authors who studied the developmental and diagnostic relevance of this mechanism. *[F. De Bei]*

Sublimation

A behaviour aiming at coping with stressful situations and/or conflicts by channelling, rather than inhibiting, potentially maladaptive feelings or drives into socially acceptable behaviour. Examples of sublimation are sports and games used for conveying aggressive drives, or artistic creations that express conflictual feelings. In this way the original drives may be expressed, and at the same time the activity or the resulting product can be a source of social approval or reward. *[F. De Bei]*

Suppression

An attitude that implies an active and intentional avoidance of disturbing thoughts, desires or feelings. Through this mechanism, problematic elements are kept in mind, but their solution is postponed. It may appear when someone is facing a problem that cannot be resolved in the immediate future ("I was certainly upset, but I knew that things would have improved if I had waited"). It may also appear as a reaction to stressful situations not depending on one's own will ("What else could I do? I had to accept the bad news and move on"). The possibility of recalling the suppressed memory distinguishes this mechanism from others where the elements of denial and repression are more evident. *[F. De Bei]*

DEFLECTION

In Gestalt therapy, a mode of communication that avoids direct I–thou → contact in favour of indirect or partially avoidant modes of communication such as: generalization, the use of impersonal pronoun, metaphorical allusions, circumlocutions, change of topic, etc. This "indirect" communication can also have a potentially positive aspect in that it is able to convey messages to a third party in cases where direct communication is not possible. *[R. Zerbetto, S. Bergomi]*

REFERENCES. Polster E., Polster M., *Gestalt therapy integrated: Contours of theory and practice*, 1973.

DEFORMATION → DISTORTION

DEHUMANIZATION

A perceptual distortion due to the suspension of identification and → empathy processes with other people. This leads a person to act towards other individuals "as if" they do not belong to mankind but to other animal species or to the world of inanimate objects. Dehumanization would be at the basis of all the expressions of extreme physical or psychological violence not justified by an immediate need for self-defence or by a → desire for revenge for being a victim of injustice. It would be determined by a dissociation from other people's pain that cancels out the inhibitions that normally prohibit the inflicting of pain on another human being and causing their death. This dissociation enables the exclusion of the conscious processes of feelings of guilt and the empathic feelings of pain that are normally generated by the simple observation of violence suffered by another human being. Persecution, social discrimination, torture acted on the individual level (for example, in the case of violence or sexual abuse) or on the social level (for example, perpetuated by military institutions in war scenarios, or by institutions such as mental hospitals), can be facilitated by or fully based on the phenomenon of dehumanization. Many individual psychopathological variables can also encourage the implementation of dehumanizing behaviour. However, the so-called "situational" variable should not be underestimated.

A classic example of this is the "Stanford Prison experiment" conducted by the American psychologist P. Zimbardo in 1971. In psychotherapy, the phenomenon can be detected as a crucial factor in certain disorders, such as post-traumatic disorders, or as a relational expression of the disorder, for example in case of severe forms of paranoia and perversion. *[R.]*

DELETION

In neuro-linguistic programming, one of the three processes of the → meta-model, along with generalization and distortion. It is the process by which, selectively, people pay attention to only some information of their own experience. It is a "violation" of verbal language, highlighting how, in the passage of information between the deep/unconscious and the surface/logic part, some elements of a person's experience can be deleted, compared with the complete experience actually lived. Useful in everyday talk, in inventing metaphors and in hypnotic language, deletion is, however, a reduced perception of reality, which can be a source of inconvenience and misunderstandings. With the help of neuro-linguistic programming, through the meta-model – also called precision language – the "deleted" parts of a person's experience are retrieved by using simple questions. As it is an impoverished model of a person's experience, deletion implies a restriction of behaviour options. There are several types of "violations": simple deletion, appearing, for instance, the expression "I fear . . ." deletes the reason for the fear of the person who speaks, and this increases the perception of their emotional state; in comparative deletion, for example "he is better!", the term of comparison is deleted; in nominalization, – "education today is certainly not common" – the focus of the situation is missing, that is, who the receiver is and what is meant by "education"; in unspecified name – "these things are not interesting" – the subject, who the interest refers to, is missing; in unspecified verb – "you hurt me" – the way in which the action took place is missing and one need only think of the ambiguity between being hurt by words or physically. *[L. Bracciodieta]*

REFERENCES. Bandler R., Grinder J., *The models of the hypnotic techniques of Milton H. Erickson*, 1975; Erickson M.H., *My voice will go*, 1983; M. Hall, *The GNP and the magic of language*, 2007.

DENIAL → DEFENCE MECHANISMS

DEPRESSIVE POSITION → PARANOID–SCHIZOID POSITION

DEPRESSIVE SCHEME

In cognitive-behavioural psychotherapy, depression is characterized by a → cognitive triad: the depressed subject has a negative vision of himself, of the world and of his future. The subject perceives himself (→ self-concept) as being inadequate, abandoned and worthless. The → beliefs of the subject regard the existence of what he perceives to be objectively unsurmountable obstacles and inadequate personal resources. The world appears devoid of pleasure or of gratification, whilst the perception of the future is pessimistic because the individual thinks that his actual problems cannot be resolved. This desperation can lead to suicidal ideation, where the desire to commit suicide reflects the desire to flee from problems that are perceived as being unsurmountable. Many motivational, behavioural and physical symptoms typical of depression arise from this kind of cognitive configuration. *[A. Meluzzi]*

REFERENCES. Beck A.T., *Depression*, 1967.

DEREFLECTION

In logotherapy, a psychotherapeutic technique conceived by V.E. Frankl and published under this name in 1946. Dereflection aims at facilitating the de-centreing of a person from their problematic experience and their orientation towards something outside themselves: a task, a value to be realized, someone to love. Within the franklian view of the → dimensional ontology, it refers to the typical human competence of → self-transcendence, a resource inherent to the spiritual level of a person. This technique, elective in the treatment of anxiety and sexual disorders, has the merit of having anticipated similar techniques, which can be found in Masters and Johnson's cognitive-behavioural approach to sexual disorders. *[D. Bellantoni]*

REFERENCES. Bellantoni D., *L'Analisi esistenziale di Viktor E. Frank*, 2011; Frankl V.E., *Man's search for meaning: An introduction to logotherapy*, 1946; Id., *On the theory and therapy of mental disorders*, 2004; Id., *The unheard cry for meaning*, 2011; Id., *The will to meaning*, 1988.

DESIGNATED PATIENT

Within the of the systemic approach of the → Milan School of Family Therapy, the member of the → family who presents, or is presented by the family seeking therapy, as being the person who is the bearer of the → symptoms in the family. The main reason a family seeks therapeutic intervention is usually the presence of symptoms or problematic behaviour in one of its members. The designated patient, however, is not necessarily the family member that an objective observer would consider to be the person with the most obvious problem. From a systemic perspective, the pathology of the individual can only be understood within the → context of the family. The symptoms can play an important role in posing an obstacle to changes in the life cycle of a family. On one hand, the symptoms can maintain a pathological → homeostasis; on the other hand, they may give the family an opportunity to → change from the moment they are addressed in therapy. *[R.]*

REFERENCES. Simon F.B., Stierlin H., Wynne L.C., *The language of family therapy: A systemic vocabulary and sourcebook*, 1985.

DESIRE

A term denoting the experience of attraction towards a subject or an object. It consists of a volitional impulse directed to something that one wants to possess (or use) or to a goal one wants to achieve. According to Freud, it is the fundamental libidinal drive (→ libido) towards pleasure, a sensation characterized by the reduction of psychological tension (→ drive) and it appears in a disguised form in → dreams. It is distinguished from the concept of → need, which is understood as a state related to specific physiological needs (such as hunger or thirst) or needs related to specific developmental stages. In psychoanalysis, desires always refer to an → unconscious desire related to early childhood, which left a memory trace, and it is the latter that, connecting with the present desire, provides charge and intensity that may result in symptoms or express themselves in dreams.

In psychoanalytic treatment, the distinction between needs and libidinal desires is important: Casement distinguishes between "growth needs", which need to be satisfied in the course of a therapy, otherwise they would prevent the psychological growth of the patient, and "libidinal demands", which need to be frustrated, as a therapist's collusion with the latter would not allow the patient an appropriate processing of intense and often painful feelings. Other psychological and psychotherapeutic approaches, on the contrary, use the terms need and desire as synonyms and they theorize the various stages through which each individual needs to go to reach the satisfaction of the higher need, namely → self-actualization. In this sense, desire is the → motivation that drives a person to move from the current situation to the desired one. For psychotherapists, therefore, desires can be an important lever to use to introduce the desired change, but they can also become a source of resistance (→ resistance to change) whenever therapeutic interventions require a person to give up – or postpone – something they desire, in order to achieve the therapeutic objective. *[R.]*

DESTRUCTIVENESS

It represents man's tendency to destructive violence. This term was used by Fromm in a well-structured investigation, from the primitive age to present time, where he clarified the existence of cultural, conventional, political and more generally socio-historical facts that influence the so called "sadistic instincts" and the multiple forms used by man to express their destructive tendencies. There are two types of aggression: the defensive "benign" type, in the service of the survival of the individual and the species, and the aggressive "malignant" type, that is, cruelty and destructiveness specific to the human species and absent in most mammals. To explain man's destructive tendency, S. Freud developed, starting from 1920, a new theory based on the dualism between life instinct (→ Eros) and death instinct (→ Thanatos). Death instinct represents self-destruction, the dissolution of the unity of the organism, the return to the primordial inorganic state. *[L. Isardi, E. Benelli]*

REFERENCES. Fromm E., *Anatomy of human destructiveness*, 1973; Id., *On disobedience and other essays*, 1981.

DETERMINISM

An epistemological assumption according to which every psychological phenomenon is the result of an antecedent or concomitant cause or set of causes. The principle of causality is searched for, depending on theoretical orientation, in unconscious factors (psychoanalytic determinism), in previous conditioning and learning (behaviourist determinism), in the biological substrate (psychiatric determinism). This term is also used in opposition to that of intentionality of action (→ will), freedom of conscience and free will. Over the years, the deterministic approach realized the impossibility of controlling the infinite causal variables surrounding mental phenomena, as well as the importance of recursive and → feedback processes in shaping human behaviour. In psychotherapy, referring only to the deterministic principle to understand mental manifestations poses a risk of "hyper-simplification". For example, this happens when a psychopathological situation is explained only by mentioning the presence/absence of unconscious conflict, erroneous learnings, poor production of a single neurotransmitter in the brain. This approach can therefore give rise to diagnostic biases. *[R.]*

DETRIANGULATION

In systemic-relational psychotherapy, an intervention technique used when a relational dynamic of → triangulation occurs (M. Bowen, S. Minuchin). This can concern one or more family members and the therapist themself. Detriangulation concerns the possibility of facilitating the transformation of this dynamic in a more functional way, for therapeutic change. During a session, the therapist can activate detriangulation through different modes of intervention: explaining the relational dynamics characterized by triangulation; talking about the ongoing communication mode (meta-communication); redefining the relational position of the "triangulated" subject (→ redefinition); highlighting the characteristics of triangulation and providing a relational prescription (→symptom prescription); activating the triangulation with one or more family members, highlighting the reactions (amplification of symptom). *[M. Menafro]*

REFERENCES. Bertrando P., Toffanetti D., *Storia della terapia familiare*, 2000; Cancrini L., *Guida alla psicoterapia*, 1982; Hoffman L., *Foundations of family therapy: A conceptual framework for systems*, 1981; Loriedo C., Picardi A., *Dalla teoria generale dei sistemi alla teoria dell'attaccamento*, 2000.

DEVALUATION → DEFENCE MECHANISMS

DEVELOPMENT STAGES (ERIK ERIKSON'S)

Erikson was the first to provide a comprehensive view of the life cycle. His scheme is focused on the concept of identity, whereas S. Freud's is focused on sexuality. This scheme outlines the growth and crises of a healthy personality by dividing it into eight stages. Each stage is characterized by specific tasks that any individual would face. Erickson argues that mental structures don't originate as much from the Freudian libido that invests the organs, but rather from the work of an organ that generates typical structures. The oral, anal or genital work generates "organ modes" that result in psychic functioning modes that go beyond the use of a specific body area. The crisis of the oral stage, in the second part of a child's first year, derives from simultaneous physiological, psychological and environmental development. Erikson underlines that anal drives are properly understood only within the interpersonal and family context. Concerning the oedipal phase, he argues that Ego psychology has directed the attention to the family structure more than to the oedipal components themselves. He divides the latency phase into three sub-periods: six to eight years, eight to eleven and eleven to puberty, each with different characteristics. In conclusion, the question is to analyze the influence that a specific zone produces on the mentalization process and on the sequence of the different type of processes. It is about how to establish a sort of chronology of operating priorities of the various zones of the body or of the various sensory functions at specific ages. *[L. Longhin]*

REFERENCES. Erikson E.H., *Childhood and society*, 1950; Id., *Identity and the life cycle*, 1959.

DEVELOPMENT STAGES (MARGARET S. MAHLER'S)

In the context of psychoanalysis, Mahler identified six stages of child development. The first is the normal autistic stage, which Mahler placed in the first month of life. In this stage, the newborn seems to "function" mainly as as a biological organism. In fact, during the first weeks of life, infants are dominated by tensions or unpleasant sensations coming from the body. However, this primary → narcissism is not to be considered as a fixed and static entity, but as a process that is subject to a gradual and steady acquisition of satisfaction of needs from maternal care. In this stage, there is a first psychic investment on tactile, visual and auditory organs. This enables the transition of the child from the primary perceptual form towards both a gradual inclusion of the mother in the protective shell of the newborn and the beginning of a new relationship stage with the object-mother that satisfies the child's needs.

According to Mahler, at around two months of age, the child moves from the autistic stage to the normal symbiotic stage. The term symbiosis is used by Mahler in this context as a metaphor to represent the mother–child unit, which she called the "symbiotic membrane". Maternal care offers a constant support to the child while waiting for the development of a fully functioning → Ego. The normal symbiotic stage is characterized by an increased affective and perceptive investment, coming from the mother–infant relationship. However, a strong differentiation between the inner and outer world is still missing; moreover, the mother figure, which is the main conquest of the child, still represents a partial object in the formation of the infantile → Self. Within the organizing and structuring process of the primitive relationships of the newborn, the mother figure represents the driving force in a common symbiotic orbit. The third stage is that of separation-individuation: it represents the specific mode of adaptation and organization of the Ego during a child's growth. In the first stage of psychic development, children experience needs, impulses and behavioural patterns that are continuously adapting and organizing. Clinical experience indicates how the Ego normally develops towards a greater and gradual adaptation to reality. In turn, this process was divided by Mahler into four sub-stages. The first sub-stage ranges from four to five months to ten to twelve months and is characterized by differentiation in the development of the child's body image. The second sub-stage, called practicing, ranges from ten to twelve months to sixteen to eighteen months. The early stage of this phase is characterized by the child's ability to create a physical distance from the mother by walking on all fours and by trying to re-establish a standing position by themselves, although with the need of some help. After that, a proper practicing stage can be identified, which is characterized by autonomous upright walking. In this stage, the child returns to the mother for "refueling" after "the amorous adventure with the world". The practicing stage takes place during the last months of the first year of life, when children move away from their mother and need her help to learn to walk upright. In this period, children are also interested in playing with inanimate objects. The third sub-stage is characterized by the ability to dominate reality and by autonomy and it takes place between fifteen months of life and the end of the second year of life. Children experience the difficulty of modifying reality, their fragility and the separation from the mother. The "crisis of rapprochement" is the search for the mother and it represents an important evolutionary step to develop an optimal distance from the mother. Finally, in the fourth sub-stage, there is the consolidation of individuality. According to Mahler, the process of separation, individuation and differentiation of the body image of the child begins in the fourth to fifth month of life. Among the many signs of this change there is the attention of the child to their own body and to the symbolic orbit. This is due to the fact that, in the process of separation-individuation, the evolution of the symbiotic stage is marked in particular by the progressive consolidation of a lived experience of separation. Without a preliminary experience of separation, the ability to develop a relationship, as well as the ability to develop dialogue, cannot be structured. Psychic development is crucial, as it represents the ability to relate to reality, but practicing physical separation is also necessary for the development of a psychological separation. The ability of a good mother is to give sufficient security to the child and to encourage autonomy at the same time. This clarifies the meaning of the child's attention to the mother; the child remembers the experiences of satisfaction received and they are more inclined to tolerate the absence of the mother because they hope for her reappearance as a source of gratification of their needs. In this stage, the "specific smile" and an ability to compare the mother and the unfamiliar also appear. The ability to distinguish the self from objects is preceded by the ability to distinguish objects. It is important to remember how the child can be little interested in exploration if the mother is not involved in the symbiosis due to personal or family problems that force her to look after them mechanically and unaffectedly. The child remains attached to the mother in an abulic way, devoid of real satisfaction. This gives rise to a type of personality development that D.W. Winnicott defined as → false Self. The image of the child's own body changes due to the contributions of new experiences that enable a growing enrichment of the child by creating a "memory" full of states of satisfaction or frustration. In this stage, the child acquires the first "not-me possession", an object that they can handle and bring to the mouth; the relationship with food becomes important. Moreover, this represents the initial experience of the differentiation between the representations of the Ego and external reality. *[L. Longhin]*

REFERENCES. Mahler M.S., *On human symbiosis and the vicissitudes of individuation: Infantile psychosis, volume 1*, 1968; Mahler M.S., Pine F., Bergman A., *The psychological birth of the child*, 1975.

DEVELOPMENT STAGES (JEAN PIAGET'S)

According to J. Piaget, development is an evolution driven by the need for balance in an open system. From a dynamic point of view, balance is a mechanism that allows people to build their representation of reality, the link between object and subject, and which regulates their interaction. The source of knowledge lies in the interactions between subject and object. The concept of intelligence (cognitive ability) is closely related to the concept of → adaptation to the environment. Intelligence is an extension of human biological adaptation to the environment. Piaget distinguished between two processes that characterize each type of adaptation during the developmental age: assimilation and accommodation. In the early stages of development, assimilation is predominant. It consists in the incorporation of an event or object without modification in a behavioural or cognitive schema that has been already acquired (for example, the grasping reflex brings infants to grasp new objects with their hands). Then accommodation starts to prevail. Accommodation is the modification of a cognitive or behavioural schema to accommodate new objects or events (for example, if an object is difficult to grasp, children need to change the way they grasp it). A good adaptation to the environment is realized when assimilation and accommodation are well integrated with each other. A child's cognitive development process can be divided into three consecutive stages. In turn, each of them can be divided into sub-stages, where three main structures appear and develop. The first to develop are the sensorimotor structures. These are systems of concrete actions involving real objects (from birth to 2 years). Then, the structures of concrete operations appear, that is, systems of actions that are mentally performed but based on real data (2 to 11 years). Finally, formal operations become possible. These are based on logic and on hypothetical-deductive reasoning (11 to 15 years).

The sensorimotor stage is the period of a child's life that precedes the development of language, when their behaviour is based on the coordination of perception and movement. This stage is divided into six sub-stages: innate reflexes (the first month of life); primary circular reactions (1 to 4 months), when a child repeats an action initially produced by chance to find interesting effects; secondary circular reactions (4 to 8 months), when the distinction between objectives and means can be observed for the first time; means–ends coordination (8 to 12 months), when children discover the means to achieve an objective; tertiary circular reactions (12 to 18 months), when new means are discovered through active experimentation; the symbolic function (from 18 months onwards), when children are capable of acting on reality with their thought. During this period, cognitive development is extremely fast because there is a real revolution at the mental level: the child begins to perceive the world as external and objective. During the next stage, children develop concrete operations. The pre-operational stage (from 2 to 7 years) is characterized by an increasing internalization of behaviour and by the appearance of inner mental activity. Thanks to the development of language, reasoning becomes possible with the help of → imagination. Piaget calls language "representative intellect", and it plays the role of knowing and narrating the truth. An example of this is creative play, in which children use objects to represent other objects. After the radical → egocentrism of the sensory-motor stage has passed, an intellectual egocentrism persists in this stage, as the point of view of others is not differentiated from one's own. At this stage, reasoning is neither inductive nor deductive but it is trasductive or precausal. At the stage of concrete operations (7 to 11 years) not only do children use symbols, but they can manipulate them logically. An important achievement of this period is the acquisition of the concept of reversibility, that is, that the effects of an operation can be undone by an inverse operation. In the next stage, the representative intellect is structured.

The formal operations stage starts from 12 years of age onwards. At this point, the child becomes able to reason with hypotheses that describe different possibilities, to check them and to choose the one that best matches the present situation: knowledge becomes hypothetical-deductive. Piaget considered the concept of operational intelligence as fundamental to understanding the evolution of the human intellect in various historical periods and in different areas of knowledge and he proposed an approach to research called "genetic → epistemology". *[R.]*

DEVELOPMENT STAGES (RENÉ A. SPITZ'S)

Spitz needs to be credited for having conducted research on child psychoanalysis and on the progressive and reciprocal formation of the → Ego in relation to the → object. His attention was focused on the role of the first object relations in the psychic life of infants. Spitz reduced the difference between behavioural psychology and psychoanalysis by paying attention to the stages of child development, by expanding the investigation methods with the use of reactive tests and by using recordings and film footage. He conducted the first psychoanalytic research on object relations between infants and mothers, starting from direct and monitored observation of infants and their mothers for long periods of time. He documented the transformation of the adaptive biological bond between infant and mother, thus redefining the fundamental concept of libidinal object. Spitz described the development of the child as a transition from the physiological to the psychological component. He identified that mother and infant develop very complex interactive patterns, a kind of dialogue that allows the child to turn, gradually, meaningless stimuli into very significant signals. Children are receptive to the signals expressed by their mother; therefore, they are soaked in the sense of the maternal message that is rich in affection. Spitz divided child development according to stages or phases that correspond to the appearance of three psychic organizers. The first stage comes into play when children are two to three months old, with the appearance of the "smiling response". The second stage is "the stranger anxiety", which appears between the eighth and the fifteenth month after the formation of a clear distinction between the mother and other people. The third organizer is the appearance of "negativism", first as an attitude and then also as a word. This is an aggressive investment that appears at around the fifteenth month. The "pre-object" stage is characterized by the complete undifferentiation between outer and inner reality. The development is aimed at achieving a state of rest. In this stage, a psychological object does not exist, because the ability to mentalize the outside world has not been developed yet. Spitz claimed that much importance should be given to the affective climate in which the mother–child relationship takes place, because these first experiences are the basis for the formation of the "libidinal object". From the perspective of affective development, the libidinal object is the person onto which the individual pours the first form of affection. In psychoanalysis, the word "object" is used to describe a real person, for example a mother, or to indicate that person's representations settled in the mind. The process leading to the formation of a libidinal object is longer and more complex than the "cognitive" process and its different phases can be identified. A libidinal object should not be seen as a "libidinal discharge", nor as a result of defensive internalization, but as the fundamental and essential human bond through which the whole psychological development is actualized. Around the eighth month of life, a child not only recognizes the mother's face as different from everyone else, but it also reacts anxiously when seeing the face of a stranger and expresses a behaviour called "stranger anxiety". The presence of a stranger communicates the mother's absence to the child and this causes acute suffering that generates escaping attempts and withdrawal. Spitz shows that every aspect of the early psychological development in children is mediated by the relation with the mother figure. The third "organizer" is the appearance of "negativism" around the fifteenth month of life. This stage is characterized by the word "no". This activates semantic communication, as the word "no" is the first chance to introduce a negation in the outside world. The "no" represents an aggressive investment due to unpleasant experiences. According to Spitz, a child understands the intentions of the mother through a process of → identification, because, by identifying with the mother, a child assumes the "no" from her with the meaning of prohibition, but also with the affective value that is linked to it. The research on children's early development, developed by Spitz, was resumed by M.S. Mahler, a child psychoanalyst, who clarified the normal and abnormal features of this process and used the theoretical framework developed by Spitz to explain the deepest and most disturbed components of psychotic children. Mahler, like Spitz, observed the importance of human environment, as the mother provides the child's immature Ego with the "mirroring function". This function is instead compromised by an anxious, hostile, unstable, unpredictable and especially non-affective mother. *[L. Longhin]*

REFERENCES. Spitz R.A., *No and yes: On the genesis of human communication*, 1957; Id., *A genetic field theory of ego formation*, 1959.

DEVIANCE

A behaviour that violates a rule and does not comply with a socially accepted "model of normality". Foucault argued that society gives judgement on deviance on the basis of what it knows about the deviant subject, his/her life and the relationship between the same society and his/her offence, making inferences about what one may expect from the same individual in the future. Judgement, thus, becomes not only a categorization of the individual but also of his/her becoming. The social meaning of deviance, coming from labelling theorists (→ labelling theory), is expressed by Foucault as an existential redefinition. In later years, through the contribution of systems (→ systems theory) about the study of behaviour, the circular causality and the deterministic link between cause and effect, the analysis of the whole → context was proponed, in its entirety and circularity, without arbitrary punctuations and static identifications of a starting or an end point. The analysis shifts from the deviant individual to the deviant action: the individual isn't labelled as inherently dangerous, and moreover attention is paid to a study unit – the deviant action – more useful for understanding the nature of events, so as to be able to intervene, both in a preventive and a rehabilitative way. De Leo Patrizi analyzed deviance as a path, an organizing process that is not the sole effect of factors or antecedent causes, but has an active and constructive role, where the social actors organize connections between situational, relational, temporal, symbolic dimensions. *[P. Meringolo]*

DIAGNOSIS-INTERVENTION

It is the application of the methodological principle of → research-intervention to the area of psychological diagnosis. In diagnosis-intervention, no diagnostic *a priori* classification preceding the therapy is used (such as those provided by the main manuals of classical diagnostic based on signs and symptoms; → medical diagnosis), as the diagnostic process develops more as the effect than as the start of a therapeutic intervention: each diagnosis assumes the value of a continuous process of discovery, which auto-corrects itself during the intervention of the therapist, who measures the outcome. Therefore, in a diagnosis-intervention, a problem is known by its solution. An evolved typology of diagnosis-intervention is represented by → operative diagnosis, which is used in the context of the most recent strategic therapy models (see also the interactional-strategic paradigm, in the opening chapter, "The eight paradigms and their respective theoretical-applicative models"). *[R.]*

DIAGNOSTIC MANUALS

The various psychotherapy approaches favour an operational approach to → nosology, where the formulation of a case and diagnostics knowledge are strictly functional to therapy and intervention rather than being an abstract and formalized definition of the diagnostic framework. However, psychological studies have consolidated a widespread tradition of psychometric diagnoses using → psychological tests aimed at the study and analysis of normal and pathological psychological functioning (psychopathology tests, personality tests, psycho-aptitude tests, intelligence tests, projective tests, neuropsychological tests, etc.). This apparent contradiction is due to a different operational perspective (→ operative diagnosis) that distinguishes psychological and psychotherapeutic sciences from medical-psychiatric sciences: the first type of sciences is more idiographically patient-oriented, problem-oriented and solution-oriented. The second type is more anchored to the medical-biological principle of diagnosis-etiology-therapy. This difference expresses itself in the almost total absence, within the specialized literature, of psychological-psychotherapeutic manuals, despite the strong international proliferation of psychiatric manuals such as → DSM or → ICD-10. However, the recent publication of the first Psychodynamic Diagnostic Manual (→ PDM) has marked a trend reversal. This is a sign that the scientific community of psychotherapists of all orientations has started to feel the need for a more coherent psycho-diagnostic formulation, without clinging to nomothetic and objectifying definitions of psychological problems. Moreover, this would also prevent the flattening of intervention tools and theories of psychotherapy on medical-psychiatric diagnoses that have little to do with the true nature of psychotherapeutic interventions. *[A. Bartoletti]*

DIALOGIC RELATIONSHIP

In Gestalt psychotherapy, openness to being challenged in the development of one's convictions. The term "dia-logue" indicates the extreme distance between two lines of reasoning, in the same way as the word "dia-meter" indicates the distance between two points of a circumference, and therefore the potential overcoming of a "mono-logical" dimension in the direction of a dialectic between opposites. This opposition does not necessarily mean a conflict (evoked by the Heraclitean aphorism "conflict is the father of everything"), in that it also represents the dialectical foundation of democracy as lying in the perennial conflict between government and opposition: it can also indicate, in fact, the possibility of exploring a content from different perspectives. From here the ingenious invention of the "platonic dialogues", in which the master (Socrates) does not present himself as the holder of knowledge – but – conscious of "knowing that he does not know" – he puts it "into play" in an exchange of perspectives. The "seeking together" therefore corresponds to an intersubjective and dia-logic style that overrides the hierarchical structure precisely of those who presume to be the holders of the truth with respect to who should only accept it unquestioningly. The neurophysiological premises that refer in particular to the researches of Damasio, evidence the lack of sustainability of the dualist mind–body theory in view of the continuous dialogue between emotions and cognitions in the construction of the self. The multiplicity of the self is also explored by Jung and Hillman, as well as by Perls and Polster in the dramatization between the polarities of the self in the Gestaltic monodrama (→ enactment of the conflict). *[R. Zerbetto, D. De Marinis]*

REFERENCES. Damasio A.R., *L'errore di Cartesio*, 1994; Hillman J., *Re-visioning psychology*, 1975; Jung C.G. (1934–1954), *Archetypes and the collective unconscious*, in *Collected Works*, IX, 1969; Perls F., *Gestalt therapy verbatim*, 1969; Polster E., *A population of selves: A therapeutic exploration of personal diversity*, 1995.

DIDACTIC ANALYSIS

In the context of Freudian psychoanalysis, a psychoanalytic treatment that the candidate analyst undergoes to analyze their motivations and to overcome the "blind spots" (W. Stekel defines in this way unresolved repressions in clinical settings that create shadows in its analytical perception). In 1918, the psychoanalyst H. Nunberg proposed the introduction a brief analytic treatment for those who wanted to become analysts. This treatment then became an established practice at the Berlin Psychoanalytic Institute in 1920, with the introduction of the so-called "tripod": didactic analysis, supervision, teaching seminars. Didactic analysis has become an obligatory step since the International Congress of Psychoanalysis in 1922 (the first Conference was in 1908 in Salzburg). Didactic analysis seems to propose again the same needs that emerged during Freud's self-analysis. In fact, the discovery of psychoanalysis is linked to the personal exploration that Freud undertook on himself after his father's death. He realized that analysts can access the practice of analysis only through knowing their unconscious, an indispensable condition in order to recognize their own → countertransference and dominate it. Only later did he become convinced of the irreplaceable role of didactic analysis in respect to self-analysis. The educational value of personal analysis is anticipated in *Recommendations to Physicians Practising Psycho-analysis*. Didactic analysis is related to psychoanalytic theory; therefore the analyst "must turn his own unconscious like a receptive organ towards the transmitting unconscious of the patient". To do so, the analyst must be able to communicate more freely with their own unconscious and this should be possible, in principle, thanks to didactic analysis. Ferenczi helped to add value to didactic analysis as he considered it one of the basic rules of psychoanalysis. According to him, didactic analysis is as complete and deep as therapeutic analysis: the analyst – on whom depends the fate of many people – must know and control the most secret weaknesses of their own character, and this is impossible without a thorough analysis. The Hungarian psychoanalytic school has established the tradition that the same didactic analyst also supervizes clinical cases followed by the candidate at an advanced stage of its training. It is a unique and typical practice: in other nations didactic analyst and supervisor were, and still are, different people. A lot of criticism highlighted the therapeutic ineffectiveness of didactic analysis and even its harmfulness, accompanied by a systematic indoctrination. For a long time, according to established traditions in different countries, didactic analysts have excelled in *reporting* or *non-reporting*. That is, they could decide to report or not report the characteristics of the candidates that emerged during the didactic analysis and their progress to the training committee colleagues. The critics to this reporting mode emphasized the total control over candidates' life that emerged and that was considered harmful for their mental health, intellectual freedom and "creativity". After didactic analysis, many analysts have undergone a second personal analysis, considered by them "truly therapeutic". According to the San Francisco psychoanalytic School of Control Mastery Theory, during didactic analysis the applicant submits some test (in order to change his pathogenic beliefs) to the training institute and to several figures whom he meets during the training, even the secretaries of the institute. It is important to take this into account to avoid major alterations in the treatment results due to the interference of a third party apparently not involved in it. *[M. Casonato, S. Sagliaschi]*

REFERENCES. Ferenczi S., *The clinical diary of Sándor Ferenczi*, 1988; Strupp H.H., Binder J.L., *Psychotherapy in a new key: A guide to time-limited dynamic psychotherapy*, 1984; Weiss J., Sampson H., *The role of pathogenic beliefs in psychic reality*, 1997.

DIFFERENTIAL REINFORCEMENT

Within the field of neo-behavioural psychotherapy, intervention technique based on the premise that many → behaviours present a degree of incompatibility that is present to a greater or lesser extent with other behaviours. Therefore, by removing the → reinforcement of an undesired behaviour and at the same time positively reinforcing behaviours that are incompatible with the original behaviour, and that are more acceptable, one can achieve a reduction in the frequency of the undesired behaviour. *[M. D'Ambrosio]*

REFERENCES. Meazzini P., *Trattato teorico-pratico di terapia e modificazione del comportamento*, 1984.

DIMENSIONAL ONTOLOGY

A term coined by the Viennese psychiatrist Frankl, which refers to an anthropological vision according to which man is considered in light of three distinct dimensions: biological, psychological and spiritual. This conception, by emphasizing in particular the contribution of N. Hartmann and M. Scheler, highlights the peculiarity of the human person and takes a position against any reductionism. On this view, Frankl founded → logotherapy and existential analysis, a psychological and psychotherapeutic approach that, as an alternative and/or complement to other approaches, should avoid the risk of an inadequate fragmentation of the person, reduced to "nothing other than" his biological (biologism), psychological (psychology) or spiritual (spiritualism) component. This anthropological foundation, therefore, allows existential analysis to turn to man according to a holistic (→ holism) view, not only in clinical, but also in educational and formative settings. In psychopathology, Frankl made this conception "operational" through the two laws of dimensional ontology: 1) one and the same phenomenon projected out of its own dimension into dimensions lower than its own is depicted in such a way that the individual pictures contradict one another: for example, in noogenic neurosis the effects on the psychic and somatic do not correspond to its etiology, which is spiritual; 2) different phenomena projected out of their own dimension into one dimension lower than their own are depicted in such a manner that the pictures are ambiguous: for example, the visions of a mystic, on the purely psychological, may appear not different from the hallucinations of a psychotic. *[D. Bellantoni]*

REFERENCES. Bellantoni D., *L'analisi esistenziale di Viktor E. Frankl*, 2011; Frankl V.E., *Man's search for meaning: An introduction to logotherapy*, 1946; Id., *The doctor and the soul: From psychotherapy to logotherapy*, 1986.

DIRECT EXPERIENCE

In Gestalt therapy, the creation of knowledge through an actual contact with the world. According to the phenomenological-existential approach (→ phenomenology) of Gestalt psychotherapy, the phenomenon – in its double aspect, primary and secondary – is considered the direct manifestation of reality. Consequently, "direct experience" means specifically the phenomenal experience, that is, what a person feels when experiencing simultaneously the inner and the outer world, without going through abstract representations, which would be a mental construct. The latter, standing in the middle between perceiver and perceived, would separate rather than connect them ("thinking divides, feeling unites", said E. Pound). Making direct experience a conscious act implies that a person extends attention from the primary phenomenon, that is, the recognition of the external world, to the secondary phenomenon, namely the recognition of one's inner reaction in the face of the outside world. These are two different and simultaneous aspects. To coexist in perception, these aspects require a differentiated attention that does not give space to simplifying reductionism. In fact, experiencing the world without recognizing one's internal reaction produces, in the long run, a chronic state of disinterest, as in depression. Whereas, experiencing one's reactions without recognizing the external world produces hallucinatory states, as happens in various pathologies. In both cases, these are partial and approximate forms of knowledge that have heavy consequences for the quality of life. *[P. Quattrini]*

REFERENCES. Bowen M., *Family therapy in clinical practice*, 1978; Brentano F., *Psychology from an empirical standpoint*, 1874; James W., *The will to believe: And other essays in popular philosophy*, 1896; Merleau Ponty M., *Phenomenology of perception*, 1945; Quattrini P., *Fenomenologia dell'esperienza*, 2007.

DIRECTIVE THERAPY

In strategic family therapy, an intervention strategy where the therapist takes an active role towards the patient in order to use, also in an implicit way, interpersonal influence and suggestive communication (→ suggestion) to obtain a → change. This type of intervention, conceived in the 1960s by Haley and other representatives of the Mental Research Institute in Palo Alto, differs from Roger's non-directive therapy for its theoretical assumptions, aim and style of managing the therapy. According to C.R. Rogers, the individual tends towards self-realization and the therapist needs to stimulate their natural abilities. Therefore, the session has a quite free and unstructured style. Instead, Haley affirms that individuals live harnessed in hierarchical structures and relationships and, when they ask for a therapy, they are in a state of confusion and suffering. This prevents them exploiting their full potential (if not in a dysfunctional way). Therefore, the main task of the therapist is to take responsibility in leading the "game" (according to P. Watzlawick, "take command of the ship") to accompany the patient in the process of change. The session has, therefore, a more rigid structure and requires the client to follow precise instructions, since according to M.H. Erickson, the patient needs to receive an order to do something and this something must be connected to their problem. *[F. Petruccelli]*

REFERENCES. Haley J., *Strategies of psychotherapy*, 1963; Id., *Problem-solving therapy*, 1987.

DISAPPOINTMENT

Affective experience resulting from the frustration of expectations, desires and beliefs. Disappointment is the consequence of a broken expectation. The greater the expectation, the more intense and pervasive is the disappointment. A person may experience disappointment towards themselves, others or the world in general. In this context "world" is meant as a social and cultural value system within which the person is immersed. In psychotherapy, many depressive states are based on disappointment. These states are induced by the "deluded-disappointed" effect, that is, by having expected something that did not occur. This can be a disappointment in love, a professional failure, a perceived injustice, as well as any other situation where a taken-for-granted expectation (delusion) was broken. Disappointment is greatly intensified whenever the person's "illusory" belief was particularly rigid and central in their perception system of reality. *[R.]*

DISCHARGE

Concept that in psychoanalysis refers to the process of discharge of excitatory energy, both internal and external. The psyche in this way frees itself from its excessive tension and re-establishes a state of → homeostasis. The psyche, according to Freud, is defined by its capacity to postpone the release of physical tension (the action): "The thought was gifted with these properties that enabled the psyche to tolerate the increasing tendency of the stimuli during the postponing of the discharge". The tendency towards the discharge of energy needs to be correlated to the complementary concept of retention and of accumulation of energy, and constitutes the fundamental principle of the mechanisms of pleasure (release) and pain (tension). The purpose of the discharge is that of freeing the apparatus of the psyche from its excess stimulation and is in this sense at the origin of both the possibility of representational processes (through processes of → abreaction), as well as the malfunctioning of the same, for example in the imperative need for concrete action. This phenomenon becomes pathological in those cases of "total" discharge, when a massive disinvestment of the psyche takes place with the resultant discharge into the somatic or in the battle against even the smallest amount of excitation. *[M. Balsamo]*

REFERENCES. Freud S. (1911), *Formulations on the two principles of mental functioning*, in *The Standard Edition*, XII, 1953–1974.

DISCOUNTING

In transactional analysis, according to Schiff it is "an internal mechanism by which people minimize or ignore" aspects of reality that according to the author could be "mutually agreed" but instead are distorted due to the "frame of reference", a kind of "filter of reality" that conditions the way in which others are perceived as well as ourselves and the world, so thus confirming our own life script. Relevant information to the solution of a problem is "inadvertently" ignored and the person takes a passive attitude towards an event that could be dealt with responsibly. *[A. Ferrara]*

REFERENCES. Schiff J.L., *Transactional analysis treatment of psychosis*, 1975; Stewart I., Joines V.L., *Transactional analysis*, 1975.

DISCOURSE (LACAN'S) → PSYCHOANALYSIS (LACAN'S)

DISIDENTIFICATION

In psychosynthesis, a process through which the Ego separates from a physical sensation, an emotion, a desire, a thought, an image of itself. According to the psychiatrist R. Assagioli, we are dominated by everything we identify with and we can master and manage everything we are disidentified from. With disidentification, we create a gap between us and the contents of the psyche. We become able to observe the flow of the psyche without being involved. During disidentification we are invited to pull out our Ego from anything it identifies with, and experience it as pure self-consciousness. Disidentification is not dissociation – the defence mechanism by which people unconsciously isolate themselves from emotions that are incompatible with their self-image – but a conscious process of liberation and discovery of the Ego. This unlocks, enhances and strengthens the relationship with all the elements of personality. Disidentification may occur spontaneously during a therapy, when patients gradually detach themselves from their pathological nucleus. It can also be induced through a disidentification exercise, usually at an advanced stage of the therapeutic process. *[P. Ferrucci]*

DISIDENTITY

A principle affirming that people are not identical to themselves always and everywhere, but they diffract into multiple "replicants" in different times and spaces. It is based on the "theory of possible worlds", which postulates the existence of other worlds in addition to present reality, in each of which replicants can act. Diachronic disidentity takes place when replicants live separately at different times (this is the case, for example, of Saul of Tarsus on the road to Damascus or of the strange case of Dr Jekyll and Mr. Hyde). Instead, synchronic disidentity happens when replicants live simultaneously in different worlds (Dorian Gray and his portrait). The concept of disidentity is useful to study → transference and → countertransference and cultural and traumatic shock. *[G. Lai]*

REFERENCES. Lai G., *Disidentità*, 1988; Id., *L'eternità sulla Piazza del Mercato. Bilateral verbal trade*, 2011; Lai G., Lavanchy P., *Disidentity shock in transference and countertransference*, in «European Journal of Psychoanalysis», 2008, 26–27.

DISORDER

In psychotherapy, the term is used with two different meanings: as a synonym for a diagnostic picture and/or → syndrome, it refers to a more or less structured but organic set of psychopathological clinical manifestations (for example: panic disorder, anxiety disorders, sexual disorders, etc.); instead, as a synonym of → symptom, it refers to a specific experience of suffering reported by the patient in relation to a recognized malaise or psychological distress. The concept of disorder as a symptom, that is, what the patient explicitly complains about in the clinical setting, is central to psychotherapy. Around this concept, a debate has often taken place between the upholders of a → symbolic – and therefore hidden, → unconscious, deep – meaning of the disorder and the upholders of a more "surface" position, according to which what is reported by the patient as a symptom must, in any case, be accepted as a starting point. The clinical practice has increasingly confirmed that the hidden and figurative meaning of a disorder can be defined as primary only in some diagnostic typologies, as for example in the area of somatoform disorders, conversion disorders, as well as in many of those disorders that are expressed through delusional ideations. *[R.]*

DISPLACEMENT → DEFENCE MECHANISMS; → DREAM.

DISPUTING

A cognitive technique used in the context of → rational emotive behavioural therapy to help the patient to achieve a transformation (→ cognitive reframing) of those modes of thought that influence emotional and behavioural dysfunctional reactions. This is a rather sophisticated procedure, currently adopted in various → cognitive-behavioural therapies. The therapist who uses rational emotive behavioural therapy applies rational analysis using three lines of argument: the empirical line of argument, through which the truthfulness of a thought is verified; the logical line of argument that tests the consistency of a certain way of thinking on a conceptual level; the functional line of argument, which allows the therapist to check how a given thought helps to achieve the patient's goals and wellbeing. Despite its apparent complexity, this technique can also be used with patients with low levels of schooling as long as they have an average intelligence. *[M. Di Pietro]*

REFERENCES. Giuseppe R., *Comprehensive cognitive disputing in RET*, in M. Bernard (ed.), *Using rational emotive therapy effectively*, 1991; Ellis A., *Overcoming destructive beliefs, feelings, and behaviour*, 2001.

DISSOCIATION → DEFENCE MECHANISMS

DISTORTION

In neuro-linguistic programming, one of the three processes of the → meta-model, along with generalization and deletion. Distortion, or deformation, is a process by which individuals deform parts of their experience. It is a "violation" of verbal language, highlighting how, in the passage of information between the deep/unconscious part and the surface/logic part, some elements of a person's experience are altered, compared with the complete experience actually lived. Useful in everyday talk, in inventing metaphors and in hypnotic language, distortion is, however, a reduced perception of reality, which can be a source of inconvenience and misunderstandings. With the help of neuro-linguistic programming, through the meta-model – also called precision language –, it is possible to recover the parts that are needed to generate change by using simple specific questions. Distortion is represented by the following "violations ": mind reading, which can be found, for example, in the expression "I know that you do not like me", is an interpretation of other people's thoughts; cause/effect relationship – "you do not like me, therefore I feel bad "– carries a link between the "dislike" and the feelings of the person who is speaking; equivalence complex – "you look badly at me because you do not like me" – creates a link between an action and what the other feels for the person who is speaking; in lost performatives – "it is wrong to criticize" – the subject is missing and the sentence becomes an "absolute"; in presuppositions – "if he only knew how much I suffer, he would not talk to me like that" – the knowledge of a state presupposes a consequent action. *[L. Bracciodieta]*

REFERENCES. Bandler R., Grinder J., *The structure of magic*, 1981; Id., *The therapeutic metamorphosis*, 1980; Haley J., *Therapy uncommon*, 1973.

DIVERSITY

An essential characteristic of relations that expresses the definition and separation of one's individuality from others. At the same time, this offers the possibility of contacting and interacting with the individual or the group whose attributes are perceived as different from one's own. According to W. James, at the basis of individuality lies the differentiation between Ego and non-Ego, which Jung considered as the process leading to the development of individual → personality. Through classification and discrimination, it is possible to define who we are, recognize others as members of different groups and build one's own sense of → identity. Moreover, this process allows individuals and groups to enhance their lever of personal → self-esteem. Diversity stands as a border that draws a distinction between individuals, but at the same time it forms the connective tissue that is necessary to establish meaningful relationships. The characteristics of members belonging to different social groups due to their ethnicity, culture, physical condition, etc. can be perceived as threatening for maintaining one's own identity: in this case, processes of → labelling, prejudice and stigma can appear. Conversely, various studies have shown that the detection of characteristics of similarity – such as having similar interests, same age and same social background – represent the basis on which to construct good opinions. According to the balance theory, this effect is due to the social support that people with similar values can provide each other with, and to the greater gratification given by interpersonal interactions based on similarities. Even in a couple relationship, the diversity of the other person (for example, interests, daily commitments, future plans) can be a source of prejudice. In this case, there is a conflict when the partners try to eliminate their differences through mutual and fruitless attempts to assimilate the other person to themselves and their own needs. Building a relationship based on the mutual respect of one's individuality and diversity is an important goal of psychotherapy. *[R.]*

DOGMATISM

Dogmatism (from the late Latin "*dogmatismus*", from *dogma*) is a mental attitude or cognitive style based upon a peculiar rigidity of the system of beliefs, personal opinions considered as absolute and incontrovertible truths or dogmas. Such a rigidity is usually shown as a high degree of closure with respect to points of view different from one's own, from which an intolerance towards someone else's opinions is frequently developed, in order to maintain and consolidate one's own system of beliefs. According to the dogmatic attitude, only one's own reality exists, so realizing the "dangerous illusion that only one reality exists" (P. Watzlawick). M. Rokeach's research (1960) on personal mentality in terms of closed/open attitudes, shows a high correlation between "dogmatism" and "authoritarism", meaning an acritic way of accepting authority. Authoritarism is thus defined by "how" the subject believes, more than "what" he believes. As the degree of dogmatism increases, so does the difficulty of rationally and objectively evaluating informations, influenced by the source authority. The rigidity of the system of beliefs may lead the most dogmatic persons to the attitude of refusing groups different from their own and to prejudices or stereotyped beliefs. Following Rokeach's proposed model, E. Ponzo's studies in the evolutional framework show how prejudices and stereotypes strongly affect the capabilities of normal children in narrow-minded persons with educational dogmatism. *[R.]*

DOUBLE

In psychodrama, a "double" indicates the mental function that allows a person to understand their own feelings and communicate them with words and/or behaviour. This mode can be activated not only towards themselves, but towards others with whom a person has a strong empathic link. This is what a mother does when she "reads" the needs of her baby or, in a session of psychodrama, a member of the group who gives word to the feelings of a mate (doubling technique). Doubling technique is especially useful when it is used with people with poor self-observation skills (due to immaturity, disease or something else) or insufficient expressive instruments (for example, due to cultural poverty). *[G. Boria]*

REFERENCES. Boria G., *Psicoterapia psicodrammatica. Sviluppi del modello moreniano nel lavoro terapeutico con gruppi di adulti*, 2005.

DOUBLE-BIND TECHNIQUE

Within the approach developed by the → Mental Research Institute in Palo Alto (→ interaction-focused therapy), this expression refers to a therapeutic technique that exploits the confusing effect generated by double bind (→ double-bind theory) for the benefit of patients. By studying the work of M.H. Erickson, Haley observed that he used hypnosis techniques inspired by double bind to induce trance: if the hypnotist, having obtained the cooperation of the subject, asks them to resist him, it will become difficult for the subjects to take control of the relationship, and they will obey the hypnotist, whether they want to or not or if they try to resist. Sceptical about the concept of change as a result of → insight and self-consciousness, Haley thought that the patient's → symptoms were rather relationship-control tactics: the patient avoids doing something, or does it excessively, but affirms that this does not depend on him. Inspired by Erickson, Haley developed the use of double bind in therapy by putting the patient in a situation where it was impossible to control the relationship with the therapist through the symptom, since this was strategically prescribed (→ symptom prescription). Authorizing the symptomatic behaviour allowed the therapist to restore the control on the relationship. This tactic is like that of the analyst: offering the patients who complain about their life to lie down and keep complaining – so as to persevere in their symptom – but under the analyst's control. This technique, developed by Erickson and Haley in the contexts of hypnosis and therapy, was resumed by the therapists of the Mental Research Institute in Palo Alto and by the team of the → Milan school. *[M. Giuliani]*

REFERENCES. Haley J., *Strategies of psychotherapy*, 1963.

DOUBLE-BIND THEORY

Within the approach developed at the Mental Research Institute in Palo Alto (→ interaction-focused therapy), a hypothesis concerning the interactional origin of schizophrenia, proposed in 1956 by G. Bateson and his group. According to this theory, the subjects defined as schizophrenic have been repetitively exposed to the following situation: they are in a relationship that is essential for their survival (such as the child–parent relationship); they receive a message that expects a response (for example "I love you", with the expectation of reciprocal expressions); simultaneously, they receive a second message, at another level, which contradicts the first one (for example, a rigid and rejecting physical behaviour by parents, or "you are incapable of love", which contradicts, at a more general level, the expectation of reciprocity); they know, as they have received a disqualification, or due to previous experience, that they cannot comment on the incompatibility of the two messages (for example, "how can you think of questioning our love!"); they cannot refuse to respond to such communication nor can they run away from the context of action. When this theory was expressed, it was considered revolutionary because it joined cybernetic and communication ideas to psychiatry and to the creation of family therapy. However, over time, this theory has lost its explanatory potential and has been outweighed by more integrated biopsychosocial theories. However, it remains a pillar of communication/systemic models and perhaps as a description of pathogenic interactions. *[C.E. Sluzki]*

REFERENCES. Sluzki C.E., Ransom D.C., *Double bind: The foundation of the communicational approach to the family*, 1976

DRAGON

In the myth of the hero of analytical psychology, the dragon – who is the hero's antagonist – symbolizes the regressive tendency of libido, the devouring appearance of the unconscious, the principle of inertia that impedes the civilizing impulse of the hero. As obstacle to the autonomy of the son, the dragon expresses the concept of motherhood very well, with its emotionality and obsessiveness. It is the keeper and prison officer of the very soul of the young man. Killing the dragon symbolizes the separation of the child-hero from the mother and the process of becoming aware of one's own soul. *[M. Gay]*

REFERENCES. Jung C.G. (1952), *Symbols of transformation*, in *Collected Works, V*, 1967.

DREAM

Freud has identified the dream as being the guardian of sleep. It enacts the fulfilment of an infantile → desire that has been repressed, the return of which is favoured through the state of sleep. The oneiric fulfilment of desire blocks the emergence of conflict of which the forbidden desire is the carrier and prevents the dreamer from waking up. If this function of containment fails, the dream transforms into a nightmare and the dreamer wakes up.

The oneiric scene is the product of a triple regression (→ defence mechanisms): temporal (old psychic development), topical (to the perceptive system), formal (to a primitive language, visual). The dream does not create anything new, it limits itself to transforming pre-existing unconscious material into material that is accessible to the conscious: the manifest content (the dream as it presents itself to memory). The oneiric work is the agent of transformation, that mediates between → censorship, that supervizes the repression of the forbidden desire, and the re-emergence of repressed material. The mediation takes place through the formation of a compromise, that on one hand, satisfies the desire, and on the other, disguises the fulfilment of this desire in such a way as to render it unrecognizable to the conscious. Condensation (reduction of the represented material), displacement (transferring of the investment from one representation to another), the transformation of the representations of words into representations of things, all form part of the oneiric work, which makes ample use of modes of → symbolic representation. The secondary development of the oneiric text confers a variable degree of narrative coherence, which, in appearance, reduces its irrational character. *[S. Thanopulos]*

▷ For Jung, the dream is "a spontaneous self-portrayal, in symbolic form, of the actual situation in the unconscious", that is, the natural expression by means of which a second mode of feeling and thinking, belonging to the primary process (→ primary and secondary processes), represents the global state of the conscious/unconscious psyche in a given moment in the present. In this sense the oneiric content is not the result of any attempt at hiding or censoring, but, in conformity with Jung's theory of symbolism, represents in the best possible way contents that are unknown or incompatible with the conscious. The dream corrects and rectifies the emotional-cognitive perception of the conscious according to the more general mechanism of self-regulation of the psyche, which is → compensation, aimed at attaining the ecological rebalancing of opposites. The dream is therefore the manifestation of the imaginative and analytical function belonging to the primary process. It can represent not only the satisfaction of desires that are incompatible or incomprehensible to the conscious, but also the emergence of alternatives that were never previously taken into consideration, or the manifestation of a new attitude of the conscious, whose strength at the time is insufficient. The oneiric images are intended in a subjective sense as complex representations (personal or impersonal) belonging to the → Self or, in an objective sense, as → *imago* of objects belonging to the wold of objects. The analysis of the dream makes use of → free associations in the attempt to obtain a causal, reductionist reconstruction of the past, and of the method of amplification in order to contextualize new or impersonal oneiric images according to a search for meaning that is prospective and finalistic. *[S. Carta]*

REFERENCES. Freud S. (1900–1901), *The interpretation of dreams*, in *The Standard Edition*, IV–V, 1953–1974; Jung C.G. (1916–1948), *General aspects of dream psychology*, in *Collected Works*, VIII, 1969; Id. (1945–948), *On the nature of dreams*, in *Collected Works*, VIII, 1969.

DREAMER

In the conception elaborated by Rank, the one who expresses with his dreaming the will to be immortal. Since the dreamer's anguish of death inheres to the condition of sleep, dreaming carries out, according to Rank, the function of overcoming this anguish. In this view, dream is not equivalent any more, as Freud and psychoanalysis stated, to the (masked) fulfilment of (repressed) desire, but it is an accomplished act of will. It is the evidence of the reality of soul and must be understood in terms of an ideology of immortality. The dreamer belongs to this ideology just like the hero and the artist. *[G. Antonelli]*

REFERENCES. Rank O., *Seelenglaube und Psychologie*, 1930; Id., *Kunst und Künstler*, 1932.

DRIVE/INSTINCT

Drive (in *The Standard Edition*, the German word "*Trieb*" is translated as "instinct") is a key concept of Freudian metapsychology and it was first formulated in "Instincts and their vicissitudes", and then again in his writings *Beyond the Pleasure Principle* and *The Ego and the Id*: there are therefore two theories of drives.

FIRST DRIVE THEORY. In his work "Instincts and their vicissitudes", Freud defined the drive as a concept that forms the border between the psychic and the somatic; it serves as the interface between the psychic and somatic life. This interface function is clear through the four terms that are related to drives: pressure, aim, object and source. Pressure is the engine of the drive, the "sum of forces" that it represents. Aim is constituted by satisfaction, that is, the suppression of the state of stimulation generated by the pressure; there are many different paths to satisfaction. Object is the thing through which the pressure is able to achieve its aim, that is to say, satisfaction, and is the most variable element of drives. Last, the source refers to the part of the body where the somatic process represented by the drive in the psyche takes place. The concept of source is important for differentiating between the different drives, which are defined on the basis of the somatic zone from which they originate (oral drive, anal drive, etc.), and leads to the Freudian definition of "erogenous zone", that is to say, a zone capable of generating sexual pleasure. The first of these drive theories is characterized by an opposition of drives led by Ego or by self-preservation, whose psychic energy is referred to by the word → "libido". The former designates needs or functions that are indispensable to preservation of the individual. The latter is a multiple category, originating from a variety of organic sources. Initially they are independent of one another; only subsequently do they achieve a more or less complete synthesis. This moment of synthesis places sexual drive at the service of the reproductive function. The distinction outlined here is between partial drives (the pre-genital stage) and genital organization, which define psychosexual development through their diachronic articulation.

THE SECOND DRIVE THEORY. This theory was formulated in 1920 in *Beyond the Pleasure Principle* and in Chapter 4 of *The Ego and the Id*. The opposition that characterizes the universe of drives is now no longer between sexual drives and the drives of the Ego or self-preservation, but between the death drive and life or sexual drive. The libido remains in this latter category. There is, however, a partial correspondence between the first drive opposition and the life drive. These latter drives synthesize some elements from the preceding opposition. Indeed, they contain a portion of the sexual drives – those destined for reproducing the species – and part of the self-preservation drives, that is to say, those associated with survival of the individual. From this standpoint, the life drives bring an end to the oppositional nature of the two types of drives put forward in 1915. It is the death drive, on the contrary, that prompts the organism to reduce excitement. Although it may initially seem to be at the service of the pleasure principle – pleasure generated from the removal of tension – Freud views it as an expression of death, in as much as it is a return to a zero degree of excitement, which corresponds to the organism's tendency to return to an inorganic dimension. Although he maintains the oppositional nature between these two types of drives, Freud says that there is a blend (→ drive fusion) between the drivess in these two groups – a blend that exists in every part of the living substance, albeit in varying proportions. Despite the fact that it remains enigmatic how this blend occurs, its characteristic of being functional to life is not in any doubt. Indeed, it enables the life drives to neutralize the death drives and divert destructive forces towards the outside: in this manner, the death drive, as a destructive drive, is directed "against the external world and against other living creatures". One example of this blend of drives is the sadistic aspect that operates in sexual drives. Having postulated this blending of drives, it is necessary to also allow the possibility that drives might be completely "unblended". If the sadistic aspect of the sexual drive serves as an example of drives blending, sadism becomes autonomous – that is to say, a perverse form – and represents a model of unblended drives. At this point, the question arises: as it is not possible to perceive these two drives as such, what data allows us to infer their existence? Freud has no doubt: this opposition between the two types of drive may be perceived in the polarity between love and hate. The love–hate polarity demonstrates not just the opposition between these two types of drive, but also their blending, as may be seen from the fundamental ambivalence of love in life: hatred always accompanies love, and the former can easily transform into the latter and vice versa. *[P. Valerio, M. Bottone, R. Vitelli]*

REFERENCES. Freud S. (1915), *Instincts and their vicissitudes*, in *The Standard Edition*, XIV, 1953–1974; Id. (1920), *Beyond the pleasure principle*, in *The Standard Edition*, XIV, 1953–1974; Id. (1922), *The Ego and the Id*, in *The Standard Edition*, XIX, 1953–1974.

DRIVE FUSION

This term is used as opposed to "drive defusion" to describe qualitative and quantitative relations between life and death → drives and it indicates the mixing between these two groups of drives. After 1920, Freud links the various expressions of normal sexual life, "in which there is always a hint of sadism and masochism", to the fusion of life and death drives. Also, he considered the aggressiveness that characterizes the clinical manifestations of sadism and masochism a direct expression of the death drive that follows "drives defusion". *[F. Ortu]*

REFERENCES. Freud S. (1922), *Two encyclopaedia articles*, in *The Standard Edition*, XVIII, 1953–1974; Id. (1932–1936), *New introductory lectures on psycho-analysis and other works*, in *The Standard Edition*, XXII, 1953–1974.

DSM

It is the acronym of *Diagnostic and Statistical Manual of Mental Disorders*, a nosographic classification of the main psychological disorders developed by the American Psychiatric Association (APA). The DSM is now in its fifth edition (DSM-5). It follows the criteria of → psychiatric diagnosis and it classifies pathologies in diagnostic categories organized according to a medical model of absence–presence of disease. The previous edition of the DSM (DSM-IV) considered symptomatological, epidemiological and functional aspects developed within a multi-axial system composed of five axes: I) Clinical Syndromes / Disorders; II) Personality Disorders / Mental Retardation; III) Medical Conditions; IV) Psychosocial and Environmental Stressors; V) Global Assessment of Functioning. In the DSM-5, this system has been replaced with a more simplified, nonaxial documentation approach. Essentially, the former first three Axes (I, II and III) have been combined, with separate notations for the other two former Axes, covering psychosocial and environmental factors (IV), as well as disability (V). The classification of each disorder is conventional, being based on sets of criteria that are conventionally estabilished every time to classify a disorder within a specific diagnostic class. This theoretical-diagnostic agreement represents a great advantage both for specialized communication and research. However, it is important to avoid giving a → reification value to it, that is, to represent psychological problems in "real" nosological entities, as happens with medical diseases. *[A. Bartoletti]*

REFERENCES. APA, *DSM-5*, 2013; Caputo A., Milanese R., *Psicopillole*, 2017.

DYSFUNCTIONAL BALANCE → FUNCTIONAL BALANCE

E

EARLIEST MEMORIES

In Individual Psychology, one of the first "best approaching ways to explore personality" together with the role of the child in the family (→ family constellation). Earliest memories "enlighten some events, real or imaginary, exact or manipulated, which refer to the stage of creative elaboration of the lifestyle". Earliest memories, more than masks of repressed experiences, allow the therapist to explore the lifestyle of the subject, whether *in fieri* or the current one. As prototypes of → "lifestyle" they represent the headline of one's own personal biographical novel, the name of one's own personal myth. More than concealing the repressed contents, they reveal the grounds upon which the subject has psychologically placed himself, in the world. *[L. Cerioli]*

REFERENCES. Adler A., *The practice and theory of individual psychology*, 1920; Adler K.A., *Adler's individual psychology*, in B.B. Wolman (ed.), *Psychoanalytic techniques: A handbook for the practising psychoanalyst*, 1967.

Eclectic paradigm → Please refer to the opening chapter, "The eight paradigms and their respective theoretical-applicative models".

ECLECTICISM

The attitude of someone who does not follow a single method, but combines different methods from multiple positions or schools. It is important to distinguish between theoretical and technical eclecticism. The first, in clinical practice, contemplates the use of different techniques imported from different orientations, which can help in the management of a specific issue, or in a specific phase of therapy. In this case, therapeutic procedures and techniques from other schools will only be added to one's own reference theory. The aim is to increase the treatment → efficacy, which is better built around the needs of the patient. The therapy suits the patient and not their problems, which are treated in a rigid and orthodox way according to the therapist's specific reference model. Instead, theoretical eclecticism involves the integration of different theoretical models. Eclecticism is a much-discussed subject in the field of psychotherapy. Technical eclecticism, supported and used by many professionals, is criticized, as it can be exasperated and utilized out-of-context. This may lead to superficiality and inconsistency in the treatment because the individual techniques often follow therapeutic principles related to the theory of reference. A bigger criticism concerns clinical-theoretical eclecticism. It is accused of a lack of theoretical clarity, which could produce confused interventions and unclear objectives, for both the patient and the therapist. *[R.]*

EFFICACY

In psychotherapy, the ability to obtain the desired effects through a therapeutic intervention. The evaluation criteria of efficacy can vary greatly depending on the type of reference paradigm and the theoretical model adopted by the therapist (see also the opening chapter, "The eight paradigms and their respective theoretical-applicative models" and the Appendix, "Empirical research in psychotherapy"). *[R.]*

EFFICIENCY

In psychotherapy, the amount of means and resources used to achieve a successful treatment. Efficiency indexes can be many, including suffering and efforts made by individuals or their social system in the attempt to manage or resolve their discomfort. Time, meant both as length of intervention and number of sessions needed to achieve the therapeutic goals, represents one of the main characteristics in the evaluation of a therapeutic model's efficiency. The different importance attributed to efficiency is one of many aspects that differentiate brief and long-term therapies. *[R.]*

EGG DIAGRAM (ASSAGIOLI'S)

The first stage of the psychosynthesis journey, that is, self-knowledge, implies first of all knowing how we are from a psychological point of view. We have to familiarize ourselves

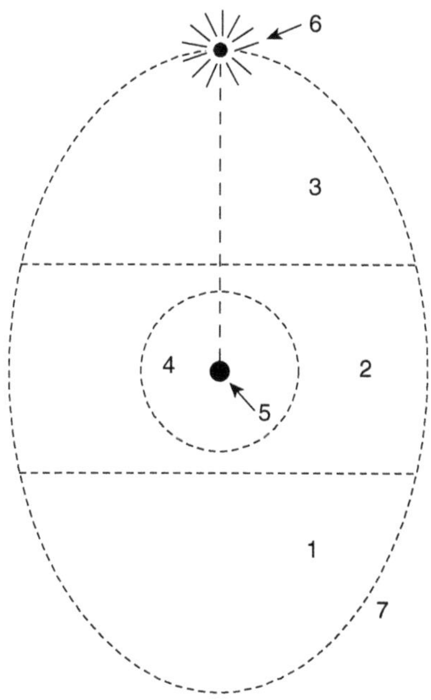

Figure 1 Egg diagram.

with the structure of the psyche that Assagioli – following the saying "one image is worth more than a thousand words" – represents with the "egg diagram". This diagram illustrates the *anatomy* of the psyche and it is subdivided into seven parts.

1) The lower unconscious
2) The middle unconscious
3) The higher unconscious
4) The field of consciousness
5) The conscious self or "I"
6) The higher Self
7) The collective unconscious

All the lines are dotted to indicate the possible and continuous passage of the psychological elements from one part to another, continuously, from inside the egg to the outside (in connection with the collective unconscious). *[D. De Paolis]*

REFERENCES. Assagioli R., *Psychosynthesis, a manual of principles and techniques*, 1965; Assagioli R., *Per l'armonia della vita*, 1966.

EGO

A term first used by Freud to indicate a psychic instance with perceptual, behavioural and cognitive control functions, of which the individual tends to be conscious (the Ego is guided by the reality principle and it is the foundation of personal identity), but also with defence functions, which the individual does not use consciously. Genetically, the Ego is formed due to a person's need for an ongoing confrontation with external reality. However, it must pragmatically take into account not only adaptive needs, opportunities and external threats, but also the instinctual needs of the → Id and the strict reminders and impositions of the → Superego (→ topographical model of the mind). As the Ego is the mediator between conscious, preconscious and unconscious (→ topographical model of the mind), it is characterized by processes and mechanisms that relate to all these systems. Among the mechanisms related to the Ego, unconscious → defence mechanisms are particularly important. The main mechanisms are: removal, identification, idealization, dissociation, rationalization, reaction formation, projection, denial, sublimation. Aspects and terms closely related to the Ego are: → egocentrism and → narcissism. The Ego can be characterized by external conflicts (for dominance and control of the environment) and internal or intrapsychic conflicts. Within and beyond the Freudian view, important characteristics are ascribed to the Ego. These express themselves at multiple levels of communication and relationship: need for coherence, of recognition, of affirmation and realization, need for contact and social interaction, need for knowledge (→ need). Psychosocial perspectives usually adopt terminological variations, which best highlight the relational and group dimension of the Ego. In particular, these are: the Self (the image of the Ego that is reflected and recognized in the interaction with the Other); the Me (the Ego that acts as a proper object of observation); personal and social identity, as narratological constructions and reconstructions and foundation of the system of interpersonal and group relationships. *[S. Smiraglia]*

▷ In the view of the psyche formulated by Jung, the Ego is a → feeling-toned complex. Like all complexes, it consists of three components: a perceptual dimension, an ideational dimension and the feeling-tone, the function of which is to keep perceptive and ideational aspects together. However, the Ego-complex has some special features that distinguish it from all the other psychic complexes and allow it to perform specific functions. "The Ego-complex in the normal person," says Jung,

> is the highest psychic instance. By it we understand the ideational mass of the Ego which we believe to be accompanied by the potent and ever-living feeling-tone of our own body. The feeling-tone is an affective state which is accompanied by bodily innervations. The Ego is the psychological expression for the firmly associated union of all general bodily sensations. The personality proper is therefore the firmest and strongest complex, and asserts itself (provided it be healthy) throughout all psychological storms. It is for that reason that the ideas which directly concern one's own personality are the most stable.

As it refers to one's own body, the Ego-complex has a greater representative and perceptive stability than other complexes. It is the centre of consciousness and it tends, unlike the other complexes, to possess a high degree of stability and time-space continuity of feeling and self-perception, despite the continual flow of perceptions and representations to which individuals are subjected during their psychological evolution. As it is more stable and consistent than the other complexes, the Ego has a hierarchical function (that is, an organizing function) compared to other complexes and it guarantees a normal, not a chaotic, psychic functioning. The Ego works also as a mediator between consciousness and the unconscious. In this way, it ensures the psychic tension underlying the "symbolic function", the true engine of inner life of an individual. Since the Ego-complex is the centre of the field of consciousness and not of the totality of the psyche, it must be distinguished from the Self (*Selbst*). By dialoging with the → Self, the Ego constitutes a psychic axis (Ego-Self) which, according to Jung, realizes the possibility of the individuation process that constitutes the true and deeper existential task of an individual and the realization of their deeper potential. In its functional expressions, the Ego can be specifically characterized and adjectivized in relation to the function performed in a precise moment: for example, one can speak of oneiric-Ego in dreams or of affective-Ego within the sphere of affections. *[L. Aversa]*

REFERENCES. Freud S. (1921), *Group psychology and the analysis of the ego*. In *The Standard Edition*, VIII, 1953–1974; Id., *The ego and the id*, in *The Standard Edition*, XIX, 1953–1974; Jung C.G., *The psychology of dementia praecox*, 1907; Mead G.H., *Mind, self and society*, 1934.

EGO PSYCHOLOGY

A branch of psychoanalysis born in the heart of the New York Psychoanalytic Society as a result of the work of a number of psychoanalysts who came from various countries of central Europe. Hartmann is considered as being the founder of Ego psychology and was its greatest theorist in the period following World War II; he contributed more than any other to the formulation of the programme of this branch of psychoanalysis, but also collaborated with other psychoanalysts: R.A. Spitz, Kris, Lowenstein, Rapaport and E.H. Erikson. After having worked at the Institute of Psychiatry and Neurology at the University of Vienna he moved to the United States, where he was the first director of the therapeutic clinic of the Institute of Psychoanalysis of New York, and where he subsequently took on the role of the president of the International Psychoanalytic Association. Hartmann was psychoanalyzed by Freud from 1934 to 1936 and in 1938 emigrated to the United States. The diverse social and cultural context in the USA contributed to his departure from a classical Freudian position, due to the opportunity he was given to work in important cultural associations, associated with the university. Within this context, Hartmann was confronted with two new demands: the first was the opportunity to establish a dialogue with academic experimental psychology; the second was the pressure exerted by social demands of a psycho-diagnostic nature aimed at orienting the individual according to the demands of society. Human society is the environment in which individuals must survive, therefore, according to Hartmann, the → Ego adapts the organism to the environment in a balanced way, keeping in mind the demands of the components that are biological and those that are made by society. The functions of the Ego were discussed by Freud in his last body of work; however, many problems related to the relationship between the instinctual → drives and the external world had remained unresolved. The ambiguity of Freud's theory in this regard consisted in the fact that, at times, the drives were described by him as being the only forces that motivate the choices made by the individual, while at other times, the autonomy of the "Ego drives" was explicitly asserted. The fundamental thesis of Hartmann's theoretical work was already present in his essay of 1939, considered as being the manifesto of this new formulation. In it, in fact, one can find, even though in a concise form, the fundamental hypotheses of his work.

HARTMANN'S FUNDAMENTAL HYPOTHESES. According to Hartmann, an autonomous "sphere of the Ego exists, that is free from the conflicts that arise from instinctual drives". Not all the activity of the psyche is involved in conflict; there is also another sphere, or component of the Ego, that is free from conflict. This is innate; it does not derive from the → Id, as was proposed by Freud; it develops and has a precise neurophysiological base. In Hartmann's theory psychic processes need to be understood from different points of view: from that of adaptation to the environment to that of its origin and development, from a dynamic-structural conceptualization of the psyche, not limited to the notions of conscious and unconscious, to the attention and value given to the relationships between different parts of the brain that are associated with the functions of the psyche. Hartmann gave particular importance to the use of scientific rigour in psychoanalysis, even if this was according to the neo-positivist epistemological conception that was dominant in the first half of the last century, the science of the so-called "hard" sciences: chemistry, physics, mechanics, etc. The second fundamental intuition of Ego psychology present in Hartmann's theory is with regard to the problem of the Ego and adaptation, correlated to processes that lie in the realm of reality. The process of adaptation is not straightforward, as it involves many problems that can vary from the field of biology to that of psychoanalysis. In fact, we assert that an individual is well-adapted to his environment if his organism and his psychic equilibrium are not overwhelmed by the external world in which he lives. This psychophysiological and environmental adaptation starts from the first moments of life. In addition, according to Hartmann, there also exists a → reality principle, according to which the relationship with the latter tends towards the seeking of equilibrium and therefore needs to be constantly modified. It is not possible to consider as being adaptive a relationship with reality where we become aware of it only to the extent to which this reality causes us pain. This relationship can be also pathological, and therefore becomes itself the source of pain; however, one cannot consider the relationship with reality as being adaptive only if pain exists. According to Hartmann, in the field of psychoanalysis the innate adaptive capacity for adaptation of the human individual as a guarantee for the achievement of positive results in the relationship with the external world is not given enough importance. Another theme that was also very important to Hartmann is that relative to the autonomy of the Ego. He asserted that autonomy cannot derive from the drives, in that there exists an autonomous development of the various functions of the Ego that highlights the strength and the weakness of the Ego itself.

According to Freud, an Ego is strong if it is successful in accepting the Id, if it can confront itself with the → Superego and if it can deal with reality. Vice-versa, the Ego is weak if the individual, when faced with these tasks, is not able to fulfil them in a successful manner and lapses into self-destructive pathology or in repetitive behaviour. Therefore, the "Ego" is weak if it has not had a healthy development. Hartmann refers to various research studies that have dealt with the process of the development of the Ego. The weakness of the Ego corresponds to a particular type of pathology in that important aspects of the personality can fail to develop or else regress. The merit of Hartmann's research consists in the fact that he shifted the focus onto the healthy functioning of the Ego and not on its pathological functioning, contrary to Freud's formulation that was focused on revealing the unconscious content of the drives, and for this reason was described as the "psychology of the Id". This new tendency gives attention to the adaptive process and to → defence mechanisms that allow the patient to see first of all what is functioning well, even in the presence of a pathology. The analysis of the defences is important in Fromm's formulation; he believed that they were to be changed and not destroyed, with the intention of capturing their profound meaning.

OTHER CHANGES. Rapaport's contribution also merits particular attention, as he attempted to give a theoretical organization to the concept of the psychology of the Ego as proposed by Hartmann. With the aim of developing the training programme of Ego psychology, Rapaport put together a historic research group that worked on meta-psychology and on psychoanalytic theory at the Menninger Foundation, which was considered to be the largest centre for psychiatric-psychoanalytic training in existence at the time. The work was focused on the organization of psychoanalytic theory, even if this was done according to the criteria of the epistemologic-neopositivistic conceptualization that was dominant at the time. Rapaport formulated a conception of psychoanalysis that extolled meta-psychological themes and neglected both semiotic and hermeneutic problems. In this formulation one can see an attempt to reconduct psychoanalysis to general psychology, in a privileged relationship with the cognitive psychology of Piaget and with the Gestalt theory of K. Lewin. This relationship is aimed at bringing about an overall vision of the structure of the psyche that is able to integrate not only the Ego and the environment, but also emotions and thoughts. In fact, Rapaport is considered to be the most important writer on the meta-psychology of affect.

A well-known researcher of the stages of development of the infant ascribing to the theory of Ego psychology is, without doubt, Spitz. His formulation relative to the three stages of development of the infant with reference to the mother–child relationship, has allowed the formulation of a psychoanalytic psychology relative to the first year of life based on experimental methods. *[L. Longhin]*

REFERENCES. Freud S. (1901), *The psychopathology of everyday life*, in *The Standard Edition*, VI,1953–1974; Id. (1938), *An outline of psycho-analysis*, in *The Standard Edition*, XXIII, 1953–1974; Hartmann H., *Principles of psychoanalysis*, 1927; Id., *Ego psychology and the problem of adaptation*, 1939; Id., *Essays on Ego psychology*, 1947; Hartmann H., Kris E., Loewenstein R.M., *Comments on the formation of psychic structure*, 1946; Rapaport D., *Emotions and memory*, 1942; Id., *The structure of psychoanalytic theory*, 1960; Id., *The conceptual model of psychoanalysis*, in «Journal of personality», 1951, 20(1); Rapaport D., Gill M.M., Schafer R., *Diagnostic psychological testing*, 1945–1946.

EGO-STATE

A central concept in the construction of Berne's theory of transactional analysis. An Ego state is a whole organized by cognitive and behavioural styles, with the respective emotional models associated. This is the framework of Berne's intrapsychic theory. He describes three Ego-states, centred on: 1) the exteropsychic origin of different styles and models (→ Parent); 2) the archaeopsychic origin (→ Child); 3) the neopsychic origin (→ Adult). Each one of the three Ego states provides the Ego with different adaptive capabilities: 1) an automated system of survival and of self-protection (Parent); 2) an intuitive function (Child); 3) an analytic function (Adult). In contrast to the corresponding Freudian needs (for example, → Ego and → Superego), the Ego-states can be diagnosed inductively and not only deductively. The Ego-states can be assessed in their scope only if understood in their structural dimension and not merely in their behavioural one. In the presence of unresolved conflicts between the need for drives by the Child and need for protection by the Parent, impasses will remain at the adult age, which will influence the analytic capacity of the → here and now of the Adult, with consequent "symptoms", both intrapsychic and relational. The analysis and the therapy of the so-called impasses are confronted with different methodologies: cathartic in the Re-decisional School of B. and M. Goulding and in the Integrative School of R.G. Erskine, and interpretive in the Roman Psychodynamic School of M. Novellino and C. Moiso. *[M. Novellino]*

REFERENCES. Berne E., *Transactional analysis in psychotherapy*, 1961; Novellino M., *Psicoanalisi transazionale*, 2004.

EGOCENTRISM

The tendency to place oneself at the centre of each situation. Egocentrism characterizes the first stage of each individual's life: from 0 to 3 years old, children place themselves at the centre of the world and give great importance to the things that surround them in relation to the distance from them. The Swiss psychologist J. Piaget described this as a physiological phase where children use the information at their disposal to satisfy their needs, as if they had an absolute and universal value (→ development stages (Jean Piaget's)). What is subjective becomes objective for children who do not consider points of view and knowledge different from theirs. The acquisition of adequacy and efficacy in communication is a step in a process that takes time and proceeds gradually, in harmony with cognitive development. In adulthood, a certain inclination to egocentrism persists. In some people this inclination manifests itself only in extreme situations with high emotional involvement (for example, strong anger or pain), while in others it may lead to pathological manifestations (i.e. narcissistic disorder, pathological perfectionism) that negatively affect social life. In this context, the goal of psychotherapy becomes to replace (or place for the first time) the patient in a position where they are able to relate and functionally communicate through active listening and to consider other people's points of view. *[R.]*

EGOTISM

In Gestalt psychotherapy, "positive" egostism indicates a defensive constraint, a block, on the limit between outer and inner world, which is favourable because the organism/individual refuses potentially negative environmental elements. Instead, "negative" egotism expresses a rigid and chronic attitude of constraint, a resistance to receive potential positive elements from the outside world. *[R. Zerbetto, G. Erba]*

REFERENCES. Perls F., Hefferline R.F., Goodman P., *Gestalt therapy: Excitement and growth in the human personality*, 1951; Zerbetto R., *Gestalt: la terapia della consapevolezza*, 1998.

ELABORATION

In psychoanalysis, a psychical work that allows the patient to assimilate → interpretations and constructions proposed by the analyst through the overcoming of resistances. The term was coined by S. Freud alongside the concepts of → interpretation and → insight that, together with → therapeutic relationship, represent the main therapeutic elements of psychoanalysis. Freud acknowledges that turning an unconscious content (a memory, a fantasy, a thought) into a conscious one through an interpretation by helping the patient to reach an insight is not enough. It is necessary to introduce the time dimension and work on resistances in the treatment. Patients can only change over time by incorporating in their history new awareness and experiences. The change of a patient's structures can only be achieved if the new awareness is emotionally connoted and it does not appear only as new intellectual information. The concept of elaboration introduces a conceptual leap that, by achieving specific awareness about oneself and about one's own past, leads to the development of that function or ability related to the acquisition of awareness. This concerns the acquisition or repair of a structure rather than a simple resolution of intrapsychic conflicts. Patients must be able to identify their (and others) past and present thoughts, feelings, motivations and intentions, and verbalize and place them in an ordered and concatenated timeline up to the construction of an alternative history of their life. The concept of elaboration can be placed at the boundary of the caring theory that considers the achievement of insight as the main therapeutic factor. Some authors affirm that the insight should be necessarily truthful (and obtained by the therapist using identification, → empathy and → countertransference. That is, the analyst is supposed to correctly identify real events removed by the patient, which typically would be traumas). Conversely, other influential psychoanalysts and philosophers of science argue that the therapeutic element consists in the construction and reconstruction of appropriate and adaptive narratives made by the patient (or co-construction made by patient and therapist), a rewrite of the patient's autobiography that becomes more accessible and full of different perspectives about themselves and about others. Freud himself anticipated this concept in the late 1930s. Recently, elaboration has been considered a better articulation among memory systems (declarative and procedural), among sensory, cognitive, emotional and symbolic elements and between affective and cognitive processes (connection between emotional tone and abstraction). Elaboration can be considered as a factor common to all psychotherapeutic processes. *[S. Blasi, M. Casonato]*

REFERENCES. Blasi S., Casonato M., *I fattori terapeutici delle psicoterapie*, 2005; Frank J.D., Frank J.B., *Persuasion and healing*, 1991; Freud S. (1914), *Remembering, repeating and working through*, in *The Standard Edition*, XII, 1953–1974.

ELECTRA COMPLEX

This concept was proposed by Jung in 1913 by utilizing a mythological legend. Electra persuades her brother Orestes to avenge the assassination of their father Agamemnon by killing those responsible: their mother Clytemnestra and her lover Egist. Through this legend, Jung described his view of the psychological development of females: girls, after having reached the genital stage (→ libidinal development stages), develop the wish to have a penis; they consider their mother as responsible for this lack and drift away from her; they direct their attention towards the father, who possesses the desired object; they feel attracted by him and they want to replace the mother. They start imitating her, they wear her clothes and affirm that they will marry the father. The falling in love with their father will push them into considering the phallus, which represents him, an object of love. The failed resolution of the Electra complex will facilitate the birth of neuroses in adults. In 1920, Freud criticized the usefulness of the Electra complex and in 1931 he affirmed that this is not analogous to the → Oedipus complex: it is only in the male child that it is possible to find the fateful combination of love for one parent and a simultaneous hatred for the other, as a rival. *[G. Fossi]*

ELICITATION FREQUENCY → RESPONSE FREQUENCY

EMDR → EYE MOVEMENT DESENTIZATION AND REPROCESSING

EMOTION

A psychophysical experience characterized by high intensity, immediacy in the onset and short duration, in relation to the exposure to an internal or external stimulus. The dimensions involved in the emotional phenomenon concern: the physiological-visceral sphere, with changes in breathing, blood circulation and heartbeat, in muscles, and in other somatic functions; the expressive-motor sphere, with changes in facial expressions, gestures and behaviour; the psychological sphere, with a decrease in reasoning ability, concentration and critical reflection. The most widely used classification distinguishes between primary and secondary emotions. Primary emotions are defined as being universally and cross-culturally recognizable in facial expressions. These are joy, pain, fear, anger, etc. Instead, secondary emotions are more complex combinations of the basic emotions and are influenced and modulated by culture: examples of these include shame, blame, contempt, admiration, despair, cheerfulness, resentment, etc. Although there are some differences between the various scholars, nowadays the primary emotions described are: interest, admiration, anger, surprise, fear, joy, sadness, disgust, shame.

In psychotherapy, the theme of emotions seems to be of absolute importance, since a lack of ability to effectively manage one's own inner states seems to underlie many psychological disorders. It seems clear that work on the emotions of the patient, as well as on those of the therapist, cannot be avoided by any psychotherapy approach, since any kind of therapeutic change passes obligatorily through emotions and produces their activation. The different therapeutic schools interpret differently, but always in line with their assumptions, the assessment and intervention on emotions. *[R.]*

EMPATHY

From the Greek "*empátheia*", passion, affection; in German, "*einfuhlung*"; in Italian, "*empatia*". Empathy is the ability to understand the feelings of another person by putting oneself in the shoes of others in order to share their emotional and cognitive states. Psychology has long been divided between two approaches regarding empathy: the first approach, the more dated, considers empathy as a faculty-dimension, meaning the ability of → interpersonal identification; the second approach defines empathy as a set of cognitive and emotional roles related to specific situations. Empathy is an integration of cognitive and affective components. For some writers, the two components are designed separately. Hoffman divided the construct of empathy into three different forms: affective, cognitive and motivational. Psychoanalysts, psychotherapists and social psychologists bring attention to the affective component of empathy and consider it as "the process of emotional activation, more or less voluntary, innate, involved in sharing/participating in the experiences of others" (P. Albiero). The concept of empathy is linked to emotional and social intelligence. Most psychotherapists believe empathy is essential to building trust between therapist and client. The literature reflects strong evidence that empathy is an essential component of the therapeutic alliance across theories and that empathy is necessary in the counselling process (→ empathic understanding). The concept of empathy continues to be a central component of new forms of counselling and therapy. *[R.]*

▷ The concept of empathy has been variously adopted by numerous psychoanalytic approaches. In 1959, it also became the core of the psychoanalytic perspective of H. Kohut and his Self psychology.

In post-Kohutian Self psychology, the expression "long-term empathic immersion" is often used to describe a state in which the therapist tries to be and to remain constantly and continuously empathetic towards the patient, in spite of the inevitable difficulties of the therapeutic relationship. *[G. Nebbiosi, S. Federici]*

EMPATHIC UNDERSTANDING

In a phenomenological and existential perspective: a way of perceiving the presence of other subjects and feeling their lived experience. The term empathy was taken from the aesthetics and psychology of the nineteenth century and mostly used to indicate the intuition of the other's experience in its emotional connotations and meaning. It differs from projection and identification, and from interpretation as well, as it represents an intuitional process whose aim is not to explain symptoms but to comprehend one's way of being in the world. For this reason, empathic understanding constitutes the methodological criterion of phenomenological psychopathology (Jaspers, Binswanger). In Rogers' client-centred psychotherapy, empathic understanding represents one of the "necessary and sufficient conditions" of an effective therapeutic relationship, together with congruence and unconditional positive regard, and it is one of the most important forces in the process of becoming and of personality change. The empathic therapist, focusing completely on their client and giving attuned answers, perceives their "internal frame of reference" and allows them to evolve towards a deeper self-understanding and self-accepting attitude. *[D. Bruzzone]*

REFERENCES. Bruzzone D., *Carl Rogers*, 2007; Haugh S., Merry T. (eds.), *Rogers' therapeutic conditions: Evolution, theory and practice*, 2001; Rogers C.R., *Client-centered therapy*, 1951; Id., *A way of being*, 1980.

EMPIRICAL OBSERVATION METHOD → SCIENTIFIC METHOD IN PSYCHOLOGY AND PSYCHOTHERAPY

EMPIRICISM

Theoretical and methodological perspective according to which, knowledge can only be achieved through systematic and controlled experience. In psychology and psychotherapy, this research method adopts systematic behavioural observation, interviews, tests or experiments. In particular, empirical research in psychotherapy is characterized by studying a phenomenon through the use of a standardized methodology. This methodology consists in the experimental identification of relationships between independent variables (i.e. the variables manipulated by the experimenter, for example a specific psychotherapeutic technique) and dependent variables (i.e. the responses of the subject/patient). *[R.]*

EMPOWERMENT

A process that leads to acquiring power, that is, increasing an individual's or a group's capability to have control over their own lives, and permitting disempowered people to emancipate themselves from a lack of opportunities. The term "empowerment" defines both the process and the outcome of a proactive action aimed at acquiring power, meant as the possibility to control events and an individual's or a → group's potentiality.

It requires a multilevel construct working at the individual, organizational and community level. It is characterized by three dimensions: control, understood as a group's and community's capability to influence decisions concerning themselves; acute awareness about decision-making processes and structures; the degree of involvement of the people committed to making the desired change.

When using an empowerment perspective, the viewpoint of deficit and illness is abandoned: the aim is not to cure but rather to activate skills and promote the capability to use internal and social resources. Therefore, the role of professionals is to encourage and support knowledge and skills that are blocked and latent. The goal is to look for the resources and strengths of individuals and groups instead of focusing on and analyzing the causes that brought about the difficulties and diseases. The main aspect is not the illness, the symptom or the disease, but the ability of a person to contribute to the promotion of their own health and the management of their problem. From this standpoint, the term empowerment defines the optimal condition of a patient that allows them to partake in decisions about their treatment, which consequently allows them to assume co-responsibility in managing their → wellbeing. *[P. Meringolo, M. Chiodini]*

ENACTMENT

A psychoanalytic concept applied to the context of cognitive psychology. Initially, it spread into the intersubjective approach and then into all other relational approaches. It represents a different conception of enactment than that adopted by other therapeutic approaches. This concept is used to identify any conduct through which the patient activates a particular previous relational style, relevant to his pathology, in the analytical relationship or in a current attachment relationship. The concept tends to reuse typical clinical events identified by classics psychoanalysts, such as → transference, acting-out, projective identification (→ defence mechanisms), in the new relational theoretical context. However, acting out implies the meta-psychological concepts of energy → discharge and primary process (→ primary and secondary processes). Transference is a much more general concept and also includes other clinical phenomena. Projective identification, in its various Kleinian and Bionian forms, is not a fully relational concept and refers to mental elements that could be moved to an external space of the mind. *[M. Casonato]*

▷ In strategic family therapy, a technique through which a → family is induced to experience a new → relational pattern within the session. This technique, applied in structural family therapy and built on N. Ackerman's methods, was formally "labelled" by S. Minuchin, who introduced it into the literature and expanded it further. After the evaluation of the family pattern, the therapist restructures the interaction through the introduction of a new pattern. For example, mother and daughter are helped to communicate while the father is blocked by the interaction. This is not simply assigned as a task, but it is built to take place during the session. In this way, the family has a new experience, the previous structure is reviewed and new options become available. The elicited pattern can be assigned as a task or it can take place outside the session. *[R.]*

REFERENCES. Atwood G., Stolorow R., *Structures of subjectivity: Explorations in psychoanalytic phenomenology*, 1984; Simon F.B., Stierlin H., Wynne L.C., *The language of family therapy: A systemic vocabulary and sourcebook*, 1985; Stolorow R., Atwood G., Brandchaft B., *The intersubjective perspective*, 1994.

ENACTMENT OF THE CONFLICT

In Gestalt therapy, to act and interpret the parts of the Self, rather than simply describing them. The Greek term *drama* meant "action" and was intended as acting out (*jouer* in French) a theatrical representation through which the viewer's emotional catharsis could take place in the → projective identification (*mimesis* according to Aristotle) with the actors. It was a literary form (but also a liturgic form, when there was a sacred representation) that was not referred to as "talking about" (→ aboutism), as in epic, but as "to make an experience happen" in the → here and now. The therapeutic intervention takes place in this acting perspective, as well as in that of understanding and interpreting. It offers the opportunity to undertake an experiential process that facilitates the exploration of a paradigm that is alternative to the stereotyped and unusual one that a person wants to overcome. The Ego is not a unitary structure. According to S. Freud, there is a conflictual dynamic between a driving dimension (*Es*) and social adaptation (Superego). The parts of the Self are traced by C.G. Jung in a multiplicity of "complexes" reflecting archetypal "transpersonal" dimensions (the *Puer*, the *Senex*, the Shadow, the Mother, etc.). As affirmed by J. Hillman, the psyche is an iridescent and multiple dimension which tends by its nature to "personify" such entities and make them interact in the "theatre of the mind", as happens in dreams. From this derives the Jungian technique of "active imagination" where dreamlike psychodrama revives in the therapeutic action. This technique was later amplified by "monodrama", introduced by F. Perls in Gestalt therapy and more commonly referred to as "empty chair". Enabling a dialogue (→ dialogic relationship) between Dr. Jekyll and Mr. Hyde (who, as everyone knows, never meet) can produce unexpected results in terms of integration of split parts of personality. *[R. Zerbetto, G. Ratti]*

REFERENCES. Perls F., Hefferline R.F., Goodman P., *Gestalt therapy: Excitement and growth in the human personality*, 1951; Zerbetto R., *Gestalt: la terapia della consapevolezza*, 1998.

ENANTIODROMIA

A term of Greek origin (literally, "race to the opposite"), used by Heraclitus to indicate a trend reversal (from a direction to its opposite); that is, one of the possibilities of being in constant metamorphosis, in constant becoming. Analytical psychology uses this term to indicate a sudden change of personality from one attitude to another. According to the perspective of Jung's *Psychological Types*, a one-sided attitude, that can be identified with the dominant function, can turn into its opposite (for example, the function of thinking into that of feeling). Also, an identity with the → persona can turn into an identity with the soul. It is an abolition, a repression of complexity that can go from an identification with God, meant as ideal and highest good, to a resemblance to an archaic God with a sensual and violent nature. About this passage to the opposite, one can refer to St. Paul's conversion on the road to Damascus, to Nietzsche who, when ill, passed from an identification with Dionysus to one with Christ, or Swedenborg, who suddenly turned from a scientist into a mystic. *[M. Gay]*

REFERENCES. Jung C.G. (1921), *Psychological types*, in *Collected Works*, VI, 1971; Id. (1912–1928), *Two essays on analytical psychology*, in *Collected Works*, VII, 1967.

ENCOUNTER

Within the humanistic-existential paradigm it is an existential dimension. In their encounter with the therapist, which is unique and unrepeatable, clients process meanings that are functional for their change process; in the relationship that ensues, they enhance their own resources and create the conditions for mental and physical → wellbeing. This process helps them to accept their problems and to resolve them through emotional growth. The resulting therapeutic relationship develops a personal → insight; it constitutes the phenomenological field where the tendency to self-actualization is stimulated, modifying dysfunctional frames of reference (→ functional balance) and promoting appropriate integrated behaviour. An optimal encounter is characterized by congruency, → empathy and unconditional acceptance, which is developed by active listening that satisfies the need for → self-actualization. *[C. Montanari, F. Barbuto]*

REFERENCES. Giusti E., Romero R. (2005). *L'accoglienza;* Rogers C.R. *Client-centered therapy*, 1951.

ENCOURAGEMENT

In individual psychology, it is the empathetic proximity in facing life's challenges with greater autonomy, trust and social awareness. Encouragement is a process of sharing and stimulation aimed at testing the ability to act and express one's own personal characteristics and potentials by cooperating with others. The peculiarity of the Adlerian → setting allows subjects to rethink the dynamics of escape, avoidance, recrimination, self-pity and lamentation typical of neurotic fictions. This setting can stimulate in subjects the desire to experience progressively social, emotional and professional conduct in a more active, creative, autonomous and personal way, and to take pleasure in it. Aspirations to improve, social feelings and desires to be "vital" together with other people, find the possibility of being discovered and confirmed in this process. *[L. Cerioli]*

REFERENCES. Adler A., *Heilen un bilden,* 1914; Dinkmeyer D.C., Dreikurs R., *Encouraging children to learn*, 1963.

ENDOGENOUS

In modern psychiatry, a term used to refer to pathologies for which no organic causes or psychological reasons can be identified. On the contrary, the term exogenous indicates a mental illness caused by non-psychological factors, such as a physical illness or events originating from the outside world. In psychology, not only the world but also the *soma* is considered as exogenous. In accordance with the theory of degeneration, connected to the theory of heredity, the scientist and German neurologist Möbius applies the meaning of congenital disposition to the term endogenous, that is, what predisposes to the development of a disease:

> when we can prove or suspect the existence of an underlying cause that comes from the outside and penetrates the individual causing a disease, we have an exogenous disease. When only variable quantitative conditions are available, the underlying cause must reside in the individual and consists in the congenital disposition and therefore we speak of endogenous disease.

The German psychiatrist and philosopher Jaspers contextualizes the concepts of endogenous and exogenous at a different level of complexity, distinguishing their meaning depending on their application to physical or mental illness. According to Jaspers, the term endogenous may also apply to a "psychic disposition" and proposes a further distinction between acquired and congenital, visible and invisible disposition: "All the factors that are exogenous for physical illness (poisons, bacteria, climate) are also exogenous for mental illness, but as regards the psychic disposition, we call exogenous all physical illnesses and the somatically endogenous cerebral disorders." Finally, Tellenbach goes beyond the endogenous–exogenous contraposition, identifying as endogenous "what is stable [. . .] what emerges as a unit of fundamental character in everything that happens in life". *[R]*

REFERENCES. Jaspers K., *General psychopathology*, 1913; Möbius P.J., *Die migrane*, 1894; Tellenbach H., *Melancholia*, 1961.

ENERGY

In psychology, a term used in a metaphorical sense that draws its meaning from the context of physics and applies it to the human psyche. However, the metaphor needs to be abandoned when it becomes dysfunctional or misleading. In fact, physical energy is very different from psychic energy: the more the first is used, the more it gets exhausted, while the more the second is used, the more it increases. Some forms of psychotherapy consider psychic energy as the focus of their intervention; others consider it as a vehicle to produce changes or desired developments. For other perspectives, the construct of psychic energy represents an outdated concept. *[R.]*

ENMESHMENT

In systemic-relational therapy, Minuchin and Bowen highlighted two similar concepts: enmeshment (Minuchin) and fusion and indifferentiation (Bowen). According to the structural model (Minuchin), enmeshment represents a lack of boundaries both on a personal and generational level. In subsequent structural authors (Green), enmeshment represents a form of family cohesion, which can turn into intrusion. In family-strategic therapy, fusion represents a lack of differentiation between the various members of a family system. A fusional → family is like a tumour that grows without specializing, an undifferentiated mass inside which no individual peculiarities can be identified. This prevents the development of the various actors: "everyone must do the same thing together", "everyone knows everything about everybody". Some authors define these as open-doors families, that is, families characterized by lack of privacy. Enmeshment is like a vase with grown plants, whose roots are intertwined and suffocate each other without the possibility of re-potting. In enmeshed systems, people have no internal boundaries and have permeable boundaries towards external reality: this generates a sort of "Siamese connection" in which even the smallest personal desire constrains others. Enmeshment takes to disengaging problems, since the "myths" of one's family of origin establish heavy obligations in terms of loyalty. These prevail on and overshadow new relations. *[F. Bruni, P.G. Defilippi]*

REFERENCES. Bowen M., *A family concept of schizophrenia*, 1960; Green R.-G., Kolevzon M.S., Vosler N.R., *The Beavers-Timberlawn model of family competence and the circumplex model of family adaptability and cohesion: Separate, but equal*, in «Family Process», 1985, XXV; Green R.-G., Werner P.D., *Intrusiveness and closeness caregiving: Rethinking the concept of family "enmeshment"*, in «Family Process», 1996, XXXIII; Klugman J., *"Enmeshment" and "fusion"*, in «Family Process»,1976, XV; Minuchin S., Montalvo B., Guerney B.G., Rosman B.L., Schumer F., *Families of the slums*, 1967.

ENTELECHY

In Aristotelian thought, entelechy indicates what, in its fulfilment, implements its aim, realizes its nature, by remaining what it is. Jung uses the term *entelechy* in reference to the individuation process, which consists of an integration of personality, a synthesis over time of its dissociated parts. The Aristotelian term argues the existence of an *a priori* presence of wholeness with its own "natural" dynamic. Therefore, the use of the term by Jung paradoxically indicates a symbolism of the Self, pre-existing to its effective implementation, that can be witnessed in therapeutic practice. *[M. Gay]*

REFERENCES. Jung C.G. (1934–1954), *Archetypes and the collective unconscious*, in *Collected Works*, IX, 1969.

ENVIRONMENT

A living space within which each person develops relationships with others, the world and themselves. The social environment, as defined by human sciences, is the space within which individuals build their network of relational experiences; it includes different typologies: from the family to the professional and community environment. Therefore, the environment is not separable from the life of the individual since it is made not only of its observable characteristics but also of the subject's representations of these characteristics. Frequently, the term is associated with that of → context, although the construct of environment is extended to all factors and not just to relational or cultural ones. In view of that, the environment within which a person lives is an essential subject of study, both to understand psychological disorders and to develop intervention strategies in psychotherapy. Some forms of therapy are directly focused on changing the environment to affect the individual. However, even interventions strictly directed towards individuals will lead to an inevitable change of their living space. *[R.]*

EPISTEMOLOGY

A branch of philosophy that studies the conditions under which it is possible to have a scientific → knowledge and the methods to achieve that knowledge. The term is used in two different meanings: the first, prevalent in Anglo-Saxon culture, identifies epistemology with gnosiology or theory of knowledge, the discipline that deals with the study of knowledge in general. The second, in a more restricted domain, indicates the philosophical inquiry on scientific knowledge and it is therefore synonymous with philosophy of science. The Swiss psychologist J. Piaget named as genetic epistemology his research on the mechanisms through which knowledge is created, highlighting the original link between cognition and sensorimotor activity. He emphasized that cognitive development is divided into several phases (→ development stages (Jean Piaget's)), which may vary in duration, but always maintain the same sequence even in different cultures and historical periods. In psychology and psychotherapy, epistemological reflection is crucial, since the "objects" and events studied by these disciplines are not only the result of the mental activities and behaviours of those who produce them, but also of the concepts and theories adopted by the psychologist or psychotherapist. Therefore, the way the patient's situation is configured, the type of diagnosis and → treatment proposed will vary enormously depending on the epistemological perspective of the paradigm of reference adopted by the therapist. *[R.]*

ERICKSONIAN HYPNOTHERAPY

M.H. Erickson is recognized as the one who, more than any other, has transferred the use of hypnotic techniques (→ hypnosis) to the field of psychotherapy. His practical work can be distinguished from the tradition of studies on hypnosis for having transposed it into the therapeutic field (→ Ericksonian psychotherapy). Three types of phenomenology are involved in Ericksonian hypnotherapy: the phenomenology of the problem, of → hypnosis and of the solution. In the initial evaluation phase, the therapist analyzes the patient's symptom (the problem), in its specific phenomenological components. For example, a depressed patient presents a phenomenological experience composed of: internal focusing of attention, negativity, orientation to the past, inactivity, lack of hope, lack of purpose. At this point, the therapist constructs a new phenomenology, that of hypnosis, consisting of positive features. Hypnotic induction acts as a bridge between the problem and its solutions. In fact, through hypnosis the specialist offers patients a chance to move into a "neutral zone" where they experience the phenomenology of change or overcoming. In this way, the "gears" set in motion will give patients the drive to increase their satisfaction and their ability to activate resources in everyday life. During hypnotic therapy, the therapist works to help patients build the phenomenology of the solution. For example, the phenomenology of contentment is different from that of depression, as its features are: extroversion, positivity, activity, hope, ability to create constructive and future-oriented goals.

MAIN PHENOMENOLOGICAL FEATURES OF HYPNOSIS. The main phenomena described by hypnotized patients who have been asked to describe their experience, can be grouped into four categories: first, alteration of → attention, which turns inward and becomes focused; changes in intensity of perceptions, which may increase or decrease: some people report more vivid sensations, like a deep sense of relaxation or other strong sensory experiences (changes in tactile, visual, auditory, proprioceptive perception and in the chemical senses of taste and smell), the sense of the passing of time, etc.; second, other patients report a remarkable absence of experience in every sensory sphere; they have not seen or heard anything that happened around them, nor perceived smells, tastes, tactile sensations or the position of their arms in space. The third group of phenomenological features of hypnosis concerns feelings of dissociation, which cover two aspects: the feeling of being, at the same time, "part of" and "out of" an experience, and the feeling that this happens automatically (it is common for hypnotized patients to declare: "I was in the office, but in fact I was elsewhere, absorbed in my fantasies"); the automaticity of an experience can be mental as well as physical: it can regard images, memories or movements, as in the case of arm levitation. The final group consists of changes in responsiveness; patients under hypnosis commonly react to the mildest suggestions: allusion and implication. This kind of behaviour has been named "responsiveness to minimum suggestions" (for example, if the hypnotist warns the subject that during trance their head could move forwards, the subject in a state of hypnosis, by the action of the suggestion, might in response move their head forwards). In addition, patients in a state of hypnosis often activate an intense search for meaning and find in the hypnotist's injunctions profound meanings related to their inner lives and their own experience (for example, if the therapist tells an ambiguous story, subjects in a state of hypnosis tend to personalize it more than they would in a waking state).

THE HYPNOTIC INDUCTION. To build an effective induction, the hypnotherapist must understand the patient's own hypnotic phenomenology (structured in the four phenomenological features indicated above). Therefore, the task of the hypnotist is to place suitable material on the patient's "psychosocial stage" so that the patient, while "playing" with it, may stimulate their own hypnotic phenomenology. To induce the first hypnotic trance, the therapist places on "the patient's scene" the material related to the four specific phenomenological areas, providing suggestions for each of them. At this point, the therapist will observe which of the "games" proposed are more irresistible to the patient. The first two phenomenological categories – alteration of attention and variations in intensity – can be evoked by direct → suggestion. Instead, for the other two categories, indirect suggestion is more effective. in fact, it is not possible to tell the patient to "raise a hand" and expect an involuntary movement; it takes some degree of non-directivity to promote an automatism. To facilitate replies to minimum suggestions, increasingly indirect suggestions need to be provided. The therapist can range from integrated orders (such as "You can . . . raise your hand"), to the narration of situations that have something to do with the act of raising one's hand (like a student who wants to ask a question in class or a child who wants cookies placed up on a sideboard) until the response of arm levitation is obtained. Erickson created a large sample of indirect suggestions, which have been organized into four types by E.L. Rossi and his colleagues: 1) the Yes Set: this is built by formulating a sequence of evident truths (for instance: "You can hear sounds from the outside", "You can notice how sounds change when you focus the attention inside yourself"). This method of indirect suggestion is particularly recommended to stimulate phenomenal responses of guided attention; 2) embedded commands: these can be created through a pause and by modulating the voice after a modal verb indicating permission. This works especially in the English language, where the verb that follows is imperative. Therefore, the wording "You can go into a trance", in the form of embedded command becomes "You can . . . go into a trance". Embedded commands can also be used to elicit the phenomenon of variation in intensity, for example: "You can . . . live fully the feeling of comfort"; 3) statements of dissociation: they occur in many forms, such as: "Your conscious mind hears my voice, while your unconscious mind can fluctuate, it is so interesting to create different experiences"; with this kind of statement it is possible to orient the phenomenon of dissociation, whereby things "happen automatically" and people are both actors and spectators of an experience; 4) the implicit causative: this is the logical connection contained in sentences with the structure "when X, then Y", where X can be a behaviour and Y a state, or vice versa. For example: "When you take a deep breath, then you can get into trance", or: "When you are entering into trance, you can take a deep breath." Implicit causative is used to activate responsiveness, one of the four main phenomenological features. These four examples of indirect suggestion represent in a way, the language of hypnosis. To better understand how to use the language of hypnosis, it is possible to examine the structure of hypnosis used at the Milton Erickson Foundation, which has been called "ARE model" ("Absorb", "Ratify", "Elicit").

THE ABSORPTION. It is mainly the indirect techniques to stimulate absorption or involvement. A possible stratagem of absorption is to involve the patient in: a hypnotic phenomenon, a fantasy, a memory or a feeling (such as body heat). Numerous techniques can be used to stimulate absorption. The main techniques include: the use of the present tense, the choice of particular words, the completeness of the details provided (for example: "As soon as you close your eyes, and you concentrate, you can feel heat sensations. I don't know if you will feel this heat in the front or back of the body . . . and these sensations of warmth could be so interesting. And you could notice how these feelings of warmth start to change . . ."). The secondary techniques include: voice changes, pauses and the tone of the voice. Redundant repetitions in the absorption phase help patients to focus their attention, to direct it towards the inside and to experience sensations in a more or less vivid way. When a patient is activated in the direction of the suggested phenomenon, hypnosis is reached. Moreover, thanks to absorption, therapeutic guidelines can also be offered. In fact, the stage of absorption is not simply a means of establishing the trance (as in traditional hypnotic induction), but it already acts as a form of therapy. During the stage of ratification, the hypnotist uses a series of simple declarative sentences to ratify the trance by recapping the changes occurring in the patient from the beginning of the process of stimulation (for example: "While I was talking to you, some changes were occurring: your breathing was changing, your pulse was changing, your reflex of swallowing was changing, your perception of your body may be different").

THE STIMULATION. Stimulation benefits from indirect techniques and consists of three aspects. The first is activation of dissociation, which can either occur through suggestive techniques, such as dissociative statements, or it can be stimulated through hypnotic phenomena, such as arm levitation, catalepsy, positive and negative hallucinations. The second aspect is activation of responsiveness: after stimulating dissociation, the therapist further develops responsiveness; for example, in the style of Erickson, the specialist might suggest: "As soon as I utter the word 'now', you can take a deep breath now . . ."; in this way, by stimulating the patient's response to an unexpected suggestion, the therapist can build specific answer modes to his/her direct and implicit instructions. In fact, the main aim of hypnosis is to establish a climate of cooperation in responsiveness. The third aspect is the activation of resources: once the therapist has stimulated responses, especially to the minimum suggestions, the induction process is concluded. Activating resources is the purpose of hypnotherapy. In general, the therapist can use indirect suggestions, such as anecdotes and metaphors, to stimulate the latent resources of the patient. For example, patients with a specific phobia, such as fear of flying, have many other resources that enable them to live positively situations that would be difficult for many others; for example, they can be people skilled at public speaking. In general, the job of the therapist is to help patients access their latent resources through experiencing and investigating them, up to a point where these can be used to solve or address the issue requiring treatment. *[J. Zeig]*

REFERENCES. Nardone G., Loriedo C., Zeig J., Watzlawick P., *Ipnosi e terapie ipnotiche*, 2006.

ERICKSONIAN METAPHORS

A therapeutic communication mode used by Erickson during clinical interviews, in or out of the hypnotic trance, whereby the hypnotherapist can communicate messages and/or suggestions through the identifications and projections typical of the listening of a narration. This form of communication minimizes resistances to change, as patients are not directly judged on their behaviour, nor are subjected to direct requests to change their ways of thinking or behaving. Through the evocative power of metaphors, the message is subtly conveyed, producing emotions and inducing different → behavioural patterns. This intervention could be defined as a backward dream: what was expressed by Erickson could be interpreted by patients as a dream in which barely tolerable or completely intolerable material, expressed in figurative language, could elude the censorship of consciousness. However, a dream can only be a passive reproduction of a present conflicting condition. Instead, metaphors allow the therapist to intervene in an active way. In addition to the use of stories and anecdotes drawn from literary or mythological works, Erickson also used episodes taken from everyday life or from his personal history of physically disabled individual (due to poliomyelitis, colour-blindness and tone deafness). *[I. Bonzanini]*

REFERENCES. Erickson M.H., *My voice will go with you*, 1982; Nardone G., Watzlawick P., *The art of change*, 1993.

ERICKSONIAN PSYCHOTHERAPY

M.H. Erickson's therapy can be described as a technological approach to psychotherapy designed to solicit the responsiveness of a patient through therapeutic injunctions, in order to elicit dormant resources. In Ericksonian therapy, therapeutic work is directed towards the construction of responsiveness, in order to access a patient's resources. In this sense, hypnotic induction is a process that can be used to build responsiveness to minimal cues (→ Ericksonian hypnotherapy). For example, if the therapist tells a patient: "Lift your arm" and the patient does it, that does not necessarily indicate that the patient is in a state of hypnotic trance. A different situation is when the therapist says: "I would like you to truly realize, in a way that is uplifting, that hypnosis is really an experience that is right for you in a way that you can find handy." If the patient develops a dissociated response to this injunction and raises their right arm, it is then possible to talk about hypnosis. In hypnosis, the therapist hides the cues that elicit responsiveness, so that the patient's reactions become increasingly autonomous. Responsiveness to minimal cues indicates that the resistances of the patient are suspended, that the door to the constructive unconscious is open and that the patient is ready to be led by the therapist towards change. The task of the therapist is to help the patient to develop a process of change in their routines, and this change can have both a positive and a temporarily negative direction. In both cases, the patient will be enabled to produce change and thus, a "snowball" effect could take place in a positive direction. In fact, once the rigid set of symptoms is broken, people tend to access previously underused forces, moving towards more efficient functioning conditions. This is due to the fact that, in accordance with the assumptions of Ericksonian psychotherapy, the unconscious mind tends to have a benign nature and it is generally oriented towards health. The unconscious contains already in itself the solutions to the problems and these solutions can be brought to the foreground. In general, patients describe their symptoms in clear words: "I always have X", or "I can't X", or "I am never able to X" where X is: overcoming a depression, travel by plane, having a good marriage and so on. What patients take for granted is that they are always the victims of their problems. Therefore, the therapist must provide injunctions to elicit in patients a change in their self-victimization perception, so that the structure of their communication becomes: "I can X", and finally: "I will do X". In some cases, the best result that can be reached is that the patient admits: "I will live happily despite X", as can happen in cases of painful experiences. During a treatment, the therapist utilizes therapeutic manoeuvres that have a positive injunctive influence, in order to oppose the negative self-victimizing injunction typical of symptoms. Therapeutic tasks are often symbolic social representations designed to bring out dormant, psychological and physiological resources. These are stimulated through a positive association with resources already put in place by the patient in their social and/or private life. It is assumed that subjects already have a history that contains the "bricks" needed to build a change. For example, the history of phobic patients includes elements of tranquillity, or, in the history of socially incapable people there are some elements of good interpersonal relationship. These resources, which remain inactive in the background, can be stimulated through the therapist's directives, which appeal to the constructive latent history of patients. In Ericksonian therapy, the therapeutic process can be summarized in five major operations, conducted simultaneously rather than sequentially: deciding what to communicate to the patient; deciding how to communicate it (usually this involves the use of indirect communication, but this could also involve the use of direct therapeutic manoeuvres); understanding the patient's values system, namely their "position"; dividing the solution into gradual steps (each step can be started through a therapeutic intervention); introducing the intervention within a therapeutic sequence, tailored in a manner that is acceptable to the patient, according to their value system. Usually this involves a three-step process defined as SIFT: choosing small and well-directed steps (Steps); Intervening; leading the process up to the end (Following Through). For example, if the problem X is depression, the therapist may ask: "What is the opposite of X?" (or, if X cannot be changed easily, as in some cases of chronic pain: "How can the patient avoid being the victim of X?"). Assuming that, for the patient, the opposite of depression is happiness, the therapist can divide the idea of happiness into a series of attitudes that form a process: being active, changing mood, being outward-looking, being future-oriented, being positive towards themselves and others. Each of these steps represents an idea that can be presented to the patient, for example through an indirect story or a therapeutic directive, so that the patient can, at will, stimulate such a state. Having established a goal, the therapist evaluates the patient's values and beliefs and utilizes them (→ utilization). If the depressed patient is an adventure-lover, the therapist can suggest the idea that becoming more aware of the external environment through observation is an interesting adventure, for example observing the shape of the clouds every time the patient gets in the car. In this way, values and goals are combined. However, presenting a suggestion that suits the patient is not enough. In fact, suggestions must also be placed within a precise sequence. Ericksonian psychotherapy is essentially a method through which one can move along small steps while gradually feeding motivation. The therapist follows the rhythm of patients, working to stop their mental rigidity and helping them to achieve therapeutic goals. In regard to the presentation of a therapeutic task, therapists can start by offering a direct intervention. If they find a resistance (→ resistance to change), therapists can provide the patient with the same idea in the form of an indirect order (through the use of symbols, → metaphors, therapeutic anecdotes, etc.), following the principle that non-directivity of a manoeuvre is directly proportional to the perceived resistance. In conclusion, Ericksonian psychotherapy can be considered as a psychotherapy by reciprocal associations: the therapist finds the reciprocal of the problem (its opposite); he divides this solution into accessible steps, using indirect tailored techniques; associates the patient to the various steps, until there is a sufficient number of associations so that they lead the patient to the desired functional behaviour. In this process, the work of the therapist consists in reactivating the dormant story of the patient by creating situations by means of which, the patient himself, on his own merits, is able to get in touch with his hidden strengths and bring them to the forefront. *[J.K. Zeig]*

EROS

The psychic importance that this term has in Plato's *Symposium* is well identified by S. Freud, who uses it to define a constitutive principle of psychic life in constant antagonism with the other fundamental principle, later introduced by Freud: → *thanatos* or death instinct. Unlike Freud, Jung conceives the psyche not so much in terms of opposing principles but in terms of antinomic principles, which, in their diversity are capable of creating symbolic tension. In Jungian thought, the Freudian antinomy Eros–Thanatos is not particularly taken into account. Jung tends to consider *eros* as opposed to *logos*, although it is possible to find some semantic interpretations that do not deny the Freudian meaning. For this reason, in the context of analytical psychology, *eros* is closer to the concept of → anima, that is, of deep emotionality, a feminine principle that is antinomic to the masculine principle of *logos*. Due to this, individuals are capable of sensitivity and they are not led to an excess of cold and unemotional rationality. However, as the Jungian antinomy encompasses several meanings, it is also possible to relate *eros* to the concept and theme of death, as a different antinomian pole. *[L. Aversa]*

REFERENCES. Jung C.G. (1916–1952), *The structure and dynamics of the psyche*, in *Collected Works*, VIII, 1969.

EROTICISM

According to the perspective adopted by Freud in *Three Essays on the Theory of Sexuality*, eroticism is the specific contribution to sexual pleasure provided by the different erogenous zones. This term needs to be interpreted within the Freudian theory of sexuality. According to this theory, sexuality evolves through a series of stages, which can be identified according to the organs or body functions whose stimulation produces pleasure and whose activity allows the person to relieve tension. The first manifestations of sexuality rely on other vital functions and act autoerotically using the body itself to their satisfaction. Therefore, the expressions oral, anal, phallic or urethral eroticism, are used to indicate the specific contribution to sexual pleasure of different erogenous zones, which are linked to specific character traits. Moreover, the inhibitions of the Ego are traced to the eroticization of the organs related to the execution of the functions of the Ego. According to Freud, when erogeneity (that is, the sexual significance of an organ) increases, the Ego waives the functions performed by that specific organ to avoid undertaking a new repression, to avoid a conflict with the Id. Freud affirmed:

> If writing [. . .] has acquired the symbolic meaning of coitus, or if walking has become a symbolic substitute for stamping upon the body of Mother Earth, then both writing and walking will be abstained from because it is a though forbidden sexual behaviour were thereby being indulged in.

[F. Ortu]

REFERENCES. Freud S. (1925–1926), *Inhibitions, symptoms and anxiety*, in *The Standard Edition*, XX, 1953–1974; Laplanche J., Pontalis J.B., *The language of psychoanalysis*, 1973.

ETHNOMETHODOLOGY

A school of thought founded by Harold Garfinkel in the sixties, inspired by Edmund Husserl's phenomenological theories and Alfred Schütz's work in the field of social sciences. Ethnomethodology aims to systematically describe the "methods" used by members of a socio-cultural group to understand the meaning of their own actions. Attention focuses on shared experience and on the artefacts used within a society (or within one of its subunits) in order to confer order and meaning on performed activities. This is achieved by studying the interactive and communicative processes that allow one to generate and replicate the shared presuppositions upon which the reality of everyday life lies. The fundamental assumption of Garfinkel's theory is that social order always takes shape thanks to a layer of implicit significations, which constitutes the basis of human interactions. The aim of ethnomethodology, therefore, is that of exploring these "basic structures" that can make a social situation ordinary and predictable. This is done by bringing to light everything that the involved actors tend to take for granted during their (mutual) → interactions. The privileged field of the study of ethnomethodology thus places itself at a micro-sociological level. The research programmes aim to analyze both the face-to-face interactions and everyday conversations (which constantly renegotiate social meanings), → common sense explanations and contextual norms. These contextual norms contribute to legitimate and confirmed portions of a shared reality. In the clinical field, ethnomethodology studies, analyzes and introduces new instruments in the cure of psychological disorders and difficulties that characterize specific cultural contexts. In particular, it addresses individuals who come from an immigrant environment and, therefore, belong to different cultures (→ context). It considers the individual undergoing treatment as a socio-historical entity, which continues to interact with his/her particular cultural universe while integrating into the new context. It analyzes → conflict situations, related events and psychopathological consequences by taking into consideration the social and cultural basis of the original context. It focuses on the symbolic and semantic differences that withstand every process of thought and of representation of reality, both at an individual and a collective level. It uses and anchors the treatment to the original culture by means of therapeutic levers that can activate a change in the structure of the problem experienced by the individual receiving treatment. [*R.*]

EVACUATION

Ridding the self of disturbing mental contents – ideas or feelings – in order to maintain one's equilibrium. Freud described it as an action to rid the psyche of accretions of stimuli before thinking developed (→ pleasure principle and reality principle). The mechanism by which the evacuation is done is by projective identification (→ defence mechanisms). In this the unwanted mental content is separated (split) off from the rest of the mind and evacuated out into some body or some object, or even into space. The mental action can be aided by a physical gesture such as blinking, shrugging the shoulders, coughing, etc. For Bion, the cardinal principle of mental growth is the ability to tolerate mental pain and frustration without evacuating it. *[J. Symington]*

REFERENCES. Freud S. (1911), *Formulations on the two principles of mental functioning*, in *The Standard Edition*, XIV, 1953–1974; Bion W.R., *Learning from experience*, 1962.

EXCLUSION

In the area of transactional analysis, a psychopathological Ego-state in which there is a de-energization, or rather a repression of the free energy of one or two of the three → Ego-states. Exclusion, together with → contamination, constitutes the focal point of the pathology of the Ego-states. The individual will function in a partial way, having the need to begin symbiotic relationships with another individual, who will provide a vicarious function for the excluded Ego-state or -states. The exclusion of only one of the Ego-states is present in neurotic states and personality disturbances; the exclusion of two Ego-states characterizes psychotic states. It needs to be underlined that, being de-energized, the excluded Ego-state can therefore be reactivated to render the personality autonomous and independent; the objectives of the therapeutic intervention are therefore aimed at redistributing the psychic energy in the areas of the excluded personality and at establishing autonomous relationships. *[M. Novellino]*

REFERENCES. Berne E., *Transactional analysis in psychotherapy*, 1961; Novellino M., *Psicoanalisi transazionale*, 2004.

EXCLUSIVITY OF THE RELATIONSHIP

Availability and commitment of the therapist to focus and direct their attention only to the patient during the session. It is also the ability to create a → setting in which the patient feels fully listened to by an experienced professional who is concerned with their problems. The exclusivity of the relationship also includes respect for privacy of personal data and communications that take place between therapist and patient, in accordance with the provisions of the law. *[R.]*

EXISTENTIAL A PRIORI

According to Binswanger's existential psychoanalysis, the existential *a priori* is understood as a set of fundamental existential modalities that give tone and modulation to every individual's life and coincide with the constitutive forms of all human experience and the interactive relationship between the Ego and the ones that differ from it. According to existential psychoanalysis, the existential *a priori*, also known as Self, is an experiential concept. It is a real, constitutive and native dimension, along with the body, the psyche and the freedom of decision; it contains the project and the modalities to achieving it. The Self is the healthy, energetic, planning and creative part of the human being, unlike the Self in philosophy – which is an "objectified Ego"; unlike the Self in psychology – which is one's own self-image (general psychology); and unlike the "feeling of Self", which is the "totality of the psyche". *[D. Romagnoli, S. Antonetti]*

REFERENCES. Binswanger L., *Zur phänomenologischen Anthropologie*, 1947; Binswanger L., *Being in the world*, 1963; Mercurio A., *Teoria della persona*, 1978; Mercurio A., *Antropologia esistenziale e metapsicologia personalistica*, 1991; Mercurio A., *Teoria dell'inconscio esistenziale*, 1995.

EXISTENTIAL ANALYSIS

A synthetic synonym of existential psychoanalysis. It is a contemporary orientation that derives its concepts from both Freudian psychoanalysis and Heidegger's existential philosophy. According to existential analysis, the past and the future are just mere thoughts; present is the only thing that exists and all that exists, therefore the Being is here-and-now. Both existential analysis and → analytical existential psychotherapy try to retrieve the opportunities of satisfaction of those motivations and interests that the individual believes lost; furthermore, they support individuals in seeking the meaning of life and of their existence. *[D. Romagnoli, S. Antonetti]*

REFERENCES. Mercurio A., *Antropologia esistenziale e metapsicologia personalistica*, 1991. Mercurio A., *Teoria della persona*, 1978; Mercurio A., *Teoria dell'inconscio esistenziale*, 1995.

EXISTENTIAL ANALYTIC PSYCHOTHERAPY → ANALYTIC EXISTENTIAL PSYCHOTHERAPY

Existential-humanistic paradigm → Please refer to the opening chapter, "The eight paradigms and their respective theoretical-applicative models".

EXISTENTIAL POSITION

A central concept of the humanistic-existential dimension of Berne's transactional analysis. It identifies the psychological attitude that an individual assumes from birth, towards himself and others, in terms of positive (*OK*) or negative (*not-OK*) availability. Each individual is born with a potential of → OK-ness, of constructive openness towards relationships with others, based on autonomy, spontaneity, intimacy: it is the constructive position (*I'm OK – You're OK*). This potential becomes, in various ways, distorted by neurotic childhood experiences, which lead the person to assume different basic attitudes towards the world: a projective position (*I'm OK – You're not OK*), a depressive position (*I'm not OK – You're OK*), a destructive or "futile" position (*I'm not OK – You're not OK*). In reality, each individual presents, to some degree, each one of the four aforementioned positions, and it is under pressure that the "basic" one can be identified. In psychotherapy, the basic position, which the patient tends to assume when they are involved in the problem, is identified, and the objective consists of helping them to recuperate their basic OK-ness in that environment. The psychotherapist has to be competent in maintaining a constructive position of OK-ness towards the patient, and in elaborating his own → countertransference when he relives emotional situations which reactivate his *not-OK* positions. The constructive position is to be understood as a realistic availability towards others, so as not to slide into an illusory *I'm OK – You're OK,* and therefore a maniacal one. *[M. Novellino]*

REFERENCES. Berne E., *«Hello!» . . . and then what?*, 1972; Moiso C., Novellino M., *Stati dell'Io*, 1982.

EXISTENTIAL PSYCHOANALYSIS → ANALYTICAL EXISTENTIAL PSYCHOTHERAPY

EXISTENTIAL TRUTH

In existential psychoanalysis, a term used by M. Heidegger to state an ontology based on the concept that man is essentially → being-in-the-world. Man's nature is precariousness, instability, limit, deficiency: therefore, he needs the world, and the world, to which he belongs, is the necessary element of his constitution. He is not the being, nor does he possess being, but is related to being. The being is never given as identity or as firm or total possession, because the being does not constitute a possession, rather a possibility. The being is not a stable structure but an event, it is the "take-place". The self, as it is conventionally conceived, is devoid of an intrinsic reality. *[F. Ioppolo]*

EXOGENOUS → ENDOGENOUS

EXPERIENCE

An effect on the level of sensations, emotions and thought and on the involvement of a subject in a specific activity. In psychotherapy, experience is the main instrument adopted by the more pragmatic approaches to produce change: in fact, the "new" experience allows patients to perceive their own situation differently and, consequently, to react in a more functional way (→ corrective emotional experience). In this case, experience is considered a vehicle of change. On the contrary, the more intrapsychic approaches consider experience an effect of change, that is, what must be produced by virtue of → insight and awareness concerning one own's inner dynamics. *[R.]*

EXPERIMENTAL METHOD → SCIENTIFIC METHOD IN PSYCHOLOGY AND PSYCHOTHERAPY

EXPERIMENTATION

In psychotherapy, the capacity of the individual to seek out and to expose himself to new perceptive, emotional, cognitive and social experiences. The capacity to experiment can involve many areas of experience (the relationship with one's peers, sexuality, nutrition, etc.), as well as the exploration and/or states of consciousness that had been previously unknown to the individual. A therapeutic objective that is transversal across many models of psychotherapy is that of encouraging phenomenon of experimentation that lead the patient to widen and render more flexible his behavioural, cognitive and emotional repertoire. Very often, in fact, in the psychotherapeutic context, the phase of experimentation is experienced by the patient as a moment of emotional unblocking, that changes a previous equilibrium experienced as being excessively rigid or dysfunctional (→ functional balance). In this sense, the experimentation can be assimilated with – even though it cannot be completely superimposed with – the concept of → corrective emotional experience.

The term is also used with reference to the type of empirical research characterized by the use of statistical instruments to compare the → efficacy of the techniques and models of psychotherapy (→ research; see also the Appendix, "Empirical research in psychotherapy"). *[R.]*

EXPERIMENTING

In Gestalt psychotherapy, working on an imaginary or theatrical plane, hypothetical situations aimed at allowing the person to experiment with emotional states that have previously been avoided, and to develop attitudes that are functional to his existential needs. Gestalt psychotherapy is an approach based on experience, in the sense that it considers the process of awareness primarily as being experiential and only subsequently as being cognitive. For this reason, experiments are fundamental to this therapy, after one reflects on that which he has experimented with; when something new is discovered about oneself and about the world, it can then be put into practice in other experimental situations in order to verify their functionality. Experiments take place in a space that lies between what is inside and what is outside, the transitional space of Winnicott: a space where one can experiment with behaviours without any existentially problematic consequences; the purpose of the experiment is to enact problematic situations with imaginary personalities on an empty seat (→ hot seat) or with other members of the group. In this situation, the individual is able to experience himself in relation to the world in new areas, acquiring new knowledge, which in turn is tested in other experiments specifically constructed with the therapist. An experiment can consist of asking questions such as, "If this person with whom you are having difficulties told you this what would be your answer?", or in asking the individual to imagine a difficult situation to which he has to find a solution, and so on.

The experiment brings to light the patient's difficulties, which requires processes of development, or resources, that the person did not know he possessed. Difficulties are led back to the needs of the organism, pain, fear, aggressiveness and sex, and from this base, always through the use of experiments, more adaptive forms of behaviour are looked for that are more congruent with the individual's ethical, aesthetic and functional needs. *[P. Quattrini]*

REFERENCES. Moreno J.L., *Psychodrama first volume*, 1946; Perls F., *Ego, hunger, and aggression*, 1942; Id., *Gestalt therapy verbatim*, 1969; Id., *The Gestalt approach and eye witness to therapy*, 1973; Winnicott D.W., *Playing and reality*, 1971; Zinker J., *Creative process in Gestalt therapy*, 1977.

EXPLICIT ANALOGUE INTERVENTIONS (EAI) BRIEF THERAPY

Explicit Analogue Interventions in Brief Therapy (EAI Brief Therapy) is an approach that is based on Watzlawick's, Weakland's and Fisch's concept of second-order change (→ first- and second-order change): when the (unsuccessful) → attempted solutions keep the problem alive, it is useful to interrupt the problem-maintaining pattern and shift the direction. New and central in the approach developed by Ilka R. Hoffmann is that the concept of second-order change is re-introduced from a "non-expert" stance: instead of interrupting the client's unsuccessful attempted solution through therapeutic expertise, the client's internal images are activated for change. In EAI Brief Therapy the attempted solution is interrupted through explicit analogue resource activation. According to this model *explicit* resource activation involves accessing the client's resources directly, in a way that is transparent to the client, while *implicit* resource activation involves therapeutic interventions, which access the client's resources indirectly. The client is not aware of which resources are activated and how the intervention works. *Digital* resource activation involves therapeutic communication on a rational-intellectual level, while *analogue* resource activation uses analogue language.

EAI Brief Therapy defined seven phases of therapy: defining the presenting problem, identifying a problem focus, identifying the attempted solution, preparation phase, body-focus meditation, analogue presentation, problem reassessment. Phase I, defining the presenting problem, entails obtaining a clear definition of the problem from the client's perspective. Phase II, identifying a problem focus, is applied in those cases when the symptom is experienced as an insurmountable, overwhelming obstacle in the client's life and entails the question: "Where is it [the symptom] in your way the most?" Besides eliciting smaller and more achievable goals for therapy, this question also shifts the perspective of the problem. In Phase III the main pattern of the client's attempted solution is identified. The goal of this phase is to pinpoint where exactly the client is blocked and which vicious cycle is perpetuating the problem. Phase IV is a preparation for phases V and VI. This short phase entails condensing the experience and information of the previous phases for the client and setting the stage to try something different, by inducing curiosity for a new experience. When the client agrees, phase V, a body-focus meditation, is applied in order to focus the client's awareness and induce a relaxed state to facilitate the following phase of analogue presentation. Phase VI entails interrupting the (unsuccessful) attempted solution through explicit analogue resource activation. The therapist assists the client in shifting the perspective from the rational to the analogue level. While the client remains in a relaxed state with eyes closed, the therapist gives an impulse for an analogue presentation of the main → pattern of the unsuccessful attempted solution. Most frequently an impulse for a visual image is given. However, an impulse for an analogue presentation can also entail other modalities, such as kinaesthetic (e.g. a body posture) or auditory (e.g. a sound), or a combination of modalities. When the client describes the internal image of the attempted solution, the therapist gives an impulse to evaluate this analogue presentation. Usually the image of the unsuccessful attempted solution is evaluated as negative. The client is then given an impulse to modify this internal image until it feels "comfortable". The new image is again evaluated by the client. A positive evaluation is followed by questions from the therapist to clarify the transition of the first image into the new image. A negative evaluation is followed by an impulse from the therapist to generate alternatives. The mentioning of a problem is followed by an impulse of the therapist to shift the perspective again. The process of analogue presentation ends when the client comes to a positive evaluation and feels the new image is "complete". After returning from the relaxed state, the client is encouraged to draw the new image, focus on it for one minute per day until the next session and draw it again from time to time. In EAI Brief Therapy the client's image is not analyzed, since this is not viewed as useful. Analogue presentations are solely used to shift the client's perspective in order to access the client's *implicit* knowledge for change. In the session following the phase of analogue presentation, the problem is reassessed (Phase VII). Reported change is identified together with the client and consolidated. Therapy ends when the client perceives the presenting problem as resolved. The duration of each phase is variable. Some of these seven phases fill a whole session or even more; others are only part of a session, such as the preparation phase, which only occurs together with phases V and VI. Each session is followed by certain in-between-session tasks for the client. *[I. R. Hoffmann-Bisinger]*

REFERENCES. Hoffmann I.R., *Changing perspective – changing solutions: Activating internal images for change in systemic brief therapy*, 2007; Feldmann J., *Subliminale Wahrnehmung und Informationsverarbeitungstheorie*, in «Hypnose und Kognition», 1988, 5, 74–86.

EXPRESSION

In Gestalt therapy, a manifestation of one's inner world. Expression differs from action, which implies the intrusion into the privacy of the interlocutor (for example, talking about one's own experiences is an expression, judging the other person is an action). As long as the existence of external or internal spaces are only considered at the level of psychic reality, the alternative is just to give action to an impulse or repress it. However, words create a third space, which Winnicott called transitional. The objects that inhabit this space have an external dimension, but they become relevant only according to the importance that the internal world gives them: for example, toys are transitional objects (which resemble external experience enough to support the experience of playing); the backdrop in a theatre (which resembles a panorama sufficiently to make a drama credible to the spectator); and, above all, there are words, which have enormous importance in human existence, but only due to cultural conventions. Words form, and at the same time inhabit, a huge transitional space, which accommodates most of the life of the majority of people. In fact, when people do not talk to each other, they often listen to the television or read, or in some way deal with words. The access to this space is provided by expression, which differs from action particularly due to its lesser impact in the external space. Expression has more manageable effects in social action: action has often problematic or even dangerous consequences, whereas the right to expression is now indisputable in democratic regimes. For example, the Italian law considers that saying "criminal" to a person as illegal, even when there has been a final judgement on this person, whereas it considers it criminally irrelevant to express a bad omen such as sending someone to hell. *[P. Quattrini]*

REFERENCES. Baxandall M., *Patterns of intention*, 1985; Cardinal M., *The words to say it*, 1975; Darwin C., *The expression of the emotions in man and animals*, 1872; Eibl-Eibesfeldt I., *Human etology*, 1989; Heidegger M., *On the way to language*, 1959; Turner V., *From ritual to theatre*, 1982; Winnicott D.W., *Playing and reality*, 1971.

EXPRESSIVE TECHNIQUES – REPRESSIVE TECHNIQUES

In Gestalt therapy, specific modes of intervention that can increase the intensity of → expression or reduce the evasive effect of defences. Gestalt therapy derives many expressive techniques from the Stanislavski method, a drama school based on the practice of evoking a → direct experience, similar to that represented on stage. In fact, even in the Gestalt approach people are asked to describe the scene that they are evoking, to dwell on the details and the sensations induced by the parts and the whole and to feel the sensations and emotions that the imagined interlocutors are living in the representation, by putting themselves in their shoes. As defences lead to a fixity of expression, techniques such as the amplification or attenuation of voice and gestures are used to overcome it. Considering that the right and the left hemisphere of the brain govern different areas of the mind, it is also possible to ask people to express themselves by singing, or at least by using a rhythmic base, to activate the right hemisphere: sometimes this gives voice to parts of oneself that are immobilized by the left hemisphere. At the same time, for technical reasons, what leads out of the sense of communication is repressed: for this reason, people are invited to clarify their intentions and to verify their choices. In this way, they are not lost in abstractions or generic discourses that revolve around themselves. Also, the mechanisms of resistance are repressed (→ introjection, → retroflection, → deflection, → projection and → confluence) to allow the re-establishment of the contact, without which, according to the Gestalt perspective, the sense of life is not truly experienced. *[P. Quattrini]*

REFERENCES. Faber A., Mazlish E., *How to talk so kids will listen and listen so kids will talk*, 2001; Lankton S.R., *The answer within*, 1983; Naranjo C., *Techniques of Gestalt therapy*, 1973; Perls F., *The Gestalt approach and eye witness to therapy*, 1973; Id., *Gestalt therapy verbatim*, 1969; Quattrini P., *Per una psicoterapia fenomenologico-esistenziale*, 2011; Sini C., *Il silenzio e la parola*, 1989; Sperry R., *Organizzazione e comportamento cerebrale*, 1961; Stanislavski K., *An actor's work: A student's diary*, 1983.

EXPRESSIVE THERAPY

A specific type of psychodynamic clinical intervention that utilizes pictorial and/or bodily graphic language along with verbal language – both with children and adults – to allow the most hidden and unheard parts of the Self to express themselves, to be recognized and to access symbolic transformation processes. As Shakespeare says in *Macbeth*, to "give sorrow words" is the mission of every psychodynamic therapy. However, sometimes the word is a distant shore, unable to give immediate sense and conceivability to human experience. Along the way, the mind can resort to the silent metaphors of the aesthetic production. Aesthetic knowledge has an anticipatory character and, according to the American philosopher Langer, art work is "a non-conversational symbol capable of articulating what appears inexpressible in verbal terms; it expresses direct consciousness, emotion, identity, the mental matrix". Artistic expressions offer anyone pre-logic symbolic structures to develop symbolic abilities and languages that are appropriate to communicate inner experiences. Sounds, signs and gestures are an archaic alphabet and the creative experience has been a possible dialogue since the beginning, or since new beginnings made necessary by the vicissitudes of mental illness. Arieti recalls that, in human beings, the need to create may persist even when pain is so intense as to impede access to consciousness, when thoughts are so dispersed to be no longer understandable, when the most vital contacts with the outside world are cut off. Playing with the creation of images and gestures can help to pick up the threads of a conversation that can sometimes be suspended or broken. The richness, complexity and intensity of nonverbal expressive codes facilitate access, in a transformative way, from the dimension of the "signifier" to that of its possible "meanings". The theoretical-methodological reference point of expressive psychotherapy was initially the perspective of M. Klein and, later, the object-relations theory developed by members of the British Independent Group of psychoanalysts such as Milner, Bion and Winnicott. The latter introduced and deepened the functions of creative play and drawing. These are seen not only as indicators of conflicts or developmental needs, but especially as communication channels that can enrich the exchange, even in the preconscious, between patient and therapist and facilitate integration of mental and bodily experiences. According to Benedetti, expressive activities, which in the view of institutional psychiatry were considered an expression of psychopathology, can become a part of psychotherapy. In fact, patient and therapist can experience the phases of their common inner process through images and gestures. In a theoretical framework widely shared with other psychodynamic-oriented psychotherapies, expressive psychotherapy finds its specificity in the use of tools and methodologies resulting from art therapy and dance-movement therapy developments. These disciplines were formalized in the 1940s by M. Naumburg and M. Chase, based on Freudian (the concept of sublimation) or Jungian (active imagination) conceptualizations. They invited the use of motor and figurative instruments in a specific way. These disciplines were initially adopted to support interventions in serious situations considered not suitable for psychotherapy, or as complementary therapies to verbal psychotherapy. Later, thanks to the refinement of clinical experience and the expansion of its application fields, the need to systematize these disciplines at a theoretical and methodological level has arisen. Moreover, there was a need to integrate the specific instruments of art therapists and dance-movement therapists with the skills and responsibilities of psychotherapists, traditionally equipped in terms of verbal exchange. In the late 1970s, thanks to Robbins and the Institute for Expressive Analysis in New York, the specific perspective of expressive psychotherapy was gradually consolidated through an integration of the theoretical model of object relations and the technical apparatus of art therapy and dance-movement therapy. This orientation is supported by psychoanalytic and non-psychoanalytic research on human development, on the relationship between psyche, bodily experience, artistic expression, aesthetic communication and unconscious, and on the correlation between creativity and mental health. In this perspective, the act of creating an image or a dance does not mean distancing from a task, attacking a cognitive process and the setting that supports it, but represents an integral part of the therapeutic process. During the therapeutic work, the profound experiences, although remaining, initially, far from being conscious, express themselves in creative acts, finding their own working-through. In expressive therapy, the aesthetic production, in terms of graphic or motor signs, becomes a third focal point that mediates communication between therapist and patient, allowing them to find new ways to interact. These include: the relationship between patient and product, in which patients gradually learn to recognize themselves and see reflected parts of themselves, difficulties, unconscious defences, fantasies or needs; the relationship between patient and therapist through the product, in which transference and countertransference dynamics take shape and support the relationship; finally, the direct interaction between patient and therapist that facilitates the therapeutic intervention and the verbal and nonverbal exchange in the transitional area, instead of, or with, the transference field. The coexistence of these three dimensions of communication allows the work to proceed at multiple levels as the presence of the object is inscribed in a context of symbolic significance. The aim of the Expressive Psychotherapy Institute is to prepare future therapists by refining their ability to communicate with patients not only through words, but also through graphic signs and body movements. These are mute yet powerful metaphors, "primordial cells", "construction materials" capable of supporting, even in particularly difficult situations, a vital co-evolution, directed towards a reflexive knowledge of the potential and limitations of "human prose", its recognition and enrichment. *[R. Boccalon]*

REFERENCES. Adler J., *Offering from the conscious body*, 2002; Arieti S., *La sintesi magica*, 1974; Belfiore M., Colli L.M. (ed.), *Dall'esprimere al comunicare*, 1998; Id. (ed.), *Tra il Corpo e l'Io*, 1998; Benedetti G., *Segno, simbolo, linguaggio*, 1971; Bion W.R., *Transformations*, 1965; Boccalon R., *Dall'agire al pensare: esperienze creative e percorsi psicoterapeutici*, 2007; Della Cagnoletta M., *Arte Terapia: la prospettiva psicodinamica*, 2010; Di Benedetto A., *Prima della parola. L'ascolto psicoanalitico del non detto attraverso le forme dell'arte*, 2000; Govoni R.M., *Emozione-espressione-cura. Movimento e danza: modalità espressive nel processo psicoterapeutico*, 1998; Langer S., *Philosophy in a new key: A study in the symbolism of reason, rite, and art*, 1942; Luzzato P., *Arte Terapia: una guida al lavoro simbolico*, 2009; Milner M., *On not being able to paint*, 1950; Robbins A., *Expressive therapy*, 1986; Winnicott D.W., *Playing and reality*, 1971.

EXTERNALIZATION OF THE SYMPTOM

In narrative psychotherapy, a technique invented by White aiming to objectify (→ objectification of a problem) and personify the problem of an individual. A person with a problem – for example, an encoprectic child – is usually identified by the family or group with the problem itself; they are rejected and marginalized. The past attempts to solve the problem are considered as personal failures. Externalization has the power to establish that the problem is not the person, "the problem is the problem". The therapist proceeds by excluding diagnosis and medical definitions of the problem from the conversation, as well as the search for causes, starting instead from the description of the clients. Through questions on the influence that the Sneaky Poo, or Sense of Guilt, Bad Habits have on their lives – and the influence that they, in turn, can have on the problem – the symptoms are described as treacherous but grotesque characters and the therapy becomes the story of the victory over them. The work of M. Foucault has inspired the ideas of White on dominant cultural practices and narratives: externalization legitimates marginal stories such as those carried by the individual, who is stigmatized because of a socially intolerable problem. *[M. Giuliani]*

REFERENCES. White M., Epston D., *Narrative means to therapeutic ends*, 1990.

EXTEROPSYCHE

In the area of transactional analysis, one of Berne's three "psychic organs", hypothesized as psychobiological structures whose phenomenology expresses itself in the three → Ego states. In particular, the exteropsyche would be that organ "assigned to the assumption and the management of different experiences through which the child relates to and interprets the parental models with which he comes into contact". In the different evolutionary phases, the mechanisms of the assumption go from introjection to imitation and to identification. Its phenomenological expression, in terms of the patterns of thought–emotion–behaviour, leads to the activation of the corresponding Ego state → Parent. *[M. Novellino]*

REFERENCES. Berne E., *Transactional analysis in psychotherapy*, 1961; Novellino M., *Psicoanalisi transazionale*, 2004.

EXTINCTION

In the behavioural paradigm, a decrease in response strength in operant interactions (→ behavioural model of operant conditioning) or its disappearance in respondent interactions (→ behavioural model of classical conditioning) as a result of the disappearance of the → reinforcement. In respondent interactions, if a → conditioned response is elicited but is no longer followed by a reinforcement (→ unconditioned stimulus) it progressively disappears. In operant interactions, if a behaviour no longer produces reinforcing consequences, it becomes progressively less likely and less frequent. The word "extinction" indicates both the result (disappearance) and the principle according to which it happens. As with all natural laws – such as, for example, gravity – the principle of extinction acts independently of the awareness of the subject. *[P. Moderato, C. Copelli]*

REFERENCES. Catania A.C., *Learning*, 1997; Moderato P., *Interazioni umane*, 2005.

EXTROVERSION

In Jungian analytical psychology, one of the two fundamental attitudes of consciousness, together with → introversion. While introversion subtracts → libido to the object, extroversion behaves positively and gives wide importance to the object; indeed, it tends to steadily increase its relevance: it is characterized by openness, kindness and sociability. According to Jung, this type of attitude would have an instinctual and unconscious basis, it would be rooted in biology and it would realize itself in a rich productiveness, unlike the tenacious self-preservation of the introvert, in its quest for power and security. Healthy extroverts do not look for protection, their interest flows smoothly in the outside world, as a kind of gushing energy. People and external events attract them unreservedly, without spasmodic control needs. They move according to the objectivity of the environment, they are chameleon-like in their adaptability to life's circumstances. Obviously, the power of their subjectivity fades in front of the evidence and attractive power of the outside world, which takes the confident trait of benevolent objectivity. An historically determined environment may lose touch with the natural laws of life. In turn, the extrovert does not stop and is wrecked by their world, as they are well integrated and not simply adapted, because they are too compliant with the environment. Adaptation requires the observance of laws that are more general than local and temporary conditions. When normality is pursued in this way, it does not take into sufficient account subjective needs and necessities. The weak point becomes the subjective background formed by one's own body with its basic needs, starting with sleep, food and the need for movement. From there, the abnormal symptoms of the somatic sphere: somatization, circulatory aliments, especially aliments of internal organs, disposition to cancer, excesses in generativity and fertility. In this case, the extrovert needs to stop and give space, willingly or not, to their subjective dimension; they must exercise self-control. On a psychological level, the excess of the conscious position finds its clear expression in hysteria, with its dramatizations and exaggerations, imitative tendencies, exhibitionism and individualism, suggestibility and infantile and exaggerated fantasies concerning sexual activity. *[M. Gay]*

REFERENCES. Jung C.G. (1921), *Psychological types*, in *Collected Works*, VI, 1971.

EYE MOVEMENT DESENTIZATION AND REPROCESSING

Eye Movement Desensitization and Reprocessing (EMDR) is an integrative psychotherapeutic approach that uses eye movements to treat inappropriately processed memories of disturbing or traumatic experiences.

The theoretical framework that guides EMDR clinical practice, including the rationale for its wide range of therapeutic applications, is referred to as the Adaptive Information Processing (AIP) model. According to this model, the goal of EMDR is to address the experiential contributors to present psychological dysfunction, which can include not only major traumas but the more ubiquitous and chronic experiences of rejection, abandonment, humiliation and the perceived blame and failure that often underlie negative self-beliefs, negative self-esteem, self-efficacy issues and attachment difficulties. Unprocessed memories of disturbing etiological events and other experiential contributors are posited to set the foundation for a wide range of diagnoses and clinical complaints. The AIP model postulates that there is an information-processing system inherent in the brain that is intrinsic, physical and adaptive. According to this model, experiences are stored in associative memory networks, which provide an important basis for the interpretation of new experiences and significantly influence current perception, behaviour and feelings. The innate information-processing system of the brain is geared to integrate new events within the larger memory networks of previous experiences. Along with the elimination of the previous stored disturbing sensory information and overt symptoms, there is a spontaneous emergence of new perspectives, adaptive behaviours, → resilience and an enhanced sense of self. It is this processing, the forging of new associations within and between memory networks, that is at the heart of EMDR treatment.

EIGHT-PHASE TREATMENT APPROACH. EMDR utilizes an eight-phase approach to address the full range of clinical symptoms caused or exacerbated by past negative experiences. Phase 1 is *client history*, in which the clinician obtains background information, identifies client suitability for

EMDR treatment and identifies processing targets from events in the client's life. Phase 2 is *preparation*, in which clients deemed appropriate for EMDR treatment are prepared to process the targeted memory experiences by strengthening access to positive memory networks. Phase 3 is *assessment*, in which the target memory to be processed by EMDR is identified, accessed and baseline measurements of current reactivity are obtained. Phase 4 is *desensitization*, in which past experiences and present triggers are processed. The goal of this phase is to address the dysfunctional aspects of the memories and allow their full integration within adaptive experiential networks. Phase 5 is *installation,* in which the client's most desired positive self-belief (initial or emergent) is identified and enhanced to increase its connection with currently existing positive cognitive networks and facilitate generalization effects within associated memories networks. Phase 6 is *body scan*, in which the client identifies and processes residual physical sensations to complete resolution. Phase 7 is *closure*, which may incorporate methods to return clients to equilibrium, if needed, and ensure client stability. In this phase, clients are briefed about what to expect between sessions and are instructed about what to do in case of disturbance. Phase 8 is *reevaluation*, in which clients are assessed at the beginning of a session regarding their current psychological state and the thoughts and feelings that may have emerged since the previous session. This information is used to guide the direction of treatment.

THREE-PRONGED PROTOCOL (PAST, PRESENT, FUTURE). The generic therapeutic protocol underlying comprehensive EMDR treatment includes a three-pronged approach subsequent to appropriate therapeutic stabilization and client preparation. The client is first engaged in (a) processing the past experiences contributing to present dysfunction, (b) processing present triggers that elicit present disturbance and (c) incorporating positive patterns of behaviour for future adaptive actions. The initial targets may include the earliest memories, as well as more recent problematic situations. Then, to handle any remnants of second-order conditioning that would prevent complete generalization, the client imagines and processes the current situations that trigger symptoms (e.g. negative emotions, beliefs, sensations, behaviours). After processing the past memories and present triggers that have kept the client from learning adaptive patterns, the clinician needs to assess whether he or she lacks the education necessary for adaptive functioning. To overcome any skill or developmental deficits, the clinician first provides appropriate information and interactive experiences. Then a future template for adaptive behaviour is integrated through the additional processing of imagined positive cognitive, emotional and behavioural responses. Real-world experience and interaction provide feedback to determine what else may need to be processed. This three-pronged approach is augmented by the knowledge of various specialty areas in order to address problems as diverse as addictions, personality disorders and somatoform disorders. In essence, the application of the protocol is used cross-diagnostically to address the experiential contributors of dysfunction. In summary, EMDR views most clinical complaints as resulting from dysfunctionally stored memories. Past experiences that have not been adequately processed are directly targeted and rapidly integrated within adaptive networks. When adaptive networks are inadequate they are enhanced through education and additional processing. The EMDR integrative psychotherapy approach utilizes an eight-phase, three-pronged (past, present, future) protocol with the goal of liberating the client from the experiential contributors that set the foundation for the current pathology and incorporating the full range of experiences and stored memories needed to bring the client to a comprehensive state of mental health. *[F. Shapiro, R.M. Solomon]*

REFERENCES. Balbo M., *Emdr: uno strumento di dialogo tra le psicoterapie*, 2006; Shapiro F., *Eye Movement Desensitization and Reprocessing: Basic principles, protocols, and procedures*, 2000; Shapiro F., Forrest M.S., *EMDR: The breakthrough therapy for overcoming anxiety, stress, and trauma*, 1998.

F

FALSE SELF

A construct developed by Winnicott (→ psychoanalysis (Independent or Middle Group of British analysts)) to indicate a split-off part of personality which protects the → true Self by hiding it. Based on the identification with the parent, the false Self allows a compliant adaptation to the environmental requests, but it hampers a person's capability of living an authentic life and of establishing and maintaining close relationships. Frequently, the false Self is associated with an increased development of intellectual activity, which ends up replacing imagination, and physical and emotional life. In order to promote the development of the true Self, caregivers must protect the baby from unpredictable environmental stimuli. Moreover, they have to encourage the continuity of experience and help the baby to relate to psychic and physical states, accepting his natural acts and his own personal ideas. Instead, a false Self is fostered by unpredictable and chaotic contexts, far from his needs, that prevent the baby from having the illusory experience of being the creator of his living environment. *[V. Lingiardi]*

REFERENCES. Winnicott D.W., *Ego distortion in terms of true and false self*, in *The Maturational Process and the Facilitating Environment: Studies in the Theory of Emotional Development*, 1965, 140–152.

FAMILY

A family is a highly complex social entity that actively interacts with the social and cultural context. Both historical and cross-cultural research has documented the presence of various family forms: it is thus difficult to individuate the invariant aspects of families that persist throughout their different manifestations. Over the course of psychological thinking, definitions of the family have referred, first of all, to the lewinian concept of the → group, then to that of the → system. Both approaches, while having been useful tools for understanding the family, have undergone profound revision: if, on the one hand, research on the family as a natural, primary group has increasingly underscored the family's peculiarity as compared to other natural groups, the focus on the totality of the family system has revealed itself to be a partial perspective because the subject's role has increasingly been put between parentheses, although it remains the origin of and setting for psychic events. The concept of → relationship, instead, has revealed itself to be a useful and fruitful way to take into account both the role of family members and the outcome of their interactions. The family can thus be defined as an organization of kinship relations that has a history and that creates a history. In particular, the symbolic-relational paradigm has attempted to delineate the distinctive characteristics of the family, taking into due consideration invariant aspects as well as the different meanings that various cultures ascribe to these characteristics. Specifically:

1) the family is an *organization* in that it is an organized system with an internal hierarchy that permeates its relations – in particular, intergenerational relations – and that interacts in a dynamic way with the cultural context in which it lives;
2) the goal of the family organization is to give life to or to raise new human beings;

3) the typical characteristic of the family as an organization resides in the fact that it organizes *primary* relations, primary in that they connect the fundamental differences of the human being, the differences of gender and generation, and primary in that family relations cannot be substituted in any way. According to how its members are interconnected among themselves, the organization produces either positive or negative functioning. That gender difference is constitutive of the family has been called into question lately by recent changes occurring in several countries of the industrialized West, in which the conjugal bond has been weakened by the high frequency of separation and divorce, and where juridical recognition of unions between persons of the same sex has been granted. This has led several anthropologists to identify the *basic core* of the family in the intergenerational relation and, in particular, in the mother–child relation. *[E. Scabini]*

FAMILY CONSTELLATION

Within the framework of individual psychology, it represents the set of relationships between family members. The exploration of the ways used by subjects to "narrate themselves" within their original family system is one of the first steps of Adler's psycho-diagnostic intervention. This redefinition of the main key figures and of the original intra- and inter-familiar relational plots is not aimed at a schematic anamnestic classification. Instead, it represents the start of a reimmersion in the psychological situations that have gradually structured (especially in the first four to five years of life) patients' lifestyle and pretences. Their narrative (order of presentation, space given, emotional underlining, censorship, etc.) represents an important start from which to understand and amplify a hypothesis on how the subject is – then and now – oriented in life. *[L. Cerioli]*

REFERENCES. Adler A., *The neurotic constitution*, 1917; Id., *Understanding human nature*, 1927; Dreikurs R., *Fundamentals of Adlerian psychology*, 1950; Pagani P.L., *L'utilità diagnostica delle notizie raccolte nel corso del "primo colloquio" e nelle sedute dedicate alla "costellazione familiare" e ai "primi ricordi d'infanzia"*, in «Rivista di Psicologia Individuale», 2001, 50, 13–18.

FAMILY NETWORK MODEL

The concept of→ family as a network refers to and is deeply related to a systemic view of family relations. The social network in which the individual is embedded is considered as his "cocoon". Such a network does not include only the family, but also the extended reference group (the relatives, the clan) and the overall community context. Therefore, we are referring to a deep integration of all the relationships that are considered relevant for the self. All these issues contribute to shape one's sense of identity and affect the personal and relational wellbeing. As happened in the studies of social psychology on the Self, the individual occupies the centre of the network; in the inner circle there are the family and intimate relations; the intermediate circle is occupied by groups and associations; whereas the outer circle contains the relationships with neighbours and those with the services. Thanks to this network perspective, it is possible to understand the structural (width, density), social (presence of emotional and practical support, guidance), and functional characteristics of ties. The clinical interventions that adopt a "true" network perspective originate from these notions and always imply a thoughtful consideration of the mutual relationships between the individual, his extended family and the community context.

This perspective assumes a particular relevance in the case of migrant families or in the encounter between different cultures. *[V. Cigoli, S. Molgora]*

REFERENCES. Sluzki C.E., *Migration and the disruption of the social network*, 1998; Sluzki C.E., *Migration: The social network perspective*, 2008; Speck R.V., Attneave C. L., *Family networks*, 1973.

FAMILY SEMANTIC POLARITIES THEORY

Within the systemic-relational paradigm, meaning-making is the fulcrum of Valeria Ugazio's psychopathological model. Besides formulating an explicative hypothesis of some of the main psychopathologies, this model lays the foundations for a systemic theory of → personality development. Her family semantic polarities (FSP) theory embraces a social-constructionist frame and maintains that each developing family member construes her/his experience around a number of premises, values and personal meanings co-constructed in social relations. This represents a shift beyond the individual–family dualism: both the individual and the → family without the → behavioural "pattern that connects" them are void abstractions: out of the relations in which he or she is embedded the individual dissolves themself and the family cannot exist other than as as the "co-positioning" of individuals in a given socio-cultural context. Thus, Ugazio's model rediscovers a new interest for the individual within Gregory Bateson's interactionist and contextual conception of the mind, the systemic approach's original core. The centrality of the contextual subject is combined with George Kelly's attention to personal-meanings systems and with Vittorio Guidano's post-rationalist cognitivism. The FSP concept is very similar to Harry Procter's Family Construct System, as it hypothesizes that conversation in each family revolves around opposed meanings – the so-called family semantic polarities – which are fed by specific emotions. These polarities – along the lines of just/unjust, closed/open, attractive/repugnant – form a sort of shared plot that circumscribes the repertoire of specific narratives and storylines within which the family constructs its reality. These opposed meanings define what is relevant in each social group: only a few semantic polarities among all the ones that are present in the broader cultural context will be relevant for a given family at a certain point of its family life-cycle. Coherently with a constructionist framework, this concept takes into account both the individual's specificity and his interconnection with the other members of the relational system he belongs to. In any case, every family differs from others and therefore develops its own identity and uniqueness; similarly, each family member constructs the conversation and the episodes in his own way, differently from all the others. In this perspective, meaning is co-constructed through dialogue (especially on a tacit level) among people occupying different positions: the duality, or better the plurality, does not lie inside the single subjectivity; it is rather co-constructed in the social matrix. Indeed, although the notion of opposition may evoke two polar terms, the concept of FSP is essentially triadic in nature. Each polarity assumes at least three positions in the conversation: beyond the two extreme poles, it covers a range of intermediate positions, which can be synthesized in the median position. Ugazio's theory focuses on the semantic aspects of communication and on the conversational processes through which members of the family (or any other group with a history) construct their subjectivity within the broader socio-cultural context. It claims that each family member presents his/her own way of participating in the conversation, of co-positioning with others and of organizing the reality. Nevertheless, the way in which each individual constructs the reality is coherent with the specific position she/he takes in her/his relational system and it is interdependent with the position of the other family members. Conversation forms the primary or founding process. All the other processes, such as emotions, perceptions, memory, belief systems, goals and so on, are secondary, i.e. the outcomes of coordinated practices that organize conversation among people. This does not reduce the importance of these processes, but it anchors them to conversation: they are an aspect of how each one "composes" himself with the other family members. The FSP are discursive phenomena that Ugazio likens to the properties of conversation: from a narrative-conversational stance, also, the Self is a position in the conversation. Through these inevitable positionings, conversational partners anchor their story and therefore their identity to those of the other members of the group. The shared nature of subjectivity is consequently assured by the polar structure of the meaning, and the selves become as multiple as the positions generated by polarities. This is the nucleus of the theory: no one can avoid taking a position along each relevant semantic polarity of his/her group and everybody – to preserve his/her identity – needs somebody taking another positioning along the same semantic dimension. Ugazio's model maintains that some of the most recurrent psychopathologies develop in family contexts characterized by a specific semantic polarity. The semantics of "freedom", of "goodness", of "power" and of "belonging", typically shows a prevalence in conversational contexts where one member features phobic (PD), obsessive-compulsive (OCD), eating (ED) and mood (MD) disorders respectively. The "semantics of freedom" are typically characteristic of the conversation of clients with PD (agoraphobia, claustrophobia, panic attacks, specific phobia). Its core emotions are fear–courage, sensations of being lost and disoriented when solid and stable relational references run out, and sensations of constriction embedded in dependency from the others. The main semantic polarities are freedom–dependence and exploration–attachment: free, independent, tie-intolerant, sometimes daring individuals position themselves with dependent, fearful people who cannot cope on their own. The "semantics of goodness" centralizes the conversation of clients with OCD. The basic emotions of this semantics are innocence–guilt, disgust for the people and the instincts that embody evil, sensation of interior mortification of those who abstain and sacrifice themselves and, at the opposite pole, enjoyment and sensual pleasure. The main semantic polarities of this semantics are: goodness–evil and dead–alive. "Goodness" has an "ascetic/abstemious" connotation: "good" people renounce to their self-assertion and to the expression of their own desires and instincts. On the contrary, "bad" people set out to achieve their own pleasure and self-satisfaction. Sexuality and self-assertion are seen to be bad because their expression is felt as being violent, cruel and perverse. The "semantics of power" prevails in family conversation of clients suffering with ED (anorexia, bulimia, obesity). The core emotions of this semantic are boast–shame, a sensation of self-efficacy when people get the better of them in a competition; a sense of inadequacy, uselessness, impotence when you feel a loser. The semantics of power features two distinctive polarities: winner–loser, strong-willed–yielding. The latter is hierarchically subordinated to the first: you are a winner if you are strong-willed, whereas you are a loser if not able to fight and you give yourself up to difficulties and to the others. The winner–loser polarity has a specific difference in to respect to the other polarities: it can never be perceived as an individual trait, it is purely relational, it is always the result of a comparison. Winners and losers fight for supremacy, and competitive conflicts prevail in the conversation, as the struggle for defining the relation is crucial in this context. The topic of the struggle is not important: it is a matter of relational supremacy. The "semantics of belonging" prevails in family conversation of clients suffering from MD (major and bipolar depressive disorder). The core emotions of this semantics are joy and anger, gratefulness for having been accepted or desperation, anger and resentment for having been rejected. The two main semantic polarities are: inclusion–exclusion and honour–disgrace. The feeling of belonging is very important to the family, the kinship, the lineage, to the community and, on the other hand, exclusion and banishment are the worst things that can happen, experienced with disgrace and infamy. Some members feel excluded, rejected, abandoned whereas others feel loved, honoured and respected. The prevalence of one of these semantics is a necessary but not sufficient condition for the onset of its related psychopathology. Indeed, taking distance from the cognitivist genetic-evolutionary hypotheses, the FSP theory explains the transition from "normalcy" to psychopathology by the reciprocal positioning that the individual and the persons meaningful to him/her take within the critical semantics (which normally express also a conflict embedded in the broader cultural context). It is through these positionings that a person could experience a conflicting situation defined as dilemma or "strange reflexive loop". When this happens, the person is no longer able to construct any stable positioning along the critical FSP and he/she oscillates between mutually exclusive positionings that cannot be integrated into a shared storyline. The onset of a psychopathology – with its recourse to an "illness" – is an extreme attempt to contain the oscillation and to preserve one's self-esteem. The interpretation of meaning summarized in the FSP concept maintains that everyone's experience is never semantically closed; this has obviously major clinical implications. A given semantic may prevail in a family conversation, but it will never deplete the individual's conversational possibilities: his ability to interact along different semantics will always make other stories possible. Therapeutic change will therefore aim to facilitate a repositioning of the client within the prevalent semantics, but also to broaden his repertoire of permitted narrative plots. On the contrary, Guidano conceived personal organizations of meaning as closed: an "epistemological constraint" from which the individual cannot escape. Empirical contributions and methods – some of which have been built ad hoc to gauge FSP in therapeutic conversation – have supported Ugazio's clinical hypothesis, showing how, in therapeutic conversation, clients tend to centralize these FSP and to position also the therapist along their relevant FSP. Similar results have been reached in other studies conducted with different instruments. The FSP concept has been also applied by Campbell and Groenbaek to the analysis of organizations and of literature by Tim Parks and by Harry Procter. *[L. Fellin]*

REFERENCES. Campbell D., Groenbaek M., *Taking positions in the organization*, 2006; Castiglioni M., Contino L., Villegas M., *Tra libertà e costrizione: il dilemma dell'agorafobia*, 2011, 31; Castiglioni M., Faccio F., Veronese G., Poiana Mosolo A., Bell R.C., *Disturbi alimentari e costruzione del significato* in «Psicologia della Salute», 2011, 3; Cronen V.E., Johnson K., Lannamann M., *Paradoxes, double binds and reflexive loops: An alternative theoretical perspective* in «Family Process», 1982, 20; Guidano V.F., *Complexity of the self*, 1987; Guidano V.F., Liotti G., *Cognitive processes and emotional disorders*, 1983; Harré R., Van Langenhove L., *Positioning theory: Moral context of intentional action*, 1999; Kelly G.A., *The psychology of personal constructs*, 1955; Parks T., *Semantic polarities in the writings of T. Hardy and D.H. Lawrence*, 2009, XX; Procter H.G., *The family construct system*, in Kalekin-Fishman D., Walker B. (eds.) *The structure of group realities: Culture and society in the light of personal construct theory*, 1996; Procter H.G., *Constructs of individuals and relationships*, 2002, 59; Procter H.G., Procter M.J., *The use of qualitative grids to examine the development of the construct of good and evil in Byron's play "Cain: A Mystery"*, in «Journal of Constructivist Psychology», 2008, 21; Ugazio V., *Permitted and forbidden stories, semantic polarities and pathologies in the family*, 2012; Ugazio V., Negri A., Fellin L., Di Pasquale R., *The family semantics grid (FSG): The narrated polarities: A Manual for the semantic analysis of therapeutic conversations and self narratives* in «TPM – Testing, Psychometrics, Methodology in Applied Psychology», 2009, 16.

FAMILY THERAPY

A model of psychological intervention referring to psychoanalysis, child-development psychotherapy, group therapy and systemic-relational therapy theorizations. This is based on the assumption that individuals do not develop problems in isolation, but as a response to their social environment. The goal of the clinical intervention is to encourage a better adaptation to the environment and to promote new relational pathways. Family psychotherapy was born

> as a polycentric movement with many points of origin, many developments, sometimes interconnected, but more often independent, and many – though not definitive – points of arrival. [. . .] It is not simple to identify neither the first real family therapist, nor the early school of relief. Family therapy was and has always been eminently plural.

[E. Molinari, G. Pietrabissa, G. Castelnuovo]

REFERENCES. Bertrando P., Toffanetti D., *Storia della terapia familiare. Le persone, le idee*, 2000; Cigoli V., Galimberti C., *Terapia familiare: L'orientamento psicoanalitico*, 1983; Gurman A.S., Kniskern D.P., *Handbook of family therapy*, 1981.

FANTASY

A term used in two different meanings: the first one indicates simple and creative imaginative activity (→ imagination); the second meaning indicates the ghost as described in Freudian psychoanalysis, that is, the (normal or pathological) condition in which subconscious desires are fulfilled (→ unconscious fantasy). In general, the fantasy production of mental representations and images (derived from reality and then transfigured) is of fundamental importance in children's cognitive development. Piaget defined this stage of cognitive development as "animism" (→ development stages (Jean Piaget's)). Animism represents an expression of → egocentrism in childhood thinking, it is interpreted as a failure to distinguish between inner and outer worlds, and it would take place through an assimilation of objects to one's own activity. In adulthood, a fantasy can take the form of "daydreaming" or reverie, which may concern retrieving a pleasant experience from the past, altering a present experience or imagining a future one. In psychotherapy, a fantasy is considered an important resource of the patient. The therapist must take advantage of it, depending on the case, and orient it on a time–space axis that is adequate for the defined target. In fact, some therapeutic manoeuvres require the subject to orientate their imaginative perception towards scenarios that can lie "beyond" the problematic situation (for example, the → miracle prescription or the → "as if" technique) or refer to the situation itself (for example, the → worst fantasy technique). *[R.]*

▷ In the specific context of analytical psychology, the term fantasy refers to a complex and intricate psychic manifestation of the individual. Jung distinguishes between two meanings of the term. The first one is basically the resumption of the concept described by S. Freud in his theory of the ghost. This is a set of mental representations that are not necessarily linked to any external reality, although it is often possible to identify in them mnestic traces of recent faded or repressed past events. Jung says:

> As fantasy in the sense of ghost, I mean a set of representations that stands out from other complexes due to the fact that it does not correspond outwardly to any real situation. Although a fantasy might originally be based on mnestic images of true events, its content does not correspond to any external reality, but it is essentially a pure emanation of the creative activity of the spirit, an action or a product of a combination of elements mentally endowed with energy.

In addition to this meaning of fantasy, where there is a significant participation of consciousness, Jung mentions a second one, which may more appropriately be called "imaginative activity", where consciousness has a more passive role and there is a prevalence of the unconscious. This activity has strong similarities with the "psychic automatisms" illustrated by P. Janet (these are mental mechanisms, which, when the normal level of consciousness – *niveau mental* – is low, tend to emerge and establish themselves automatically and incongruously in respect to the normal stream of consciousness).

The characteristic of this fantasy activity is to break, spontaneously and with a strong emotional charge, in situations of "*abaissement du niveau mental*", that is, of a decrease in the level of consciousness of the Ego. This aspect of imagination can often lead to alterations of the normal state of consciousness and trigger real pathological states. Sometimes, it can also allude to deep and planned situations of ordinary consciousness.

> Causally interpreted, a fantasy seems like a symptom of a physiological or personal state, the outcome of antecedent events. Purposively interpreted, it seems like a symbol, seeking to characterize a definite goal with the help of the material at hand, or trace out a line of future psychological development.
>
> (Jung, 1921)

Dependending on the ability of the consciousness, this can actively seize and guide these psychic phenomena or suffer them passively. Therefore, the Ego can use fantasy creatively or suffer its effects with devastating consequences. Moreover, according to Jung, a fantasy can also constitute a "second form of thinking" different from rational and logical thinking. It is more linked to poietic ability and more productive in terms of images than in terms of concepts and therefore it is important in creation and individuation processes. *[L. Aversa]*

REFERENCES. Jung C.G. (1921), *Psychological types*, in *Collected Works*, VI, 1971.

FEARFIGHTER

Fearfighter is a form of computer-aided self-help (→ self-therapy), as part of cognitive behaviour therapy, which panic/phobia patients use on the internet at home or elsewhere with an internet link. With guidance from Fearfighter, patients identify the triggers for their panic and phobia and their avoidant and frightening thoughts, find out how to work out personalized goals to overcome these and learn to do self-exposure and cognitive-therapy homework exercises to overcome their panic and phobia. Fearfighter users also get up to one hour in all of brief human support by phone and/or email. Improvement guided by Fearfighter has been as great as that from face-to-face cognitive behaviour therapy, so NICE (the National Institute for Health and Care Excellence in England and Wales) recommends Fearfighter for the management of panic and phobia throughout the National Health Service. Fearfighter is now used widely by panic/phobia sufferers throughout England. *[I. Marks]*

FEEDBACK

According to both the interactional systemic therapy and the general systems theory (→ system), the term "feedback" indicates the action-return effect on the cause from which it originated, with possible change in retrospect of the cause itself. The information rebound increases or decreases the activity at the back, respectively in the presence of a positive or negative feedback. N. Wiener affirmed → communication and self-regulation as necessary in enabling systems to work: the information involved in the system and concerning past activities' results influences the future. Wiener named the scientific investigation of self-correcting phenomena → cybernetics. G. Bateson applied cybernetic principles to human interactions (first- and second-order → cybernetics). *[G. Castelnuovo, G. Pietrabissa, E. Molinari]*

FEELING-TONED COMPLEX

In Jungian analytical psychology, "feeling-toned" complexes are psychic molecular factors "affectively" characterized. They express themselves automatically and their content is repetitive. Affect is a psychic feeling and a somatic state (of body innervation). The sum of these two inseparable components enables the activation of the complex. If complexes pass the threshold of consciousness, they can put the Ego in a state of "unfreedom". Complexes are relatively autonomous and prove the separability of the psyche. This happens especially when they temporarily or permanently take control in the absence of the hegemonic and organizing function of the Ego (as in psychopathological disorders). However, their activation does not just concern psychopathology, but it represents normally a trait of the psychic process, as complexes are minimal entities of the personality of any individual. In this perspective, the Ego is, for Jung, one of the many complexes that form the psychic wholeness. Its centrality stems from the fact that the Ego is not only the focus of consciousness, but also the reference point of conscious and subliminal somatic perceptions that ensure continuity in the representation of one's own body, that is, the relationship between somatic and psychic factors that underlies a specific proprioceptive structure. The theory of feeling-toned complexes is perhaps Jung's best psychodynamic and psychopathological model and it can be used in clinical practice independently of the doctrine of archetypes, to which it was connected. *[E.V. Trapanese, S. Fossi]*

REFERENCES. Aversa L., *La teoria generale dei complessi e il problema della malattia*, in Id. (eds.), *Psicologia analitica. La teoria della clinica*, 1999; Ruberto A., *Teoria generale dei complessi: fondamenti e sviluppi*, in L. Aversa (eds.), *Fondamenti di psicologia analitica*, 1995; Ruberto A., *Teoria generale dei complessi: il complesso come la più piccola unità bio-psico-sociale concepibile*, in L. Aversa (eds.), *Psicologia analitica. La teoria della clinica*, 1999.

FEMININE

In C.G. Jung's analytical psychology framework, it is an entity expressed by the archetype of the → anima, in a continuous dynamic relationship with the archetype of the → animus, where the former is the psychic equivalent of the feminine, the latter the equivalent of the masculine. The feminine expresses the urge for the → *eros*, or psychic relatedness, whereas the masculine represents the principle of *logos*, or rationality. Masculine and feminine are meant as relative moments of human existence, both at an individual and at a collective level. Masculine and feminine behaviours do not refer to structural differences in the Ego, but rather to aptitudes present both in men and in women. It is therefore possible for the subject (man or woman) to retrieve and reinstate their counter-sexual functions, that is the Feminine expressed by the →anima (*eros*) for men and the Masculine expressed by the → animus (*logos*) for women. *[G. Antonelli, S. Putti]*

REFERENCES. Carotenuto A., *L'anima delle donne. Per una lettura psicologica del femminile*, 2001; Neumann E., *The fear of the feminine and other essays on feminine psychology*, 1953.

FICTIONS

The set of the unconscious psychic functions that are aimed to compensatively adapt to the ideals of the subject. The natural drive towards improving and overcoming difficulties stimulates in every person the structuring of subterranean ideals and goals to be achieved in order to feel better and more adequate. These are characterized as personal inventions and constructions, as ways of being "as if": a kind of attempt to recreate themselves to build a personality with a stronger and more respected appearance. These are therefore "convenient psychic representations" (Ansbacher), that can help a person to grow and evolve or – if taken dogmatically and literally and without understanding their symbolic significance – turn into traps into which a person can neurotically sink. In these cases, "the neurotic is nailed to the cross of his fiction" (Adler), instead of being helped to take on the basic tasks of life. *[L. Cerioli]*

REFERENCES. Adler A., *The neurotic constitution*, 1917; Ansbacher H.L., Ansbacher R.R. (eds.), *The individual psychology of Alfred Adler*, 1956.

FIDEISM

A dogmatic support of a belief system organized around the worship of a deity. This belief system includes an *a priori* and indisputable vision of the characteristics of the divine (dogmatics), of the characteristics of human nature (anthropology) and of the right and wrong behaviours that man must implement (morality). Historically, the word fideism was born in Paris in the late nineteenth century to indicate the orientation of the reformed Christian theology, according to which faith would be reached only through conviction and the "complete offer of one's heart", that is, before any conceptualization and regardless any historical and theological reflection. People characterized by a fideistic attitude show a serious mental rigidity that leads them to recognize and confirm only what fits their beliefs. *[R.]*

FIELD THEORY

In Gestalt therapy, the field theory was formulated by K. Lewin. In the "field", he identifies the "vital space" within which operate all the psychological factors that influence the individual behaviour in the → here and now. The person and the psychological environment compose the vital space that is externally permeated by the world. The various regions in which this space is articulated have positive value if they contain a desired object; they have negative value if they contain an object to be avoided. Different forces of attraction and repulsion correspond to this, which are described by means of specific vectors. The psychic energy that is developed within the field tends constantly towards the balance of the entire system. The emerging of a new need necessarily activates a dynamic process that then leads to a new further balance of the field. In the clinical context, the field theory has been taken up particularly by Gestalt therapy, for which the organization of the field is powerfully connected not only to the emerging need or to the interrupted task, but more generally to the experience that arises from the organism–environment relationship. However, whereas Lewin sees the field as an interior mental "representation", Gestalt therapy understands it above all as "experience" of the → contact boundary between organism and environment. From these two differing conceptions of the field, two different epistemological models emerge: one is founded on the principle of "representability" of the real, the other is centred on the "boundary" as a place of the mind, an interface between the world of meanings and the physical world. *[M. Spagnuolo Lobb, P.A. Cavaleri]*

REFERENCES. Cavaleri P.A., *Dal campo al confine di contatto. Contributo per una riconsiderazione del confine di contatto in psicoterapia della Gestalt*, in M. Spagnuolo Lobb (ed.), *Psicoterapia della Gestalt. Ermeneutica e clinica*, 2001.

FIGURE-GROUND DYNAMIC

In the context of Gestalt therapy, as in Gestalt psychology, the flexible emergence of interest from the perceptive possibilities of the experience. Both terms are an integral part of the perceptive dynamic studied in the 1920s by Gestalt psychology and subsequently applied by the founders of Gestalt therapy, in the 1950s, to the relational dynamic between organism and environment. Just as Gestalt psychology introduced a revolutionary concept of perception, which from passive acquisition of unconnected stimuli became an active, creative process carried out by the subject, so Gestalt therapy introduced a revolutionary perspective on the dynamics of human relationships, no longer determined by unconscious factors, but considered a phenomenic reality experienced in the → here and now of the organism–environment contact, regulated by the figure–ground dynamic. For Gestalt psychologists, the ground is that with which the figure is in relationship in order to emerge; it is the perceptive condition that permits the dominance of the figure, whereas the "organized", significant figure is "the unit of measurement of perception", which answers a series of laws, the most important of which is the law of pregnance. In Gestalt therapy, the formation of the figure is a creative adjustment, based on the principle of self-regulation of the relationship: the figure, which we call Gestalt, emerges from the experiential ground as the best possible organization of the energies perceived in the self and in the environment and of the intentionalities of contact; the figure is the co-creation of the → contact boundary, the place of the shared experience in which the self of the subjects involved takes form, being differentiated and acquiring novelty. The formation of the figure is supported by a vital strength (a creative aggression, which Perls identified with the child's ability to bite, acquired in the developmental phase, to which he gave the name "dental aggression") that enables the deconstruction and reconstruction of reality in an absolutely creative, unique manner. For both schools of thought, the figure–ground dynamic does not constitute a return to the conscious–unconscious dichotomy. The unconscious has been removed, while the ground is defined as what has been assimilated, possibly forgotten, and as the support system necessary to the establishment of new perceptions (for Gestalt psychology) or of new contacts (for Gestalt therapy). The ground, in the sense of the infinite current possibilities of creation in a given situation, has emerging properties that have nothing to do with mechanisms of → repression, although with motivation for contact, hence for growth.

Gestalt therapy considers two kinds of ground; one is the ground of taken-for-granted contacts, consisting of psycho-bodily learnings that contribute to the sense of safety; this support system was described by Perls as what "derives from free primary physiology which implies the experience's assimilation and integration". One example is sitting on a chair taking it for granted that the chair will hold us up. When this kind of ground is called into question, a profound existential or psychotic → anguish is experienced. The other type of ground is that of → direct experience, which highlights the figure and enables it to emerge brilliantly and clearly. Faced with a novelty of the field (→ field theory), only a part of the ground is mobilized – that part that is necessary to the creation of the new figure. For Gestalt therapy, when there is no contact between organism and environment, no figure can emerge from the ground. *[M. Spagnuolo Lobb, P.A. Cavaleri]*

FINALISM

In philosophical sciences, a concept, according to which, every natural phenomenon occurring in the universe tends to an aim. Plato and Aristotle were exponents of this thought. Pre-Socratics and epicureans took position against them with their mechanistic theories. These claimed the absolute randomness of everything that happens outside of the human will. Subsequently, various religious theories have resumed finalistic theories by identifying one or more gods as the external element that govern the world, affecting in this way some traditions of modern philosophy (I. Newton, G.W. Leibniz, I. Kant). Finalism was criticized by the English philosopher F. Bacon, who saw it as an obstacle to experimental research. In the same period, G. Galilei and R. Descartes defined as illusory the claim of finalism to be able to explain reality. In the wake of these thinkers, modern science has excluded the pursuit of the "final cause" from their scopes. Finalism reappeared during the nineteenth century in the vitalism theory, a school of thought that exalts and interprets life as a spiritual phenomenon and a vital force, beyond the biological and material aspects. Also, many psychotherapeutic currents were influenced by finalism. For instance, in Freudian psychoanalysis, the framework of the psychic apparatus is explained through the concept of sexual → drive, and everything revolves around the satisfaction of this drive. Starting from the concept of inferiority, A. Adler formulates a finalistic version of mental dynamics: individuals are driven to fight against their own limits to achieve a goal of superiority and safety. From this point of view, all human activities would move from a basic force that starts from a feeling of "inferiority", from which originates the effort aimed at reaching one's own self-affirmation. According to the Swiss analyst C.G. Jung, every psychological phenomenon can be analyzed through a causal and finalistic point of view. For example, from a finalistic perspective, dreams can have various functions: compensatory, which offer psychological balance, prospective (anticipatory of future conscious actions) or reactive, in case of traumas. Finalistic elements can also be found in J. Bowlby's thought: for example, in the concept of the human being as a "teleonomic" system, in other words, a system physically organized and programmed to learn, to receive information and to establish connections with the environment. *[R.]*

FIRST- AND SECOND-ORDER CHANGE

In the context of → brief psychotherapy MRI model and of → brief strategic therapy Nardone's model, two different types of → change may occur in a → system: a first-order change, which takes place within the system itself and leaves it unchanged, and a second-order change, which is introduced from the outside and produces changes in the system. When a system, be it an individual, a group or family, is facing a problem to solve, only the second-order change represents a concrete and effective solution, requiring a logic-level leap (that is, the exit from the system). It follows the impossibility for any system to generate the conditions for such a change from the inside, and the need for an external element to intervene in the system. In the strategic model, a second-order change is induced by working on → attempted solutions taken by the individual (or by everyone involved in the system) to solve the problem. These solutions, as first-order changes, tend instead to maintain the problem and complicate it. To obtain a second-order change, which may appear illogical or bizarre, it is usually necessary to use non-ordinary → logics of intervention. *[R. Milanese]*

REFERENCES. Nardone G., Watzlawick P., *The art of change*, 1993; Watzlawick P., Weakland J.H., Fisch R., *Change: Principles of problem formation and problem resolution*, 1974.

FIRST- AND SECOND-ORDER REALITY

In → brief psychotherapy – MRI model and in → brief strategic therapy – Naardone's model, Watzlawick distinguished two different orders of what is usually defined as "reality", departing from the constructivist presupposition (→ constructivism) that an absolute reality does not exist, but that there are only subjective conceptions of reality. The "first-order" reality refers to the purely physical properties of things, in other words, to those aspects of reality that are strictly correlated to the correct sensorial perception or to experimental confirmation that is repeatable and verifiable. The "second-order"reality consists instead of the attribution of meaning and value that one gives to the reality of the first order, and is based on communication. From this one can deduce that any psychotherapeutic intervention can only deal with change in the "second-order" reality, in other words in that world of meaning and values that the person attributes to his own first-order reality (→ strategic reframing technique). *[R. Milanese]*

REFERENCES. Watzlawick P., Watzlawick P., *How real is real? Communication, disinformation, confusion*, 1976.

FIXATION

A particular organization and compliance with specific rules. This term is used to indicate something that is immanent, that is, not temporary, and that repeats itself systematically and recurrently. A person with a mental fixation tends to emphasize an idea and to repeat it strenuously and rigidly. Being focused exclusively on a particular object generates the idea or the "obsession", that is, an obstinate and mostly morbid thought, aimed at the creation of something, or focused on misinterpreted or even non-existent facts. When a fixation reaches psychopathological levels, it can turn into obsession, compulsion or delirium. In psychotherapy, this term was introduced in the late nineteenth century by S. Freud to indicate the inability to progress beyond a certain stage of psychosexual development. According to psychoanalysis, a person has a fixation when the partial drive, the erogenous zone, the libidinal phase or the object relationship become the source of a too gratifying or too frustrating libidinal experience; fixation is followed by → regression, a → defence mechanism that interferes with the expected evolution process. Instead, according to existentialists, fixation is an unconditional support to an ideal that is no longer able to adhere to the normal flow of experience, but bends the experience to the necessities posed by the fixed ideal. As the subjects with a fixation are unable to let things be as they are, they seek to impose a sort of order in the attempt to find a foothold in the disorder and inconsistency of their own experience. *[R.]*

FLOODING

A particular exposure technique (literally "immersion") through which the patient enters into contact with the feared situation in an intense and not gradual way (→ graded exposure). Commonly, the cognitive behavioural therapy uses some intervention techniques aimed at the → extinction or rescheduling of behavioural and psychophysiological answers. In particular, the main idea of this behavioural technique – flooding – is that during exposure to an anxiety-inducing stimulus, for a sufficiently prolonged time, a spontaneous attenuation of the anxiety reaction will occur until its complete extinction. *[B. Rainieri]*

REFERENCES. Galeazzi A., Meazzini P., *Mente e comportamento. Trattato Italiano di psicoterapia cognitivo-comportamentale*, 2004; Meazzini P., *Trattato teorico-pratico di terapia e modificazione del comportamento*, 1984.

FOLKLORE

In the context of analytical psychology, folklore is – like myths and religious phenomena – the expression of intrapsychic issues related to the symbolic representation of the contents and the forces of the

→ collective unconscious. Therefore, → tales, legends and folkloristic practices would concern the psychic process becoming conscious and could be subject to amplifications and similarities capable of sending (referring) individual psychic experiences to the collective dimension. In short, folkloric materials would be used to connect the individual psychic "facts" (like dreams), which can vary from individual to individual, to the typical forms of the collective imagination. However, this would not allow therapists to draw any generalizations from clinical records: in fact, dark psychic constants would be expressed in folklore and it would be appropriate and even necessary to listen to them carefully. This psychologistic conception of folklore lacks organic consideration of the role played by culture in the formation of the expressive forms coded in it. Moreover, the scarce attention given to man's ability to transcend the normative forces that limit and shape him, translates into a tendency to discredit the pragmatic function of the → symbol in favour of a merely semantic function. *[E.V. Trapanese, S. Fossi]*

REFERENCES. Jung C.G. (1921), *Psychological types*, in *Collected Works*, VI, 1971.

FOLLOW-UP

A check carried out some months after the end of the therapy to assess the medium and long-term effect of the therapeutic intervention. Generally, to obtain statistical validity, the follow-up must be carried out at least six months after the end of the therapeutic treatment. Normally one or more moments of follow-up are scheduled, for example 1, 3, 6, 12 months after the end of therapy. The assessment of the follow-up consists of a measurement of outcomes performed by psychometric tests and/or a clinical interview. *[R.]*

FORECLOSURE

It is the exclusion of a → signifier (the Name of the Father: the signifier that ensures symbolization and repression processes and therefore sexual significance) that is at the basis of psychosis. The term is the Lacanian translation of the Freudian term *Verwerfung* ("rejection"). Foreclosure differs both from the mechanism of neurotic repression and perverse disavowal. What has been foreclosed from the symbolic level can return but it remains excluded from this level. This means that it can return in "reality" (for example, the phenomenon of hallucination). Differently, what has been repressed from the symbolic can return to the symbolic. Lacan shows how foreclosure can be identified in patients' narratives: their speaking appears without limits and without any meaning that could indicate a sexual significance. Language disorders such as neologisms, stereotypes and absence of metaphor can develop from this issue. *[M. Drazien, C. Fanelli]*

REFERENCES. Lacan J. (1955), *The seminar of Jacques Lacan: The psychoses, III*, 1993; Id. (1955–1956), *On a question preliminary to any possible treatment of psychosis*, in *Écrits: A selection, VI*, 1977.

FOUR DIMENSIONS

In psychosynthesis, the complex and articulated image of the person is represented through a multifaceted view that includes different levels. Each one of them has specific characteristics that can be integrated with the other dimensions: physical, emotional, mental and spiritual. Each dimension acquires significance in connection and resonance with the other dimensions. Each time, according to the different approaches, the reciprocal inter-dimensional contributory cause is underlined, as also the co-presence of the four dimensions in each existential moment and the expressive function of the body, emotions and mind. The spiritual dimension is the transpersonal level of the psyche and does not represent psychic functions in the same way as the other dimensions. It expresses itself through them but not vice-versa, even if, in order to express the spiritual dimension, it may be necessary for the other dimensions to find a certain degree of integration and reciprocal organization. *[M. Rosselli]*

REFERENCES. Assagioli R., *Transpersonal development: The dimension beyond psychosynthesis*, 2007; Rosselli M., *An introduction to psychosynthesis*, 2000.

FREE ASSOCIATION TECHNIQUE

In psychoanalysis (→ Freudian psychoanalysis), a method of expressing ideas that come to patients' minds and that, through a chain of subsequent links, leads to a content that is believed unconscious or repressed. It is also referred to as the "fundamental rule" of psychoanalysis; with the free association technique, patients are encouraged to let themselves go and say what comes to mind, suspending the critical and logical selection that is normally active in social relations. Freud replaced aspects of the hypnotic technique with free association, considering it as the primary method of psychoanalysis. The term "free" indicates the related suspension of the conscious control that patients must put in place, overcoming conscious feelings of embarrassment, shame, guilt and fear; their cooperation is partly motivated by the knowledge of the purpose of the analysis (that is, to solve and overcome their conflictual problems). Free association allows patients to verbalize their mental life and unfold it before the analyst complements the experience in the analytical process. The analyst's interventions, including silence, facilitate the maintenance of balance between the patient's expression and reflection. Within the analytical context, the nature of the associations allows the therapist to deduce what determines the sequences and the "material "contained in them, including the unconscious influences and conflicts between them. In addition, the therapist's interventions (the interpretation of the unconscious elements in particular) aim to expand the freedom of association of the patient, that is, the interpretation and control of resistances expressed in different ways. Free association is also influenced by resistance that may indicate what the analysed wants to avoid knowing or omitting. The concept of free association partly derives from studies developed by W. Wundt and then resumed by C.G. Jung, who developed a list of inducting words from a clinical perspective: through free association it would be possible to reach the "complex" of the patient. *[M. Casonato, S. Sagliaschi]*

REFERENCES. Bucci W., *Psicoanalisi e scienza cognitiva*, 1997; Freud S. (1920), *A note on the prehistory of the technique of analysis*, in *The Standard Edition*, XVIII, 1953–1974; Imbasciati A., *Fondamenti psicoanalitici della psicologia clinica*, 2007.

FREE-FLOATING ATTENTION

Technique recommended by Freud that identifies the analyst's specific listening position in front of the patient's → free association. After half a century, it was redefined by Bion as a condition of lack of memory and desire. The free-floating (or equally-floating) attention is intended to get both what the patient is saying with words or with silences and the nature of feelings transferred from the patient to the analyst. It consists of two components: a regression to a state of consciousness close to that of the dream, or even to a state of trance, which allows the unconscious material of the analyst to emerge through → countertransference, and observation that is in some way detached from this material. On the one hand, the analyst surrenders to a preconscious and unconscious associative flow; on the other he/she remains alert. It is a form of non-selective and non-guided attention, which is used to keep the analyst free from preconceived ideas and allows him/her to follow what the patient verbalizes without any conscious attempt to remember. According to Spence, this state is a myth of psychoanalysis; by adopting a different epistemological perspective, the author argues that instead, the analyst has a selective attention that chooses the data according to criteria dictated by the psychoanalytic theory in order to construct an expressly psychoanalytic narrative using and modelling this flow of free associations; to listen in an effective way, the analyst should pay attention also to their emotional responses, that is, to their countertransference reactions. In Spence's perspective this activity would also be driven by expectations dictated by psychoanalytic theory; the attention of the analyst is aimed towards a particular way of constructing reality and the therapeutic effect would derive from the restructuring of the patient's "reality", stimulated by the interaction with the analyst. *[S. Sagliaschi, M. Casonato]*

REFERENCES. Bion W.R., *Second thoughts: Selected papers on psycho-analysis*, 1967; Freud S. (1903), *Freud's psycho-analytic procedure*, in *The Standard Edition*, VII, 1953–1974; Id. (1912), *Recommendations to physicians practising psycho-analysis*, in *The Standard Edition*, XII, 1953–1974; Spence D.P., Narrative truth and historical truth, 1982.

FREQUENCY

In the context of cognitive-behavioural therapies, the evaluation of the behaviour that is to be modified ("goal" if the behaviour is to be increased and "target" if it is to be decreased) is an important part of all intervention schedules. In order to evaluate behaviour, one should observe it with great attention and record one's findings. One of the parameters used for measuring behaviour is its frequency or how often it reoccurs during the period of observation. *[V. Poerio]*

REFERENCES. Foxx R.M., *Increasing behaviours of severely retarded and autistic persons*, 1982; Martin G., Pear J., *Behaviour modification: What it is and how to do it*, 2007.

FRUSTRATION

A psychological condition resulting from an unsatisfied or inhibited → desire or → need due to → endogenous or exogenous reasons. This concept was introduced in 1912 by S. Freud who thought that frustration is useful for the development of the Ego and its adaptation to reality. The higher the incentive-motivation, the greater the tendency to persist in achieving the gratification that is prevented by the presence of an obstacle. A well-balanced and well-oriented frustration can activate behaviours, increase the overall level of motivation to learn (as long as it is not too intense or too prolonged) and can enable collaborations among those who are experiencing it. Beyond a certain threshold, a prolonged lack of → gratification can trigger an aggressive response. In particular, experimental psychology focuses on three factors that can lead to such a reaction by combining with each other: the nature of the frustrating event, the strength of the underlying motivation and the → personality of the frustrated subject. This reaction can be directed both outwards and towards themselves. When the extent of the frustration is so high as to exceed tolerance limits, states of → anxiety, psychomotor agitation, → anguish or apathy can develop. *[R.]*

FUNCTION

In analytical psychology, Jung used this term to mark a dynamic psychic activity, grounded in biology, partially managed by an individual within innate limits. In this sense, also sexuality, nutrition and religion have to be considered psychic functions. The term is used in three principal expressions, too. *Fundamental function*: Jung defines it as "a certain form of psychic activity that remains constant in principle under varying circumstances". He distinguishes four fundamental psychic functions, two of which are abstract or rational – *thinking* and *feeling* – and two perceptive or irrational – *sensation* and *intuition*. All individuals have recourse to these functions in relation to their psychological "type". The → Ego identifies itself with one of them and uses it spontaneously, shaping a predominant adaptation to relationships whether in the external or internal world. The "thinking" function allows people to know the meaning of what exists, organizing and relating representations; the function "feeling" permits the establishment of a qualitative hierarchy among the contents of consciousness; the "intuition" function captures subliminal perceptions through the unconscious, showing possibilities and purposes in a given situation; the "sensation" function establishes what is actually present and is expressed through the perception of the senses. *Superior/inferior function*: even if all the functions are commonly used by a person, it may happen that one of them becomes preferential to others, so more differentiated and *superior* in adaptation. Mental functioning laws, according to the Jungian model, conceive the *inferior* function as the latter and the neglected one, even more primitive or archaic, sometimes totally unconscious and not integrated. The two couples of opposite functions, around the axes thinking–feeling and sensation–intuition, can't mix with the others and act in a compensatory way (→ compensation). The analytical work activates the differentiation and the progressive balance of the different functions in order to promote the free circulation of the psychic energy, aiming to reach a conscious ability of maintaining the strain between the opposite points of view created by the different (active) functions. *Transcendent function*: it is the symbolic function *par excellence*, thanks to whom psychic elements previously characterized as distinct and opposed are fitted together in a whole synthetic unit. The attribute "transcendent" is not used by Jung to underline a metaphysical feature, but it is used to declare the ability in transcending the border that discerns and joins the conscious and the unconscious or the element of the couple in the psychic dialogue. The direction of the consciousness in achieving a goal, necessary for the psychic development of the human being, can produce the tendency to eliminate non-matching (conflictual) parts into the unconscious. The one-sidedness of the newborn conscious position causes an intrapsychic conflict and a reduction in energy and a turning inwards of the → libido: this process leads to a loss of capacity for symbolization. The analytic process, instead, activates the transcendent function; through the → transference relationship, it is possible to recover the symbolic capacity and allow the re-establishment of the balance between the conscious and the unconscious dimensions, setting the direction towards a new and vital situation: the clear understanding of the Self. *[V. Lingiardi, M. Luci, N. Fina]*

▷ According to Bion, the mind consists of a series of activities such as the ability to feel, to think, to relate. Bion's psychoanalytic function of the personality embraces a hierarchy of functions, some, like alpha function, at the very foundation of the personality and others of a higher grade, such as the ability to remember, to imagine, to relate, or to abstract. Each function is composed of a number of factors such as love, hate, greed, envy, which are deducible from observation of the function, e.g. "X's relationship with his associates is typical of a personality in which envy is a factor". [*J. Symington*]

REFERENCES. Bion W.R., *Learning from experience*, 1962; Jung C.G. (1921), *Psychological types*, in *Collected Works*, VI, 1971; Id. (1940), *The psychology of the child archetype*, in *Collected Works*, IX–I, 1969; Id. (1947), *On the essence of psyche*, in *Collected Works*, VIII, 1969; Id. (1951), *Aion: Researches into the phenomenology of the self*, in *Collected Works*, IX/II, 1969; Id (1916), *The transcendent function*, in *Collected Works*, VIII, 1969.

FUNCTIONAL ANALYTIC THERAPY

A type of therapy that makes the relationship between the client and the therapist the pivot around which all the specific → change levers that can be obtained from everyday life problems rotate. Functional analytic therapy shares its foundations with Skinner's operant conditioning behavioural therapy, emphasising in particular the importance of using the relationship with the client as a tool to obtain and provide new learning opportunities. Great importance is therefore given to the study of → reinforcements arising from natural contingencies of the patient–therapist relationship. In particular, the work of the psychologists R.J. Kohlenberg and M. Tsai has revealed an interesting result: some of their clients, treated with traditional → cognitive-behavioural methods, exceeded all expectations, showing significant improvements that had persisted over time and reaching additional objectives that had not been contemplated. When analyzing these cases, researchers have realized that they were characterized by a high involvement in the therapist–patient relationship, which was not voluntarily created. For this reason, Kohlenberg and Tsai started to use behavioural concepts as an interpretative key to those relationships. They focused on the connection between improvements and intense relationships and they built a series of steps to recreate the bond that was generated in those specific situations. In this way, they gave birth to functional analytic therapy.

In this type of therapy, the preferential techniques used to accelerate the process of change are types of learning taking place in natural settings. These are considered more valid than → role-playing and simulations, which often represent the main focus of behavioural therapy. *[R.]*

REFERENCES. Kohlenberg R.J., Tsai M., *Functional analytic psychotherapy*, in M. Hersen, W. Sledge (eds.), *Encyclopedia of psychotherapy*, 2002.

FUNCTIONAL BALANCE

It is the degree of adaptation of individuals to their personal, → interpersonal, working and cultural-life context. In addition, functional balance requires people's ability to stay in contact with their own emotional and psychological intimacy. The category functional–dysfunctional has been often – and wrongly – overlapped with the category healthy–pathological. Generally, the concept of functional–dysfunctional balance does not have any nosological value (→ nosology) in psychotherapy. On the contrary, it implies a reference to both the → coping ability of an individual (response strategies to → stress) and the more general ability to produce and maintain a stable psychological → adaptation to the internal and external → environment. When feelings of → wellbeing with low general levels of anxiety are predominant, therapists talk about functional balance; instead, the term dysfunctional balance is used when emotions of pain and discomfort prevail and when these are associated with people's desire to change some aspects of their own behaviour. The degree of functional–dysfunctional adaptation (balance) is the most widely used empirical criterion in psychotherapy to assess how incapacitating a disorder or a pathology is. It should also be noted that dysfunctional behaviour is exactly what subjects put into action when facing a difficult situation, as they consider it the best or the only possible reaction to face the problem. Strategic therapy defined this concept as → attempted solution, that is, a solution that maintains the problem, instead of solving it. This process is often responsible for the structuring of dysfunctional and chronic balances. The overall goal of psychotherapy is not to "heal" a pathological condition, but rather to help the person to change dysfunctional and painful balances and make them acceptable and functionally endurable. *[R.]*

FUNCTIONAL FAMILY THERAPY

Functional family therapy (FFT), developed by James Alexander and Bruce Parsons in 1982, is an integrative systemic and cognitive-behavioural intervention that helps build new family interaction patterns to reduce and eliminate adolescent behaviour problems. FFT does so by systematically addressing, in specific phases of treatment, relevant risk and protective factors associated with each → family. Studies conducted by numerous researchers, including teams led by James Alexander, Don Gordon and Holly Waldron have demonstrated the efficacy of FFT for youth with disruptive behaviour problems across different ethnic cultural groups, and for service providers with diverse backgrounds. Also, FFT helps prevent problem behaviour for younger siblings.

CLINICAL MODEL OVERVIEW. As described by Alexander and colleagues in 1998, FFT consists of five components: 1. Engagement; 2. Motivation; 3. Relational assessment; 4. Behaviour change; and 5. Generalization.

Engagement Phase. Engagement includes activities that facilitate a family's willingness to attend treatment or create a context of respect. Activities are driven by the concept of "matching" to the family and include simple strategies, such as wearing appropriate clothes or (if possible) matching therapists to families concerning ethnicity and gender.

Motivation Phase. Families of troubled youth typically present with → conflict, which interferes with effective problem-solving and behaviour change. As such, decreasing conflict is essential prior to initiating behaviour change. Two domains of interventions are used to create a working context: *Change Focus* and *Change Meaning*. Change-focus techniques disrupt family conflict by stopping or redirecting interactions. The most basic change-focus techniques are divert and interrupt. Therapists *divert* when they intercept a negative speech act made by a family member instead of allowing the family member to whom it was directed to answer. Therapists *interrupt* when they do not allow a family member to complete a negative statement. Therapists can also disrupt conflict by commenting on the process of how family members relate to each other in a non-blaming, strength-based manner. By *pointing process*, therapists are able to shift the focus from adolescent problems to relational aspects that underlie, but are hidden from, the family. Another technique, *sequencing/circular questioning*, is used to create depth of knowledge about a problem sequence, including the actions each person took, and their meaning. Finally, *strength-based relational statements* ascribe a positive attribution about one person's efforts towards another. This includes seeing the positive side of apparently negative relational patterns.

Change-meaning techniques disrupt family conflict by changing the meaning of how family members understand themselves, each other and their histories. The goal is not to create cognitive change by challenging "maladaptive" cognitions or providing interpretations. Rather, the focus is to provide a non-blaming and more hopeful viewpoint as a basis/context for change.

Relabelling interventions are reflections that use similar, but less harmful explanations. Relabelling often involves using a "softer" relational focus (e.g. concern versus nagging) to create a less negative tone in the family. → Reframing, defined by Watzlawick and colleagues in 1974, involves a change of "the conceptual and/or setting or viewpoint in relation to which a situation is experienced and to place it in another frame . . . and thereby change its entire meaning". In FFT, reframes include an acknowledgement of the negativity to establish that the therapist understands the relevance of the problem, but go beyond this reflection to offer an alternative benign *motive* for the behaviour. In FFT, therapists work to create new themes for understanding family interactions. Behavioural themes involve identifying sequences of problem interactions in which all of the negative elements are identified but reframed in a more positive way. *Relational themes* switch the focus to relationships rather than behaviours. Relational themes maintain the basic elements of reframes, but provide new perspectives on the relational meaning of events or behaviours.

Relational Assessment. Family members relate to one another based on their own inferred internal motivations. In FFT, the focus of assessment is not on the inferred internal process, but rather on the patterns that emerge from family interactions. The goal is not to change the relational function, but rather to change the cognitive, physiological, emotional, and behavioural strategies which the youth or parent uses to meet relational functions. If a child acts out to "get attention", FFT does not work to eliminate their need for attention! Instead, FFT changes the *means* through which attention is elicited, and how the attention is given.

Contact/Closeness versus Distance/Autonomy. The first category of assessing *relational functions* is the degree of interpersonal connectivity expressed in behaviour patterns, ranging from "close" and highly interconnected to "distant" and quite independent. These dimensional anchors are not viewed as fixed invariant points on a dimension, but instead the central tendency that best characterizes each relationship.

The Second Dimension: Relational ("Relative Power") Hierarchy. FFT examines the balance of control and power in the family. In many ways, parents experience power as the most salient aspect in raising adolescents; however, FFT asserts that primarily what parents want is a sense of being able to control and help their youth. When therapists provide alternative ways to influence youth, hierarchy itself becomes less salient. In fact, many parents are quite pleased when children begin to comply after the parent–adolescent relationship has been repaired and the youth now wants to maintain a positive relationship with the parent(s). Power and consequences have important roles, but are often more difficult to change, and certainly less positive than relational changes that motivate youth to develop positive behaviours.

Behaviour-Change Phase. The goal of behaviour change is to ease the emergence of new adaptive and productive behaviours that meet the family members' functional needs. This may include building new skills or refining existing skills. Many behavioural intervention strategies are used in FFT. Some of the most common examples are included below.

A common behaviour change technique is communication training. Key elements of communication training include enhancing *source responsibility* ("I" statements), *source directness* ("you" statements), *brevity, specificity, congruence,* and *presenting alternatives*. Therapists help family members to be more effective *active listeners* by instilling guidance about how to use cues during and after the time someone else communicates. In addition, therapists guide family members to provide *impact statements* that offer feedback about one's personal reaction and require no justification from either party. FFT borrows from numerous parenting experts to tailor *parenting skills*, building interventions to families. Interventions often include positive and negative → reinforcement, limit-setting with consistent follow-through, contracting and parental monitoring. A number of *technical aids* are also frequently used to facilitate behaviour change. Examples include (a) tape recordings of sessions and handouts, (b) reminder cards, post-it notes, charts and message centres, (c) school–home feedback reports, and (d) answering machines, texting and cell phones. These examples represent common techniques used in FFT. However, just about any structured activity can be useful, *as long as the behaviours they create and maintain are consistent with relational functions*. Over the years, FFT therapists have utilized a wide range of cognitive-behavioural techniques, trauma and experiential techniques, and already established cultural practices (e.g. preparing meals together) as contexts for change. Once they become comfortable with the core construct of "matching" interventions to family functions, therapists have an almost limitless supply of techniques to utilize in creating change.

Generalization Phase. Families are connected in a web of social, legal, cultural, economic and community systems. FFT incorporates specific principles, which govern the inclusion of these systems in the treatment planning process. Unlike generic treatment planning, which at times wraps services around the family with little consideration of family dynamics, FFT focuses on each family's interpersonal needs when considering adjunctive support services. Before an intervention is implemented, it is necessary to establish the validity of the intervention for the family, and tailor the intervention to the family's relational needs. For example, job training for a sixteen-year-old may be valuable in providing necessary skill building. However, the mother may not support participation in such a programme if it replaces the father's role and enables the father to further disengage from the family. By facilitating appropriate links to adjunctive services, treatment effects can be generalized to new contexts and sustained over time.

Summary of the FFT Model and Core Elements. FFT is an integrated systemic and cognitive-behavioural intervention that produces change through a phase-based process. Each phase is informed by core concepts of matching, non-blaming relational focus, and respect. FFT therapists are trained to be clear on the overall principles and perspectives that guide the integrative process, with a default mode that is relational and respectful, but is accommodating enough to utilize other perspectives as long as they are consistent with the FFT model and to help intervene with *this particular family, effectively, at this particular time. [M. S. Robbins, J. F. Alexander, M. E. Guadagno]*

REFERENCES. Robbins M.S., Alexander J.F., Turner C.W., *Disrupting defensive family interactions in family therapy with delinquent adolescents*, in «Journal of Family Psychology», 2000, 14, 4; Robbins M.S., Szapocznik J., Alexander J.F., Miller J.R., *Family systems therapy with children and adolescents*, in M. Hersen, A.S. Bellack (ed.), *Children and adolescents: Clinical formulation and treatment*, in «Comprehensive Clinical Psychology», v, 1998.

FUNCTIONS OF EGO

Within the psychoanalytic orientation called "Ego psychology", a set of functions in connection with reality, which does not represent a frustrating limit but a stimulus for the growth of the Ego. Hartmann – considered, together with other psychoanalysts, the founder of this orientation – believes that it is possible to conceive psychoanalysis as general psychology by focusing on the Ego and by reformulating the psychic structure identified by S. Freud and centred on the psychic → conflict. According to Freud, if man does not adapt to reality, he becomes ill. Instead, Hartmann argues that reality is a human construction and it is not imposed: through individual and social development, man builds his environment and changes it. Adaptation is interpreted as a process of modification of oneself and reality. Freud claims that adaptation consists of being able to endure the frustration resulting from the fact that reality denies the fulfilment of desires. Differently, Hartmann thinks that adaptation consists in being able to obtain satisfaction and pleasure in modifying oneself and the relational and environmental reality. Pleasure should be understood as non-instinctual "energy", proper to the Ego, free from the conflicts arising during the interaction processes with reality, which is the place where the Ego is built and where pleasure originates. The Ego is a set of functions in connection with reality, which in turn does not represent a frustrating limit but a stimulus for the growth of the Ego. If reality could totally and easily "accommodate" man's wishes and needs, man would not reach happiness because he would be denied the possibility to grow. Hartmann proposes, in a clear way, the necessary assumptions to allow psychoanalysis to intervene significantly in all branches of psychology. *[L. Longhin]*

REFERENCES. Hartmann H., *Ego psychology and the problem of adaptation*, 1939.

FUNDAMENTAL RULE

It is the rule that marks the beginning of the psychoanalytic treatment and it lies in asking the patient to say everything that comes into his mind without omitting anything, however meaningless, ridiculous or painful it may seem to him. Based on the → free association technique, its equivalent, in the analyst's behaviour, is → free-floating attention. Therefore, not only the patient, but the psychoanalyst, too, has to free associate. Freud comes to establish the fundamental rule – cornerstone of the so-called "passive" technique – after having gone through → hypnosis and suggestion. From the criticism to the fundamental rule, the → active technique, introduced by Ferenczi, originates. Respecting this rule would not, indeed, allow overcoming what the Hungarian psychoanalyst calls "dead points in analysis". The same associative freedom can indeed be used by the patient as a → resistance: an obsessive patient may, for example, resist analysis by associating inanities. The matter has been resumed by H. Racker, for whom the futility of associations can even express a deeper past: the patient's dead and empty side. The establishment of another rule, considered equally fundamental, has followed the fundamental rule of free association: the analyst's analysis. Ferenczi talks meaningfully about the "second fundamental rule". The idea, suggested at the time even by C.G. Jung, was forwarded by H. Nunberg, with Freud's support, in 1918 and adopted by the International Psychoanalytical Association during the 1925 Bad Homburg Congress. *[G. Antonelli]*

REFERENCES. Ferenczi S., *The elasticity of psycho-analytic technique*, in *Final contributions to the problems and methods of psycho-analysis*, 1928; Lacan J. (1958), *The direction of the treatment and the principles of its power*, in *Écrits*, 1977

FUSION

In psychoanalysis, it is the fantasy of spontaneous sharing with an external or internal "object". This fantasy can be present at the developmental stage, but also at any age and at any stage of normality or pathology. Understanding the "state of fusion" in children means bearing in mind that their primitive knowledge of reality is dictated by the "affections" attributed to the objects with which they fuse. In the early stages of their life, the only way to know the outside world is through their "internal objects". The good object is experienced as a part of the Self and gratifications do not derive from an object that takes care of them (their mother), but from a "natural" reality belonging to the Self. They live the good object as a reality "con-fused with the Self". The first psychic distinction between Self and not-Self arises when children feel the discomfort of suffering caused by the lack of something. This absence establishes in them as a "bad" presence. Only at a later stage, will it be identified as separated from the Self. *[L. Longhin]*

REFERENCES. Imbasciati A., *Fondamenti psicoanalitici della psicologia clinica*, 1994.

G

GAME

In everyday language, it is an activity that can have different purposes (recreational, educational, therapeutic, etc.). Games define a context in which it is possible to distinguish between "playing" and "being serious" and between fiction and reality. In game theory, the notion of "game" depicts the set of behaviours that are considered admissible in an interactional system. J. von Neumann is considered the founder of the modern game theory. He wrote the article "Toward a theory of social games" (1928) in which he enunciated the basic ideas of the strategic games theory, meant as the theory of interpersonal conflict and decision. The application of this theory to family processes is the result of the application of cybernetic concepts (→ cybernetics). A family is a system in which behaviours are determined by family roles. This behaviour can be compared to a game in which all family members (players) try to satisfy their personal needs or to achieve their individual goals. This tension towards different needs and objectives leads inevitably to conflict. Each family member has to develop a strategy to win or at least to lose as little as possible. The therapeutic approaches of strategic therapy can also be seen in the light of game theory. Therapists must develop strategies to achieve therapeutic goals with respect to → resistance to change of individuals and/or families. *[R.]*

▷ The word "game" is used by the Milan school (→ Milan School of family therapy) as an intuitive metaphor indicating how subjects, included into a relational network or system (a family), act affected by rules and express their degree of freedom in their communication. These "games" have been studied by Selvini's team to describe the pathogenic relationships of families that develop a psychosis in one of their members. These games were investigated in the late 1980s to build models that connected the symptomatic behaviour of a child (the patient) with the problems of the parental/conjugal couple and with the relationship between brothers. Among these, the most significant games are: the "couple impasse", the "fraud of affections" and the "incitement", that is, patterns of relationships that govern family malaise. *[A.M. Sorrentino]*

▷ Psychological games are one of the supporting pillars of transactional analysis. These represent the main type of dysfunction in interpersonal communication and consist of a communicative dynamic tied to the transmission of two parallel levels of messages between the two "players": a social level, tied to the verbal conversation, that is, to what the two players in good faith mean to say (→ Adult Ego state); and a psychological level, connected to an implicit and unaware communication (→ Child and/or → Parent Ego state). This communication dynamic leads the two players to "recite", unwittingly, dramatic roles (Persecutor/Saviour/Victim). This leads towards an unforeseen outcome, called "exchange", which makes the psychological level emerge with a conclusive "payoff". The latter reinforces, in the two players, both the "→ script conviction" constructed in childhood and ancient emotions, called → *rackets*. The game, therefore, is an unconscious strategy to confirm, in a neo-Freudian → repetition compulsion, the individual's script. In transactional psychoanalysis, the game is analyzed for its transference value. The classic example of a game is that of "Why not? Yes, but . . .". In this dynamic, the first player (Victim) shows himself needy without asking anything in a direct way; the second player (Saviour) begins to propose ideas and solutions, which are constantly rejected by the first, until the second loses patience from the frustration caused by the uselessness of his good intentions, going in this way from the role of Saviour to that of Persecutor: the payoff consists in the anger and in the disappointment of both players, who confirm to themselves the script conviction about the non → *OK-ness (*feeling of inadequacy) about himself and others. From a methodological point of view, the analysis of psychological games highlights the different proposals of the therapeutic approach of the different schools of transactional psychoanalysis: in the "classic" and "re-decisional" schools, the aim of the therapy is that of interrupting and/or analyzing cognitively possible games in therapy; in psychodynamic transactional analysis and in transactional psychoanalysis, the intra-therapeutic game appears at a central moment in the emotional analysis of the transfer and countertransfer dynamics. *[M. Novellino]*

▷ In Winnicott's thought (→ psychoanalysis (Independent or Middle Group of British analysts)), a game is an activity that creates a communication between a person's internal world of fantasies and desires and the external reality. This creates a "transitional space" where a process of maturation can take place along with a gradual integration between the perception of one's needs and the awareness of the objective external conditions.

In particular, these conditions refer to people's relationship with other human beings, who can make the achievement of one's needs possible. In this view, games are not considered as a result of the processes of sublimation of → drives, nor a reactive formations effect (→ defence mechanisms). Instead, they are considered a direct expression of love and creativity, which are seen as a manifestation of a child's vitality. Aggressiveness itself can be freely expressed in an environment that, without answering with hate and violence, is able to contain it without being destroyed by it. During a child's development, the ability to play is an activity that facilitates the structuring of the Self, identity and the ability to interact with others. Moreover, it expresses and enriches creativity and the ability to gain control over the real world. The therapeutic process is fulfilled if the ability to play of a patient and of a therapist meet in a shared area, and give rise to a creative experience that promotes the maturation and transformation of the patient. If the patient is unable to play, the therapist must foster the formation of a transitional space that enables a "highly specialized form of play", as it was called by Winnicott. In this way, profound transformations and possibilities of communication can be produced. These do not depend on interpretations, but are rather their prerequisite. This conception of therapy emphasizes the importance of creating a shared mental space. Two elements can be promoted in this space: the expression of the patient's vitality and the continuation of the developmental processes that had been lacking or missing in the history of the patient's psychological growth. *[P. Cruciani]*

REFERENCES. Berne E., *Games people play*, 1964; Novellino M., *Psicoanalisi transazionale*, 2004; Selvini Palazzoli M., Cirillo S., Selvini M., Sorrentino A.M., *Family games*, 1989; Selvini M., *Reinventare la psicoterapia*, 2004; Winnicott D.W., *Playing and reality*, 1971.

GENERAL ADAPTATION SYNDROME → STRESS

GENERALIZATION

In neurolinguistic programming, it is one of the three → meta-model processes called "language of precision" – along with → deletion and → distortion. It is a procedure whereby an element of an individual's world model tends to represent an entire category. Generalization is a, so-called, "violation" of verbal language, highlighting how, in the passage of information between the deep/unconscious part and the surface/logic part, some elements of a person's experience are altered, compared with the complete experience actually lived. It is a reduced perception of reality, a cause of discomfort and misunderstandings, that reports a single experience to a whole category of experiences. The excessive use of generalizations involves the risk of losing many details of an experience. This causes a significant depletion of one's mental map and a consequent restriction of an individual's possibilities of choice (for example: "all men are traitors"). Generalizations can be negative or positive and are accompanied by the following "violations": universal quantifiers (always, all, never, no, anyone, everyone, etc.) and modal operators (I must, I can, I want) which express needs, opportunities and will. *[D. Poggiolini]*

REFERENCES. Hall M., *NLP and magic of language*, 2007.

GENERATIONS

From its very beginning, the field of family psychotherapy has developed a branch of research and clinical intervention that can be referred to as "generational". Within this branch of research, contributions with different matrices of clinical thinking and different backgrounds can be found; however, they all connect the wellbeing and the psychopathology of family members to the dynamics of the intergenerational ties. In particular, the paths for the transmission of constrains (losses, abuses, faults) and resources (benefits of ties) are highlighted. The → setting of this type of therapy is characterized by joint sessions, attended by different generations, and by the revisitation of family matrices by the members of a couple. Specific techniques are applied, such as family genogram, kinetic sculptures and joint drawing. *[V. Cigoli, S. Molgora]*

REFERENCES. Andolfi M., Angelo C., D'Atena P., *Families' account of therapy: An intergenerational research perspective*, 2001; Boszormenyi-Nagy I., Spark G. M., *Invisible loyalties: reciprocity in intergenerational family therapy*, 1973; Bowen M., *Family therapy in clinical practice*, 1978; Eiguer A., *The intergenerational: An approach to psychoanalytic family therapy*, 1997; Framo J., *Family-of-origin therapy: An intergenerational approach*, 1996; Cigoli V., Tamanza G., *The clinical generational interview*, 2009; Racamier P. C., *The genius of origins: Psychoanalysis and psychoses*, 1992.

GESTALT PSYCHOLOGY

Also known as "psychology of form", due to the fact that the German word "*Gestalt*" means "form", in the sense of a whole that is made up not only from its parts but also of the "effects" produced by the way in which they are organized. The origins of Gestalt psychology can be traced to the work of Brentano, who invented the theory of the primary and secondary phenomenon and the intentionality of perception: von Ehrenfels, considered to be his precursor, in order to demonstrate that the whole is not identical to the sum of the parts, organized the same group of notes in different orders and so created different melodies. At the beginning of the twentieth century, Koffka, Kohler and Wertheimer developed phenomena related to perception – the processes of which it is made up – and its laws (law of similarity, of good form, of proximity, of closure, of good continuation, of simplicity), departing from the presupposition that the whole is greater or is at the very least different from the sum of its parts. Wertheimer highlighted the tendency to intentionally perceive a coherent whole: he who is perceiving guides himself towards those objects that are congruent to the emergence of the needs of the organism in the moment in which they appear, whilst the rest remains in the background (→ figure–ground dynamic). In the formulation of the figure–ground hypothesis according to Rubin, perception is the result of an inexorable relationship between the picture in the foreground and that in its background (for example, from the photograph of an unknown animal it is impossible to tell its size if there is no familiar object next to it). In Koffka's theoretical viewpoint, the concept of totality acquires a meaning that is even more significant: the world is "what appears to us" in the very act of perception itself, and appearance therefore is no longer in opposition to reality.

Kohler introduced the concept of → insight, the sudden awareness of a new way of understanding a situation: "insight" is the discovery of new relationships between the different elements, different to those that were formerly perceived as being present. Gestalt psychologists highlight the way in which what we perceive does not simply reflect the summation of several different sensations but is the result of an "organized" totality, that is, through processes of organization that build the sensory data into a complex unit. The data chosen are those that are required for the completion of a "Gestalt", that is to say, a total that has a certain meaning to the organism. In the same way as physics has shown that perfect insulators do not exist and that everything is in the force field of the rest of the universe, similarly fundamental to Gestalt psychology is Lewin's → field theory that explains behaviour by inserting it into a relationship with the context within which it is taking place: reasons for behaviour are not to be pursued by looking into the past, but by focusing on the relationship between the individual and his environment in the present. *[P. Quattrini]*

REFERENCES. Brentano F., *Psychology from an empirical standpoint*, 1874; Koffka K., *Principles of Gestalt psychology*, 1935; Köhler W., *The mentality of apes*, 1921; Lewin K., *Principles of topological psychology*, 1936; Rubin E., *Visuaell wahrgenommene Figuren*, in S. Yantis (ed.), *Visual perception: Essential reading*, 2000; von Ehrenfels C., *Über gestaltqualitäten*, in «Vierteljahrsschrift für wissenschaftliche Philosophie», 1890, 14; Wertheimer M. (1924), *Über Gestalttheorie*, in «Social Research», 1944, 11.

GESTALT PSYCHOTHERAPY

Gestalt psychotherapy has never been a technical elaboration model, and this allowed it to remain a living thing instead of stiffening in a static "true" theoretical vision. However, to protect the survival of the "Gestalt organism", this must be supplied with solid theoretical roots by placing it in one of the science-of-knowledge approaches. For this reason, both in America and Europe, some schools use the phenomenological-existential approach as the main reference paradigm, whereas others use a pragmatist background. In a sense, Gestalt psychotherapy is what remains of psychoanalysis once it has discarded the idea that in the psychological world, as in the world of atomic physics, the many aspects of reality arise from the transformation of the same primary basis: that is, what S. Freud called → libido. Perls, the main founder of this approach, replaced this vision with existentialism, phenomenology and Gestalt psychology. To the latter belong the concepts of intentionality of perception, the principle that the whole is not equal to the sum of the parts, the figure–ground theory (→ figure–ground dynamic) and the → field theory, which places individuals at the centre of their present time. Other authors have developed various theoretical frameworks, which have not always been universally accepted. Goodman theorized the concept of → contact boundary: a place of encounter between the inner and the outer world and a moment of generation of the Self, understood not as a structure but as an interactive entity. According to the existentialist view, "contact" represents a proximity between therapist and patient, where proximity is enough to make something happen, but where, at the same time, distance is enough for it to happen. During the encounter of a subject with another subject, the phenomenological basis of Gestalt psychotherapy gives importance to the action of "feeling", which is considered a co-creation tool of intersubjective knowledge, not forced by the mediation of conceptual interpretations. Here, therapy happens in a space inhabited by therapist and patient through the production of new meanings. This approach is focused on the self-regulating ability of organisms through the surfacing of needs, which offer solutions to conflicts through organismic abilities such as aggression, that can resolve a "Gordian knot" with a simple stroke of the sword. The Ego is considered here only a behavioural style, and therapy is not meant as a transition from being ill to being healthy, but as a transition from a locked state to a state of flow, with the prospect of a life that takes its course instead of being stuck in immobilizing conflicts. In an existentialist view, a person's will is the extreme limit of psychological investigation, beyond which this is no longer legitimate: Perls considered this position a pillar of Gestalt psychotherapy. Instead, he did not embrace the conception of pain of Existentialist philosophy. From Schopenhauer to

Kierkegaard and J.P. Sartre, this conception is considered an absolute truth, while Perls emphasizes the biological sense of it:

> man is a biological event, society itself is part of nature, and responsible actions and conscience are therefore biological functions. The process of reintegration of different parts can only have success if all human activity, so much deliberate as spontaneous, thoughts and instincts, are considered and treated like a biological process.

Pain is simply an alarm bell, which alerts one's body about the need to take action on the ongoing situation. Husserl considered phenomenology a strict observation of phenomena, with a suspension of judgements and theories. Instead, Heidegger's phenomenology became the theory of disclosing, the only place where "beings" become "being". Thus, the "disclosing" does not appear simply as a phenomenon to investigate with scientific rigour, but as something to give value to: being a phenomenon is the maximum that can be asked of a being, and for this reason, this is worthy of the deepest respect, without the need to put it on a level of reality considered as superior, as is done when it is interpreted. In this view, perception is considered intentional, that is, people perceive what they need: this is not only an inclination, but also a necessity of organisms. This is how Perls explains the so-called neurotic fixations, which are represented as unfinished Gestalts, which resurface continually with the intention of reaching a conclusion. In the United States, Perls came in contact with pragmatism through Goodman. This was a philosophical point of view underappreciated in that period by European academia, but that was useful to his approach. At the time, James, one of the leading exponents of pragmatism, had remarked that theoretical assumptions are limited by the existential conditions of the person who processes them: there are live hypotheses and dead hypotheses, that is, hypotheses that are highly valued by some, but are out of reach for others. In a pragmatist sense, knowledge is self-knowledge, with an interchangeable object of knowledge. That is, it is knowledge taken out of context (abstracted): knowledge outside the "event horizon", a very important knowledge of a part that would remain unknowable if the focus was limited to the phenomenon, in its strict sense. In fact, we would remain "imprisoned in the present", according to Polster, one of the great masters of Gestalt psychotherapy. In this view, interpretation is also linked to a person's experiences; however, translation, that is, "this corresponds to that", is still the fundamental operational instrument of pragmatism, which risks, in this way, to lose contact with the phenomenon. Although maps are useful for orientation, they should never be confused with territory. Understanding can never replace experiencing if the goal is to stay consistent to the phenomenological-existential perspective, where the "hermeneutic circle", the infinite unfolding of the rebounds of intersubjectivity, cannot be nullified in the name of objective knowledge. Just as interpretation is common to all Freudian schools, expression is the reference point of all Gestalt psychotherapy approaches, both pragmatists and phenomenological-existentialists: however, people can express themselves functionally, to understand, or existentially, to live, and this is what separates the paths of the two approaches. This difference is not explicated in the clinical work, but this does not mean that it is not important: the functionality of an expression does not necessarily correspond to the pleasure of the experience. In the classical world, the concept of *phýsis* (nature), unlike in modern scientific meaning, not only indicates a "naturated" nature object of knowledge, but also a "naturating" nature, that is an active nature, a subject that creates while it exists and produces the sense of the world. A phenomenon is not a simple object that must be known: it is an active and creative event, that "makes" the world, which contains existential meaning in itself, that is, sense and reason for existence. This was described by Merleau-Ponty as the scar that the knife of the world leaves on the skin of people who perceive it. Expressing themselves, which means giving action to a phenomenon, is certainly functional, but it is, above all, life, a mystery that does not need to be solved, but to be contemplated, lived, as said by Kierkegaard. Technically, the existential-phenomenological approach leans against the cornerstones of responsibility and secondary phenomenon, namely the act of "feeling": to intervene in the patient's experience, the therapist can call attention to the fact that, since a person necessarily feels, at any time we feel something, and for physio-biological reasons, this act of "feeling" is delimited by the polarity pleasure–displeasure. People are responsible for the conduct of their lives, that is, for the choices made moment by moment. However, their possibility to choose is limited by their ability to identify their choices: broadening the range of possible choices is an integral part of therapy and supporting this development is part of a Gestalt therapist's job. What the patient wants to do → here-and-now is the leitmotiv of a Gestalt therapy session, since there is no other place to do something if not the here-and-now or the there-and-then, that is, a place and a time where a person can work on reality. The implementation of decisions may refer to a time in the future, but the decision itself can be taken in the here-and-now of the session, no matter if it may be changed at a later time. Although life is, in a way, diachronic, that is, it unfolds with the passing of time, it is synchronic in relation to sense; that is, it exists all at the same time, and it is the architecture of sense that is built over the course of a lifetime that supports the ephemeral and fundamental experience, which is the meaning of life. *[P. Quattrini]*

REFERENCES. Goldstein K., *The organism*, 1939; Heidegger M., *Being and time*, 1962; Husserl E., *Ideas : General introduction to pure phenomenology*, 1913; James W., *The will to believe: And other essays in popular philosophy*, 1896; Kierkegaard S., *Fear and trembling*, 1843; Id., *Either/Or*, 1843; Merleau-Ponty M., *Phenomenology of perception*, 1945; Naranjo C., *Techniques of Gestalt therapy*, 1973; Perls F., *Ego, hunger, and aggression*, 1942; Id., *The Gestalt approach and eye witness to therapy*, 1973; Perls F., Hefferline R.F., Goodman P., *Gestalt therapy: Excitement and growth in the human personality*, 1951; Polster E., *Every person's life is worth a novel*, 1987; Rovatti P., *Abitare la distanza: per un'etica del linguaggio*, 1994; Schopenhauer A., *The world as will and representation*, 1819.

GESTALT PSYCHOTHERAPY (SPAGNUOLO LOBB'S)

Since 1979 Spagnuolo Lobb has been contributing to the development of the theory and method of Gestalt therapy in hermeneutic line with the basic texts of Perls, Hefferline and Goodman. Developing the thinking of I. From, Spagnuolo Lobb presents a model centred on the unitary nature of the phenomenological field and on the co-creation of the → contact boundary in the → figure–ground dynamic. The contact boundary is defined as the place in which the self unfolds, that is to say the shared figure of the process of contact that emerges from the ground of possibilities of the phenomenological field. It is the place and time where it is possible to experience both the anxiety that gives rise to the unease and a new perception of the self in relation to the other. Spagnuolo Lobb moves the focus of the therapeutic operation. Going beyond the more famous technique of Gestalt therapy – the "empty chair" (→ hot seat) – she places, in the experience felt at the contact boundary between therapist and patient, the possibility of making phenomenologically evident the anxious-making relational modalities, acquired in the constitutive interactions (e.g. "Tell me, the therapist – instead of the empty chair – what you would tell your mother"). There are various consequences of this displacement; for instance, when, during a session, a patient says to the therapist: "Last night I was upset and couldn't sleep", this communication is to be read and explored, not only as an internal experience, but also as a figure that the patient creates from the ground of the relationship with that specific psychotherapist, and which includes an intentionality of contact towards her/him ("I hope you won't make me leave here upset like last time"). The perspective on the co-creation at the contact boundary enables the intrapsychic point of view to be left and a contextual experience of change to be had based on the mutual regulation of the rhythms and perceptions of the other (a dance), as the neurosciences and intersubjective theories make clear. For Spagnuolo Lobb the health towards which the psychotherapist must direct her/his work is the spontaneous vitality, the "missing gesture" visible in the aesthetic of the patient's movement, while the neurosis is the desensitization of the contact boundary, the sleeping of the senses that makes people feel bored and boring. Accepting the teachings of E. and M. Polster, Spagnuolo Lobb considers the therapeutic operation to be a sort of spotlight that illuminates the "beauty" of the subjects involved, a light that makes visible the harmonic vitality inherent in the wholeness with which each is present in the relationship and adjusts to it in a unique, creative manner. Thus, the patient will be able to awaken – looking at him/herself and feeling recognized in this light – the sense of her/his beauty and the spontaneity of being there. Spagnuolo Lobb's diagnostic model provides a map that enables one to find one's direction in what happens at the contact boundary, and acquire tools in order to read both the contributions of the past and the "tensions" towards the future, as they present themselves in the → here-and-now of the treatment → setting. The concept of the here-and-now is thus redirected in the concept of *now-for-next*. The developmental perspective of a polyphonic development of relational competences (or domains) enables access to the complexity of the patient's being-there, not comparing it with maturative tasks that belong to the developmental phases, but observing how s/he manages the complexity of situations towards a creative adjustment. On this epistemological basis, Spagnuolo Lobb has constructed models for specific clinical situations: 1) the model of couple psychotherapy, based on some experiential dimensions of the couple's functioning, which range from recognizing oneself in the mutual difference to revealing oneself to the other in one's affective vulnerability, trusting to "feel at home in foreign territory"; 2) the model of family psychotherapy, which distinguishes four stages in the session, in which the phenomenological field of the setting is developed the acceptance of the creation and manifestation of the intentionality of contact; 3) the model of support of co-parenting, articulated in six relational competences, each characterized by specific intentionalities of the experiential field. Referring to aesthetic Gestalt values, this model aims to be a support for seeing the "beauty" in one's offspring; 4) the model of psychoprophylaxis at delivery, for couples, which considers parturition to be a relational process whose competences can be applied both to the relationship of the couple and to the relationship with the offspring. The model – validated by research – distinguishes seven psychological dimensions inherent in pregnancy and delivery, and explores each of them in the learning units of the training for couples; 5) the community model for psychiatric structures, which applies the Gestalt hermeneutic to treatment of seriously disturbed clients (in both the private and the institutional setting), distinguishing relational experiences that enable the construction of the "ground of taken-for-granted certainties" necessary for the structuring and differentiation of the self; 6) finally, the model of training for groups and for → stress in organizations, which identifies the group's functions of contact: free-flowing leadership, the presence of the members at the contact boundary, the "therapeutic function" that is set up with the ability to see the other. *[M. Spagnuolo Lobb]*

GOAL-OBJECT

In neo-behavioural psychology, it is the purpose of any behavioural action. Tolman explained in empirical terms the intentionality of behaviour on the basis of the following considerations: there is a purpose in any behaviour identified as goal-object (or goal-situation); to achieve or back away from if it is a condition of discomfort. The relationship between behaviour and goal-object is: behaviour ceases when the goal-object is reached; the goal-object is the same over time (constancy of the goal-object); behaviour is directed to the goal-object in terms of its position, in spite of changes in adapting to intervening obstacles. Reaching or breaking away from the goal-object is characterized not only by the features of the goal-object and by the persistence in going "towards" or "away from", but also by the fact that it always implies a specific pattern of relationship with certain means-objects as ways to reach the goal-object. These interactions with the means-object lead to the selective identification of the shortest (easiest) paths to achieve or move away from the goal-object. *[G. Lo Savio, G. Papale]*

REFERENCES. Tolman E.C., *Purposive behaviour in animals and men*, 1932; Id., *Cognitive maps in rats and men*, in «Psychological Review», 1948, 55, 4; Id., *Essays on motivation and learning*, 1951.

GOOD BREAST/BAD BREAST

The breast is the first object with which the baby establishes a specifically psychic connection. According to Kleinian theory, the breast, during the first phases of growth, is intended not only in its material and objective features, that is, as a representative of a mother who is external or separated, but as an emotional and functional object, defined by the alternation of physiological and instinctual pressures. Consequently, the breast is the prototype of the so-called → partial objects, forerunners of what will become, later on, the representation of the stable and total objects. The Ego of the breast-fed is exposed from the beginning to the push of both external and inner reality, which may produce anguish, starting from the trauma of birth; on the other hand, it may bring ease or pleasure through the warmth and the nourishment of motherly care. Not to be overcome by sensations of anguish and to maintain a relationship with agreeable and satisfactory perceptions, the Ego must perform a mechanism of splitting and projecting into the original external object (that is, the breast), with the death drive → libido, keeping them well separated. Thus, it will establish a relationship with two objects: the good breast and the bad breast. The relationship with the two is rooted in the phantasy of an ideal object, holder of nourishment and wellbeing, which is confirmed by the agreeable and protective presence of the actual mother. To the extent that the external experiences nourish such a phantasy, so the exposure of the Ego to the menace represented by the anguish and persecutory parts ejected into the bad breast is reduced. The ejection into the object, "breast", of the intolerable anguish and of the parts of the Ego containing the death drive – producing the effect of the splitting of the breast into two parts: "good and bad" – can determine the fear of retaliation by a persecutory object. The splitting and the projection into the breast of bad parts belonging to the Ego or the object create an object that is potentially menacing and that can damage or destroy the good object. The psychic dynamics of the child, during the first phases of life, are marked by the operations of splitting, ejections of menacing lived experienced and introjection of good objects. This psychic condition was defined by Klein → paranoid–schizoid position. The presence of overcoming states of anguish determines the activation of → defence mechanisms aiming at reducing the pressure towards the Ego. These are "negation" (which is connected to a phantasy of magic annihilation of the persecutor), "idealization" (which transforms the persecutory object into an ideal one) and "projective identification". The last one consists of the projection of parts of the self into the external object, in order to possess and control it as if it were a part of the self. It is relevant to notice that, on clinical grounds, projective identification is at the base of the states of paranoid suffering and hypochondria. When such mechanisms are not sufficient to dominate anguish, it may occur that, as an extreme defensive measure, the Ego is disintegrated, that is, fragmented into small pieces, thus becoming non-existent. Such an effort gives rise to the most serious anguishes of dissipation and atomization, which are present in the psychotic pathologies. *[M.L. Ricci, A. Voltolin]*

REFERENCES. Klein M., *Notes on some schizoid mechanisms*, 1946; Segal H., *Klein*,1979.

GOOD OBJECT

In psychoanalysis, an aspect of the Self that is a source of love, gratitude and generosity. In Kleinian theory (→ psychoanalysis (Klein's and Bion's)) the good object is a → partial object that supplies what is needed and evokes love accordingly; both these aspects give rise to the quality named "good". A secure establishment of the good object inside one's mind is the basis for mental stability. Usually, these good objects are experienced as internal parental figures who have the interests and wellbeing of an individual close to their heart. If these objects are damaged, for example through anger, greed or envious attacks, this will be reflected in a diminished sense of wellbeing of the Self. The threat of the loss of the good object gives rise to anxiety, whereas its actual loss leads to a sense of torment, depression, guilt and the wish to make reparation. *[J. Symington]*

REFERENCES. Klein M., *The writings of Melanie Klein, I*, 1975.

GOOD-ENOUGH MOTHER

An expression used by Winnicott (→ psychoanalysis (Independent or Middle Group of British analysts)) to describe the suitability of a mother in perceiving the vital needs of her child and in satisfying them as soon as they arise.

> The good-enough mother, as I have stated, starts off with an almost complete adaptation to her infant's needs, and as time proceeds she adapts less and less completely, gradually, according to the infant's growing ability to deal with her failure.

Winnicott meant to indicate a mother's behaviour, where the mother is considered a real human being and not the product of the idealization processes described by M. Klein, which referred instead to internal objects. The term "good-enough" expresses very well the realistic orientation of Winnicott's model, which takes for granted that perfect behaviours do not exist in reality. Moreover, it indicates that it is important for a child to learn how to endure frustrating moments, if these are properly dosed. With regard to psychotherapy, this realistic conception can be reasonably extended to the attitude and abilities of a therapist who is able to meet the needs of the patient in a timely manner but by promoting, at the same time, their ability to endure frustrations. *[P. Cruciani]*

REFERENCES. Winnicott D.W., *Playing and reality*, 1971.

GOOD MOTHER → MOTHER

GOOD-ME – BAD-ME – NOT-ME

In interpersonal psychiatry, the "good me" personification originates from the experience of a relationship with a good → mother, who can be described as such because she is free from anxiety and therefore empathically able to dispel her child's recursive tensions of need by expressing tenderness for him and by intensifying an already positive relationship through affective rewards. From the very early stages of his life, the infant builds his own experience and self-representation through interpersonal relationships, chiefly with his mother. Their interaction is built within a relational field that contains and affects both. When an infant feels that his mother positively mirrors and approves of him, he regards himself as being positive and therefore "good". In a similar way, the "bad me" personification derives from the relationship with a bad → mother who is perceived as being bad because she is unable to relax the child's tensions of need that demand immediate relief. Given that he fails to experience a positive mirroring from a mother who is either too anxious or exceedingly disturbed – and therefore not very empathetic – the infant feels that he is "bad". Thus, the "bad me" becomes associated to anxious experiences, given that the caregiver's anxiety also causes anxiety in the infant. As a result, the mother–child relationship is disturbed and it results in a growing amount of tension, which leads the infant towards behaviours that provoke maternal disapproval, rage and prohibitions and further increase the infant's tensions in a circular way. The "not me" personification emerges from the failure of the "self-system" and relates to the uncanny emotions experienced by the infant during the early stages of his life, whenever he experienced – through a significant figure – sudden, very negative and unpleasant emotions that caused the onset of a paralyzing anxiety attack. Such an occurrence is perceived as being undifferentiated, indistinct and confused, but also violent and abrupt enough to generate feelings of terror, loathing and dread. The anxiety linked to "not me" personifications is rather primitive; it may be experienced by anyone under certain circumstances and may trigger arcane and derealization-provoking emotions. However, whilst the "bad me" and "good me" personifications may be experienced and recognized by the individual as parts of his Self, as a strictly "private" and impossible to communicate part, the "not me" personification is intercepted by awareness only in few exceptional cases. *[A. Cresti, S.Brizzi]*

REFERENCES. Sullivan H.S., *The Interpersonal theory of psychiatry*, 1953.

GRADED EXPOSURE

In cognitive-behavioural therapy, it refers to confrontation in either imagination (→ imaginal exposure) or in vivo (→ in-vivo exposure) or even in virtual reality, of an hierarchy of specific feared situations or objects, put in an order of increasing difficulty. Graded exposure, historically bound to experimental studies of classical conditioning (→ behavioural model of classical conditioning) and to the principles of → extinction of the linkage between → conditioned stimulus and → unconditioned stimulus, is also based, like other exposure techniques, on processes of habituation to the stimulus and of extinction of the avoiding reactions. The most well-known and codified technique is → systematic desensitization, where the exposure to the hierarchy of stimula, is carried out in a situation of relaxation, which is a physiological and emotional state incompatible with an anxiety response. [A. Cocchi, A. Meneghelli]

REFERENCES. Barlow D.H. (ed.) *Clinical handbook of psychological disorders: A step by step treatment manual*, 2007; Borgo S., Milic S., Sibilia L., *Interfaccia medicina-psicologia: Thesarus di psicoterapia comportamentale*, 1991; Craske M.G., Anthony M.M., Barlow D.H., *Mastering your fears and phobias*, 2006; Jones M.C., *A laboratory study of fear: The case of Peter*, «Pedagogical Seminary», 1924, 31, 308–315; Leitenberg H., *Behavioural approaches to treatment of neuroses*, in *Handbook of behaviour modification and behavioural therapy*, 1976; Wolpe J., *Psychotherapy by reciprocal inhibition*, 1958.

GRATIFICATION

A condition of fulfilment that comes from achieving a goal, an object of desire. According to behaviourism, gratification can be identified as a → reward that is able to reinforce the behaviour itself and thus to foster its reproduction. Gratification is an important consequence of the relationship between individuality and the outside world and it is at the basis of many psychological and psychosocial models. In particular, the theories of → motivation have underlined the importance of rewards in relation to the → needs of an organism (physiological or primary needs) and of a person (social and self-realization needs). This term has taken on prominence also in sociological theories, as in the "uses and gratifications" theory developed by the scientist E. Katz in the early 1960s. In particular, due to this theory, the attention of researchers has gradually shifted from the characteristics of the media to the expectations of their users, highlighting the active role they have in searching for consumptions capable of meeting – in various ways – the demands of the Ego. Although gratification appears essential to prompt people to act, it is recognized that it can only exist in relation to the expression of a → desire and the consistency of effort. That is, there is no gratification if a desire is systematically satisfied with low commitment and in all conditions. In this sense, also a limited → frustration can serve to elevate the commitment by supporting and increasing the thrust of desire, or in other words, the motivation to succeed. *[S. Smiraglia]*

REFERENCES. Rheinberg F., *Motivation*, 2006.

GREAT MOTHER

A concept derived from the history of religion, which includes multiple forms of a mother-goddess figure. It is a "mother of origins", a chthonic goddess who can be good or bad, fruitful or destructive, incestuous or separating. This is an archetypal concept that, in its negative meaning, represents an archaic and pregenital development phase of mind. In this case, the regression of → libido and the comparison with the great mother underline the numinous and fascinating nature of the great mother herself, who can crush the individual psyche and pose a serious danger to the psyche, as demonstrated by the studies of Jung on schizophrenia. Moreover, his research on the archaic contents of the psyche show that his assumptions about this mythical figure can well adapt to patients with → borderline and narcissistic pathologies. In its positive meaning, the great mother highlights the unconscious dimension and supports the psychological development of a person by promoting a process of psychic integration. *[N. Fina]*

REFERENCES. Jung C.G. (1938–1954), *Psychological aspects of the mother archetype*, in *Collected Works*, IX, 1969; Neumann E., *The great mother*, 1955.

GRID (BION'S)

A tool used to classify statements or thoughts of the psychoanalyst or the patient in order to shed light on their meaning. The horizontal axis comprises the ways in which thoughts/statements are utilized in the context of the relationship: whether the statements are made to further clarify what is happening between the two, and thus increase intimacy (column 1), or whether there is an attempt to mislead and bypass the painful truth (column 2). The vertical axis classifies the stages of development of thoughts, from unthought beta elements, to thought alpha elements, which underlie dream thoughts, preconceptions, conceptions and concepts. In particular, the purpose of the grid is to sharpen the analysts's understanding of what is happening in the session. For example, it can make the therapist more aware of how the patient is reversing the perspective of the interpretation, or of how either the analyst or the patient is avoiding the truth. *[J. Symington]*.

REFERENCES. Bion W.R., *Elements of psychoanalysis,* 1963.

GROUP

Kurt Lewin developed a theory regarding groups both as a dynamic phenomenon and as a factor of social change. Some elements may be found in many other studies: in a group, members have a "destiny" or a common task; the group has a structure of roles and status in relation to each other, provides face-to-face interactions, and may be identified on the basis of a self-categorization. Brown argued that a group exists when two or more individuals are defined as its components and when its existence is recognized by at least one other person, and it is said, resuming the thought of Asch and Sherif, that being part of a group has psychological consequences even when others are not physically present. Membership is at the base of social identity: one of the main consequences is, therefore, the change in the way we perceive ourselves, which influences the self-assessment and the → self-esteem. The bias in favour of their own group (ingroup) is an indirect way to strengthen self-confidence, even though by means of the devaluation of the external group (outgroup). The choice of the group to which individuals may belong is never random, but based on costs and benefits they believe to meet with, on the basis of their past experiences in similar situations, and finally, according to Hogg, on the degree to which an individual perceives himself as a "typical" member of the group. This concept becomes a factor orienting their participation.

In therapeutic contexts, the group → setting was firstly applied by E.W. Lazell in 1919. He started to gather and treat psychotic patients in groups by using "word therapy"; at a later time, the group setting was developed by Bion as a context and an intervention instrument. Nowadays, group therapy refers to different theoretical approaches (Rogersian, existential, dynamic, gestaltic) and adopts different intervention techniques: expressive, elaborative, supportive (→ group techniques). Among the most important forms, it is important to mention T-group, group meeting, group analysis, Gestalt group, sensory/body awareness group and → psychodrama. *[P. Meringolo]*

▷ Bion (→ psychoanalysis (Klein's and Bion's)) distinguishes two types of group activity. The first is the sophisticated or work group in which the group members work towards achieving the goal of the group, as, for example understanding their emotional problems. This work-group activity is continually being interfered with by the powerful → group mind which appears to act on certain → basic assumptions. This group conflict is also manifest in the Establishment, the analytic pair and in the inner world of the individual. It is a matter of whether a creative intercourse between the two can take place leading to growth or whether mutual destruction will ensue. The Church and the Army both use the work group to contain creatively the basic assumptions of the group-mind, respectively the basic assumption of dependency and basic assumption fight–flight. *[J. Symington]*

REFERENCES. Bion W.R., *Experiences in groups*, 1961; Brown R., *Group processes*, 1988; Hogg M.A., *The social psychology of group cohesiveness: From attraction to social identity*, 1992; Lewin K., *Resolving social conflicts*, 1945; Sherif M., *Group conflict and cooperation*, 1966; Tajfel H. (ed.), *Human groups and social categories*, 1981; Turner J.C., *Towards a cognitive redefinition of the social group*, in Id. (ed.), *Social identity and intergroup relations*, 1982.

GROUP ANALYSIS

A type of psychotherapy practiced by the group and for the group, including the leader that focuses his specific attention on the internal/external group world of the single individuals.

The term group analysis was created by T. Burrow but it was S. Foulkes that founded group analysis as a therapeutic method as well as a group clinic. Foulkes' thought was not complicated but complex, often contradictory, influenced by S. Freud, K. Goldstein and N. Elias. Foulkes started work at a particular historical moment (the 1930s and 1940s), in which new epistemological paradigms undermined the old positivist framework. Later, in parallel with the birth of the complexity paradigm, the past-dominating dichotomies waned – as did those between nature and nurture, intrapsychic and interpsychic, mind and body, individual and group; a deviation from the classic object relationship theories, as postulated by psychoanalysis, became dominant. The complexity paradigm had, first of all, the merit of teaching how the internalization of relationships was not limited to the family environment, but involved the whole social and cultural environment. This, and other teachings, have been translated by Foulkes into clinical work. Inspired by Goldstein's intuitions (e.g. the vision of the central nervous system as *network*, in which the single neurons were nodal points), Foulkes imagined human relationships as networks in which the individuals, connected with each other, represented nodal points. These networks had horizontal ramifications (plots of present relationships) as well as vertical branches (biological and cultural past). There was a primary network – or plexus (the family): the most intimate network connected to the individual.

Foulkes believed that only inside this perspective was it possible to fully understand the human mind and psychopathology. This view represented turmoil as seen through the lens of psychoanalytical thought in the past, which considered the individual to be driven more by instinctual than relational needs. As Foulkes wrote: "what is inside is outside, the 'social' is not external but internal and it penetrates the most internal essence of individual personality". And:

> every individual is essentially and inevitably determined by the world he lives in, by the community, by the group, of which he constitutes one part. (. . .) The old contrast between internal and external world, nature and nurture, individual and society, phantasy and reality, mind and body, cannot be maintained.

Group analysis found fertile ground especially in some European countries. In England, for example, numerous contributions developed on the grounds of group analytic theory and practice. Particularly relevant is the creation of the Group Analytic Society by Foulkes himself in London, as well as the first anti-psychiatric community inspired by Jones and Main in Great Britain too. In Italy, numerous theoretic and epistemological developments allowed group analysis to become a theory of personality, psychopathology and clinical methodology, deserving the status of science. Fabrizio and Diego Napolitani were the founders of, respectively, the Institute of Psychoanalysis in Rome in 1963 and the Association of Analyst of Group in Milan in 1968, later known as the Italian Group Analytic Society (1982); these were the first Italian therapeutic communities where group analysis became the main therapeutic instrument. In those years, important contributions came from L. Ancona, F. Vanni, J. Linares and others. Inspired by Foulkes' intuitions, Napolitani founded the "internal groups theory" and he underlined the importance of intentionality as "the way the subject gives his sense to the world and, at the same time, he wants it to accord with the sense he gave it". In other words, the individual is disposed to learn (to assume that they were originally his signs) the signs of intentionality, affection and relational ways that his own environment intends to transmit to him, literally, to teach. There does not exist an individual that is not part of his environment; the individual inhabits a social environment that, in turn, inhabits him. Particularly over the last decades, many branches evolved within/from Italian group analysis. Just think about the family group analysis (in particular by Menarini and Pontalti), the institutional field (A. Correale and F. Fasolo), the social field (Di Maria) and the clinical-epistemological one (Lo Verso). Lo Verso aimed to build a model (subject-relationships group analysis) in order to emphasize the intersubjective dimension and to get over the old and well-known object-relationship model, being more interested in the intrapsychic dimension of individual development.

One of the most interesting theoretical formulations of Italian group analysis is the "transpersonal" defined by Menarini (1989) as the collective impersonal that goes through our most intimate identity without any possibility of conceptualization by our cognitive apparatus. In Lo Verso's formulation, it has been divided into five levels: biological-genetic, ethnic-anthropologic, transgenerational, institutional, socio-communicative. Further developments by Di Maria and G. Lavanco integrated the eco-socio-political aspects, conceptualizing a sixth level called political-environmental. Group analysis is a theoretical and operational instrument whose aim is the cure and transformation of psychic suffering and a better understanding of own internal worlds; it uses a socio-anthropologic view of human events in their multi-individual or transpersonal aspects, in order to constitute a psychology of the personality based on the anthropologic paradigm, whic considers human nature as coincident with his/her culture. From this perspective, transpersonal is considered a psychic dimension of the culture and psychopathology and its symptoms are based at the invisible levels. A group analysis focused on the reading of psychopathology implies the concept of family "intention" (and psychic field), because the family, on one side, ensures the subject growth, containing the individual immaturity; on the other side, it has the duty to leave the spaces of significance of his/her own existence open to the subject. Fundamental is the concept of family matrix, human organization and elemental transpersonal unit that creates, within the care relationship, the mental and psychological dispositions in the baby, and allows her/him, during the following stages of development, to give sense and significance to new events, categorizing and transforming them in mental events and making unsaturated the meaning connections. The family matrix is unsaturated when it allows the cultural themes transmitted by the family to be reviewed and rethought, allowing openness to the new and unknown. The saturated matrix, instead, consists of a worried and occlusive fulfilment from the family (real and/or internal) that does not conceive (does not allow the birth of) the autonomy of its own son. From a therapeutic point of view, the main instrument is the group, but it is possible to work in individual and familial → settings, because the group analyst has to have in mind different settings. Fundamental is the moment of foundation of the group that precedes the leadership. In this sense, Lo Verso's parameters of different settings are really helpful, and they represent a valid instrument to help the clinician to think about different variables of the work he is going to start. Group-analytic–oriented therapeutic groups are in general small groups (five to nine patients), with a non-directive leadership, of medium-long (at least three years) duration. The duration of this kind of therapy is justified by the ambition of the proposed goals, which aim to a symptomatic remission as well as to a transformation of the *self*, to a maturation of psychic structures, to a comprehension/distance from the own internal groups, to an integration of the mind–body relationship. *[G. Lo Verso, I. Formica]*

REFERENCES. Foulkes S.H., *Therapeutic group analysis*, 1964; Id., *Group analytic psychotherapy: Method and principles*, 1986; Id., *Introduction to group-analytic psychotherapy*, 1983; Foulkes S.H., Anthony E.J., *Group psychotherapy: The psychoanalytic approach*, 1965; Di Maria F., Formica I., *Fondamenti di gruppoanalisi*, 2009; Lo Verso G., *Clinica della gruppoanalisi e psicologia*, 1989; Id., *Le relazioni soggettuali*, 1994; Menarini R., *Presentazione*, in G. Lo Verso (ed.), *Clinica della gruppoanalisi e psicologia*, 1989; Napolitani D., *Individualità e gruppalità*, 1987.

GROUP EXPOSURE

In cognitive-behavioural therapy, it is a method of intervention that is not frequently found in literature, based on a confrontation of a hierarchy of localized and feared situations or objects, laid out according in order of increasing difficulty. Since it is carried out in groups of selected individuals and not singly, it allows consistent advantages in terms of beneficial costs and it can take place as → graded exposure or → in-vivo exposure *[A. Cocchi, A. Meneghelli]*

REFERENCES. Gould R.A., Buckminster S., Pollack M.H., Otto M.W., Yap L. *Cognitive-behavioural and pharmacological treatment for social phobia: A meta-Analysis.* «Science and Practice», 1997, 4, 291–306*;* Heimberg R.G., Dodge C.S., Hope D.H. *et al., Cognitive-behavioural group treatment for social phobia: Comparison with a credible placebo control.* «Cognitive Therapy and Research», 1990, 14, 1–3

GROUP PSYCHOTHERAPY

A specific type of psychotherapy whose main aim is to cure; it is performed in a group → setting, in the presence of (one or two) therapists and a limited number of patients. Group psychotherapy was created in 1904 by the pioneering work of Dr. J Pratt with a group of patients with tuberculosis, the aim of which was to think both about medical and psychological aspects of the illness. He noticed that the sessions had a positive impact on the mood of the patients and on the course of their illness. Potential mechanisms underlying these psychosomatic improvements are based on: the possibility of sharing the condition of illness with others; of coming out of psychic isolation; the major attention given to cure and compliance with treatment; and the feeling of being supported by other patients.

Several years later, around 1930, a group of psychotherapists and psychoanalysts started to use the group as a therapeutic instrument with psychiatric patients. In the psychoanalytical field, the main group orientations were commonly defined as analysis *in* group, analysis *of* group, analysis *through* the group. These definitions had a more historical and educational value than a clinical one.

Important contributions to group psychotherapy came from authors such as W. Bion and H. Ezriel. During World War II, Bion developed his interest in groups while he was working in the psychiatric ward of the military hospital in Northfield and, after the end of the war, he conducted groups at the Tavistock Clinic in London. He was considered more a theorist than a clinician and treated the whole ward as a big group, using a non-directive leadership style in order to stimulate in the participants, who appeared quarrelsome and unmotivated to recover, the responsibility for their own recovery. Bion considered the group as a whole, and not the single patients, as the recipient of his therapeutic intervention. Focusing on the group he noticed that there were unconscious drives acting in it that were in opposition to the conscious therapeutic project agreed on by the group. Bion identifies the existence of a psychic reality that catalyzes the emotional life of the group, repeating itself in a typical way and expressing itself through three → basic assumptions (pairing, fight–flight and dependency), which represent → defence mechanisms activated by the group; they are unconscious and often they appear opposite to the rational ideas of the participants. Other important contributions to group psychotherapy come from authors like Whitaker and Lieberman, which had the merit of developing a model of the therapeutic group – called "focal conflict of group" – that could be considered an attempt to integrate the group dynamic of lewinian origin with psychoanalytic theory and practice. The group, in fact, is considered a totality that acts on individuals and on their unconscious conflicts. The focal conflict of the group is an unconscious conflict, shared by its participants, and it develops slowly. Therefore, individual behaviours, expressed in succession on the phenomenology of the group, can be considered as an associative chain referring to an underlying theme on the situation of the → here-and-now in the group. Actually, the conflict is due to the contrast between a disturbing element – a wish – and a reaction – the fear – which pervade the group and orient its energies. The focal conflict solution seems to be a compromise between opposite forces. Further relevant contributions on group psychotherapy come from J.L. Moreno, Yalom, K. McKenzie and S.H. Foulkes, who is a fundamental author in terms of the clinical methodology of the group (→ group analysis). Moreno is known as the inventor of the → psychodrama, a psychological approach that allows the person to express, acting on the scene, different dimensions of his life and to establish links between them. Thanks to its representation on the scene, the psychodrama helps to build a harmonic plot within intrapsychic needs and the requests coming from external reality, and it leads to the discovery and development of one' own spontaneity and creativity. Yalom and McKenzie referred in particular to the study and investigation of "short" groups, focused on symptoms, limited in time and aims: they are groups that activate therapeutic effects based on interpersonal interaction and supportiveness. Particularly important are Yalom's studies on therapeutic factors in group psychotherapy, which he identified as: instillation of hope, universality, imparting information, altruism, corrective recapitulation of primary family group, development of socializing techniques, imitative behaviour, interpersonal learning, group cohesion, catharsis, existential factors (→ therapeutic factors in group psychotherapy). Today there are various "formats" and settings of groups, used in a wide range of areas. There is an increased interest in using groups in psychotherapy because this instrument, if there are the required conditions of aims and specific training, has the same efficacy as individual psychotherapy, and it allows strong experience and relational growth to develop, with reduced costs compared to individual psychotherapy. There are experiences with groups coming from different models than the psychodynamic approach, such as cognitive and systemic approaches. In terms of indications and counterindications of group therapy, it is important to underline that criteria for a correct indication are not easy to identify because they cannot be reduced to a simple classificatory psychiatric diagnosis. Today the problem is not to establish "which patient for which group" but "which group for which patient"; by looking beyond the symptomatology horizons, there is always a group where also the most counterindicated patient for group psychotherapy can find a space for the cure in which he/she can start to feel better. It means that a good psychotherapist, before establishing and conducting a group, has to have the mental flexibility to think about the different settings it depends on. For this reason, we have to take into consideration P. Dell's challenge when he states: "We must stop to ask to ourselves if the patient is suitable for our treatment; we should start to study if our treatment is suitable for the patients". In this regard, Lo Verso highlighted the importance of "going for groups", and particularly the moment of the foundation of the group, which requires a lot of time (metaphorically nine months) and an adequate and competent moment of thought exercised by the psychotherapist that will conduct it.

Therefore, starting a group must be preceded by a series of preliminary questions from the clinician, like: Which group would I like to do? Which are its aims and methods? Will I choose a public or private setting? Is it a homogeneous or heterogeneous group? What is its timing? Will I conduct it by myself? Will I have supervision? etc. These initial questions are fundamental conditions for professional correctness and clinical efficacy in order to define, at a foundation phase, the group, its procedures, as well as its limitations and its possibilities. Groups can be of different types: open, half-open, closed (it depends if it is planned to work with the same patients or with a continuous recycling), as well as homogeneous groups, mono symptomatic and heterogeneous groups, short-terms or long-terms groups, groups for children, adolescents or family, and for different types of disorders (eating disorders, personality disorders, neurosis). Moreover, there are other types of groups (counselling groups, self-help groups, rehabilitations groups) which are not strictly therapeutic, but can offer psychological help anyway. In contrast with the past, today we assist in an extension of empirical research on therapeutic groups, as demonstrated by Lo Coco, Prestano and Lo Verso in a recent study. Empirical research, if considered not merely in a strictly scientific way, can: help to understand differences of methods and results between group psychotherapies and individual psychotherapies; identify the efficacy of groups, what exactly happens in them and what the results are; look at the real complexity of the work of the group where the real variables are the patient and his internal and external world, the therapist (in terms of training, experience, specific competences, personality, etc.), the interaction between them, the group and the socio-institutional context. *[G. Lo Verso, I. Formica]*

REFERENCES. Bion W.R., *Experiences in groups,* 1961; Lo Coco G., Prestano C., Lo Verso G. (eds.), *L'efficacia clinica delle psicoterapie di gruppo,* 2008; Lo Verso G., *Le relazioni soggettuali,* 1994; Whitaker D., Lieberman M.A., *Psychotherapy through the group process,* 1965. Yalom I.D. and Leszcz M., *The theory and practice of group psychotherapy,* 1970.

GROUP TECHNIQUES

The techniques aimed at influencing and directing the processes taking place within a → group of people of small (3 – 20 elements) or large (up to hundreds of elements) dimensions, gathered together for recreational, work, educational or psychotherapeutic purposes. The expression is a contraction of the more complete definition "Group dynamics theories and techniques" (in which the term "dynamics" does not have a psychoanalytic meaning, but indicates the processes taking place in the group). Different "families" of techniques are derived from different theories and their diverse possible modelizations of the dynamics happening in a group (e.g. of its spontaneous and/or of its ideal functioning). Inside those techniques families (e.g. in the physical actions technique) single manoeuvres are identified (e.g. the physiological activation); in their turn, manoeuvres can be inflected in different forms, which in literature are called group's "games" or "exercises" (e.g. walking in a circle at a sustained speed). Some authors and operators tend to wrongly reduce the group dynamics techniques to a set of more or less curious and unusual exercises to be submitted to the group. However, exercises that may appear similar can be in fact employed with very different aims, significance and effects depending on the theory/modelization adopted by the subject proposing them to the group. Nowadays, as far as group techniques are concerned, the most consistent and significant literature and practice refer to the psychosocial and humanistic-existential group theories. *[R.]*

GROUP MIND

According to Bion, a group mind becomes manifest when the individual members of a group anonymously evacuate into the group aspects of themselves for which they take no further personal responsibility. There follows a striking group resistance to any attempt by the group leader to make an interpretation of group dynamics. Thus, the group mind is against mental growth. Bion describes the group mind as operating under one of three → basic assumptions: (i) dependency – when the group needs a leader on which it can be totally dependent, (ii) fight–flight – when the group faces a common enemy and has to prepare to fight it or flee from it, (iii) pairing – when two members form a pair which the group supports in the belief that the pair will produce the solution – the baby – to the group's problem. *[J. Symington]*

REFERENCES. Bion W.R., *Experiences in groups,* 1961.

GUIDED IMAGINATION

Within the cognitive-behavioural approach, a technique in which the patient is asked to imagine situations, sounds, scents, and moods related to stimuli. During this "fantasy" path, the therapist suggests to the patient, step by step, the situation to imagine (for example, a place), actions to be taken and other details considered fundamental for a good psychotherapeutic result. The goal is → relaxation and an increased sense of → wellbeing. Recordings of standard content allow the use of such technique without the presence of a therapist. *[F. Cagnoni]*

REFERENCES. Marks I.M., *Living with Fear: Understanding and coping with anxiety*, 1978.

GUILT

In existential psychoanalysis, a primitive and ineliminable ontological condition of existence due to a predefined project that sees man as "thrown in the world", in which he has no choice but to be in the world where he is. Therefore, guilt can be defined as "being responsible without being free", without having the possibility to eliminate from the world what one has committed. According to existential analytic therapy, guilt is linked to the concepts of freedom and responsibility, and these to the concept of person. The real guilt comes from the Self, both in the sense that it stems from an action that goes against one's Self, that is, against the real development of the person, and in the sense that the Self of the person brings guilt to the surface for the person's own good. The real guilt generates existential anguish and produces consciousness of guilt. It can originate from the unconscious from intrauterine life and often it can be found locked inside a sense of guilt. Guilt is formed by complex organizations of thoughts, decisions, and behaviours made of a single substance: unconscious hate. *[D. Romagnoli, S. Antonetti]*

REFERENCES. Mercurio A., *Amore, libertà e colpa*, 1980.

H

HABIT

A tendency to reproduce behaviours, actions, thoughts or emotions automatically and without any voluntary effort as a result of previously learned experiences. Such a repertoire of responses may concern very complex behaviours and can be activated even in the absence of the stimuli that initially contributed to their formation. In psychotherapy, mental and behavioural *habitus* can be the specific object of change. In particular, some forms of psychotherapy, such as those that are mainly behavioural (see the opening chapter, "The eight paradigms and their respective theoretical-applicative models"), base much of their work on changing dysfunctional habits. The term → dysfunctional is used here to indicate any strongly maladaptive behaviour that, as such, is a source of mental suffering for the subject. In any therapeutic intervention, patients' habits represent a dimension that needs to be taken into account since it tends inevitably to delineate their lifestyle. *[R.]*

HADES

Chthonic God and, by extension, underworld in Greek mythology. He kidnapped Persephone, daughter of Zeus (accomplice in the kidnapping) and Demeter (Goddess linked with motherhood of Earth and vegetation). His mother caused a terrible famine for revenge. Zeus then solved the situation in this way: Persephone would spend six months a year on Earth with her mother (these months became the months of fertility of the earth, of spring and summer) and six months in the underworld with Hades. In Jungian analytical psychology it represents the *nekyia*, the detachment from the upper world of consciousness and the descent into the evanescent and dark underworld of the unconscious. *[A. Cannavina]*

REFERENCES. Jung C.G. (1944), *Pychology and alchemy*, in *Collected Works*, VIII, 1968; Kerényi K., *The heroes of the Greeks*, 1959.

HAPPY CONVERSATION

In conversational therapy, a happy conversation is the result of a "verbal trade" that makes the maximum profits both for the "seller" and for the "buyer". It is a bilateral verbal trade, where two traders, for example, a therapist and a patient, exchange verbal goods. When the traders of words earn, there is a happy conversation. When they lose, they have an unhappy conversation. Aphasia is the catastrophic loss of the trade, the silence of the conversation. The trader of words, for example the therapist, studies and uses all the means and the appropriate incentives to pursue the goal of a happy conversation and to avoid an unhappy conversation. The application range of happy goes from disorders treated by psychoanalysis to the treatment of aphasias and conversations with company managers. *[G. Lai]*

REFERENCES. Lai G., *La conversazione felice*, 1985; Id., *L'eternità sulla Piazza del Mercato. Bilateral verbal trade*, 2011

HAVING

A term introduced by Fromm to indicate an existential condition based on a neurotic need to own things or people that has its roots in the oral stage (→ libidinal development stages). Fromm distinguishes between an "existential" having aimed at staying alive, and a "characterological" having, based on voracity, expressed by the person who is driven by an illusory but reassuring perception of permanence – of themselves and of what they manage to have – and who identifies themself with their own objects, in a non-productive and unsatisfying relationship. The lack of one's own → being is not solved and always generates the same drive to possession. This meaning of "having" defines our sick, alienating society, characterized by an insatiable hunger of consumerism and the absence of a healthy natural interpersonal communication, which belongs to the existential nature of being. *[E. Benelli, G. Rombolà Corsini, M. Zetti]*

REFERENCES. Fromm E., *The sane society*, 1955; Id., *To have or to be?*, 1976.

HEALER

It is a person who, with the help of → rituals and methodologies that are not recognized by modern science, heals or pretends to heal, and sometimes declares himself as a means of → communication with divine entities. This term is used in anthropological-religious disciplines, ethnopsychiatry and ethnopsychotherapy, to indicate people that can relieve pain and cure various disorders. The figure of the healer, although in different and distinct forms, can be found in the history of most of past and modern cultures under different names such as "shaman", "segnatore", "curandero", "exorcist", "santon", "thaumaturge", "sorcerer", "wizard", "prophet", etc. Healers do not distinguish mental disorders from other types of disorders and in some cultures their supposed powers can also be attributed to places and oracles. The cases of healing, mostly of psychosomatic and somatoform disorders, can be connected to mechanisms based on the → logic of belief and on → suggestion. Often, there is a belief that an object or a spirit has settled in the body of the sufferer. The cure must expel it through a ritual ceremony, an event that often involves a part of the community, which represents the interest of the collective in the problems of the individual. → Healing rituals are often characterized by hypnotic trance states (→ hypnosis) induced by substances or simply by ritual contexts themselves, which are marked by dances, songs, sounds or rhythmic movements that facilitate the emergence of altered state of consciousness. *[R.]*

HEALING

A positive resolution of an invalidating condition. In medicine, it means to restore the body's health according to a criterion of biological normality. In psychology, the concept of healing is more ambiguous because a mental disorder is not a disease that changes the course of existence, but it is the change of existence itself: thus, it is an experience, a piece of life, a → crisis and an event that changes a person. Considering that life is a continuous → adaptation from an earlier psychological balance to a subsequent one, an individual may come across difficulties, obstacles, crises, sometimes called "disorders" or imbalances, which can be overcome or healed through psychotherapeutic treatment. In psychotherapy, the term healing takes on different meanings depending on the paradigm of reference. Existentialists and humanists interpret healing as growth and maturation. According to psychoanalysts, healing means understanding the dynamics underlying a crisis. Behaviourists and cognitivists consider it as the result of a review of → conditioning, schemes and inappropriate behaviour. From the perspective of → constructivism, which disputes the distinction between normality and abnormality, healing can be achieved only when a patient or a → system (family, couple, school, etc.) perceive and recognize that the "evil" that troubled them is no longer invalidating. To this day, there is a great difficulty in assessing accurately the → efficacy of a psychotherapeutic intervention, as it is very difficult to obtain objective and unbiased measurements. *[R.]*

HELPLESSNESS

A temporary or permanent impossibility, for an individual, to act and use his or her personal resources to achieve his or her own goals. Helplessness can be associated with lack of confidence (lowering of → self-esteem and loss in believing in one's own success), behavioural inhibition, depression, → alienation. As stated by H. Laborit, the body is a system aimed at action and the feeling/awareness of not being able to act effectively – which can, or not, be based on real elements – represents a significant blow to an individual's vital motivations. In this perspective, M. Seligman has theorized "learned helplessness" as the basis of many forms of maladjustment and distress in adolescents (in particular, demotivation and school failure) and in adults. In a nutshell, there are social and existential circumstances in which individuals suffer from the inability to resolve a situation of impediment. On this basis, → frustration and negativity transfer people's anxiety into situations where, instead, action would be possible and decisive: people learn to think pessimistically and therefore they think and act helplessly. *[S. Smiraglia]*

▷ Freud linked the state of helplessness of newborns to their biological immaturity. He used the term *Hilflosigkeit* – usually translated as helplessness – to designate the complete dependence of newborns on their mother, who appears as "the only object that can protect from the risks of the outside world". In 1925, Freud argued that the separation or loss of the mother exposes the child not only to internal but also to external risks, causes an overwhelming state of tension and creates "the need to be loved which will accompany the child through the rest of its life". In this way, the complete helplessness of the newborn causes the omnipotence of the mother, establishes the first situations of risk and influences significantly the structure of one's psychic life. *[F. Ortu]*

REFERENCES. Freud S. (1925–1926), *An Autobiographical study, Inhibitions, symptoms and anxiety, The question of lay analysis*, in The Standard Edition, XX, 1953–1974; Laplanche J., Pontalis J.B., *The language of psychoanalysis*, 1988.

HERE-AND-NOW

As a distinction between the concept of time and that of the "here-and-now", the following platonic assumption can be applied: "was" and "will be" are part of time, even if it is only the "is" that incarnates the authentic dimension as a point of conjunction between instant and eternity. In this way, in the West, it is the basis of the connection between time and thought that proved to be a constant in philosophy and a determining factor in psychology. Given the historical dependence of psychiatric thought on the predominant current epistemological thinking, the theoretical models adopted over time in psychology vary widely in the use they make of the construct of "time". In this way, in the psychodynamic model, the here-and-now is conceptualized as the result of all the past causes, from an intrapsychic, causal and deterministic point of view, where the psychic data brought to therapy are submitted to a kind of preliminary logical examination. In the psychological models that are phenomenologically derived, on the other hand, the focus is placed on the exchange between the subject and his environment, viewed as a phenomenological unit that is based on science. This is the reality. And it is in this place that the concept of exchange of information, in other words "communication" becomes crucial. The here-and-now of being human is in fact the definition of the field of study of the theory of communication (→ pragmatics of human communication). The study of communication is the investigation of how people influence each other in a reciprocal manner through the use of messages vehicled by behaviour: more generally, one can say that it deals with the study of the → interaction in the here-and-now, between organsisms and their → environment, perceived as being the reality of the given moment. *[R.]*

▷ In the → brief therapy – MRI's model, the focus of therapy is circumscribed to the present moment, or rather on the *hic et nunc* of the conversation. During a game of chess, in fact, in any given moment, it is possible to understand the situation of the game without needing to refer to a "memory" of the past moves; it is only necessary to observe the configuration of the pieces on the chess board. Extending the metaphor of G. Bateson to the therapeutic situation (→ interaction-focused therapy), the direct observation of the communication between the individual and the persons around him that are important to him is considered as being very useful in reaching the aim of discovering models of → communication in the here-and-now; however, the contents of these concepts are not demonstrable: if it is true that behaviour is influenced by past experiences, it is also true that memory is a "construction" and therefore it is not a reliable source of information. Psychology is both a subject and an object of study: it is not possible to find an Archimedean point outside of the mind; the human mind studies itself and tends to automatically confirm itself: the intrapsychic forces are unverifiable (the mind as a "black box"). The problem of how people attribute meaning is therefore bracketed. The prospective study of psychological problems that results from this is ahistorical: intrapsychic experiences that are subjective are not studied, but the attention is focused on the behaviour within the relationship in the here-and-now. *[M. Genchi]*

▷ For Gestalt therapy, the here-and-now is the space–time dimension by means of which the psychologically healthy person puts her/himself in → contact with her/himself and with the world. From the phenomenological point of view, this dimension goes back to the experience of the person's body, her/his feelings, her/his emotions, her/his reality. By means of the "continuum of → consciousness", remaining in contact with what is occurring in the here-and-now, the unresolved situation or the unfulfilled need come powerfully to light in order to be faced. The open Gestalt, which emerges on the surface of the here-and-now, finds expression in the spontaneous movements of the body, in the voice, in nonverbal behaviours. Paying attention to the experience, which is flowing in the present, enables the support of the patient's process of awareness, to delineate her/his intentionality and orientation in the "field" (→ field theory) to integrate the polar conflicts, to recompose the unity between feeling and acting. More recently, Stern has developed interesting reflections on the "present moment", identifying it as a basic psychological experience and as the founding element of every intersubjective relationship. *[M. Spagnuolo Lobb, P.A. Cavaleri]*

REFERENCES. Cavaleri P.A., *La dialettica polare nella psicoterapia della Gestalt*, in «Quaderni di Gestalt», 1996, 22–23; Id., *Dal campo al confine di contatto. Contributo per una riconsiderazione del confine di contatto in psicoterapia della Gestalt*, in M. Spagnuolo Lobb (ed.), *Psicoterapia della Gestalt. Ermeneutica e clinica*, 2001; Id., *La profondità della superficie. Percorsi introduttivi alla psicoterapia della Gestalt*, 2003; Perls F., Hefferline R.F., Goodman P., *Gestalt therapy: Excitement and growth in the human personality*, 1951; Spagnuolo Lobb M., *The now-for-next in psychotherapy*, 2013; Stern D.N., *The present moment*, 2004; Watzlawick P., Beavin J.H., Jackson Don D., *Pragmatics of human communication*, 1967.

HERMENEUTICS

A discipline that investigates the theory and methodology of the interpretation (of texts, documents, speeches, signs or even historical periods) of past and present reality, making sense from the knowledge of the historical characteristics and cultural traditions into which the thing being investigated was born. With hermeneutics, also the concept of truth is reformulated. This is not considered stable and unchangeable any more, but relative, linked to historical epochs and different societies, apart from individual sensibility and culture. Many forms of psychotherapy, such as psychoanalysis, make hermeneutics an instrument of knowledge and action on the internal psychological world of the patient (also see → interpretation). *[R.]*

HERO

In Jungian thought, an individual who is "a bridge" between the human and the superhuman condition. Jung writes:

> The god is by nature wholly supernatural; the hero's nature is human but raised to the limit of the supernatural – he is semi-divine [. . .] The hero's supernaturalness includes the human nature and thus represents a synthesis of the ("divine," i.e., not yet humanized) unconscious and human consciousness.

A man who aspires to be a god is likely to fall into psychopathology, as he denies the nature and the necessary limits of human beings. Instead, the heroic path can, under certain conditions, be helped by analysis: on this path, facing the energy and the symbols contained in the unconscious does not exclude keeping awareness of an individual's limitations. *[G. Cavallari]*

REFERENCES Jung C.G. (1934–1954), *The archetypes and the collective unconscious*, in Collected Works, IX, 1969; Neumann E., *The origins and history of consciousness*, 1954.

HEURISTICS

It is the art and technique of searching for solutions. The heuristic process is not based on a rigid application of procedures, but on intuitive, rapid, analogical and often creative cognitive strategies. Heuristics are at the basis of most therapeutic → problem-solving methods and they can end up structuring real algorithms on processes of change in psychotherapy, starting with the application of → techniques, → strategies and → stratagems. These can simplify the complexity of a problem and have a direct impact on the variables that produce a rupture of a pathogenic balance. Therefore, structuring an algorithm of therapeutic change may be the point of arrival of a heuristic process. In psychotherapy, two opposite and extreme positions can be identified. Some scholars claim the impossibility of structuring heuristic models, such as techniques, languages, → prescriptions and formalized → protocols treatments and consider each situation as unique and unrepeatable. According to them, clinicians need to reinvent, each time, a new therapeutic solution to respect the uniqueness of each patient. Conversely, some models overemphasize heuristics to the point where they become a rigid and sometimes reductivist (→ reductivism) application of standard therapy protocols. In this case, the search for an apparent rigour runs the risk of eliminating insight and inventiveness, which are instead essential foundations of heuristics *[R.]*

HIERARCHY

In strategic family therapy, the concept of hierarchy has a triple meaning. The first describes the power and its structure in families. This aspect of hierarchy concerns the role of differentiation between parents and children, as well as the barriers between generations. The second meaning defines the organization of logical types or logical hierarchies, in which a lower order of logical types is a subset of a higher order. The third meaning indicates a hierarchy of increasingly inclusive systemic levels. For example, a single member of a → family is a system that is logically subordinated to the family system. In the same way, a family is subordinated to a "community" system and a community system to a "society". *[R.]*

REFERENCES. Simon F.B., Stierlin H., Wynne L.C., *The language of family therapy: A systemic vocabulary and sourcebook*, 1985.

HISTORICAL TRUTH

In psychoanalysis, according to Spence, it is a faithful reconstruction of what has really happened in a patient's story. Therefore, it is a report that allows the therapist to decide if what the patient is saying, as it has a place in a definite time and follows adequate rules of conformity, corresponds to a sort of exact transcription of the past. The research of an historical truth is implicit in S. Freud's metaphor of the work of archaeology, which, through fragments and associations, rebuilds an existing reality that contains elements of the real past of the patient. In historical truth, importance is attributed to the act of remembering itself. Nevertheless, Freud himself knew that also memories are transformed and reread according to the concept of *Nachträglichkeit* ("deferred action") and reorganized in accordance with personal meanings. *[A.M. Speranza]*

REFERENCES. Spence D.P., *Narrative and historical truth*, 1982.

HOLDING

According to Winnicott (→ psychoanalysis (Independent or Middle Group of British analysts)), it is the mother's ability to support her child during the development process. This term deliberately refers to both a mother's ability to physically support her children and protect them from physiological offences, taking into account their specific sensitivity and adapting to the changes that take place during their development, and the psychological ability of a → good-enough mother to contain a child's anguish. The holding process promotes integration, which allows children to build a sense of continuity in the experience of their true Self. The risk of failure in this integration is represented by disintegration, the unthinkable anguish linked to falling apart, falling forever, being without any relation with the body, being without orientation (the raw material of psychotic anguish). In therapy, the holding process is considered a specific mental function of the therapist, who can contain patients' anxieties and allow them to have a transformative experience of continuity and containment. *[A.M. Speranza]*

REFERENCES. Winnicott D.W., *Through paediatrics to psychoanalysis*, 1958; Id., *The maturational process and the facilitating environment*, 1965.

HOLISM

A philosophical theory based on the concept that the whole is greater than the sum of its component parts. The term, coined by J. Smuts, was later developed into a more exhaustive definition, which better detailed some concepts: each part is part of a whole and cannot be studied separately from the rest; each part contains the whole; the parts – i.e. the objects of study such as cells, organs, apparatuses or mental processes – are considered fractions of the macro-process of "wholeness".

According to the holistic approach in psychology, a person is considered a mind–body whole which, therefore, should not be investigated independently from the complex macro-system to which it belongs. Consequently, holism introduces three different views: subjective, which refers to the individual; ecological, which includes the ecological and planetary macro-system; energetic, which refers to the extended mind (→ mind–body model). The first concept is strictly biological and it involves the neurophysiological and biochemical processes of the human body, which are seen as interacting with each other and with mental processes; the second concept concerns the interplay between human beings and the world around them (the environment, the ecosystem, the biosphere); the third concept encompasses the process of interconnection and interdependence with the mental-energetic dimension to which we belong. *[G. Pagliaro]*

REFERENCES. Laszlo E., *Evolution: The grand synthesis*, 1987; Lovelock J.E., *Gaia*, 1979.

HOMEOSTASIS

A concept introduced for the first time in the nineteenth century by the French physicist C. Bernard, with reference to the capacity of organisms to maintain a stable internal balance, thanks to processes of regulation and counter-regulation that go into action every time there is a variation in their external environment. The concept of homeostasis within the field of psychotherapy is closely related to the concept of → resistance to change and refers to the tendency of every system, whether this be an individual, a couple or a family, to strive to maintain its own equilibrium even in cases where these are recognized by the system itself as being dysfunctional (→ functional, equilibrium). In order for an effective psychotherapeutic → change to be maintained over time, therapy has to lead to the interruption of the initial dysfunctional homeostasis and to the establishment and consolidation of a new homeostatic equilibrium. If this does not take place, it is very likely that the person (or couple or family), will revert to the old dysfunctional system when faced with a difficulty, particularly if this has been its system for a long time, as happens for example in the case of pathologies that are very serious and long-standing such as obsessive-phobic syndromes and eating disorders.

In the approach adopted by the Milan School of Psychotherapy, the term homeostasis is used to refer to the internal stability of a → system that is maintained through a process of self-regulation. Don D. Jackson was the first to apply this concept to family systems and used it to describe pathological family systems and their mechanisms, which were characterized by excessive rigidity, lack of flexibility and a limited ability to evolve. *[R.]*

HOMEWORK

Also called "tasks to be performed at home", it concerns tasks of self-observation and of mental states and/or behaviour modification, which the therapist agrees upon and prescribes to patients during a session and which patients do later outside the session itself. Homework is used, with different methods and aims, in cognitive-behavioural therapy, but also in interpersonal psychotherapy. In the strategic model, structured homework – or paradoxical prescriptions – are a decisive factor in the change process; these are of three types: direct prescriptions (clear instructions to be executed); indirect prescriptions (behavior injunctions that mask the real target); paradoxical prescriptions. Homework is mostly used in cognitive-behavioural therapy, which distinguishes behavioural, affective and cognitive homework. Behavioural homework concerns prescriptions given to patients about a behaviour to be adopted in a particular situation: for example, the shame-attacking exercises are recommended to patients with social phobia in situations of social exposure; cognitive homework refers to tasks that require the person to activate cognitive processes, as in the case of cognitive reformulation: for example, patients are asked to fill out a card with their predictions and expectations about a feared event and then they are asked to think about possible alternatives; finally, emotional homework is very useful in dealing directly with negative emotions through visualization techniques such as rational emotive imagery. This consists in making patients imagine a vivid and detailed personal experience that really happened – or that they fear could happen – and browse the emotions experienced in relation to the real or hypothetical event. Homework is important in the therapeutic process as it allows patients to acquire the necessary knowledge and the tools to control their problems, thus increasing psychological autonomy and self-efficacy. Patients, once they have completed their homework, experience a strong sense of self-efficacy, which is useful to break the vicious circle "I cannot do it, therefore I'm worthless". Also, homework influence the therapeutic → relationship: by feeling an active part of the changing process, the patient controls, operationally, task after task, what is discussed and analyzed in the sessions and this increases the credibility and reliability of the therapist from the patient's point of view; moreover, the patient can verify that psychotherapy takes care of solving concrete and practical problems, and with homework the patient learns that by inhibiting a particular behaviour (for example, social-exposure avoidance for people with social phobia), → emotions (anxiety, shame) can be faced and the associated thoughts (inadequacy, failure) changed. For the therapist, homework is an instrument to verify the results achieved through the therapy or the limits that are still present; when giving tasks, the therapist should not adopt a directive attitude with patients: "tasks", in fact, should be agreed between therapist and patient, who should discuss what might happen if the tasks are not performed, in order to prevent discouragement and lack of motivation in the patient. *[M. Procacci, C. Petracca]*

REFERENCES. Baldini F., *Homework: Un'antologia di prescrizioni terapeutiche*, 2004; Bandura A., *Self-efficacy: The Exercise of control*, 1997; De Silvestri C., *Il mestiere di psicoterapeuta: Manuale pratico di psicoterapia cognitivo-emotivo-comportamentale*, 1999; Nardone G., Watzlawick P., *The art of change*, 1993; Weissman M.M., Markowitz J.C., *Interpersonal psychotherapy current status*, in «Archives of General Psychiatry», 1994, 51.

HOMOSEXUALITY

If sexual orientation is a consequence of the object to whom the erotic and/or romantic attraction is directed, the homosexual person is the one attracted by a same-sex individual. Even if the term is commonly related to the heterosexual–homosexual continuum, the concept of sexual orientation is more complex and composed of: erotic attraction, sexual phantasies, sexual behaviours, affective and/or romantic fascination, self-definition and social representation, and the cultural context in which the sexuality is expressed. For these reasons, it seems proper to refer to homosexuality in the plural form: the homosexualities (similarly, the heterosexualities). For a long time, homosexual orientation has been considered a psychopathological manifestation of human development and only since 1970s has started to be considered as a normal variation of human sexuality. In 1973, the American Psychiatric Association (APA) eliminated the diagnosis of homosexuality from the *Diagnostic and Statistical Manual of Mental Disorders* (→ diagnostic manuals). In 1991, the American Psychoanalytic Association approved a document in which it deplores any public and private discrimination against lesbians and gay men and invites training institutes not to select candidates on the basis of their sexual orientation. The scientific community permanently disowned the so-called "conversion therapies", which have the purpose of "treating" homosexuality, and, in general, any treatment based on the thesis that homosexuality is a mental disorder and that sexual orientation could be modified by a "therapeutic" intervention. In the psychological and psychoanalytical field, many authors have contributed to constructing an approach to homosexuality free from prejudices, such as: J. Butler, N. Chodorow, J. Drescher, R. Hopcke, R. Isay, S. Mitchell, R. Roughton. Today, homosexuality is no longer considered a topic for research in psychopathology, and clinical attention is more and more aimed at investigating homophobia in its psychological, social and institutional aspects (including the "internalized homophobia", that is, when the social stigma is internalized by the homosexual person themself). *[V. Lingiardi]*

REFERENCES. Drescher J. *Psychoanalytic therapy and the gay man*, 1998. Isay R., *Being homosexual: Gay men and their development*, 1996; Lingiardi V., *Citizen gay: Affetti e diritti*, 2012; Rigliano P., Graglia M. (eds.), *Gay e lesbiche in psicoterapia*, 2006.

HOT SEAT

In Gestalt psychotherapy, the original linguistic form, *hot seat*, means chair that is "on fire", in a visual sense. But, besides being an instrument for the creation of a focal point, it is also the place where the person assumes responsibility for his communication and, for this reason, in the tradition of Gestalt psychotherapy, it has taken on the meaning of a "hot" seat in an emotional sense. In practice, it is the classical form in which the Gestalt → setting presents itself: three chairs placed in a triangular shape; the therapist is seated on one of these chairs; on the other the patient; on the third chair, which remains empty, will sit the problematic interlocuters enacted by the patient. Each chair faces the space in-between the other two chairs, as a reminder that every human being is the result of a dialectic contraposition of internal parts, and that, in order to truly understand a person, it is within this contraposition that one has to look, that is, in the intrapsychic processes that animate the emotional world. In reality, with the "hot seat" one intends a tripolar situation, where the patient present himself in his relationship with the therapist as being intrinsically ambivalent: for this reason, he talks from two separate positions, represented visually by two different chairs or simply considered as two different points of view that the person imagines taking on in an alternative manner, in such a way as to manifest the dialectical relationship with himself. In the Gestalt approach, the internal interlocuters, both those arising from dreams as well as those arising from memories, are considered to be parts of the self even when they appear as other persons, and the dialogue between these aspects is considered to be fundamental (→ dialogic relationship), from the point of view of the development of awareness and of the abilities that are necessary to manage internal conflicts that are present in every human being. In this sense the hot seat is nothing but a fundamental technical instrument that allows the creative handling of a conflict after it has been internalized. *[P. Quattrini]*

REFERENCES. Naranjo C., *Techniques of Gestalt therapy*, 1973; Perls F., *Gestalt therapy verbatim*, 1969; Perls F., Hefferline R.F., Goodman P., *Gestalt therapy: Excitement and growth in the human personality*, 1951; Polster E., Polster M., *Gestalt therapy integrated: Contours of theory and practice*, 1973.

HOW-TO-WORSEN TECHNIQUE

In → brief strategic psychotherapy Nardone's model, a paradoxical problem-solving technique (→ paradox) aimed at focusing the patient's attention on the mechanisms that further aggravate their malaise, increasing awareness and aversion towards them. In strategic terms, the technique aims to identify, correct or interrupt the usual dysfunctional solutions (→ attempted solutions) implemented by the patient in the attempt to control and/or solve their problem, but that, on the contrary, feed it. The technique can be used in two main ways: questioning and prescriptive. In the first case, the patient is given a question to ponder between two sessions, with the request to find the answers on a rational level. The question is expressed in a suggestive and redundant way. An example could be: "Between now and the next meeting I ask you, maybe dedicating five minutes a day to this task, to find all the answers to the following question: If I wanted to voluntarily and deliberately worsen, instead of improve, my situation, what should I do or not do, what should I think or not think? Bring all the answers with you". The interrogative variation of the "how-to-worsen technique" is often used for phobic and phobic-obsessive disorders during the first of the strategic therapy phases. This typically has three types of result: the person can identify the main and redundant attempted solutions implemented (usually this new awareness translates into an improvement due to the voluntary interruption of them);

the person changes their previous way of thinking in dealing with their disorder, paving the way for alternative and creative solutions; the person brings a detailed lists of their most difficult situations concerning, typically, the phobic and obsessive-compulsive area, allowing the therapist to plan, even more fittingly, the therapeutic strategies to use. In the prescriptive form of the technique, particularly used in obsessive, paranoid and/or depressive disorders, the patient is indirectly given a paradoxical prescription (→ symptom prescription, → paradox logic). This is to ask themselves every morning, before starting the day's activities, what they should do to intentionally ruin their day and/or what ways they should contrive to provoke malaises or deliberately accentuate their disorder. As can easily be understood, this reflection and this morning plan create in the patient a strongly adversarial perception towards all those pejorative behaviours or dysfunctional thoughts that typically feed the disorder. The technique has its roots in Taoist philosophy applied to the art of → stratagems, and can be found in the stratagem "twist more to straighten". *[A. Bartoletti]*

REFERENCES. Fisch R., Weakland J.H., Segal L., *The tactics of change: Doing therapy briefly*, 1982; Nardone G., *Non c'è notte che non veda il giorno*, 2003; Id., *Cavalcare la propria tigre*, 2003; Nardone G., Balbi E., *The logic of therapeutic change*, 2015;

HUMAN AGENCY

In neo-behavioural therapy, the ability to behave actively in the environment with the aim of transforming it. Bandura's social-cognitive theory considers individuals as able to exert an → influence on events. This belief, called self-efficacy, determines behaviours, which therefore do not depend exclusively on the external results of an action, as in the classic behavioural paradigm. Human agency operates through three classes of interacting causes: internal personal factors, implemented behaviour, environmental events. The theoretical construct of human agency finds application in education, health psychology, sports, work and, in psychotherapy, in anxiety, mood, nutrition and substance abuse disorders. *[F. Celi]*

REFERENCES. Bandura A., *Human agency: The rhetoric and the reality*, in «American Psychologist», 1991, 46; Id., *Self-efficacy: Toward a unifying theory of behavioural change*, 1977.

HUMAN CREATIVE IMPULSE

In the psychoanalytical framework it basically represents the yearning for immortality. Beginning with *The Trauma of Birth,* Rank stopped considering, as he had in his previous work, artistic creativeness as based on sexual drives and their repression. On the one hand, creative impulse cannot be fully equalized to the sexual drive; on the other hand, it conflicts with life. If the neurotic is "an artist *manqué*" because of his fear of experiencing a "totally merged" condition, the artist desires immortality to protect himself/herself from a true experience of life. Both "types" have to be overcome. Rank predicts the end of art (together with the end of psychoanalysis) and argues that the creative impulse is a necessary element of support in personality development. In other words, creativity cannot be strictly assimilated into either sexual impulse or artistic production. *[G. Antonelli]*

REFERENCES. Rank O., *Kunst und Künstler*, 1932

HUMAN NATURE

The etymological meaning of the word "nature" is "that which exists to generate", or rather, "the force that generates". In this respect, Aristotle asserted that everything is organized according to an internal natural principle that pushes towards the realization of one's essence (for example, the seed is oriented towards becoming a tree). Analogously, the Stoics talked about a vital and harmonic function – "the concept of the breath of life" (*pneuma*) – that penetrates the universe, that organizes the universe and that directs everything in it according to a rational and necessary order. The nature of things would therefore be an intrinsically rational principle that inherently establishes the goal of realizing one's own essence, a process described as proceeding in a harmonic manner. The application of this definition to human beings has led us to be able to describe human nature as a collection of tendencies, innate and permanent inclinations that make human beings what they are, in a philosophical, psychological, spiritual and moral sense. In this sense, the total fulfilment of human nature would be the adaptation to an ideal prototype that, although "inscribed" in man, cannot, however be ever completely attained.

In this sense, in psychology, the term "human nature" is regarded with some scepticism because it implies an *a priori*, anthropological vision that establishes what is normal and what is pathological, and what are the "true" goals to which the human being should aspire. In the course of history, psychiatric, political and religious institutions have attempted – and continue to attempt to this very day – to assert their power by trying to impose their own definition of human nature. Unfortunately, in the field of psychotherapy the concept of human nature carries with it the definition of what needs to be cured and changed, or else defines what is just, as being "natural", and what is unjust, as being "unnatural". In these cases, the "social norm" greatly influences a medical-psychological discipline. *[R.]*

HUMAN NEEDS

In the field of humanistic psychology, Maslow proposed an interesting classification of human needs – the graphical representation of which is known as "Maslow's pyramid" – and ordered them in "higher" and "lower" needs. He placed them according to their hierarchical and evolutionary relationship and in sequence by intensity and priority. All levels of need represent a transition on the path towards the realization of the Self. The hierarchy consists of five different levels, from the most elementary (necessary for the survival of the individual) to the most complex (social needs). Individuals "realize" themselves, that is, identify the most authentic Self, passing progressively through the various stages, which are: physiological needs (hunger, thirst, etc.); needs for safety, security and protection; needs for belonging (affection, identification); needs for esteem, prestige, success; and needs for self-realization (realizing their own identity and expectations and occupying a satisfactory position in the social group). Motivations are subject to constant transformation within the subjectivity and perception of the subject: a need considered crucial at a given time may be perceived differently over time, and can be differently valued by a person versus another, also in connection with the socio-cultural environment.

Also Fromm developed a fundamental theory of needs. Psychological needs are summarized in *Psychoanalysis of Contemporary Society* and developed throughout the complex elaboration of his thought. He affirms that human social order is not adequate to the real potential of man; it does not give value to his authenticity and does not go along with his natural need for self-realization. According to Fromm, an *a priori* harmony between man and society does not exist, and man's effort lies in the continuous attempt to adapt, looking for a balance between internal and external instances, social needs and individual needs: ultimately, between the way of → being and the way of → having. According to Fromm, in addition to essential needs related to self-preservation (such as hunger, thirst, reproduction), man has five equally important basic needs: relatedness, transcendence, rootedness, sense of identity and frame of orientation. These needs arise naturally in human beings and derive from the processes of their evolution. They are not disconnected from each other and constitute a multidimensional grid, more than a ladder, as they are interconnected and variously interpreted according to the different structures of → character types. Psychological needs, together with basic needs, are useful when attempting to resolve the existential paradox in a dynamic relationship between individual and society. Fromm did not follow a schematic distinction, but he used the map of psychic needs as a frame of orientation in the journey that man takes between the drive for self-preservation and the inclination towards his psychological development. Man's adaptation is therefore a complex set of elements that belong to internal and external needs, looking for a dialectic compromise in the social scenario and its organizations – above all, family. The modes of existence postulated by Fromm, → having and → being, converge on the necessity to meet needs. Both modes are potentialities of human nature: at the basis of the having mode lies the biological factor related to survival. At the basis of being lies the need to overcome isolation, which, according to Fromm, is a specific condition of human existence – the needs of being can be considered a psycho-socio-economic cost that man bears as a result of the separation from nature and his gradual autonomy – since man needs to live within an organized society as a response to the rift between his identity and that nature in which he was immersed until he became fully aware of his existence. The prerequisites of being are freedom and autonomy, which motivate the efforts towards the development of the processes of awareness and critical thinking, in which man is finally protagonist of his existence and rejoins others in a reciprocal, authentic and supportive relationship. From the perspective of humanistic psychoanalysis, the having mode concerns the possession of things and their extensions. It supports narcissistic needs and their persistence in a neverending hypothesis of gratification, to the point that things possess man and not vice versa; so much so as to affect the personal identity that winds around conflict – between individuals as well as between nations – around greed, the tyranny of time, the irrevocable acquisition of knowledge and authority, the anxious search for certainty and security. The being mode concerns a conception of needs such as those indicated by Fromm, related to creativity, transcendence, competence, dialogue, joint participation, harmony with others and with the world, shared enjoyment, the timelessness of the creative act (which transcends time) and some indescribable experiences in man.

According to Fromm, human history began when people, by becoming aware of their existence, broke the bond that kept them immersed in nature. In the same way, the individual history of each person, their path towards identification and self-realization, originates in the separation from the mother. Man comes into contact with his loneliness when, free from the physical dependency of the caregiver, the primary natural ties with the mother dissolve and this activates a process of recognition in which he feels that he has irretrievably lost the primordial union with the maternal womb and the support, the nourishment and the wealth that are ensured by it. The individual, although gradually, emerges alone and without any chance of getting back. In order to define and integrate his identity, he will have to get in touch with the anguish aroused by this condition. Moreover, the condition of isolation is generated, in a dual effect, by the organization of human life with its social structures. This organization has led to fundamental achievements, such as the supremacy over nature, the development of reason, the creation of bonds, which are socially useful for mutual survival; but it has also generated an additional condition of solitude and isolation. The need to transcend isolation finds satisfaction in the act of creation, where it is possible to transcend time, to gain experience in the → here-and-now, to exit the narrow passage between past and future. The need for transcendence is therefore man's attempt to rise through his own "creativity". This need, according to Fromm, exists even when man becomes aggressive or destructive.

Fromm develops the concept of transcendence by elaborating the complex model of humanist thought. The term refers to the ability of man, who becomes himself, to act in accordance with his own conscience. This ability is also related to the overcoming of the limits imposed by the society in which man lives. The condition of those who "transcend" is that of "cosmopolite". In the need for transcendence, love, religion and material production find fertile ground, but sometimes even hatred and aggressiveness are expressed, as secondary abilities alternative to creativity. In fact, social structures do not always allow an individual to express biophilic creativity (→ biophilia), as this does not find the conditions in which to prevail. On the contrary, according to Fromm, doing without having a purpose is a sublime manifestation of self-realization: "the greatest thing in life consists in giving expression to one's own forces, and not with a purpose, but for the love of the act itself".

According to Fromm, the need for identity is part of gaining the self-experience that is necessary to man for his self-actualization. Therefore, such a need implies an experience that can be integrated only if the typical features of the having mode are not structured in a radical way. In order to produce the experience of identity, it is necessary for this experience to penetrate into the path of identification looking for extinction, or attenuation, of narcissism and incestuous fixations, and to aim at the overcoming of destructive and necrophiliac tendencies. Within the dimension of identity, lies also the need for correlation, which can be seen as the relationship between the society in which the individual lives and the predominance of a specific character orientation in the majority of individuals belonging to a given culture.

According to Fromm, the character structure of an individual is shaped by the social-economic structure of the society in which he lives: a man cannot choose but accept the system of production of his society, and this results in a vast, complex and sometimes painful process of adaptation. The type of society influences, in various ways, relationships between people, determining the modalities of socialization and assimilation (obtaining what a person needs to meet their necessities) and shaping their personality. The social character conditions men to desire what they desire, to act according to their own will, within the structures and social networks that form society and its organizations. Among these, family is the main source of relationships, identity and rootedness, and constitutes a privileged intermediary between the economic base and the ideals of society, in addition to being the basis of the guidance system that man needs to find references and to integrate into society. The style used by man to assimilate, that is, to obtain what he needs for living, creates the orientation of the character. People with a productive orientation become independent and produce by themselves what they need. People who do not find within themselves the strength to obtain goods useful for their sustenance, lean towards the non-productive character, in its various forms. Fromm distinguishes between social character (common to several individuals in a same culture) and individual character (the set of characteristics that make the difference between individuals of the same culture).

The following orientations belong to non-productive characters: the receptive orientation (masochistic relationship); exploitative orientation (sadistic relationship); hoarding orientation (authoritarian, hoarding and based on the value of use); marketing orientation (people are seen as goods, based on exchange value and saleability of themselves, characterized by indifference, emotional anaesthesia, estrangement from relationships). According to Fromm, the marketing character has a better chance of "change" than the hoarding one. Instead, production-oriented characters are defined by the being mode and by the tendency to implement human potential in creativity, production of relationships, sharing and search for harmony. The need for a guidance system is explored by Fromm in *Psychoanalysis and Religion*, where he discusses man's need of a fundamental structure to overcome the original condition of loneliness and alienation and establish relationships with others. This need can be satisfied by an ideology, a religion or a neurosis. The disharmony of the existential condition generates in man specific needs, which are typical of his nature and distinguish him from animals. He tries to solve this disharmony of the existential condition by creating (or joining) a system of thought that can serve as a frame of orientation. Such a system must consist of intellectual and emotional aspects and must be marked by the construction of sense, and it is expressed in every field of human activity. If the need for a frame of orientation can be considered universal, its forms and its contents are diversified, and these determine, according to Fromm, substantial differences in value between systems. Frames of orientation are a good response to our needs only if they are brought back to the need for identity, transcendence, correlation and rootedness. In fact, there are frames of orientation that slow down man's process of growth and discovery, though apparently responding to his needs. In the worst case, these make man regress, tying him down to incestuous fixations, inviting him to express collective narcissistic needs, directing him towards destructive and necrofile solutions. The need for rootedness is located in this humanistic vision, that is, a man's need to feel a "member" of the world. Fromm identifies feelings of brotherhood and friendship in it and from it he elaborates the idea of peace. Peace among men is seen as the outcome of an internal change of man, regulated by an inner time, called "messianic", in which union has replaced alienation, and the fracture generated between the individual, their counterpart and nature can finally heal. From the perspective of rootedness as an expression of solidarity among people, Fromm also explores the concept of "universalism", that is, the state of peace between one nation and another, in a renewed feeling of love for the stranger and the enemy, which involves the overcoming of the narcissistic perception of qualitative difference, so that no population may consider itself superior or elected. *[E. Benelli, I. Battaglini]*

REFERENCES. Fromm E., *The sane society*, 1955; Id., *For the love of life*, 1986; Id., *Psychoanalysis and religion*, 1950; Id., *On disobedience and other essays*, 1981; Maslow A., *Motivation and personality*, 1954.

HUMANISTIC PSYCHOANALYSIS

Psychoanalytic school of thought developed from the theories of the psychoanalyst and social psychologist Fromm, that are based on the concept of "human nature", intended as being the essence of the nature of all men. This concept needs to be understood within the wider framework of his reflections and on the value Fromm gave to the nature of the human being, which he subsumed under the label of "humanism".

CENTRALITY OF THE DIMENSION OF MAN.

> The most important and fundamental thought of humanism is the idea that human nature – humanity *(humanitas)* – is not an abstraction but a reality: that in each individual we find all humanity; that every man is all men; that every individual represents all humanity and, therefore, that all men are equal, not in their talents or abilities, but in their basic human quality.
>
> (Fromm, 1964)

The idea of the concrete unity of the human race, where, therefore, every individual shares with any other human the same "nature" constituted of a collection of potentialities and essential possibilities, represents the presupposition and guiding principle of Frommian thought. Fromm's theory is also made up of a synthesis of a multiplicity of theoretical approaches (amongst which primarily sociology, but also anthropology, history of religion, ethics and philosophy) that characterize this paradigm. Three main roots of Frommian humanism can be identified. The first is that deriving from the humanistic interpretation of the Talmudic writings of the rabbi Rabinkov, from whose vision Fromm can be considered as operating; second, a particular universalization and combination with the "humanistic" matrix of the philosophy of K. Marx, of which Fromm proposes an ethical-humanistic interpretation; not least, the third root of his philosophy is to be found in psychoanalysis itself, which was considered by Fromm to have developed in the wake of humanism, within the framework of the classical tradition from which it derives: "Psychoanalysis is part of that humanistic movement that started in Europe fifty years ago".

Next to this matrix, even the sociological components, outlined in his successive work on the psychology of religion and merged with his psychoanalytic training are influenced by a humanistic perspective and converge, becoming an essential component of his psychoanalytic paradigm, in the attempt to understand man in all his different dimensions; according to Funk, "his method aims at establishing humanism as a human science, without losing the unitary essence of the human being".

Departing from the basic assumption according to which, "every single man carries humanity in himself – the human condition is one and it is the same for all men" – this kind of model takes into account the double belonging of the human being; on the one hand, inserted into a social structure that is historically determined and of which he forms part, and on the other hand, a psychological structure that is common to all the human race, a universal nature. From this originates a specific theoretical vision that aims at observing the intersection and the interaction, in the individual, between the social and cultural context on one hand and human nature – singular but at once universally shared – on the other. Fromm exposes the first version of this vision, that can be characterized methodologically as "sociological psychology" or "psychological sociology", in his brief but important contribution, *Psychoanalysis and Sociology*, in 1929. With the term "socio-psychological approach" Fromm intends to mean that "it is more appropriate to consider man *a priori* as being socialized, and therefore to conceptualize the psyche as being determined by the relationships that exist between the single person and society". Without denying the existence of a biological-natural component in the structure of the human psyche and avoiding in this way the socio-relativistic errors, Fromm arrives at developing a particular conceptualization of the influence that society exercises in modulating the conditions in which man lives.

CRITICISM OF FREUD. Fromm was able to develop his own paradigm through distancing himself from S. Freud, accomplished through the use of Sullivan's relational concept (→ interpersonal psychiatry):

> we consider man as being a social creature, and not, as asserted by Freud, first and foremost a self-sufficient being, and only secondly as needing others [. . .]. In this sense we feel that individual psychology is fundamentally social psychology or, as stated by Sullivan, psychology of interpersonal relationships;

from this conceptualization he developed, in turn, a body of work that was influenced by Marxist thought. If, in his writings regarding "method" Fromm speaks again of the "libidinal structure of a society", he successively abandoned the theory of the → libido, using, instead the concept of "passion" borrowed from B. Spinoza, to define the notion of "social character" (→ character types): "with this expression I refer to the nucleus of the character structure of the great majority of the members of the same culture". This character-structure defines, according to Fromm, the behaviour of the individual within a determined social configuration. The subjective function of character is therefore that of "moulding the human energy with the goal of allowing the functioning of a given society", orienting human behaviour in such a way that it is faithful to the model proposed by that society, "to ensure the continuity of its functioning". "The social character interiorizes the external necessities, in this way harnessing the human energy to the advantage of the goals of a determined social and economic system".

THE UNCONSCIOUS AND SOCIAL FILTERS. Fromm departs from the abandonment of the theory of the libidinal drives in favour of the concept of "passion", in other words the idea that the unconscious is formed depending on the ongoing practices of the economy and of society. The unconscious, that lies at the bottom of every social structure, is characterized as being the representation of "universal man". From him, only those components that are loyal to the continued existence of a particular type of society will surface. Therefore, the

> contents of the unconscious are neither good nor bad, neither rational, nor irrational, it is all that is human. The unconscious is the whole individual, less that part of him that corresponds to his society. The unconscious is in this way socially characterized through a dialectic relationship, that is socially mediated and historically relative, at the bottom of which lies an operation of "socially conditioned filtration" that takes place through logical, linguistic demands and social taboos.

The fact that the individual belongs to both the human race, and to the common psychological structure that binds those who belong to such a race, determines a social declination and a characterization of the unconscious as being the totality of human potential. From this, only those parts that contribute to the stability of a determined society will emerge in the conscious, as a result of the presence of social filters. The "socially produced filters" are therefore those psychological constructs that allow a good part of the human experience, individual and collective, to remain unconscious, that is, to not emerge to the level of conscious awareness. Fromm identified various types of filters. First of all, language, that with its variety of words allows us to distinguish between experiences that are described in more detail, and therefore more easily elaborated by the conscious in their multiple declinations, and descriptions described in much less detail, and that are therefore more easily relegated to the unconscious. A second filter is given by logical thought: conscious thought is permeated with a norm that regulates and "relegates" the illogical thoughts to the area of the unconscious, according to a mental attitude that discards what appears to be illogical. A third kind of filter is in regard to the social function of taboos, which regulate experiences on the basis of whether their content is more or less acceptable. Experiences that violate taboos that society has chosen for itself in order to ensure its survival contain thoughts and feelings that have to necessarily remain in the social unconscious.

HUMANISTIC PSYCHOTHERAPY AND PSYCHOANALYSIS. Humanistic psychoanalysis, departing from the widespread developments generated from the fertile thought of Fromm, can be considered as being both a conception of man as well as a methodological approach that is enriched by clinical experience. In contrast with the concept of "mental health" – which is defined by assumptions such as the absence of disease and established by sociological co-relativistic parameters, in which every person is considered to mentally sane when well-adjusted to society, to its structures, to its laws –, the humanistic prospective outlines, instead, a definition of health based on the concept of → self-actualization. A healthy individual is one who is able to develop his interests and his potential, who becomes what he really is, not someone who has merely "adapted". From a humanistic perspective, society has to be useful to man, who cannot be defined only from an anatomical and psychological perspective, but also "psychologically and mentally". This is Fromm's methodological principle, and the "programme" of making the unconscious conscious becomes the project of "transforming the mere idea of the universality of man into the living experience of his universality, and the experiential fulfilment of humanity". Fromm's clinical approach favours the critical observation of behaviour and inserts this into a "historical scene", in which the emergent personal and social unconscious content is the fundamental focus of the psychoanalytic journey and of the exploration of the symbolic and behavioural language. Moreover, Fromm emphasized the importance of the analysis of fundamental aspects of the biophilic nature of man (→ biophilia), observed in its subjection to cultural conditions and in the development of his character as conceived by him, as for example in the case of → necrophilia. The rehabilitation of the individual takes place through the development of his "passions", the "experimenting with being" of these crucial themes that constitute their positive framework.

For Fromm, the value of the symptom represents the failed attempts of the patient to adapt to society, and can be considered to be the starting point from which the analysis departs in order to promote awareness of his authentic and real aspirations and desires for self-fulfilment, together with feelings of harmony and being at one with the world and with others.

Fromm's approach takes into account, develops, differentiates and integrates many of the assumptions postulated by Freud and recaptured by K. Horney, C. Thompson, W.R.D. Fairbairn, H. Guntrip, H. Kohut, regarding the fundamental elements of the analytic relationship, such as the "mother fixation", the concept of the "idol", → insight, interpretation of the → transference, developing these therapeutic factors into a completely original formulation, in which the analyst takes from the patient his emotional world to offer him not so much his self as his function, guaranteeing him a neutrality that does not exempt him from the centre-to-centre positioning (in other words of the analyst's Ego with regard to the patient's Ego) between two total humanities (two human beings that are "whole", as defined by Biancoli), distinct from the mutual analysis as advocated by radical critics of psychoanalysis.

This mutuality is to be understood as a dialogue between two totalities in the → here-and-now, in which asymmetry is provided by the capacity of the analyst to listen to both himself and to the patient, and by his ability to implement the process of the birth and development of the new Ego, which also includes those elements that the patient does not know he possesses. The interior processes of the analyst will proceed in resonance with the processes and contents of the unconscious of the patient – and in this way the analyst continues with the analytic exploration and the personal transformation, with the discovery of his own humanity through that of the other and the experimentation of the universal dimension in himself and in others. Fromm offers an alternative to the here-and-now by proposing a dialogue between "a modality of having" and a "modality of being" (→ having, → being). Fromm's conceptualization therefore translates, in an original fashion, the operative aspects of psychotherapy, deriving them, in a coherent manner, from his own radical humanism. The theoretical, technical and practical development of Fromm's psychoanalytic approach (followed in Italy by E. Benelli, I. Battaglini and their collaborators amongst others), cannot be separated from the interaction of the social sciences with the behavioural sciences, and takes into account the complex architectures and methodological and scientific instruments of Fromm, made up of psychoanalysis, anthropology, sociology, history of religion, economics, philosophy, psychology of art, of groups, of the masses, with their application, placing man in society and looking at society as an expression of human nature. According to Biancoli,

> the problem of the science of this procedure will find an answer in the internal coherence of Frommian thought, in the inductive method that is his own, with the construction of hypotheses on a clinical basis or on historic-economics and statistics, with empirical verification of the hypotheses itself and its development. [. . .] Fromm's theories in no way contradicts the science of his time.

[I. Battaglini, L. Corti, E. Benelli]

REFERENCES. Biancoli R., *Situazione umana e libertà in Erich Fromm*, in P.L. Eletti (ed.), *Saggi sull'opera di Erich Fromm*, 1983; Id., *L'idea di "uomo intero", "umanità totale", e le sue applicazioni cliniche*, speech presented at the international conference «Erich Fromm – Psychoanalyst and Supervisor», Ascona, 4–5 April 1997; Fromm E., *Psychoanalysis and sociology*, 1929; Id., *Escape from freedom*, 1941; Id., *Psychoanalytic characterology and its application to the understanding of culture*, 1949; Id., *Psychoanalysis and zen Buddhism*, 1960; Id., *The humanist concept of mental health*, 1961; Id., *Beyond the chains of illusion: My encounter with Marx and Freud*, 1962; Id., *Humanism and psychoanalysis*, in «Contemporary Psychoanalysis», 1964, I; Id., *The crisis of psychoanalysis*, 1970; Id., Fromm E., *Anatomy of human destructiveness*, 1973; Id., *To have or to be*, 1976; Funk R., *Erich Fromm: The courage to be human*, 1982; Id., *Radikaler Humanismus – humanistischer Radikalismus*, in J. Speck (ed.), *Grundprobleme der großen Philosophen: Philosophie der Gegenwart*, 1984, VI; Id., *Erich Fromm's concept of social character*, in «Social Thought & Research» 1998, 21, 1–2; Id., *The Jewish roots of Erich Fromm's humanistic thinking*, 1988; Id., *Erich Fromm: His life and ideas*, 2000; Schiavone M., *Antropologia, sociologia e psicoanalisi in Erich Fromm*, in *Incontro con Erich Fromm. Atti del simposio Internazionale su Erich Fromm: "Dalla necrofilia alla biofilia: linee per una psicoanalisi umanistica"*,1988; Sullivan H.S., *The Interpersonal theory of psychiatry*, 1962; Id., *The fusion of psychiatry and social science*, 1964.

HUMOUR

A form of communication and interpretation of events that can arouse pleasant emotional reactions, laughter and social affiliation in oneself or in the interlocutor. This reaction is a result of the use of a specific linguistic structure and/or a caricatural use of verbal and nonverbal communication.

The second aspect has been particularly investigated by authors who are interested in the phenomenon of humour in theatre (for example Aristotle and L. Pirandello), but even richer is the literature concerning the linguistic structure that characterizes humour. However, it seems that in both cases, the golden rule underlying humour is the rupture of expectation, the surprise effect, the violation of a shared rule. The investigation of the typical linguistic structure of humour has led to the identification of numerous humour techniques, including, for example: repetition, that is, the recurrence, in the same form, of circumstances or words at different times; shift of emphasis, where importance is given to a marginal element of the sentence by putting it in the foreground and by generating, as a consequence, a shift in the contextual meaning ("Alcohol kills slowly," says the first; "Well, I'm in no hurry," replies the second); paronymic distortion, that is, replacing a word with another word that resembles the first one in form but that differs in meaning ("We are overweighted with work"); paradoxical oscillation (→ logic of paradox), where there is a change of level, which, however, also restores the previous level, since it excludes and includes it at the same time ("What is a sadist? One who is kind to a masochist": if the masochist receives kindness, wanting instead to be tormented, he takes pleasure; but if he takes pleasure, he suffers; but if he suffers he takes pleasure . . . in a continuous oscillation). All the authors who have studied the phenomenon of humour have proposed different distinctions and have attributed different meanings to humour, on the one hand, and to wit, comedy, satire and parody, on the other.

In psychotherapy, the use of humour contributes to creating and maintaining a profitable relationship with the patient; it also provides the possibility of making new points of view pleasantly acceptable to the patient through observing and perceiving their problematic condition. Moreover, laughing brings benefits to the body by facilitating the oxygenation of blood, the renewal of the reserve of air in the lungs, the stimulation of the production of serotonin, endorphins and antibodies; it also increases blood circulation in the internal organs, skin and facial muscles. On the other hand, an imbalance of the phenomenon of laughing (that is, a hypertrophy or its absence) is an indicator of the presence of a mental disorder. In psychoanalysis, humour is considered a → defence mechanism. *[R.]*

HYPNO-SYSTEMIC THERAPY

Within the systemic-relational paradigm, it is a model oriented to resources and focused on solutions. Hypno-systemic therapy is based on → systems theory, communication theory, hypnotherapy aimed at autonomy and focused on competences, neurobiology, modern brain research and on research concerning → autopoiesis, memory and → priming. The term "hypno-systemic" was introduced in 1982 by Schmidt and since then it has found wide resonance in the field of systemic therapy of → Ericksonian hypnotherapy. Not only is it adopted in professional psychotherapy contexts but also in numerous clinics and hospitals, with great results (as demonstrated by evaluation research).

HUMAN EXPERIENCE AS THE RESULT OF THE FOCUSING OF ATTENTION. Experience is the result of the focusing of attention (at a visual, auditory, olfactory, gustatory, kinaesthetic level) on a voluntary-conscious level and an involuntary level. Involuntary processes are faster and stronger than the voluntary ones. The brainstem and the medium brain/limbic system have more influence on experience than the neocortex. The processes that create the experience (even daily) show a resemblance to the processes used during hypnotic inductions. Hypnotic inductions are similar to the processes of daily communication; they are part of a natural experience. For example, dreams show how these processes work: human beings produce imaginative processes at an involuntary level, combined with a high intensity of associations in these processes (the "inner observer" is so immersed in his associative processes that these fantasies appear to him as the only "real reality"). Therefore, the body produces emotional, physiological processes and processes of thoughts corresponding to these images (for example, blood pressure, heart rate, muscle reactions, hormonal reactions, immune system changes, gene activations). The body literally expresses one's own reality according to the processes of imagination that are produced at an involuntary level. This reality is constantly changing and, in order to appear stable, it constantly needs similar processes of focusing of attention. A shift of attention also changes the experienced reality and also what is called "Ego" or "my Ego". The everyday consciousness is constructed in a similar way. Communication and interaction processes in families and in other systems work in an almost hypnotic way and they induce experiential processes that adapt to their rules ("systemic rule-based trance") as, for example, was showed in the research of J.A. Bargh on priming.

DIFFERENT "EGO-STATES" (MULTIPLICITY) AND COMPETENCE HYPOTHESIS. As shown by research on dreams, hypnotherapy and therapy of trauma, it can be stated that human beings possess not only one but several "Ego-states". Each of these Ego-states is associated with different patterns of cognitive, emotional, physiological and interactional processes and contains different types of competences and limitations. If someone is suffering from severe symptoms (usually defined as pathological deficiency), this does not prove that he does not have the skills that would make him capable of solving the problem. Normally, it is discovered that each person owns all the necessary competence models if the episodes showing competence models, which are useful for creating healthy and constructive solutions, are looked for in a systematic way. In symptomatic states, these behaviour patterns are dissociated and not available. In such states, subjects strongly identify themselves with the Ego-states that express helplessness and inability. Through the systematic exploration of internal processes, it is usually possible to access all the necessary competence models. This was clearly showed by Erickson, with strategies such as "pseudo-orientation in time", "age progression", "age regression focused on competence", etc.

SYMPTOMS AS "PROBLEMATIC TRANCE PROCESSES". These symptomatic Ego-states express psychophysiological patterns or networks learned in specific contexts. According to research on the brain that refers to the Hebbian theory on neurobiological plasticity, "cells that interact are bound". In this way, human beings build psychophysiological networks in each episode of life that is experienced as emotionally intense (in research on memory: "episodic memory"). If, in the context of a person's life, there are some redundant "trigger-levers" (context markers) associated with symptomatic networks, these levers can reactivate symptomatic processes. A similar mechanism comes into play when someone uses an intense hypnotic imaginative process to self-induce a specific experience, but in a symptomatic process this happens unconsciously and against one's will. As shown by Gilligan and Schmidt, a symptomatic status involves the same processes of a self-induced trance state. The only difference between a "solution-oriented trance" and a "problematic trance" is that in the second type of trance one fights against unwanted and involuntary experiences, with the result that the Ego loses the battle and feels like a victim (involuntary processes are always faster and stronger). On the other hand, in a "solution-oriented trance" there is synergy between the conscious processes of the Ego and the involuntary processes.

SYMPTOMS AS ATTEMPTED SOLUTIONS IN CONFLICTING SYSTEMIC CONTEXTS. In a systemic perspective, these processes can be also considered as a form of competences built into relationships and as → attempted solutions in relational contexts, since each process, including symptomatic processes, produces results/effects in relationships (even unintentionally). Conversations with patients clarify that, at an unaware level, people have fearful fantasies about what would happen if they used their competence to find a solution for their own benefits. These fantasies express the fear that this may produce negative effects in relationships, especially those that are emotionally intense. In addition, it can be demonstrated that the suffering caused by symptoms is not an expression of incompetence, but rather an unconscious attempted solution to avoid conflicts of loyalty and other conflicts related to one's objective. This has important implications for interventions, since it is not sufficient to try eliminating a symptomatic process, but it is important to take into account what effect this action would have on the patient at a relational level. Patients must be helped to find balance between their functional and healthy development and the aspects of loyalty that they consider important.

RECOMMENDATIONS FOR THERAPEUTIC INTERVENTIONS. The application of the hypno-systemic construct expresses itself through a constant introduction of differences in patterns of problem stabilization (internal patterns and/or interactional patterns). As claimed by G. Bateson, information is represented by a dynamic that continually creates differences; similarly, a therapeutic intervention should introduce new alternative visions into a system. The patterns of a problem show a split of the experience system into at least two parts (the process of the Ego against the involuntary process of the "happening"). For this reason, all interventions should support the constructive cooperation between the conscious Ego and the involuntary processes of a person within a system. For this reason, the therapist should try to make the terms of the intervention very clear and provide persuasive explanations to support the construction of a meta-observer position. This would allow the patient to integrate and guide the experiential processes (by establishing awareness and leading to competence and to the possibility to choose). In order for a change to be effective, it is sufficient to introduce differences in just one or a few elements of the pattern, because each element influences, circularly, the others. Clients are encouraged to develop their observation from a meta-position (dissociated from the problematic experience, that is, a safe observation point), where they can observe/reconstruct the processes of their problem. The hypno-systemic approach provides a broad range of structured descriptions of the problem and of solution patterns, which are offered to patients in such a way as to create a systematic learning of how they work. Subsequently, these structured types of construction of reality can be used to: make changes in patients' patterns of behaviour; find useful experiences in their past, that is, in their existing competences "tank"; compare, systematically, the problem and the solution patterns. Discovering the existence of problem and solution patterns generates the possibility of introducing the view that a patient "owns" a variety of Ego-states. This also means that only one Ego-state experiences the problem, not the "person" in general. In this way, it is possible to create effective possibilities to mitigate the problem (the so called "dissociative interventions": "It is not the whole of me, but a part of me, that suffers from the problem; there are also other functional sides in me . . ."). After these types of comparisons have been built, the patient can be led to give a positive connotation to the symptomatic reactions that result from unaware reactions in relation to what the organism needs. In this view, the symptoms may be used as messengers of useful information that come from inner knowledge of what is needed for a healthy solution. In this way, people can develop more self-esteem, but also greater personal responsibility in respect of the promotion of their own health. Starting from these comparisons and from all the structured descriptions of the patterns (internal and interactional), various tasks, experiments and assignments can be developed, which strongly direct the focus of attention on the pattern of competence put in place during one's everyday life. In addition, many processes of imagination can be developed in which customers are put in active contact with their own "dormant", latent competences. This is done by using techniques known as "revivification" and "reactivation" in → Ericksonian hypnotherapy. In this way, the client can effectively and lastingly be brought into contact with competent Ego-states.

Since involuntary and automated problem patterns are very powerful and faster than the desired solution processes, hypno-systemic therapy offers many interventions through which clients can identify the "levers trigger" of their problem patterns in their usual systemic contexts (in line with the Hebbian theory of plasticity, these levers can induce the problem) and interrupt these patterns. Also, they can use the levers that trigger the problem as useful signals to enable solution responses (using the leverage of the problem as a sort of "alarm clock" that triggers the solution pattern). This facilitates an effective and durable transfer of competencies in one's everyday context. Clients are advised to check what effect would produce the use of their competencies in their relationships. If conflicts are found in the objective (e.g. conflicts of loyalty), hypno-systemic therapy offers a variety of interventions to help them achieving an optimal balance between their diverse needs (for example, to obtain benefits for themselves and the chosen objectives of loyalty). Family or other relevant systems are often included in the cooperation, but this never happens for example in a family therapy → setting, because this would imply that the family needs therapy. Generally, only a part of the family accepts this idea, and this can create conflicts in the system (second-order → cybernetics). As reality is created by focusing attention, this is analyzed through the processes that appear useful in systems of relationships, as well as through the ways in which the "problem patterns" can be transformed into useful information with respect to "what" is required and "who" requires it, in order to create functional interactions to achieve goals. Therefore, for example, family sessions become sessions aiming at the induction of experiences of competence and of cooperative interactions within the supporting system, not the problem system. *[G. Schmidt]*

REFERENCES. Gilligan S., *Therapeutic trances: The cooperation principle in Ericksonian hypnotherapy*, 1987; Hebb D., *The organization of behaviour*, 1949; Libet B., Schröder J., *Mind time: Wie das Gehirn Bewusstsein produziert*, 2007; Nijenhuis E.R.S., *Somatoform dissociation: Major symptoms of dissociative disorders*, 2001; Roth G., *Fühlen, Denken, Handeln. Wie das Gehirn unser Verhalten steuert*, 2001; Schmidt G., *Systemische Familientherapie als zirkuläre Hypnotherapie*, in «Familiendynamik», 1985, 10; Id., *Systemic-hypnotherapeutic concepts for the cooperation with clients, defined as depressed, and with their relationship-systems: From depressing to unfolding worlds*, in «Brief Strategic and Systemic Therapy European Review», 2004, 1; Watkins H.H., Watkins J.G., *Ego-States: Theorie und Therapie*, 2008.

HYPNOSIS

A procedure by which an altered state of consciousness based on a state of physical and mental relaxation, called trance, is induced in patients. This generates an enhanced receptive state to stimuli coming from the subconscious. This state can be achieved through induction, → reframing, mental images and other techniques. Through hypnosis the therapist creates the conditions to gain an easier access to the internal resources of a person and allows the person to see problems in a different and more productive way. In fact, during hypnotic trance, the right hemisphere becomes active and predominant compared to the left one. A hypnotic state is not deep sleep or a state of complete unconsciousness, but a sort of half-sleep, where rational defences are lowered. By using patients' own language, hypnotic therapy does not force subjects to change, but it makes them actors, creators of change, and evokes in them the feelings that will lead them to modify their reactions. The practice of hypnosis dates to the Sumerian civilization, although evidences of this practice were found also among Egyptians, where it was called "magic sleep", and in ancient China. In modern times, it was F. Mesmer who used hypnosis for the first time in 1770 for therapeutic purposes. A fundamental contribution to the hypnotic technique came from J.M. Charcot. Hypnotherapy makes its appearance towards the middle of last century, thanks to M.H. Erickson, who applied hypnosis to therapy, and made it an effective form of intervention. Erickson conducted numerous studies that led him to develop an intervention paradigm to understand hypnotic dynamics. There are many different types of hypnotic therapy. They can be broadly distinguished between direct forms, where a therapist proceeds with a formal induction of trance (→ clinical hypnosis, Ericksonian hypnotherapy, → hypno-systemic therapy), and indirect forms, where the induction takes place through suggestive communication (→ hypnosis without trance). *[R.]*

HYPNOSIS WITHOUT TRANCE

An altered state of consciousness without the presence of a formal hypnotic trance (→ hypnosis), which can be achieved through an ordinary communicative exchange. This state can be detected through the empirical observation of an expansion of perceptual abilities in a state of relaxation, in which people can more easily influence themselves or be influenced by others. This state of high suggestibility is produced through communicative manoeuvres that allow the subject to abandon their perceptual-emotional rigidity. People appear with a relaxed posture, with no signs of disquiet, with wide-open eyes and dilated pupils and with the possible presence of rhythmic movements of the eyelids; their voice is clear and has a slow pace, their attention is focused on the topic under discussion or the action in progress, without any sign of distraction. This dimension of pleased suggestibility allows subjects to overcome their resistances and blocks. The construct of hypnosis and hypnotherapy without trance was introduced into psychotherapy by Watzlawick. The author used this definition to refer to the whole series of hypnotic communication techniques that can be used during therapeutic communication without the need of a hypnotic induction ritual. In particular, Watzlawick refers to the part of the work of M.H. Erickson concerning how to give prescriptions to patients by using an evocative/hypnotic language. *The Art of Change* is the first text where this construct was explained in detail. In fact, starting from this work, many techniques of hypnosis without trance have been developed and refined within the framework of strategic therapies. These are techniques of strategic communication directed towards the production of specific changes in the interlocutor. In particular, the studies and research carried out by Nardone and his collaborators over the last 30 years (→ brief strategic therapy Nardone's model) have helped to identify and refine several techniques of hypnosis without trance, both verbal and nonverbal, which showed high levels of efficacy. The most important are: the tune-in (→ tuning technique), the → strategic dialogue, the use of an evocative language and the use of communicative redundancies. Unlike the "indicative" language used by most therapies, hypnotherapy without trance refers to "performative" and → injunctive language, which does not describe but "prescribes", that is, it allows a person to experience different realities.

Due to these characteristics, hypnosis without trance is the privileged communication mode used in the early stages of strategic treatments. It is capable of generating real → corrective emotional experiences, bypassing the natural → resistance to change of patients. *[R. Milanese]*

REFERENCES. Nardone G., Loriedo C., Zeig J., Watzlawick P., *Ipnosi e terapie ipnotiche*, 2006; Nardone G., Salvini A., *The strategic dialogue*, 2007; Nardone G., Watzlawick P., *The art of change*, 1993.

HYPOCHONDRIAC CHECK-UP TECHNIQUE

In the context of → brief strategic psychotherapy Nardone's model, a → symptom prescription technique used to treat hypochondriac disorders. In this technique, patients are asked to perform a ritualized task consisting of a voluntary search of all symptoms/indicators that could indicate the presence of possible diseases. The paradoxical request is highly structured and communicated in a suggestive way. Patients can, for example, be required to inspect their body at specific moments of the day – when they have just got up, after lunch and after dinner – and search for potential indicators of disease and to write down in detail all the identified symptoms. The prescription is a typical application of the stratagem "sail the sea without the sky's knowledge". In fact, this is presented at a communicative level as a kind of detailed diagnostic check-up, which aims to identify any pathogenic processes in progress. Instead, the real goal is primarily therapeutic: modifying the patient's hypochondriac perceptions/reactions. The rationale for this requirement follows a classic mode of intervention of M.H. Erickson, who often tended to turn a symptomatic behaviour into a voluntary and forced one. In this way, the behaviour assumes, for the patient, the status of an "ordeal" – an extremely tiring, strenuous or annoying task. The strategy is to "lead the enemy up the attic and then remove the ladder": the prescription is initially perceived by patients as positive, appropriate, healthy, but it turns quickly into its opposite and they are forced to abandon their symptoms. Diagnostic self-monitoring has the disruptive effect of changing the perception of patients, increasing their sense of familiarity with the normal bodily physiological alterations/fluctuations that were previously perceived as threatening. *[A. Bartoletti]*

REFERENCES. Haley J., *Ordeal therapy: Unusual ways to change behaviour*, 1984; Nardone G., *Brief strategic solution-oriented therapy of phobic and obsessive disorders*, 1996; Bartoletti A., Nardone G., *La paura delle malattie*, 2018.

HYPOCONDRIASIS → DEFENCE MECHANISMS

HYPOTHESIS

It is a statement on facts, that needs to be proved through → observations or experiments. When a hypothesis is adopted by an individual regardless of evidence, as in → heuristics or as an assumption, it may give rise to (and justify) unverified and unproved deductions, and can control dysfunctional behaviours. Psychotherapy tends to give an attribute of temporariness to hypotheses, until verification or falsification, which need to be obtained through evidence of behaviours. *[R. Mosticoni]*

REFERENCES. Blackledge J.T., *An introduction to relational frame theory: Basics and applications*, in «The Behaviour Analyst Today», 2003, 3(4); Ellis A., *Rational psychotherapy and individual psychology*, in «Journal of Individual Psychology», 1957, 13.

I

ICD

It is the acronym of International Classification of Diseases, a → diagnostic manual developed and edited by the World Health Organization reporting the "international statistical classification of diseases and related health problems". The manual has reached its tenth edition and Chapter V is dedicated to mental and behavioural disorders. The ICD-10 introduces a classification of psychological disorders based on a nosographic and descriptive diagnostic logic (→ psychiatric diagnosis) similar to the one adopted by → DSM. The differences between these two types of diagnostics systems can be found only within the set of criteria that were established to include specific psychopathological phenomena within a given diagnostic class. Unlike the DSM, ICD-10 is composed of two different diagnostic manuals depending on whether one's objectives are clinical or diagnostic. In the first case, the diagnostic criteria are more descriptive and flexible, while in the second case they are more specific and stringent. *[A. Bartoletti]*

ID

A term introduced by Freud after 1920 to indicate the psychic instance constituted by unconscious drives (→ drive). Within the psychic economy, the Id is, therefore, considered the true reservoir of psychic energy. It is distinct from the other two instances of the personality, that is, the → Ego and the → Superego, which are genetically derived from the Id, and are in conflict with it. After 1920, Freud amended his conception of the psyche expressed in *The Interpretation of Dreams*. The fullest example of this change regards the Ego and the Id. In this text, the three "systems" of the first topography – conscious, pre-conscious and unconscious (→ topographical model of the mind) – are joined by three "instances": the Id, the Ego and the Superego, moving in this way from the dynamic hypotheses of the psyche to a structural hypothesis. Indeed, whereas in the former, psychic phenomena are the product of a conflict between the systems, in the latter the conflict is placed in relation both with the position that the instances occupy in the structure of the personality, and with the way in which they fit together. In the original German, the word chosen by Freud for Id is "*Es*", the neuter third-person pronoun. The choice of this term highlights the fact that rather than being the lead actor in their lives, individuals are determined by extraneous forces that inhabit them, and about which they know nothing. The Id is, therefore, the most intimate and extraneous part of each of us. Taken together, these forces make up the system of drives characteristic of the unconscious. Unlike the unconscious in the first topography, which was predominantly constituted by repressed experiences, in this new conception the unconscious becomes much broader (as a matter of fact, this approach was at least partially present in the first dynamic conception of the unconscious). The Id ultimately encapsulates both what Freud defined as the unconscious in the first topography, that is to say, predominantly the repressed contents, and the chaotic reservoir of drives that is subject to repression and other defensive processes (→ defence mechanisms) predominantly arising out of the Ego, which is acted upon by the Superego. Taken together, these drives are determined by the opposition of the life instinct and the death instinct. Freud expanded the concept of the unconscious by asserting that the instance that undertakes censorship and repression (the Ego) is itself unconscious. But how is it possible for part of the Ego to be unconscious if the Ego exists specifically in opposition to the unconscious? In effect, if on a dynamic level both the Ego and Superego enter into conflict with the Id, on a genetic level, that is to say, as regards their formation, they are merely differentiations of the Id, which explains why a portion of them is unconscious. Nevertheless, unlike the other instances, the Id does not have its own specific organization; indeed, Freud indicates that it is chaotic, not determined by any "general will"; in other words, its activity is not directed. *[P. Valerio, M. Bottone, R. Vitelli]*

REFERENCES. Freud S. (1900–1901), *The interpretation of dreams*, in *The Standard Edition*, IV–V, 1953–1974; Id. (1920), *Beyond the pleasure principle*, in *The Standard Edition*, XIV, 1953–1974; Id. (1922), *The ego and the id*, in *The Standard Edition*, XIX, 1953–1974.

IDEAL MODEL

In psychosynthesis, it is a central technique, concerning one's self-image, conceived beyond the current limitations and pathologies. Patients are asked to imagine what they want to become. The ideal model emerges only after the false models have been examined (for example, a lower self-concept, or an inauthentic self-image imposed from the outside). It is also important to pay attention to unrealistic, grandiose or moralistic self-images. The visualization of the ideal model should be as vivid and concrete as possible, remembering the psychosynthetic law affirming that images tend to evoke corresponding thoughts, emotions and behaviours. The ideal model can cause temporary adverse reactions: these are useful indications, which it is important to examine and understand. *[P. Ferrucci]*

REFERENCES. Assagioli R., *Psychosynthesis: A manual of principles and techniques*, 1965; Id., *The act of will*, 1973.

IDEALIZATION → DEFENCE MECHANISMS

IDENTIFICATION

A process by which individuals model themselves according to the behaviours, thoughts and feelings of another person. Identification is a process that accompanies the whole evolution of a person: the earliest form of identification can be observed between babies and their mother. Then, the process evolves to include characteristics of both parents and of other family members. This enables children to meet their own needs, acquire habits and pursue goals and ideals. Identification involves people with whom one comes into contact (significant others): parents and teachers for a child; the peer group in adolescence; a loved one in the process of falling in love; public figures (for example show business celebrities); and other figures that are considered important in people's lives and who become a model or who are idealized. An identification with prosocial values can be considered as a protective factor in the psychosocial development of an individual. Conversely, the identification with values carrying a negative social connotation may predispose to delinquency. Another example of identification with potential psychopathological outcomes is the identification with projects and ambitions that are above one's capabilities, so much to bring a person to develop feelings of inadequacy, guilt and inferiority. Identification can lead to serious pathologies due to social alienation when it expresses itself as a detachment from reality with psychotic (→ psychosis) and delusional features. *[R.]*

▷ Freudian thought distinguishes between two types of identification: primary and secondary. The primary one is an act of love; it is the first act of love. When babies hatch out of their autoerotic egg, where they exist in an all-powerful isolation, without the presence of anyone else's needs, they meet others and turn to them in their need for subsistence. According to S. Freud, the first feeling experienced in that moment is a feeling of hatred. In fact, the appearance of the other unveils, for the infant, the illusion of being self-sufficient. The next movement, in which the infant appreciates the other as a helper, is an act of love: identification. Infants identify with people who guarantee the fulfilment of their needs and somehow reconstruct the original perfection. Secondary identification is the psychological process by which infants, who have just left behind autoerotic self-sufficiency and the absolute confusion between subject and object (→ symbiosis), hold the other person in their own mind when this is absent. This becomes the "picture" of the other that dwells within an infant: a role model. According to Freud, this is the dynamic that leads to the development of the → Ego and → Superego. *[S. Panizza]*

IDENTIFICATION WITH AGGRESSOR → DEFENCE MECHANISMS

IDENTIFICATION WITH PERSONA

Jung attributes to → persona the role of enabling and promoting individuals' adaptation to the environment. Persona is considered by Jung a *mask*, that is, the set of roles that people "interpret" and act in their life. A fluid and not totally absorbing → identification with persona facilitates adaptation and social integration, while maintaining a sufficient level of originality and autonomy in the expression of the psyche and its functions. Instead, a too rigid and absolute identification with this psychic instance, although ensuring a good adaptation to reality, penalizes the expression and realization of the deeper inner components of individual personality. According to the Jungian concept of dialectic of opposites, when the conscious attitude is dominated by a too strong identification with persona, a compensatory movement is activated. This movement, pushes the subject, at an unconscious level, towards forms of identification with → anima or → animus. In fact, the function of these two instances is a form of adaptation to one's own inner life. *[N. Fina]*

REFERENCES. Jung C.G. (1916), *Adaptation, individuation, collectivity*, in *Collected Works*, XVIII, 1977; Id. (1928), *The relations between the ego and the unconscious*, in *Collected Works*, VII, 1967.

IDENTIFICATION WITH SHADOW

Jung defined → shadow as the most obscure and unacceptable part of our personality, something that alters our ideal self-image and that, for this reason, we are reluctant to tolerate. The conscious recognition of the existence of a personal shadow enables its integration. Differently, the unconscious identification with it gives rise to a personality dominated by pathological traits of various degrees of severity, incapable of true ethical responsibility. This condition can lead to behaviours of inadequate social adjustment. *[N. Fina]*

REFERENCES. Jung C.G. (1916–1952), *The structure and dynamics of the psyche*, in *Collected Works*, VIII, 1969; Id. (1921–946), *Practice of psychotherapy*, in *Collected Works*, XVI, 1966.

IDENTITY → PERSONAL IDENTITY

ILLUSION OF ALTERNATIVES TECHNIQUE

The great hypnotist M.H. Erickson was the first to use this technique in psychotherapy. Subsequently, this has been used in all the models of strategic therapy, such as the brief strategic therapy MRI model and the brief strategic therapy Nardone's model. It is a communication technique that can be used when a therapist needs to prescribe a task or an exercise considered too difficult or demanding by the patient. Typically, the latter usually comes up with excuses or impediments to avoid the assigned prescription. Operationally, the therapist prescribes the patient the possibility to choose between two tasks: a "therapeutic" task, which the therapist considers would be rejected by the patient, and a second task, much more worrying and which the patient will feel is almost certainly impossible to perform. By rejecting the most demanding task, the patient is induced to choose the other one as, by contrast and comparison, it looks easier. This choice could not have been made if the first option had been presented as the only possibility. *[I. Bonzanini]*

REFERENCES. Watzlawick P., *The language of change*, 1978.

IMAGE

In analytical psychology, it is a concept associated with → archetype. Image, triggered by the psychic energy of archetypical behavioural patterns, expresses the autonomous activity of the psyche. That is, it expresses the product of the symbolic activity that gives meaning to unconscious affective contents and makes them accessible to consciousness. According to Jung, image is the expression both of "the specific activity of the unconscious" and "the momentary state of consciousness". It concentrates together personal and affective contents and universal symbolic forms of human mental activity, such as mythological themes. For this reason, images (especially primordial or archetypical images) exert a numinous power (→ numinosum) on the individual psyche: the charm of the unknown that scares, but that at the same time attracts the consciousness towards the search for meaning. *[M. Tibaldi, A. De Coro]*

REFERENCES. Jung C.G. (1921), *Psychological types*, in *Collected Works*, VI, 1971; Id. (1936), *The concept of the collective unconscious*, in *Collected Works*, IX/I, 1969.

IMAGINAL EXPOSURE

In the context of cognitive-behavioural therapy, a coping strategy of dysfunctional phobic responses based on → anxiety. Imaginal exposure characterizes both → flooding and desensitization techniques. Helped by a therapist, the subject virtually re-experiences the situation that causes anxiety and looks for new and functional responses (→ functional balance), lowering the level of activity and worry. However, in flooding, the immersion in the anxiety-provoking situation is abrupt, whereas in desensitization it is gradual. This strategy is supported by the idea that the mental images experienced in a relaxed clinical setting could have a specific effect on reality. That is, managing anxiety through imagination would help to manage it in real feared situations. *[A. Tamburello, E. De Monte]*

REFERENCES. Beck A.T., *Cognitive therapy and the emotional disorders*, 1975; Reber A.S., *Dictionary of Psychology*, 1985; Schuyler D., *A practical guide to cognitive therapy*, 1991.

IMAGINARY

In Lacanian clinic, it is one of the "essential registers of human reality", together with the symbolic and the real. The function of analysis is to decipher the complex layering of the analysand's discourse. The dimension of the imaginary is structured in progressive developments that start from the theory of the → mirror stage. This describes the illusory nature at the basis of the "the development of the function of the Ego" and it represents the original way used by Lacan to formulate the problem of narcissism. It refers to an experience that determines, at an early stage of a child's development (between 6 and 18 months), an essential moment in defining a child's psychic structure. This is the recognition of oneself through one's own image reflected in the mirror. On the one hand, this experience enables subjects to identify themselves as an "I" but, on the other, it puts them on an illusory line. In fact, the image reflected by the mirror and captured by children, gives them the illusion of a maturation and a mastery that do not correspond to reality because, on this side of the mirror, the subject is still under conditions of dependency and motor incoordination. Hence, the dimension of the imaginary develops within a system of notions related to the mother–child relationship as a model of every imaginary relationship, since it is characterized by specular reciprocity. These notions have also the function of highlighting the theme of the paternal function in its eminently symbolic value. This dimension is further debated in terms of the function it assumes following the mediation made by language on desire and it finally finds its theoretical foundation under the systematization of the categories of the real, the symbolic and the imaginary. *[S. Guido]*

REFERENCES. Di Ciaccia A., Recalcati M., *Jacques Lacan: Un insegnamento sul sapere dell'inconscio*, 2000; Lacan J. (1936), *The mirror stage as formative of the function of the I as revealed in psychoanalytic experience*, in *Écrits: A selection*, 2004.

IMAGINATION

It is the ability to evoke, produce and manage mental representations in the absence of the object to which they refer. Imagination is influenced by the emotional sphere; therefore, it can be interpreted either as an activity directed towards a neurotic alienation from reality or the ability to start creative processes (→ creativity). In Freudian thought, imagination is a compensatory representation of reality, in the sense that it provides substitutional satisfaction when desire is frustrated by an adverse reality. In parallel with the development of the psychic apparatus, the fantastic activity is replaced by a more mature perception and by actions that affect reality with the aim of changing it to obtain satisfaction. In this sense, according to Freudian psychoanalysis, even an artistic production appears as a mere substitute of an artist's frustrated desires. On the contrary, C.G. Jung gave also positive value to imaginative activity by distinguishing between neurotic imagination, understood as a daydream with regressive meaning, and creative imagination, which is able to integrate and organize perceptive contents in original representations. He also described → active imagination as an important therapeutic technique for analytical psychology.

Hypnotic approaches assign a pivotal role to anticipation and imaginative manipulation of reality to achieve therapeutic change. These approaches also focus on exploring how imaginative activity is accompanied by muscle or neurovegetative responses, which can prepare and facilitate the body to cope with the imagined situation when it occurs. Imagination, meant as the ability of projecting oneself beyond contingent reality, represents, directly or indirectly, the source from which both patient and therapist can draw during the process of therapeutic change, so much so that many psychotherapeutic techniques are based on imaginative processes. *[R.]*

IMAGO

A Latin term introduced by Jung about the representations of one's parents: the parental *imago* consists of a set of characteristics of personal experiences with mother and father and their archetypal images. Maternal *imago* conveys emotional meanings linked to being "kept within" and fed, while paternal *imago* is connected to expectations of protection and spiritual guidance. The task of psychotherapy is to promote the withdrawal of projections of unconscious contents – archetypal and personal – from the real parents. However, as these representations have been built since early childhood, the distinction between "subjective" and "objective" representations in parental *imago* is relative. By extension, Jung defines the representation of all psychic entirety as *imago Dei*. *[A. De Coro]*

REFERENCES. Jung C.G. (1934), *The practical use of dream-analysis*, in *Collected Works*, XVI, 1966; Pieri P.F., *Dizionario junghiano*, 1998.

IMMEDIATE EXPERIENCE

In Gestalt therapy, it is the experience of memories, desires, emotions, feelings, movements, before these are mediated by their respective names, that is, by the concepts that signify them. According to Wundt, immediate experience is a complex phenomenon that can be broken up into simple elements by following a behaviourist perspective. Analyzing the experience of an emotion one could conclude that an emotion is nothing more than the sum of: how memories are put together, the weight of the contingent physical status, one's own ideas about the world, etc. Instead, from a Gestalt perspective, the whole is not identical to the sum of the parts: immediate experience cannot be reduced to its parts, but it is meaningful in respect to these, that is, it composes a unique and peculiar experience. Although this experience implies the existence of an event that can be analyzed, it transcends it in an unpredictable way. In this sense, it is possible to speak about an holistic approach: each experience is a whole that must be considered as it is and that can be managed but not analyzed, as reducing it to its components would cancel its uniqueness. In Gestalt therapy, the main issue is how to manage experiences. For this reason, it is important to take into account the biological function of emotions. In this context, emotions are meant as psychic organs whose function is to perform activities that are essential to the survival of the individual and of the species (nutrition, escape, territoriality and sexuality). Keeping in mind the goal of one's emotions, many behaviours can lead to achieving this goal, and this plurality offers behavioural alternatives that allow for changes without having to dismantle the specificity of experience. *[P. Quattrini]*

REFERENCES. Cantor G., *Contributions to the founding of the theory of transfinite numbers*, 1915; Lorenz K., *The foundations of ethology*, 1981; Perls F., *Ego, hunger, and aggression*, 1942; Quattrini P., *Fenomenologia dell'esperienza*, 2007; Smuts J., *Holism and evolution*, 1926; Wundt W., *An Introduction to Psychology*, 1973.

IMPULSE

A psychological need that pushes a living being to take action to achieve a particular goal through innate action patterns. An impulse is an automatic drive, not the result of learning or a personal choice. Impulses are rather strict in respect to what they want and what they aim to, and they hardly obtain gratification from a different object. The → DSM-5 includes "impulse control disorders" in a new chapter (not available in DSM-IV) on Disruptive, Impulse-Control, and Conduct Disorders covering disorders "characterized by problems in emotional and behavioural self-control". This chapter also includes Impulse-Control Disorders Not Elsewhere Classified, which encompasses intermittent explosive disorder, pyromania and kleptomania. *[G. Palmieri]*

REFERENCES. American Psychiatric Association, *Diagnostic and statistical manual of mental disorders* (5th ed.), 2013; Cassano G.B. *et al.* (eds.), *Trattato italiano di psichiatria*, 1992.

INCEST TABOO

In the field of classical psychoanalysis, incest constitutes prohibition by antonomasia, underlying the → Oedipus complex that regulates the normal sexual development of the child. The so-called theory of → seduction gives a pre-psychoanalytic aetiological explanation of hysteria departing from an incest that has really taken place or an episode of childhood molestation by a person outside of the family. During self-analysis, Freud remembered having been subjected to incestual abuse by his father, but he soon convinced himself that it was the effect of self-suggestion, and that the pseudo-memory was an artefact that did not find correspondence in events that really took place. In a letter dated 1897 to his friend W. Fliess, Freud stated that he no longer believed the explanation of traumatic seduction or that of incestuous seduction. Starting from the end of the nineteenth century, the incestuous attraction would become, however, the prime subject of psychoanalytic reflection (Oedipus complex), precisely because it is tied to the nucleus of the concept of the affective family that developed in that historical period, and that constitutes the implicit skeletal structure of Freudian psychoanalysis. Following a complex interaction of historical phenomena, amongst which the crusade against masturbation of the eighteenth and nineteenth centuries and the consequent forms of control over the body, the politics against the extended family in the middle class and the more rigid structuring of the proletarian one, a new type of nuclear family emerged, one that would invest affection to the parent–child relationship, predicting a more intimate type of contact between them and presenting itself as a cell that is relatively isolated from wider social networks.

For Freud the incestuous → drive is the foundation of the patriarchal system, pushing the sons and daughters, or the primordial horde, to kill the father, to then, overcome by feelings of guilt, interiorize the figure of the father and his norms. Analogously, at an individual level, the oedipal situation of the family progresses as a result of the internalization of the paternal figure in the form of the → Superego.

Starting from 1912, Jung moved the incestuous desire and the taboo attached to it onto a decidedly symbolic plane, to indicate the possibility of the conjunction of different components of the psyche. During the course of the 1980s, the nineteenth-century fear of incest was relaunched by radical feminism, which wanted women to be emancipated from the oppression of the patriarchal family, claiming that men are intrinsically abusive, based on the ideology that he who has a penis is intrinsically an abuser.

For this very reason in this period a revisitation took place that was stimulated by Masson's research into the history of psychoanalytic theory of seduction, in which the eighteenth-century theory of traumatic seduction, nowadays renamed "child abuse", contradicted the aetiological knowledge of psychiatric science prevalent at the time, which did not take into consideration childhood trauma as a possible cause of psychological disorder, with the possible exception of post-traumatic stress disorder.

Biological science believes that incest produces genetic damage and therefore, from an evolutionary point of view, the taboo associated with it constitutes an adaptive defence mechanism in the species that have a limited number of children. In the herds of primates, as in different primitive tribes, exogamy is prevalent whereby females that have reached sexual maturity are pushed towards leaving their group of origin to couple with males of other tribes. Precisely on the basis of these genetic presuppositions (that have, moreover, recently been contested on a biological plane), a recent German Constitutional Court judgement affirmed that the incrimination of the crime of incest between brothers, above the age of consent, is justified on the basis of the "supposition" of the negative psychological consequences of the eventual offspring of the parents or of the other members of the incestuous family. From a psychiatric point of view, psychological disorders in these hypothetical cases could derive however, for genetic reasons, from the incestuous procreation; there are, however, many doubts about the fact that the incestuous relationship that does not produce offspring can produce psychological disorders; if anything the contrary is true, that is, as a result of antecedent mental illness, an incestuous relationship is established that is therefore a symptomatic manifestation of the antecedent disorders and not an effect caused by the incestuous relationship itself. In the field of literature some rare cases exist of siblings that have maintained an incestuous sexual relationship all their life, even though they had a normal family life in parallel, apparently without any negative psychiatric consequences (even though they appear to fall under the contemporary definition of 'ego-syntonic paraphilia'). It is important to note, however, that in the course of evolution, behaviour related to a diminished sexual drive has been selected in the case of precocious cohabitation, that frequently inhibits, mainly for biological reasons and through the use of pheromones rather than as a result of a cultural taboo, any form of explicit sexual behaviour between adults and children and between siblings. This lack of inhibition increases the risk factor for incest that is inherent in the reconstituted family, that is, those families whose members have not been living together from a young age.

Incest is however a very rare phenomenon: a Finnish study showed that the prevalence of father–daughter incest to be around 0.15 per cent (the prevalence in the case of schizophrenic fathers is ten times greater) whilst the risk for the daughters that live in reconstituted families or non-biological families increases up to 30 times more. In literature, however, cases exist of siblings separated at a young age and adopted by different families, that, upon meeting in adulthood, have fallen in love without knowing about the blood tie existing between them. *[A. Bella, M. Casonato, G. Fossi]*

REFERENCES. Breuer J., Freud S., (1893–1895), *Studies on hysteria*, in *The Standard Edition*, II, 1953–1974; Foucault M., *Abnormal*, 1999; Freud S. (1900–1901), *The interpretation of dreams*, in *The Standard Edition*, IV–V, 1953–1974; Id. (1912–1914), *Totem and taboo*, in *The Standard Edition*, XIV, 1953–1974; Jung C.G (1912), *Symbols of transformation*, in *Collected Works*, 1956; Malcolm J., *In the Freud Archives*, 1984; Masson J.M., *The assault on truth*, 1984.

INDIVIDUAL

The etymology of this word highlights the indivisible nature of living beings and their irreducibility to other beings of the same species. Jung's psychotherapeutic model embraces the perspective of phenomenology and conceives human individuals as the outstanding and unique outcome of a combination between biology and historical and social environment influences. Individuality has a dimension of singularity, which expresses itself in the particular and unrepeatable character of each person. However, at the same time, it implies a plurality of different levels (for example, personal, suprapersonal or collective) and a multiplicity of centres of consciousness. The goal of psychotherapy is the full expression of individuality, defined as a process of → individuation, which involves the recognition of differences and of the deep relationship between the self and the whole. *[A. De Coro, E. Iberni]*

REFERENCES. Jung C.G. (1921), *Psychological types*, in *Collected Works*, VI, 1971; Pieri P.F., *Dizionario junghiano*, 1998.

INDIVIDUAL PSYCHOLOGY

The result of the creative genius of Alfred Adler within the psychodynamic paradigm. Originally trained as a doctor, he was a keen observer of the dynamics of the psyche and in the close to four decades of his career as a scholar, formulated a new and original model that is aimed at the understanding of the functioning of personality. He identified the fundamental dynamics that organize what he defined as the "lifestyle" (expression chosen to designate the uniqueness of every individual); he studied childhood development, with particular focus on the factors that favour the development of a healthy personality and those that orient a person towards the development of a pathological organization of the personality. He tried to explain the nature of deep-rooted psychological disorders that can affect human beings at any age. He formulated his own method for diagnosing the lifestyle and experimented with therapeutic techniques to correct its deviations. Having discarded the rigid determinism imposed by classical psychoanalysis, he treated adolescents, neurotic and psychotic adults and criminals; he believed that man can always be helped to develop in new and healthier directions in their live; he considered therapeutic optimism to be not only an encouraging prospective, but a natural consequence of the knowledge inherent to individual psychology.

A little more than a century has passed since the final formulation of the therapeutic model by Adler; since then a succession of scholars have used his teachings in various settings for both prevention and intervention, in the clinical setting, in the school setting, in organizations, in research. The cardinal principles of this model have not been eroded by time and have conserved their explicatory potential, in spite of the profound socio-cultural transformations that have changed human beings' way of life. Adlerian psychologists, in many parts of the world, work using the theories and methods that, to a large extent, mirror his original conceptualizations. The considerable similarity between the original Adlerian model and the current one is due to two main factors. The first is with regard to the presuppositions, of an anthropological nature, that are the foundation of the entire conceptualization of individual psychology; these are presuppositions that are well articulated and far-reaching, which constitute the thread utilized by Adler to weave the body of his theory; the second is with regard to the fact that he placed at the heart of his theory dynamisms that contribute directly to the lifestyle, which Adler employed as the yarn used to complete the pattern of his theory.

ANTHROPOLOGICAL PRESUPPOSITIONS AND MOTIVATIONAL SYSTEMS. The anthropological presuppositions on which the theory of individual psychology is based can be subdivided into three groups, of equal importance, but each articulated in a different manner. The first group relates to the "principle of movement", according to which all the activity of the psyche cannot be considered as being static but as being in constant movement; man is in constant movement towards something, towards "goals that he imposes on himself". Adler highlighted the double levels, conscious and unconscious, on which the choice of the direction of the movement is based. The intentionality constitutes the base of this teleological vision, as opposed to causal determinism. The second group articulates the "principle of unity": it is a nucleus that is conceptually richer because it is composed of three dimensions. The first is the unity of the functions of the psyche: it concerns the fundamental unity of the psyche and the synergy of the mind with the body. Man is a biopsychological unit and the conscious and unconscious dimensions are not separate from the lifestyle. The second dimension relates to the unity of the person–environment system: the individual cannot be conceived as being isolated from the context in which he lives. The unit of analysis used to understand man cannot be solely intrapsychic; the web of influence that, with different degrees of intensity, arises from the social groups to which one belongs shape the form of the lifestyle. Finally, the third dimension relates to the unity of the functioning of the psyche: sensations, perceptions, images, memories, fantasies and dreams are organized along the trajectory established by the goals, conscious or unconscious, towards which the lifestyle of the individual is oriented. Every function of the psyche contributes in a congruent manner, and finds expression in harmony with the unified needs of the lifestyle. Finally, the third group of anthropological presuppositions relates to the principle of the harmony of the individual with the community. For Adler, man is essentially a social creature and has to function in the continuous research of equilibrium between the satisfaction of his personal needs and the expectations of the community in which he lives. Adler believed in the existence of an ideal norm that would guide and inspire the creative research for a functional "life project" aimed at the achievement of "self-fulfilment". Neurosis, psychosis and criminal behaviour are always based on a private logic, as opposed to a sense of the community. In developing his theory, Adler used concepts that were connected to two innate motivational systems that are an integral part of the human being: these being cooperation and competition. According to Adler, the motivational system of competition originates from innate aggressive drives, vital energy that orients the individual towards self-affirmation and the search for a sense of security. The aggressive drive feeds the irrepressible need to compete in order to be able to find one's place in the world, in order to be recognized by others, to assert one's value, in order to live. On the other hand, the motivational system of cooperation originates from the innate need to give and ask for help and protection: its prototype can be seen in the instinctive drive of the mother to feed the newborn, that then progresses to the care given to the baby in its infancy, ultimately leading to the forming of a sense of belonging to the community where cooperation is the dimension at the service of life.

THREE STAGES OF DEVELOPMENT. The definitive formulation of this theory engaged Adler in successive revisions and elaborations, of which three distinct periods can be identified, characterized by the specificity of events and by the underlying operative logic.

The first period starts with the initial developments in which Adler manifests a philosophical orientation, theoretical ideas and areas of research that were very personal. His first interests regarded two specific strands of thought: social medicine (he wrote extensively about how the conditions of work influence the physical and psychological health of the workers) and the effects of the conditions deriving from a state of organ inferiority. Around 1902, he started a period of collaboration with a group of scholars led by S. Freud; in this context he maintained and developed his own ideas, and during the renowned "Wednesday nights" he proposed points of view that were different to those that were more closely allied with psychoanalysis. He was, however, influenced by many of the ideas of the group; nevertheless, in 1911 he distanced himself from Freudian thought, based on concepts that were not congenial to him, and declared the autonomy of his theoretical-methodological system that he made known under the title of "comparative individual psychology". Because of their evident differences, Adler's psychology remained for decades in the shadow of psychoanalysis, an effect that only appears to have dissipated in recent times. However, the ideas absorbed by Adler from the "psychoanalytic period" cannot be considered trivial. He welcomed the idea of the exploration of unconscious drives that underlie conscious behaviour, and considered it as necessary in order to be able to explain the origins of neurotic symptoms; he also agreed with the idea that the first years of life are very important in the structuring of personality, and he accepted the idea that it was not necessary to think of a method in order to understand the principles through which the psyche of the man is expressed. He rejected Darwinian determinism, welcomed by Freud as the key to the understanding of psychological phenomena, and substituted the concept of causality with that of the goal to be pursued, of a teleological nature. He was interested in the study of dreams, but he re-dimensioned its importance and formulated other criteria of interpretation of a teleological nature: he was convinced that the dynamic organizing principle of personality was aggressiveness and not a libido of a sexual nature, as was advocated by

Freud. Adler also had the opportunity to refine his ideas regarding the origin of neuroses; he believed that these were caused by repeated psychological trauma caused by situations of organic inferiority, real or imagined, and not, as Freud believed, from an unresolved oedipal complex. In spite of the diversity of their respective theories, his partnership with Freud lasted for a long time, and gave Adler the opportunity to carry out an exercise in "the creative contrast" through which he could refine, in an accurate manner, his theories.

Adler's departure from the psychoanalytic movement made this second period of his work a fertile one with regard to the structuring of his theory; during the "period of theoretical definition", started in 1911, he dedicated himself to capitalizing on the ideas he had collected, and organizing them to form a new theory that was able to explain the origin of neurosis. He retained the concept of inferiority at the centre of this theory; however he amplified its first conceptualization, which was limited to exclusively organic aspects: he worked on the experience that arises from subjective perception, and paired the concept of inferiority with social experience, in particular those of early infancy. The observation that the life of the psyche develops from the natural inferiority of the infant, and that the social context in which he grows can help us either "overcome the sense of inferiority" or else further entrench it in its psyche, led Adler to study, in an attentive manner, the primary figures with which the baby establishes a relationship: parents, siblings, the school environment, peers and social groups. The emotional traces that are the result of these experiences, and that are deposited in the depths of the soul, remain active, and, for the larger part, unconscious: these were considered by him to be the first permanent factor in the development of the psyche. This factor cannot but be combined with a second, in an ongoing dynamic interaction, intuitively conceivable as the push towards the overcoming of the inferiority that Adler defined with the expression "striving for superiority". All human beings, according to Adler, are equipped with an aggressiveness from which they are able draw the strength to orient themselves towards security; the aggressive drives lead to self-fulfilment following a line of research that identifies a sense of security with the position of superiority. Adler also postulated the presence of a third factor, dynamically related to the first two factors, which he identified as the "creative Self", the organizing centre of the personality that allows the psyche to orient itself towards the development of the lifestyle by choosing ways in which to overcome inferiority and to achieve superiority. The creative Self has the task of developing the impressions that develop as a result of experience, together with that of directing the strategies for moving between pairs of opposites: inferiority–superiority, high–low, triumph–defeat, strong–weak, virile–feminine. Every individual is able to develop a lifestyle that is healthy if the opposites make up a unitary vision: neurosis, instead, originates in the entrenchment of interior experiences around only one of the two poles, particularly that of inferiority.

The third period of Adler's work started after 1920 and it was during this time that his social interests were given concrete expression through "practical experimentation". The training carried out according to the principles of individual psychology generated considerable interest; he opened clinics for parents and teachers as well as schools that were inspired by the principles of his theory. The practical application of this theory led to the development of another important dimension of the theory, already implied in his previous work: the concept of "community feeling". According to Adler, the real nature of man is social and he was convinced that man has to position himself within his community as a united and indivisible entity, in movement from states of inferiority to conditions of superiority. These movements should not only follow the logic of personal interest, but also need to be inspired by the interest of the collective: the striving for superiority has to take place in harmony with the interests of the community. Adler was convinced that a healthy lifestyle is one in which the individual is able to work on personal goals that have objectives that are in harmony with those of the social context in which he operates. According to him, psychopathology, deviations, the pathological expressions of individuals or of social groups take root when social reasoning is lost and when a private logic that ignores or neglects the interests of the community prevails. This point of view guided Adler in the experiences of the last part of his scientific life, that was characterized by the fact that he combined his role as a doctor, therapist and educator, with that of the promoter of his theories in various parts of the world.

CARDINAL CONCEPTS. Individual psychology is a complex system of ideas, but some of the concepts that have been mentioned above – that play a fundamental role in his theory of human psychology – are particularly significant. These are: the lifestyle, emotion and inferiority complex, striving for superiority and will to power and social interest. The expression "lifestyle" is used to indicate the unity of personality. It is the result of the creative dimension of the individual that, during the course of his life, combines the hereditary components with the stimuli coming from the environment. In the construction of the lifestyle the "objective" qualities that are inherited, as well as those coming from the environment, are not as important as the meaning the individual attributes to them; these assume the function of predisposing factors that the individual uses to create his "lifestyle", which is unique and unrepeatable, and that will make up the way he relates to himself, to others and to the world. According to Adler, the lifestyle is formed in the first four to five years of life; patterns of behaviour and of reactions become habitual with experience, and the lifestyle develops enduring characteristics. In adulthood, the different aspects of behaviour become more cohesive and more complex, but continue to adhere to the modes of behaviour established in the first years of life. The components of the lifestyle include both the perceptual dimension and an operational dimension. The former refers to the perception that the individual has of himself, of his ideal Self, the way he perceives others and the world, and of his ethical and aesthetic beliefs. The operative dimension refers to the evaluation that the individual makes of his possibilities, of his aspirations and of the way in which he sees the world, that lead him to choose the goal that he wants to achieve and the ways in which to achieve it. The final goal that the individual establishes always relates to the concept of superiority; in the reality of daily life the striving for superiority is expressed in an infinite variety of concrete goals. Sometimes these can appear to be in contrast with each other, but they are always dominated by the same theme. Once the final goal is established, all the individual's tendencies will contribute in a unified manner, towards moving in the pre-established direction. The theme of inferiority, for Adler, represents a central characteristic that is interwoven into all his work. The idea of inferiority of the "organ" represents its first formulation and is based on the idea, known to clinicians from ancient times, that all human bodies have a part that is more vulnerable than others. The perception of weakness causes the individual to become sensitive and to pay particular attention to the inferior organ; this activates the mechanism of "compensation" that is aimed at overcoming the frustration experienced as a result of the inadequate functioning. The inferiority of the organ can refer to any part of the body and the psychological processes that develop from it will vary in their intensity, and do not necessarily relate to the objective degree of inferiority but rather to the perception that the individual has of it. In the absence of organic pathology, the sense of inferiority may arise from any physical or psychological function. In this case a morbid degree of sensitivity may develop that reinforces the individual's concentration on himself, and the mechanism of compensation will consist of the same processes as seen in the case of organ inferiority. The study of the psychological states that result from organ inferiority led Adler to extend his study of the nucleus of inferiority to other conditions. He considered the inferiority of the infant as being a natural condition of the human being who appears to be very vulnerable in the face of educational errors. A child that grows in an environment that is frustrating, rejecting, indulgent, discouraging or violent is at risk of developing the perception of being inadequate to cope with the demands of life and of developing a profound feeling of inferiority. The experience of inferiority is fuelled by repeated attacks: the individual will measure his perception of his own abilities and resources against his image of the difficulties that he feels are connected to a task that he has to face. The fear of being unsuccessful, the anticipation of failure, the fear of the collapse of the image he has of himself, will fuel this feeling of inferiority, which then leads to avoidant behaviour, to the devaluing of the task or to justifications that will mask the underlying lack of courage. The different degrees to which experiences of inferiority may be present require different designations to describe experiences that can be located along a continuum that varies from a mild condition that is not particularly complicated, to more serious and disabling conditions. At the first level one can find the "sense of inferiority", made up of perceptions that are annoying, but bearable and easily managed; indeed, they are desirable because they contribute towards the cementing of a realistic perception of the Self and help the individual take precautions from the risks of an excessive sense of security, orientated towards feelings of omnipotence. The "sense of inferiority" then follows, which constitutes a significantly more annoying presence and requires the use of coping strategies that are more elaborate, but restricted, however, to dynamics that take place at a conscious level, such that they do not lead to the development of neurotic symptoms. When the feeling of inferiority increases in intensity to a degree to which it inhibits, hinders or changes behaviour, it can then be described as being an "inferiority complex". This consists of a condition marked by a profound sense of discouragement: the individual who has an inferiority complex has lost his faith in himself and lacks the energy to try to assert himself. The neurosis develops from the attempts of the individual to free himself from his inferiority complex by using maladjusted coping strategies that inhibit the growth of the individual and push him towards adopting repetitive and unfruitful behaviour.

According to Adler, the aspiration towards superiority is an irrepressible desire; it is an innate drive that manifests itself at all ages and in every condition. All human beings experience a basic need for security that can be satisfied through the different ways of achieving a sense of superiority: the striving for success, for self-fulfilment, for recognition, for excellence. In all contexts and situations that man faces, the striving for superiority is the dynamic process that permits the overcoming of feelings of inferiority. Only the inferiority complex is able to remove the dynamic value of superiority and to block its expressive possibilities. A form of striving for superiority is the research of personal power. Adler denominated the tendency to seek power as being the "will" to power", a term that has generated much misunderstanding as a result of its immediate association with the work of F. Nietzsche. In reality, with this term, Adler intends to describe a pathological form of striving for superiority; he considers it to be a pernicious tendency that fuels the neurotic who, when operating in the world, ignores the needs of others and is not able to develop feelings of empathy towards his peers.

Finally, the concept of social interest: Adler considers it as originating from the innate potential of the individual and ascribes to it the important function of tying the individual to the community. The social interest can take the form of love towards one's peers, their productions and towards nature, but also the pleasure experienced in belonging to a community. The primary relationship with the maternal figure is considered to be very important for a healthy development of the social interest that forms the basis for the development of the capacity to collaborate with others, to understand others and in achieving empathic relationships. From infancy, the social interest also serves to balance out the striving for superiority. According to Adler, if the social interest is able to develop in a healthy manner, it leads to the good management of the need for superiority of the individual, leading him to take into account the needs of others and the harmonization of legitimate personal aspirations with the interest of the collective. This is such an important concept of individual psychology that it is considered as being the measure of the usefulness of life projects; the expression the "barometer of normality", coined by Adler, is even more precise and effective in describing this concept. The importance attributed by Adler to this concept reiterates the idea that man is part of society and that the feeling that ties him to it becomes a personality factor that one cannot disregard. Considering man as an isolated reality, detached from the context in which he lives, does not make sense; the life of the psyche acquires meaning only within the dynamics of the community. To evaluate a personality, one needs to therefore observe his behaviour in the world, to evaluate the degree of interest exhibited in others and the degree of social interest he exhibits when dealing with the problems of the world. *[G. Mazzoli]*

REFERENCES. Adler A., *The neurotic constitution*, 1917; Id., *The practice and theory of individual psychology*, 1920; Id., *Menschenkenntnis*, 1921; Id., *The problem child*, 1930; Id., *Individual psychology*, 1931; Id., *What life should mean to you*, 1931; Ansbacher H.L., Ansbacher R.R. (eds.), *The individual psychology of Alfred Adler*, 1956.

INDIVIDUATION

A process of differentiation, that is, of shaping and characterization of individuals. This concept represents the most meaningful psychological idea of the whole of Jung's work. The individuation process enables the emergence of characteristics of personality that are potentially existing since birth. It coincides with the evolution of one's consciousness from the original state of identity and begins with the psychological birth of a child, that is, with the emergence of the consciousness of the Ego. The final goal of the process is the psychological development of the individual as distinct from the generality, of a conscious wholeness, where Ego and Self are combined while each retains their peculiar qualities. This implies a continuous movement of differentiation from, and adaptation to, the outside world. In the second half of one's life more attention is paid to the requirements of the internal world; there is a push towards a differentiation from the collective psyche, to become an individual able to distinguish one's own peculiarities from the constraints of the unconscious and cultural collectives. Individuation is realized as an internal process of integration of repressed unconscious parts to adapt to reality, and as a development of a critical consciousness that, once distinguished from the "person" and the collective culture, can face the latter and provide new creative contributions. Individuation is not to be confused with individualism or egoism, because it does not generate separation from relationships, but it helps a freer personality to emerge within the normal world in which a person lives. *[A. Benvenuti, G. Kaufman]*

REFERENCES. Jung C.G. (1928), *The relations between the ego and the unconscious*, in *Collected Works*, VII, 1967; Id. (1939), *Conscious, unconscious and individuation*, in *Collected Works*, IX–I, 1969.

INDUCTIVE PROCESS

This term refers to a thought process that, departing from in one or two particular cases, arrives at a logical conclusion that goes beyond the particular cases taken into consideration. This process is manifested through the identification of regularities in the functioning or in the intrinsic characteristics of objects, individuals or particular events, which are then generalized to other events with characteristics that are considered to be similar. Inductive reasoning is the foundation of that form of thought that is described as → common sense, and it is characterized by the tendency to derive from the observation of a limited number of incidents the prediction that these will repeat themselves in similar situations. According to classic cognitivist authors, the process of inductive thinking can constitute the basis of the mental constructions of phobias, obsessions, paranoid ideas, depression, obsessive-compulsive disorders. This happens because the individual intensifies the unpleasant thoughts associated with experiences that took place in particular circumstances, applying them also to other situations through a process of mental associations. This form of "naive realism" is at times also present in the process of psychotherapy, when some authors generalize the results of experiments or therapies carried out on a small number of individuals to the entire human race. As a result of their characteristic of immediacy, inductive processes can also be utilized as instruments of → therapeutic change. *[R.]*

REFERENCES. Salvini A., *Pluralismo teorico e pragmatismo conoscitivo: assunti metateorici in psicologia della personalità*, in E. Fiora, L. Pedrabissi, A. Salvini, *Pluralismo teorico e pragmatismo conoscitivo in psicologia della personalità*, 1988.

INFERENCE

A logical deduction made from one or more premises. It may concern a specific conclusion or a generalization. In logic, the principles that allow a conclusion to be considered valid are called "rules of inference". "Arbitrary" inference consists in drawing an unjustified conclusion, for example without evidence or in the presence of contradictory evidences, which leads to an incorrect perception or interpretation of reality and events (→ cognitive distortions). *[R.]*

INFLATION

In the context of analytical psychology, a term used to define a catastrophic phenomenon, resulting from an assimilation of the Ego to the Self or from an assimilation of the Self to the Ego, which interrupts the dialogue between consciousness and the unconscious, blocking in this way one's development. In the first case, the space of the Ego is cancelled by the invasion of the unconscious and it feels helpless towards the collective dimension. In the second case, the Ego is "deflated", it identifies with unconscious contents and feels omnipotent. Inflationary phenomena, to which human personality is subject due to its inherent weakness caused by the separability of the psyche, manifest themselves with different degrees of intensity: they can be temporary moments that mark one's psychic development and analytical processes or psychopathological situations of narcissistic type. *[A. De Coro, E. Iberni]*

REFERENCES. Jung C.G. (1951), *Aion: Researches into the phenomenology of the self*, in *Collected Works*, IX/II, 1951; Pieri P.F., *Dizionario junghiano*, 1998.

INFLUENCE

It is the ability to change perceptions, thoughts, and behaviours of others through → interaction and → communication. As stated in the first axiom of the → pragmatics of human communication, according to which "one cannot not communicate", any communication contains elements of influence directed to the receiver, such as to assert that "it is not possible not to influence". In psychotherapy, it is essential for the therapist to understand the various phenomena of mutual influence between therapist and patient, and how to use them consciously to obtain significant results in terms of reduction of suffering. The factors affecting influence are related to: the therapist's → personality; that of the patient; their → interaction;and the specific techniques used by the therapist to induce change during the treatment. *[R.]*

INHIBITORY STIMULUS

In the behavioural paradigm, it is an inhibitory stimulus through which an inhibitory response to → anxiety in the presence of stimuli that evoke it can be manifested, to weaken the stimulus–response link (→ stimulus–response relationship). The usual procedure consists of the development of a conditioned inhibition by means of "reciprocal inhibition". The method is based on the idea that anxiety is a → conditioned response dissociable from the stimulus that caused it, through the evocation of a more intense → antagonistic response. When, in the presence of an anxiogenic stimulus, an antagonist response to anxiety can be elicited, between the two competing stimuli the strongest will inhibit the weaker with the progressive decrease of anxiety until → extinction occurs. → Relaxation is an excellent inhibitor of anxiety for many types of stimuli. *[E. Luisetti]*

REFERENCES. Wolpe J., *Psychotherapy by reciprocal inhibition*, 1958.

INJUNCTION

In transactional analysis, a parental message that leads the child to limit one of his areas of expression and development (feeling his own existence accepted, feeling emotions, thinking, defining his own identity). It is one of the two poles of childhood dynamics of the construction of the psychological → script; the other is the → script decision. Injunction is characterized by: transmission through a nonverbal channel, which is, therefore, essentially emotional; the unawareness of its scope, by both the parents and the child; the emotional intensity, given the young age at which it takes place (by the age of three); the unconscious aim of the parent to avoid contact with expressions of the child, which can awaken painful and unresolved areas in themselves. In transactional psychoanalysis – a "plank" of transactional analysis – the therapist analyzes the reactivation of transference emotions tied to the patient's projection of messages of injunction that are attributed to him. *[M. Novellino]*

REFERENCES. Berne E., *«Hello!». . .and then what?*, 1972; Novellino M., *Psicoanalisi transazionale*, 2004.

INJUNCTIVE LANGUAGE

Injunctive language is the linguistic form that conveys "orders". It can be considered one of the structuring concepts concerning systemic explanations of behaviour. In this conceptual frame, the members of a group are perceived as controlling each other's behaviour through information. Every behaviour is an overt or covert expression of an order given to the other members of the group. One of the most interesting types of injunction is the paradoxical one. In fact, a pragmatic → paradox consists of two injunctions where the second injunction prescribes an antagonist action in regard to the prescription of the first injunction. Pragmatic paradoxes are the basic pattern of → double binds. Performative language is used to prescribe behaviour in a direct (→ injunction) or indirect way (→ suggestion). This behaviour can be external and concrete, as it is in words and action, or it can be subtle and internal, as an emotion or a perception. It differentiates mainly from the denotative or explanatory forms of expression that are used to describe perceptions or experience. Performative language is widely used in brief strategic forms of psychotherapy (→ brief strategic therapy Nardone's model, → brief therapy MRI's model) as the therapist, in these approaches, is responsible for inducing concrete changes in the patient's perception, behaviour and feelings. Palo Alto's brief therapy is widely known for its use of therapeutic → double binds. Performative language has been described in psychotherapy literature mainly through the study of Milton H. Erickson's hypnotic work, structural and strategic family therapy models, the Brief Therapy Center model (→ Mental Research Institute) and its heirs (Nardone, Wittezaele, Garcia). *[T. Garcia-Rivera]*

INSIGHT

A term expressing a concept of pivotal importance in Gestalt psychology and later adopted also by psychoanalysis. In the Gestalt approach, the term was introduced by W. Köhler, in the interwar period, to indicate a sudden enlightenment or idea that leads to a real restructuring of the perceptive field, allowing a person to solve a problem instantaneously. Through experiments involving apes, Köhler could show that, if faced with a dilemma, apes could suddenly guess, after a period of exploration, how to use, together, the scattered objects available in their field of perception. The apes could give objects a new position in space and consequently a new function. The solution to the dilemma consisted in the possibility of reconfiguring the items available in the field, by experiencing them simultaneously and globally as organized in a new form, useful for the solution of the problem. On the other hand, the inability to perceive a different function of the items available in the field is called "functional fixedness". This concept is in line with the Gestalt theory according to which "the whole is other than the sum of the parts". It directly opposes the behaviourist theory of E.L. Thorndike, who argued that learning processes are linked to a series of "trial and error" and supported by the possibility of → reinforcement. The term is also used in psychiatry to indicate a lack of awareness in the patient concerning the presence of their own disorder. *[R.]*

▷ In psychoanalysis, insight is an experience of "mutative knowledge". As in psychology, it concerns a redefinition of the system by a subject that generates a change. This phenomenon is similar to the religious experience of enlightenment and, according to Levenson, analogous to the "eureka moment", when suddenly a long-sought solution comes to mind. More broadly, this concept is used to indicate the ability of a patient to grasp the psychic dynamic factors, acting in the solution of a conflict, as key steps for therapeutic change. The analytical → setting, with its peculiar features, facilitates this type of understanding. It is structured as a place where it is possible to exert a certain freedom of self-observation, association and discernment. This can happen on a purely intellectual level, when patients understand their own psychic dynamics from a theoretical perspective but without drawing an experience from it, or on an affective level, when patients understand the unconscious motivations behind their actions in their entirety and undergo a cognitive restructuring. Only the latter kind of insight allows patients to obtain a true and deep understanding that leads to therapeutic transformation. A. Saraval stated that insight can happen due to an interpretation or a free association during the analysis. However, it can also take place outside the analytical setting, upon awakening from a dream or due to events, emotions or simply due to a sudden free association of the patient. The main factors that can lead to an insight can be divided into: verbal interventions of the analyst and interpretations (of → transference, extra-transference, inaccurate); relationship, behaviour and attitude of the therapist (according to F. Alexander and T.M. French the → corrective emotional experience, according to J. Weiss the disconfirmation of → pathogenic beliefs, but also the internalization of the analyst's attitude and the characteristics of the setting); extra-analytical life. Any analyst–patient interaction can generate an insight. D.W. Winnicott affirmed that often a new awareness can derive from observing a different model of behaviour from others as well as from a caring silence, which offers support and consolation and which remains there even without verbal language expressions. In psychiatry, insight is interpreted as a patient's awareness of their own psychic disorder and possibly of its origin, due to intrinsic reasons. The "coming to light", the insight, would be the key to an understanding of the events that give the subject the possibility of change. Therefore, it would be pursued even in the case of → psychosis, as awareness of the disease, which is a prerequisite to the opportunity to address actively one's situation. Starting from this definition, A.S. David developed his theory on insight. He developed a model consisting of three different but overlapping dimensions: the ability to recognize oneself as ill; the compliance to treatment; the ability to correlate abnormal mental events (for example, hallucinations and delusions) to a pathological phenomenon. *[M. Casonato, M. Gaffuri]*

▷ Within the cognitive approach, there are two types of insight: cognitive, which refers to the → awareness and understanding of one's own psychic dynamics and psychopathology on an intellective and theoretical level; and emotional, which refers to the ability to detect, classify and interpret one's own emotional experience. *[G. Palmieri]*

REFERENCES. Levenson E.A., *Fifty years of evolving interpersonal psychoanalysis*, 2006; Musatti C.L., *Trattato di psicoanalisi*, 1950.

INSTITUTIONALIZATION

A long-term inclusion and hospitalization in specific facilities such as nursing homes, orphanages, prisons or therapeutic communities characterized by rigid daily routines and procedures as well as by partial restriction of personal freedom. This measure is adopted when individuals are not able to take care of their own daily needs (because they suffer from severe chronic diseases, or because too young or too old), or when individuals are endangering their own life or that of others, as in cases of severe mental disorders (violent forms of paranoia, anorexia, drug addiction, severe depression). The chronic hospitalization of patients in structures and their continual exposure to rigid, repetitive and monotonous daily tasks, often evolve into regressive and stereotyped behaviours that often tend to aboulia and catatonia, withdrawing into themselves, addiction and poor personal hygiene care. For this reason, the anti-psychiatric movement (→ anti-psychiatry) was opposed to the process of psychiatric institutionalization. In Italy, the Basaglia law (law 180) was issued on May 13, 1978. With this law, asylums and mental health services were reformed, with the aim of promoting people's active recovery paths, both inside and outside therapeutic communities, through the integrated intervention of various professional figures (psychiatrists, educators, social workers, psychologists). *[R.]*

INTEGRATED PSYCHOTHERAPY

A type of psychotherapy that makes flexible use of methods, techniques and strategies derived from various different theoretical models, in order to plan and carry out tailor-made and more personalized interaction for the client. The aim of integrated psychotherapy is to modify the client's subjective experience, adaptive functioning and quality of life. Targets are generally people who have decided to make use of psychotherapy to overcome symptomatic problems, identity disorders and /or relationship difficulties that are causing psychic pain and distressing behaviour patterns.

INTEGRATED TREATMENT AIMS AND PLANNING. The purpose of the therapeutic process is to enable the client to re-examine his past history (his sense of identity), to take energetic action in the present (mind–body connection) and to make realistic plans for his future (influencing his destiny with a new and more functional lifestyle). In order to achieve such a result it is necessary to proceed with care, carrying out a general → assessment followed by a progressive psycho-diagnostic evaluation of the results reached along the way, in the four main phases characteristic of integrated psychotherapy. The first is the assessment phase: an analysis of the demand, needs and most urgent necessities is carried out and the way in which the problems first arose is clarified. Having placed the patient in the context of his "system", he is offered a series of encounters in which the clinician tries to reassure him by arousing hope. At this point, the feasibility of taking on the client is examined on the basis of elements such as how motivated and ready for → change he is (ambivalence about starting therapy) and how chronic is the problem. The second phase is that of pre-therapy: a multidimensional assessment is performed through semi-structured clinical interviews and a set of logical → idiographic tests (identifying the specific characteristics of the subject, → psychological tests) as well as a series of nomothetic tests (standardized inventories) to evaluate the symptoms and potential resources (vulnerability, → resilience, → coping), for the purpose of formulating a treatment plan. The person receives an explanatory profile with information about the type of psychotherapeutic intervention proposed (frequency, intensity, duration). In the third phase of psychotherapy, the holistic treatment plan is activated, the aim being the reduction of overall stress levels generated by the disorder. The empathic alliance (involvement, emotional bonding and adherence to treatment) constitutes a predictive factor for the construction of a good collaborative therapeutic relationship and shared objectives. Homework is often given to modify certain thinking patterns and to facilitate the change desired by the client. Continuous assessment of treatment efficacy is applied throughout the process to measure changes in personality structure as well as the degree of symptom improvement. In the final phase, a series of questionnaires provides an evaluation of outcome, achievement of agreed objectives and stabilization of therapeutic effects. Finally, a → follow-up period is always planned in order to reinforce and stabilize outcomes (wellbeing, quality of life, an optimistic and humorous sense of values with positive emotions).

HISTORY OF THE INTEGRATIVE APPROACH AND FURTHER DEVELOPMENTS. In 1910, during an international congress, Freud declared that treatment via the spoken word and interpretation had proved inadequate for some phobic patients and would have to be modified. Later, for economic reasons, antiscientific orthodoxies prevailed and ideological approaches monopolized the scene for several years, leading to the birth of numerous psychotherapeutic models (recorded in a collection of over 400). However, an agreement was gradually reached over the recognition of certain sovereign principles, thus conferring scientific validity on the first great basic models: behaviour is determined by unconscious reasons (psychodynamics), but our actions are also influenced by environmental conditioning (behaviourism) and furthermore it is our subjective perception of self that orients our way of being in the world (humanistic, existential). In the years from 1930 and 1980 various experimental forms were created by merging together some of the principal basic models, including body work as well as systemic and hypnotic approaches. Between 1995 and 2002 important scientific research of international significance was carried out to evaluate evidence-based results in psychotherapy. Work carried out by consumers' associations and also prestigious meta-analytic research in academic contexts decreed the principle of equality: equal outcome efficacy whatever the procedures and techniques. The ability of psychotherapy to achieve real objectives and desired effects was recognized. In clinical practice the biopsychosocial model became the chosen strategy for optimal intervention, in that the key question became "which treatment is the most appropriate for this individual with this specific problem and in this particular system/context (→ efficacy) and who can carry it out in the shortest possible time at the lowest possible cost (→ efficiency)?" It follows that, taken individually, the numerous therapeutic models turn out to be partially incomplete, and so to increase the efficacy of treatments the SEPI (Society for the Exploration of Psychotherapy Integration), the movement that collects together the results of research into psychotherapeutic integration, has received increasing consensus amongst professionals. In applied clinical practice a guiding meta-model has been adopted that provides the following methods of intervention: technical → eclecticism (selecting effective procedures from different theories); theoretical integration (combining two or more different theories); change processes (trans-theoretical interventions in the various developmental phases of treatment); common factors (selecting decisive elements essential for the therapeutic relationship); assimilative integration (a central model of useful techniques taken from other models). We no longer search for the best therapeutic model, but rather for the best aspect of each approach, considering the different therapeutic priorities and depending on both the complexity of the problems (poly-symptomatic, comorbidity) and on the contextual situations of the client's life. In order to reach the objectives, always defined together with the client, ingredients considered necessary for an effective relationship (non-specific factors) have to be administered and certain active principles that are useful for directing and accelerating change have to be carefully weighed up. According to Norcross (2011) the latest scientific research of the essential variables that determine outcomes can be quantified in the following way: 3 per cent → interaction, 7 per cent the personality of the psychotherapist, 8 per cent the method of intervention, 12 per cent the therapeutic relationship, 30 per cent the client's contribution (expectations, predisposition, dysfunctional severity), 40 per cent the ecosystem of social support (favourable or adverse life events). In clinical practice the main treatment factors derive from the application of: awareness-raising psycho-educational techniques; emotionally cathartic experiences that provide emotional corrective experience through dramatization; counter-conditioning and stimulus control; reinforcement control and management; self-liberation of social context. The purpose of all these healing factors is to treat disorders, to overcome traumas and dissociated situations and to construct new adaptive behaviour patterns. The art of clinical practice consists in humanizing the encounter by harmonizing treatment method and relationship to monitor and calibrate the quality and the frequency of low-intensity or high-intensity interventions in therapy. Relational interventions during the process, which are considered "warm" (non-directive empathic understanding) and prescriptions, alternate with "cold" procedures (directive cognitive empathy). They favour both the overcoming of → resistance to change and renewed emotional mentalization through a more secure attachment style. The constitutive and essential aspects of the integrated approach are based on mapping the ethics of evidence-based best practice emerging from professional psychotherapists' experience (practical and qualitative activities), and on randomized experimental tests from available scientific evidence. They are confirmed by quantitative laboratory research data, subjective preference of user appreciation – which is formalized in the application of common fundamental elements universally shared and distilled by various comparative therapeutic models.

MOVING TOWARDS INTEGRATED METHODOLOGICAL PLURALISM. Research and professional state of the art in the field of integrated methodology are based on codified procedures emerging both from empirical standards and from scientific evidence. Pluralism saves clinicians from hiding behind a rigid professional identity that presumes that they alone possess the one and only immutable truth. Furthermore, it allows professionals to step back from ideological fideistic self-referential theories and to move towards positions of research based on scientific evidence (validity and verification). For the client it offers a chance to adhere exclusively to those technical and methodological aspects that he finds attractive and useful, leaving him plenty of free choice. In this field, scientific research advances with caution, offering useful provisional guidance without claiming to reach definitive conclusions. *[E. Giusti]*

REFERENCES. Giusti E., *Psicoterapia, in Dizionario Enciclopedico della Salute e della Medicina*, 2006; Giusti E., Germano F., Psicoterapeuti generalisti. Competenze essenziali di base: dall'adeguatezza verso l'eccellenza, 2006; Giusti E., Militello F., *Neuroni specchio e psicoterapia. Ricerche per apprendere il mestiere con la videodidattica*, 2011; Giusti E., Montanari C., Iannazzo A., *Psicoterapie integrate. Piani di trattamento per psicoterapeuti con interventi a breve, medio e lungo termine*, 2004; Spalletta E., *Personalità sane e disturbate. Un'introduzione propedeutica alla cura delle normopatie del quotidiano*, 2010.

INTEGRATED STRATEGIC THERAPY

It was, from the moment of its formulation, intended as an integrated approach, in that within in it a multitude of theoretical approaches converge (→ cybernetics, → constructivism, theories about human → communication, cognitive behavioural psychotherapy) and different modes of intervention (→ hypnosis, behavioural → prescriptions, → desensitization techniques, etc.). However, this is not a simple mix of theories and techniques, but a body of "complex" views on being human (of life and of relationships) and about therapeutic work that is always careful and aimed at a full understanding of the patient and the implementation of effective (→ efficacy) and efficient (→ efficiency) resolution of his problems.

According to Erickson, the strategic intervention reflects a kaleidoscopic vision of reality, therefore the instruments utilized are not decided *a priori*, in that there is no one well-defined technique that allows us to respect the multifaceted nature of the human being in "relation" to himself and to others. The therapist, according to the objectives of the intervention and respecting the individuality of every therapeutic situation, uses his theoretical-practical knowledge in carrying out the principal task that is asked of him, that is, the resolution of the problem brought into therapy. The totality of the theories, instruments and techniques brought into therapy, therefore, cannot be limited by a single style of approach to the patient, but rather has to draw from a plurality of these with the aim of "strategically" adopting precisely those types of interventions that are most functional to the resolution of the problem of the patient, "tailoring" the intervention to him rather than employing "prefabricated" techniques. *[F. Petruccelli]*

REFERENCES. Erickson M.H., *Collected works of Milton H. Erickson*, E.L. Rossi (ed.) 2008–2015; Erickson M.H., Rossi E.L., *Hypnoterapy*, 1979.

INTELLECTUALIZATION → DEFENCE MECHANISMS

INTENTIONALITY

In Gestalt therapy, a characteristic of consciousness that tends to something specific. In the context of the phenomenological approach (→ phenomenology, → phenomenological method), the term refers to one of the most important aspects of consciousness; it exists, in fact, only in its relating to something, in its "in-tending towards" an object, in its being transcended: it is in the act of transcending that subjectivity is constituted; it is in "transcendence" that the substantial element of consciousness is found. The notion of intentionality, as emerges from the phenomenology of E. Husserl, implies, on the one hand, the impossibility of a "reality in itself" and, on the other, the exclusion of a "consciousness in itself", incapable of perceiving the world in itself. On the epistemological level, such a manner of conceiving intentionality is a fundamental reference point both for psychology and for psychopathology. If the being is constituted essentially in being transcended, in having intentions, in entering into contact with what surrounds him, this implies the necessity that psychopathology and psychotherapy must turn to the analysis of this continual transcending, "being intended", entering into contact; above all, it is necessary to investigate how, in what forms and in what manner the being "is intended". It is to this central nucleus of research that psychotherapies of phenomenological or phenomenological-existential orientation have recourse. Gestalt therapy, in particular, puts the "self" at the centre of the treatment operation, which knowingly and actively develops meanings, produces intentions, subsists in its continual opening to the world, so as to constitute a single reality with it. It is in this relationship with the world, in this "in-tending towards" it, that the origin of mental suffering and, at the same time, the space of treatment, are to be identified. *[M. Spagnuolo Lobb, P.A. Cavaleri]*

INTERACTION

A mutual relationship between elements of a → system or between two or more systems. The nature of the relationship is circular, thus indicating a retroactive influence between the elements involved.

At a social level, interaction is a relational process between two or more people, which implies a reaction and a modification of one's own actions according to other people's conduct and mutual expectations. Interactions can be understood at different levels: within themselves, between themselves and others and between themselves and the outside world, in a continuum that moves from the → intrapsychic to the → interpersonal and social world. Every human interactional system consists of homeostatic mechanisms (→ homeostasis) that tend to keep the balance, and by positive → feedback that pushes the system towards change. Several interaction models can be described in functional terms, such as models of family, social, political and economic interaction. Symmetrical and complementary (→ complementarity) interaction models were described for the first time in → pragmatics of human communication. These are based respectively on the similarity or difference of how two or more people communicate. The first formalization of the interactional theory in relation to psychotherapy is due to Don D. Jackson, who in 1958, founded the → Mental Research Institute (MRI) in Palo Alto. The institute is devoted specifically to the study of the processes and patterns of interaction. The results obtained by MRI and the studies of J. Haley and J.H. Weakland on the body of work of M.H. Erickson contributed to the development of the → interactional-strategic paradigm. *[R.]*

Interactional-strategic paradigm → Please refer to the opening chapter, "The eight paradigms and their respective theoretical-applicative models".

INTERACTION-FOCUSED THERAPY

Interaction-focused Therapy (IFT) is grounded in communication theory set forth by Gregory Bateson, Don Jackson, John Weakland, Jay Haley and William Fry, and solidified at the → Mental Research Institute (MRI) during the 1950s and 1960. Individual behaviour, especially "symptomatic" behaviour, becomes comprehensible when one acts in accord with tenets of the interactional approach, such as, one cannot not communicate, and conceiving behavioural exchanges (analogic and digital) as proposals about the nature of the relationship, which are contextually coherent and recursively organized such that any attribution of meaning (i.e. causality) is a product of observer-imposed punctuation. IFT holds the non–blame-evoking view that we all do the best we can considering how behaviour finds its meaning in the context(s) and relationship(s) of which it is a part. Members of a system define the nature of the relationship by symmetrical and complementary transactions in the here-and-now. Symptoms emerge when consensus about the nature of the relationship cannot be achieved. Systemic therapy is

> predicated on the necessity for viewing the symptoms of the identified patient within the total family interaction, with the explicit theoretical belief that there is a relationship between the symptom of the identified patient and the total family interaction. The extent to which the therapist "believes" in family therapy will determine his emphasis on techniques that convey this orientation to the patient.

Consonant with → Milan school of family therapy, MRI Brief Therapy, Jay Haley and others, IFT adopts the systemic logic first articulated by Jackson:

> when primary focus is shifted from . . . individuals to . . . the interaction between . . . [members of a system] . . . there are no good guys or bad guys or long-suffering wives and bastardly husbands. There are patterns of interaction which have to be so conceptualized that it isn't possible to say the husband withdraws because his wife nags, nor the reverse.

Members of any interacting group with a history are understood "as a mutual causative system, whose complementary communication reinforces the nature of their interaction. The therapist looks for rules that govern this system; therapy consists of the therapist behaving in a way that the rules must change".

In IFT, the therapist is accountable for his actions and takes responsibility for behaving in such a way as to evoke constructive change. This position of accountable action is exhaustively set forth by Jackson:

> If a family is stuck in a rigid pattern, the therapist should do something to break up that pattern. There are all sorts of contingency possibilities – other behaviours, other opportunities, other people to whom family members can relate differently. Therefore they *can* change, regardless of their unconscious motivation or other psychological dimensions that have in the past prevented them from changing.

As in Haley's strategic therapy (→ strategic family therapy, → strategic directive psychotherapy), the IFT therapist identifies solvable problems, sets goals, designs interventions to achieve those goals, examines and takes responsibility for the efficacy of outcome.

With the preceding presuppositions in mind, the therapist joins the client by gathering information about the problem. Who is involved? How? When and where does the difficulty occur? What is the client(s) explanation, or "why", about the problem? When did they decide this was the best explanation for the difficulty? What are the client's language, worldview, and punctuation (causal explanation) about the problem? What are the reasons that brings the client in to talk about the problem now? In what context would the symptom make sense if the symptom (i.e. behaviour being complained of) were an unlabelled comment about the untenable nature of the relationship? How is the symptom protective of others? → Circular questions and → positive connotation are used to bring forth patterns of interaction (i.e. relational logic), which make the symptom coherent. What are the effects of the behaviour of one person on other people in the system? Exploring the *effects* of behaviour on others rather than the *motives* of behaviour quickly reveals the rules of a relationship. Who is doing what, to whom and in what way is it a problem? What happens then? What do other family members do? Who else is involved? What is going on then? Attempts to resolve often act to *maintain* the problem. How have family members tried to solve the problem? What were things like before family members settled on this explanation for their situation? Look for overt and covert coalitions. What will the future look like once the situation has changed? Questions are asked to obtain information *and* so that family members can overhear and digest the relationship ramifications of responses. Develop a relationship-focused hypothesis including all members of the family. A non-judgmental stance is maintained, adhering to the conviction that there is nothing wrong with the symptomatic person or anyone else in the relationship nexus. Positively connote *all* members of the treatment unit. Once a relationship-focused hypothesis is validated, adopt and work within the client's frame of reference/worldview to offer an alternative way of understanding the situation that allows family members to interact in ways that no longer call forth and perpetuate the problem. The objective is to develop a therapeutic reality that allows all members of the relational system to change, using therapeutic reframes, based on the emerging relationship information, that allow family members a legitimizing logic for behaving differently. Give a task to disrupt the behaviour pattern calling forth and perpetuating the symptom. How? By engaging family members to behave on the basis of a systemic conceptualization of their difficulty that makes such change plausible. In the next session obtain information on how the clients carried out the task. Use this information to either refine or solidify a therapeutic reality. In ways consonant with the client's frame of reference, emphasize the adaptive nature of responses, normalizing and positively connoting all family members. Prescribe tasks to maintain constructive changes.

Numerous therapy models have emerged in recent years, most claiming to be new, "evidence-based," effective, and supposedly unrelated to the radically relational, contextual and constructivist perspective set forth by the early pioneers of system thinking. In contrast, IFT explicitly embraces the communication theory articulated by Bateson, Jackson and colleagues in the 1950s and 1960s. IFT does not claim to be "new"; rather, therapeutic success derives from close study and application of the interactional logic set forth by early system pioneers. Outcome studies of IFT with the widest range of problems demonstrate efficacy and efficiency equal to, and in many instances superior to, results shown by *any* other therapeutic approach. Essential aspects of IFT and presuppositions on which the approach is based have been outlined as an invitation to rediscover a wealth of "new" ideas to be found in the "old" systemic literature. *[A. W. Ray]*

REFERENCES. Bateson G., *Steps to an Ecology of Mind*, 1972; Cecchin G., Lane G., Ray W., *Irreverence*, 1992; Haley J., *Uncommon Therapy*, 1973; Nardone G., Watzlawick P., *Interactional Brief Strategic Therapy Outcome research: A long term controlled study*, in W. Ray, G. Nardone (eds.), *Paul Watzlawick: Insight may cause blindness and other essays*, 2009; Ray W.A. (ed.), *Don D. Jackson: Essays from the dawn of an era*, in *Selected papers, vol. I*, 2005; Id. (ed.), Don D. Jackson, *Interactional theory in the practice of psychotherapy*, in *Selected papers, vol. II*, 2009; Ray W.A., de Shazer S., *Evolving brief therapies*, 1999; Ray W.A., Keeney B., *Resource focused therapy*, 1993; Selvini Palazzoli M., Boscolo L., Cecchin G., Prata G., *Hypothesizing, circularity, and neutrality: Three guidelines for the conductor of the interview*, in «Family Process», 1980, 19 (1); Weakland J.H., Ray W.A., *Propagations. Thirty years of influence from the Mental Research Institute*, 1995.

INTERACTIONIST MODEL AND THERAPY

A model that integrates the methods of semiotic, strategic and holistic psychology within a socio-psychological constructivist framework (→ symbolic interactionism). It can be described in reference to three complementary levels of analysis: epistemological, theoretical and clinical/methodological. The epistemological level refers to the perspectives of symbolic interactionism, → anthropomorphism, social psychology, social constructionism, → conceptual realism, radical → constructivism, which are combined with the strategic and systemic perspectives. The interactionist model assumes that psychological and social realities, also the problematic ones, are built by actions and by the cognitive processes used to describe, explain and interpret them. Accordingly, the effects of interactionist psychotherapy emerge from the communication and the relationship between therapist and client, with the purpose of creating a change and not curing. Problematic behaviours and mental states are configured through pragmatic semiotic processes—such as adaptive expedients that can, in a holistic perspective, be dysfunctional on a personal level and in interpersonal and social relations, implicating also biological or socio-psychological systems. Therefore, the processes of construction of reality, even the problematic ones, are attributable to intentional acts and actions, although not always conscious. In this view, situations and subjects are considered active and not passive in respect to events. The interactionist perspective adopts a meta-model with a strong and consistent epistemological reference, which is common to the entire strategic-interactionist paradigm. This meta-model is pragmatic, pluralistic, relativist, non-ontologising, not deterministic or normative. It differs from the traditional models of psychotherapy that are linked, instead, to a positivist, realist, medicalizing, deterministic and normative reference with an emphasis on nosology, and on the dualism between normality and pathology and between the observed and the observer.

The second level of analysis is theoretical. The interactionist perspective configures human actions and their more or less problematic, different, atypical and deviant processes, as people's attempts to adapt to different interactive contexts, whether they be intrapersonal or interpersonal. The intervention in psychotherapy aims to change how individuals represent the world, how they perceive and emotionally relate to situations in life, how they reconstruct their autobiographical experience and anticipate future events. Therefore, the way people portray and attempt to resolve their discomfort or their deviant solutions in relation to each other, plays a fundamental role. The interactionist approach considers the functional or dysfunctional way people act as the product of an active construction of meaning by actors in relation to each other and within themselves, through historically contextualized forms of social negotiation. The theoretical assumptions in interactionist psychotherapy techniques consider that: people generate actively the experience of which they suffer the unpleasant side effects, by replicating it through behaviours of avoidance and control; people think and act on the basis of the meanings they give to events, although they are not always aware of what makes these meanings to emerge; the systems of representation and constructs that make evaluating themselves or a situation as problematic, are shaped by people through social and cultural interactions, and are understandable only within the relational contexts that organize them and that tend to maintain them; people build the experience of themselves, others and the world, including when these are considered pathological, through representational systems of which language, action and communication are the most important generative elements; the biographical self-representation can be treated as if it was a narrative genre that provides schemas, scripts, rules and roles; change always involves important emotional transformations of meaning and sense through action; the problematic forms of thought and action are not right or wrong, healthy or pathological, but only → attempted solutions with adaptive purposes but with dysfunctional results.

As emphasized by interactionist methodology, in the intersubjective construction of reality particular attention is given to the role/rule of relations. This regards both linguistic and symbolic aspects, which converge in systems of thought, values and beliefs. These systems may result in dysfunctionality in the relationships that people have with themselves and with others. The narrative methodology focuses instead on discursive practices that build autobiographical systems and relational contexts through which the modes of experience, be it normative or deviant, are generated, maintained or changed. Structural relationships that create fields of interdependence between acts and actions, people and roles, problems and disorders, imply a systemic perspective, with reference to which physiological, psychological and social aspects are configured as interdependent.

The third level of analysis is clinical-methodological. With respect to the epistemological and theoretical consistency that characterizes the approaches concerning the interactional-strategic paradigm, the clinical-methodological practice adopts constructivist, narrative, strategic and holistic techniques. These include: the change of personal theories, both implicit and explicit, that organize the experience that people have of themselves, others and the world through reprocessing self-representations, multiple roles, identity and situational scripts; a perceptual and emotional redefinition through dialogic strategies (communicative stratagems), metalogic, paradoxes, evocative injunctions, logical reorganization and self-regulating and restructuring acts and actions at a somatic-sensory level; narrative and biographical reorganization and reconfiguration of constructs of sense and meaning through the splitting off or the evaluative integration of personal and relational experience. At a holistic and systemic level, the intervention involves a finalized recomposition of the conditions of → wellbeing, growth and empowerment, where the emphasis is on the implementation of the psychophysical balance rather than on symptomatic treatment with the use of specific methods derived from the most recent acquisitions of integrated medicine and focused on the mind–body relationship. The therapist's task is not to assess whether and how much the customer's constrictions are right or wrong, but to what extent they are adequate to personal wellbeing and to the relational adaptation to the world. The clinical areas specifically addressed by interactionist psychotherapy are as follows: sexual/affective and identity disorders; existential problems associated with one's self-representation, autobiographical narrative genres, role-playing situations and life cycle; the so-called "symptomatic" disorders (for example, anxiety, phobias, compulsions, depression, eating disorders, addictions, dysphorias/depressions, reactive psychosis, persecution complexes, dissociative and ego-dystonic disorders); deviant behaviour, self-harming disorders, problems of social and interpersonal adaptation and their somatic implications; promotion of states of holistic and subjective psychosomatic eurhythmy. The areas of intervention in the contexts tackled by interactionist psychotherapy (institutional, organizational, educational and territorial) are particularly relevant in the modern labour market. In this context, the promotion of change requested of therapists is not only directed to the sphere of private, individual, couple, family or group therapies, but also to the categories of meaning adopted by communities, to the organizational structure of institutions and health services, to the sphere of shared meaning at a socio-cultural level that have assimilated the historically predominant medical/diagnostic model. First, these categories of meaning and organization define the way problems of discomfort and deviance (and, conversely, of wellness and "normality") are defined at a social level and at level of services. As these are constructs, their meaning follows the knowledge modalities that are used to define them; thus, they preordain which operative strategies are legitimate to produce change. The interactionist model pursues the promotion of epistemic restructuring (meant as structural change of the theoretical position of thought or behaviour) at a collective and organizational level. This aims at facilitating the implementation of a paradigm shift that allows the categories of meaning and intervention practices based on the medical/diagnostic model to be abandoned, in favour of a more modern and efficient anthropomorphic model. Among the areas of application addressed to date by this approach, the following can be mentioned: clinical and health psychology (redefined also in a holistic perspective); psychology in educational institutions; the structuring of services and operative strategies in social, educational, legal and working contexts with adults and children. *[G. Pagliaro]*

REFERENCES. Berger P.L., Luckmann T., *The social construction of reality*, 1966; Goffman E., *Interaction ritual*, 1967; Mead G.H., *Mind, Self and society*, 1934.

INTERNAL WORKING MODELS

According to the → attachment theory, a set of conscious and/or unconscious rules that allows a person to organize information concerning attachment and to grant or restrict the access to it, in relation to experiences, feelings and ideas concerning attachment itself. These mental representations are constructed towards the end of the first year of life and start from the emotional experience that a child has lived in early relations with the caregiver. Therefore, a child forms a "working model" of the attachment figure, which summarizes the history of the affective responses and the availability of the parent towards their requests, and a complementary model of the Self. This also takes into account the behavioural skills and potentialities that the child can use to achieve a feeling of security. Internal working models are crucial for the construction of the affective reality of individuals. In fact, these models allow individuals to guide the review of their experience and their attachment behaviour, and make them able to make predictions on affective experience in meaningful relationships. Internal working models work outside of conscious awareness and provide individuals the rules through which they perceive, predict and act, especially in the context of relationships. For this reason, these models have a tendency to stability, as they tend to actively recreate experiences consistently with the history of relationships that individuals have lived before. *[A.M. Speranza]*

INTERNATIONAL STATISTICAL CLASSIFICATION OF DISEASES AND RELATED HEALTH PROBLEMS → ICD

INTERPERSONAL

In the field of psychotherapy, it is everything that becomes significant as it is shared with other people. More specifically, interpersonal → communication and interpersonal → relationship are believed to determine the contents of the → interaction with the environment. They are considered constructs capable of delineating the transitions of evolutionary stages, the construction of personality and related disorders. Many approaches have investigated the importance of interpersonal relationships. This field is still one of the most fertile and problematic in research on personality. H. Stack Sullivan was the first to develop a theory of psychiatry based on interpersonal relationships (interpersonal → psychiatry) where socio-cultural forces play a major role in the formation of mental health problems. Thanks to his contribution, attention shifted from the → intrapsychic to the interactional level (→ interaction). Later, the concept was extended to the field of communication and some observations formulated in this field revolutionized the way we think about relationships and interactions. In a different way, Sullivan's studies became the foundation that gave a start to interpersonal psychoanalysis, a psychoanalytic school that highlights the importance of interpersonal patterns in interaction with others and who had, in K. Horney, its highest expression. The same horneyan theoretical-clinical basis is reflected in the theory and technique of groups and in → group analysis. Subsequently, the term has been the protagonist of many psychoanalytic theories on mother–child relationships. However, it was the existential-phenomenological approach, more than any other, that highlighted the importance of the connection between the individual and the social sphere in relation to personal wellbeing. *[R.]*

INTERPERSONAL PSYCHIATRY

In his *Interpersonal Theory of Psychiatry*, Sullivan conceives interpersonal psychiatry as "an expanding science concerned with the kinds of events or processes in which the psychiatrist participates while being an observant psychiatrist"; he also adds that

> scientific psychiatry has to be defined as the study of interpersonal relationships, and this in the end calls for the use of the kind of conceptual framework that we now call [→] *field theory*. From such a standpoint, personality is taken to be hypothetical. That which can be studied is the pattern of processes which characterize the interaction of personalities in particular recurrent situations or fields which "include" the observer.

Sullivan was the founder and main theorist of the interpersonal theory of psychiatry, which took shape in the 1930s and developed into the neo-Freudian psychoanalytic school of thought, which included, amongst others, C. Thompson, K. Horney, E. Fromm, E.H. Erikson and F. Fromm-Reichmann. Sullivan did not personally edit his complete works but the numerous writing and notes that he wrote for conferences and lessons at the Psychiatric Institute of Washington and at the William Alanson White Institute of New York have been organized, selected and published by the White Foundation.

PRIMARY ASSUMPTIONS. The primary assumption of Sullivan's interpersonal theory of psychiatry – which Greenberg and Mitchell labelled "relational/structural model" as opposed to Freud's → drive/structure model – highlights the role played by culture in shaping personality; in fact, in

Sullivan's view, the human being is not the consequence of innate inborn drives but the result of his relationships with other human beings. By shifting from an intrapsychic to an interpersonal level, by founding a mind theory on relational bases and by emphasizing the important role played by the environment in shaping character – which, in addition, emerges from the relationships between human beings and their reciprocal communication – interpersonal psychiatry broadens the therapeutic possibilities offered by traditional psychiatric approaches and classical Freudian psychoanalysis, which had always conceived narcissistic psychoses as "untreatable disorders".

By adding an interpersonal dimension to his psychiatric treatments, Sullivan was the first to broadly apply psychoanalytic concepts to schizophrenic disorders. Because he strongly believed that both "normal" and pathological behaviour were the result of how one relates and reacts to the events of life, Sullivan turned freely to the social sciences, stressed the importance of a multicultural approach and supported psychoanalysis, which he promoted with psychiatrists as a psychiatric technique. As for the role played by communication, Sullivan embraced the theories formulated by anthropologist E. Sapir, who saw language as the main communication tool and argue that, in order to share single experiences, human beings needed to refer to a socially shared linguistic code. Sullivan's thinking was also influenced by Hungarian psychoanalyst S. Ferenczi, with whom he shared the view that the analyst plays a pivotal role in the therapeutic relationship. In fact, Ferenczi highlighted the concept of countertransference, while Sullivan developed the notion of analyst as participant observer. No one can be observed or treated without taking into account the person's very interpersonal situation. Personality can be known only through the medium of interpersonal interactions, given that it is defined by what one does within an interpersonal field.

BASIC CONCEPTS. Sullivan's theory points to psychiatry as a science studying interpersonal relationships and suggests that most mental disorders are the consequences of poor communication in which anxiety hinders all communicative processes. Individuals are the result of an interpersonal relationship in which each person is involved as a portion of an interpersonal field rather than being a separate entity in processes that affect and are affected by the field. Man is an evolving creature and the development of both personality and mental disorders is more affected by (even imaginary) interpersonal interactions with significant adults than by intrinsically individual factors; hence the emphasis placed by this perspective on the pivotal role played by the empathetical relationship with the mother. A good mother–child relationship lays the foundation of a secure base for the child's development; conversely, a poor one leads to mental disorders whereby → mentalization processes are hindered by the anxiety that develops within the relational field of the mother–child interaction, interferes with the child's development and threatens his need for security. According to the interpersonal theory of psychiatry, the human being's fundamental needs are the need for satisfaction and the need for security, which both entail engaging a human being from "the outside"; the mother is the first source of satisfaction for the needy child. The child's tensions of need cause the mother's tensions and prompt her to intervene to assuage those of her baby. The infant's calls for help (i.e. crying, motor agitation, screams) catch the mother's attention and, as soon as the need has been fulfilled, the tension drops. Once he feels satisfied, the infant returns to the previously lost state of wellbeing (euphoria). The set of tensions that require the mother's attentive intervention constitute what Sullivan called "tenderness theorem", which describe how the infant's need to be mothered and the mother's need to care are reciprocal and complementary. The infant's experience originates from the alternation of needs and satisfactions and is perceived according to three different modes: *prototaxic* (when experiences are pre-symbolic); *parataxic* (when symbols are used privately); and *syntaxic* (when experiences can be communicated). As Sullivan noted, the difference in these three modes "lies in the extent and the character of the elaboration that one's contact with events has undergone". The first mental operations are prototaxic; nonetheless, even after the self-system has structured itself to satisfy needs and avoid anxiety, the prototaxic mode may resurface again later in life through anxiety states, sleep and schizophrenic conditions. The latter, in fact, are characterized by the massive appearance of primitive operations (such as dissociation) and may lead to parataxic distortions, i.e. parataxically distorted experiences of another person. Sullivan's interpersonal theory posits that the parents' way of relating to their child moulds the latter's relationship modalities. The child's personality (the Self) is shaped by "reflected appraisal", i.e. the parents' positive responses to him. Maternal anxiety, rage or disapproval will cause distress and anxiety in the infant and turn his self-concept into "bad-me" (→ good-me) personification; thus, he will experience a growing anxiety whereas parental approval will support the child's "good-me" personification. The most anxious and painful experiences that the child tries to dissociate and to keep out of consciousness constitute the "not-me" personification, which is characterized – as Sullivan remarks – by being "manifest in certain peculiar absences of phenomena when there should be phenomena" (dissociated behaviour) and "practically beyond discussion in communicative terms". *[A.Cresti, S. Brizzi]*

REFERENCES. Conci M., Dazzi S.,Mantovani M.L.(ed.), *La tradizione interpersonale, in psichiatria, psicoterapia e psicoanalisi,* 1997; Greenberg J.R, Mitchell S.A., *Object relations in psychoanalytic theory,* 1983.; Lionells M., Fiscalini J., Mann C..H., Stern D.B.(edited by), *Handbook of Interpersonal psychoanalysis,* 1995; Mitchell S.A., Black M..J., *Freud and beyond: A history of modern psychoanalytic thought* 1995. Sullivan H.S., *The common field of research and clinical psychiatry,* in "Psychiatric Quarterly", 1927, 1, 3; Sullivan H.S., *Conceptions of modern psychiatry,* 1940; Sullivan, H.S., *The Interpersonal theory of psychiatry,* 1953 ; Sullivan H.S., *The psychiatric interview,* 1954; Sullivan H.S., *Clinical studies in psychiatry,* 1956; Sullivan H.S., *Schizophrenia as a human process,* 1962 ; Sullivan H.S., *The fusion of psychiatry and social science,*1964; Sullivan H.S., *Personal psychopathology,* 1972.

INTERPRETATION

In psychoanalysis, it is the method through which analysts express in words what they understand of the mental life of patients. This understanding, communicated to the patient, is based on the expression by the patient, even unknowingly, of desires, fantasies, fears, memories and other elements that were unconscious or which the patient knew in a distorted, incomplete, inaccurate way. Therefore, interpretation is the enunciation of new knowledge about the world of patients to patients themselves. It allows them to understand their inner past and present life in new ways and therefore, to change attitudes, behaviours and feelings. Interpretation has been defined as the main instrument of psychoanalysis. According to K. Eissler, every psychoanalytic activity should be eventually brought back to interpretation. As stated by Strachey, in order for interpretation to be "mutative" (that is, to produce change), it must be provided at the "point of urgency" of unconscious contents. According to Glover, also an incorrect interpretation may play a therapeutic part, but only through a suggestive action, that is, by reassuring or providing an explanation, no matter what this would be. The interpretation of a → symptom, a → dream, a slip, is made to determine its meaning. According to R. Schafer and Spence, Atwood and Stolorow, the "meaning", traditionally considered pre-existing, would actually be determined by interpretation itself in a process of rewriting a patient's personal history. According to the traditional psychoanalytic conception, it is crucial for analysts to provide a meaning to patients' productions and to communicate them to allow patients to make their unconscious contents become conscious. According to contemporary authors, these are, vice versa, psychoanalytic strategies of construction of personal history and "psychoanalytic meaning" of events. Several types of interpretations can be identified: *dynamic interpretations* define conflictual mental tendencies that cause behaviours, feelings and other mental activities; *anagogical interpretations* analyze the oneiric material; *genetic interpretations* connect existing thoughts, feelings, conflicts and behaviours with those of early childhood:

an example of this is the reconstruction that brings information together (collected through free associations, dreams, etc.) concerning early psychological significant experiences; *transference interpretations* clarify distortions in the therapeutic relationship based on the transference – or the projection – on the analyst of behaviours and feelings experienced originally with a caregiver or with significant figures of the past. The criteria for assessing the accuracy of interpretations are the response of the analysand and the smooth harmonious integration of interpretations within the material that has emerged. Freud noted that therapists often produce "constructions" that do not necessarily have to be "true", but nor are they arbitrary. These should facilitate a reconstruction of aspects of one's personal life in an acceptable and therapeutically effective manner. This idea was resumed and deepened by Spence, who talked about narrative → truth and stressed the efficacy of reconstruction rather than its truthfulness, which was instead a main theme among scholars in the 1950s. *[M. Casonato, S. Sagliaschi]*

REFERENCES. Atwood G., Stolorow R., *Structures of subjectivity: explorations in psychoanalytic phenomenology*, 1984; Freud S. (1900–1901), *The interpretation of dreams*, in *The Standard Edition*, IV–V, 1953–1974; Id. (1937), *Constructions in analysis*, in *The Standard Edition*, XXIII, 1953–1974; Glover, E., *The therapeutic effect of inexact interpretation*, in «The international Journal of Psycho-Analysis», 1931, 12; Spence D., *Narrative truth and historical truth*, 1982; Strachey J., *The nature of the therapeutic action in psychoanalysis*, in «International Journal of Psycho-Analysis», 1934, 15.

INTERVENTION-RESEARCH

A methodological principle that originated from the field of action-research, a term coined in the 1940s by a group of researchers that were carrying out research in the administrative field, and that was first formulated in the psychosocial theories of K. Lewin in 1946. It is a scientific process that connects theory to practice and that is focused on the resolution of problems by means of the planning of a sequence of interventions; this process develops over time and involves the continuous checking of the effects of these interventions, so as to modify them in the case in which these are not proving to be satisfactory (→ self-correctiveness). The process of intervention-research assumes that the functional knowledge of a problem can only be obtained as a result of the attempts to modify (intervention) the problem itself; according to this perspective, therefore, it is the solution that explains the problem and not vice versa.

The operational application of the principle of intervention-research in the field of psychotherapy leads to the concept of → diagnosis-intervention, that contrasts with the classical concept of → psychiatric diagnosis and of → psychological diagnosis in which, on the contrary, the phase of acquisition of knowledge regarding the problem presented by the patient takes place before the phase of intervention. Intervention-research in psychotherapy, therefore, by presupposing that the phase of therapeutic intervention and the phase of acquisition of diagnostic knowledge take place simultaneously, consists of experimentation and of the analytic study of the methods of change as a *sine qua non* condition in order to understand a given pathological behaviour. The observed changes that are the result of the intervention are what will "explain" the nature of the problem, making it possible only *a posteriori* to make a "diagnosis" of the problem itself. *[R.]*

INTIMACY

A component of the Bernean triad, together with → awareness and → spontaneity, which expresses the capacity of autonomy of an individual and which constitutes the methodological and philosophical objective of transactional analysis. In the experience of intimacy, the person enters into a relationship with another in a modality that is free from psychological → games, therefore, in a direct way, expressing the naturalness of one's own being and welcoming that of the other. Phenomenologically, the individual experiences a state of unique consciousness, in which he feels free to present himself as he is, confident that he will be welcomed in his entirety, and leaves the same possibility to the other; it deals, therefore, with an intrapsychic experience, but also a relational one. *[M. Novellino]*

REFERENCES. Berne E., *Games people play*, 1964; Moiso C., Novellino M., *Stati dell'Io*, 1982.

INTRAPSYCHIC

The term indicates a process that takes place within the psyche. For example, an intrapsychic → conflict indicates the simultaneous presence within the same person of two conflicting forces, motivations or tensions. It is the antithesis of the term → interpersonal, which designates what happens between people. *[R.]*

INTROJECTION

In Gestalt therapy, a function that allows the passage of elements from the outer to the inner world of the organism/individual. This function prevails in the early stages of development and it can represent the basis for the crystallization of "introjects" (conscious and unconscious beliefs). These can affect positively (as sense of recognition and esteem) or negatively (as disregard and lack of appreciation of the Self) the next stages of the development of personality and its consolidation. *[R. Zerbetto, A.S. Persico]*

REFERENCES. Perls F., Hefferline R.F., Goodman P., *Gestalt therapy: Excitement and growth in the human personality*, 1951; Zerbetto R., *Gestalt: la terapia della consapevolezza*, 1998.

INTROSPECTION

This term indicates the observation of the contents of one's own → conscience, which can be applied to thoughts, feelings, intentions, or to other more complex psychological processes. In psychotherapy, classical psychoanalysis has made the introspective method the main tool to obtain the therapeutic effect of → insight through the use of → free associations. Historically, the use of introspection in psychological investigation has been strongly contested by behaviourist authors. The main arguments have been based on two considerations: the data coming from the introspective action are not immediately observable and measurable and therefore they remain subjective; it is logically impossible for individuals to be simultaneously observer and observed. Both these critics conclude that the introspective method does not meet the scientific criteria, such as observability, replicability and measurability of a phenomenon. However, these arguments appear to be anchored to a neo-positivist philosophy of science. This experienced some success in the early twentieth century but it was progressively superseded by some recent constructivist developments. On the one hand, these developments go beyond a clear distinction of observer–observed and, on the other, they do not recognize the observability criterion as necessary to produce knowledge (→ mentalism). The most recent therapeutic currents of thought, except for behaviourism, all adopt introspection as a method of investigation of mental processes and psychic contents subject to change. *[R.]*

INTROVERSION

In the psychodynamic conception, it is one of the basic attitudes towards the world, consisting in the → libido, that is, the psychic energy, aiming at the inside. In this sense, when there is a well-integrated consciousness, introversion and → extroversion follow each other, in the individual, in connection with personal and environmental variables. When introversion becomes customary, it is legitimate to talk about an "introverted type". The subject's interest does not aim at the object, as it does in the case of the extraverted type, but at the inside of the very same subject. The construct of introversion has to be considered under the light of Jung's typology, which distinguishes two attitudes (introversion and extraversion), and four functions of consciousness: two rational (feeling and thinking) and two irrational (sensation and intuition). Sensation is irrational inasmuch as it receives the pure presence, the simple "what" of things, without questioning about their *why*. On the contrary, thinking poses the question of the why of things, in the same way that feeling judges their value, accepting or refusing them. The meaning bestowed by Jung on feeling deviates from the common one. Intuition, finally, is not interested in the why of things, but in their "for what", that is their openness to the unknown (intuitive-introverted types can be mystics, seers, artists). For a correct understanding of the introverted type, to have the attitude ascertained is not enough, but it becomes necessary to determine which of the functions of consciousness aims at the inside. Consequently, one can talk about introverted-thinking type, introverted-feeling type, and so on. As a rule, it can be said that the introverted type leaves, in shadow (not lived), his extroversion and, more particularly, that the thinking- and feeling-introverted types leave in shadow, respectively, extroverted feeling and intuition. The treatment of an introverted patient will consequently have to deal with proceeding in the direction of an integration of extroverted sides left in shadow; for this, the patient's dreams will be a valuable help, as they compensate the functional and attitudinal one-sidedness. *[G. Antonelli]*

REFERENCES. Jung C.G. (1921), *Psychological types*, in *Collected Works, VI, 1971*; Freud S. (1952), *Beyond the pleasure principle*, in *The Standard Edition*, XIV, 1953–1974.

INTRUSIVENESS

With reference to different areas and situations of everyday and relational life, intrusiveness can be defined as the trait of an extraneous individual who intervenes with non-requested actions and judgments in other people's intimate sphere and in behaviours of → communication or → relationship. In this sense, intrusiveness can be considered a form of invasion of privacy. This is not only unpleasant but also harmful as it represents a – not necessarily unconscious – expression of → manipulation of other people's behaviour and an alteration of personal and relational balance of people who are not able to offer effective resistance. Frequent examples of intrusiveness can be identified in the interference on the life of a couple by family members and acquaintances. Similarly, with reference to the methodological problems of psychological and social research, intrusiveness concerns the alteration of an observed system due to the presence of the researcher and the study method adopted. This condition cannot be eliminated by psychosocial research but only attenuated on a technical level. For example, a researcher can become part of a group to learn its rules of interaction rather than subject its members to instrumental investigations (interviews, questionnaires, tests). In general terms, important differences are reported in the literature, which distinguishes between experimental and non-experimental method (observation). Experimental method is based on a deliberate manipulation of situational variables, in order to highlight the relationship between the independent variable (cause) and the dependent variable (effect). It is a highly intrusive method, generally used in artificial situations. However, as it is based on standardized procedures, it allows researchers to support their theoretical assumptions in a timely manner. In non-experimental methods, it is worth distinguishing between participating observation and controlled observation. In the first case, researchers integrate themselves in a natural situation and become participants of the interactions that they want to observe; within the field of observation, they draw clear advantages in terms of knowledge since they are intimately in contact with actors' subjective perspective. However, this advantage brings a disadvantage: researchers are subjectively influenced by the relationships in which they participate. Differently, in controlled observation, researchers move to the edge of the field of observation, to limit their relational involvement. In this case, the disadvantage can be noted in the phenomenon of social desirability: people hide, more or less consciously, aspects of their behaviour that they consider less commendable and exhibit behaviours and opinions that do not represent them completely. In this sense, the alteration of the opinions and behaviour is attributed to the intrusiveness of the investigation techniques. In psychotherapy, the degree of intrusiveness changes in relation to the different theoretical-methodological approaches and consequently to the style of the therapist, which can be more or less oriented to intervene on and to manipulate awareness and behaviour of patients. *[S. Smiraglia]*

REFERENCES. Corposanto C., *Metodologia e tecniche non intrusive nella ricerca sociale*, 2004; Nardone G. (ed.), *Modelli di psicoterapia a confronto*, 1988.

INVARIABLE PRESCRIPTION

In the psychotherapeutic approach of the Milan School, a therapeutic → prescription invented in 1979 by the team formed by Selvini Palazzoli and G. Prata. For over ten years, it was prescribed to families who had sons or daughters with eating disorders or with a psychotic disorder. → Follow-up studies confirmed the extreme efficacy of the invariable prescription with anorexic patients who had parents who were over-controlling, and as being much less effective (especially in the long term) with psychotic patients. The invariable prescription consisted in dismissing the patient and his or her siblings, and nominating the parents as co-therapists of the team; the parents were then asked, upon returning home, to tell their children and any other members of the → family that may be present, that the contents of the therapeutic session were a secret, which they could not divulge to them, and to subsequently observe their reactions, jotting down their observations in a notebook, independently of each other. During the next session, they were asked to leave the home for increasingly long periods of time (one evening, a weekend, a week), leaving behind a note, and to continue writing down their observations of the reactions of the rest of the family. The therapy would be based on the information provided by the parents' observations. This technique also became a valuable instrument in the research by these authors on interactive family processes (metaphorically denominated as "pathological family games") that lead to psychosis in the son or daughter, which led to the discovery of phenomena such as "instigation" and "cheating" in these types of families. The use of this therapeutic prescription was, however, gradually abandoned, at least in this ritualistic form. *[S. Cirillo]*

REFERENCES. Selvini Palazzoli M., Cirillo S., Selvini M., Sorrentino A.M., *Family games*, 1989.

IN-VIVO DESENSITIZATION

In the context of cognitive-behavioural psychotherapy, a part of the → systematic desensitization conceived by J. Wolpe. In-vivo desensitization decreases the probability of emitting avoidance or escape responses triggered by environmental situations full of anxiety-inducing stimuli. In particular, this technique consists in approaching these stimuli through cadenced approaches (→ graded exposure). However, from a general perspective, it represents the final step of a wider methodology. The initial creation of a hierarchy of anxiety-inducing stimuli is followed by a calm and ordered presentation of the stimuli in the subject's imagination (→ imaginal exposure), starting from the least to the most feared, to facilitate an early elaboration. Finally, at the end of this process, in-vivo desensitization exposes the subject to the real feared situation, having previously already diminished its degree of psychophysical activation. The expected result is the extinction of the anxious sensitization associated to the stimuli. As a separate procedure, in-vivo desensitization can be performed without the imaginative phase while maintaining the hierarchical progression. This facilitates a gradual and immediate facing-up to the feared stimuli. The subjects measure themselves immediately against the feared stimuli without any preparatory imaginative phase. *[A. Tamburello, E. De Monte].*

REFERENCES. Beck A.T., *Cognitive therapy and the emotional disorders*, 1975; Reber A.S., *Dictionary of psychology*, 1986; Schuyler D., *A practical guide to cognitive therapy*, 1991.

IN-VIVO EXPOSURE

In the context of cognitive-behavioural psychotherapy, a technique by which subjects face feared objects and situations in their perceptual environment, without implementing distraction or avoidance strategies so as to experience their harmlessness and their progressive mastery. In its → graded exposure mode, in-vivo exposure is recognized as effective in the treatment of specific phobias, panic disorder with agoraphobia, anxiety and social phobia, obsessive compulsive disorder (accompanied by compulsive ritual response prevention) and post-traumatic stress disorder. In addition to → extinction and habituation processes, in-vivo exposure appears to work due to → cognitive reframing and new associative and/or emotional processes related to the dangerousness of stimuli. *[A. Cocchi, A. Meneghelli]*

REFERENCES. Craske M.G., Anthony M.M., Barlow D.H., *Mastering your fears and phobias: Workbook*, 2006; Franklin M.E., Foa E.B., *Obsessive-compulsive disorder*, in D.H. Barlow (ed.), *Clinical handbook of psychological disorders: A step-by-step treatment manual*, 2007; Sloan T., Telch M.J., *The effects of safety-seeking behaviour and guided threat reappraisal on fear reduction during exposure: An experimental investigation*, in «Behaviour Research and Therapy», 2002, 40.

INVOLVEMENT

A more or less intense participation to situations and relationships that characterize people's lives. In particular, involvement is a state of the → Ego that modifies the perception and evaluation of one's own and others' behaviour, of expressed positions and social situations. In this respect, the term used is Ego *involvement* and its impact on social → attitudes is widely recognized. In particular, it is identified as an element capable of influencing the degree of commitment that people bring into play to defend their ideological and moral positions. The involvement of the Ego generates significant psychological stress, both emotional and cognitive. This tends to raise people's personal coherence and identification with the social group. From the perspective of cognitive processes, involvement motivates people to elaborate centrally, and not peripherally, information and pressures to change, exerted by a persuasive source (ELM: Elaboration likelihood model). In psychotherapy, the therapist's involvement is generally understood as an element in the relationship with patients, capable of affecting the fairness and efficacy of treatment. → Transference (the projection of the patient's relational experiences on the analyst) and → countertransference (in contrast, the projection developed by the therapist towards the patient) identify dynamics that could be compromised by involvement. From here, specifically during an orthodox psychoanalytic treatment, arises for the analyst the imperative to not intervene in order to avoid any influence and to avoid losing supposed professional independence. Instead, other approaches have given value to → empathy as expressive signs of intense participation in the patient's problems and as a lever of change. *[S. Smiraglia]*

REFERENCES. Freud S. (1937), *Analysis terminable and interminable*, in *The Standard Edition*, XXIII, 1953–1974; Petty R., Cacioppo J., *Communication and persuasion: Central and peripheral routes to attitude change*, 1986; Rogers C.R., *Client-centered therapy*, 1951; Sherif M., *Social interaction process and products*, 1967.

IRRATIONAL BELIEFS

In the cognitive field, any beliefs, concepts or ideas that do not follow the principles of logic, or are inappropriate to empirical reality and rigidly dogmatic. The definition is from Albert Ellis and has become a central element of the cognitive psychotherapeutic model. Furthermore, beliefs that prevent people from reaching their goals and long-term outcomes are considered irrational. Ellis stated that, irrespective of their culture, all human beings potentially often find themselves transforming their individual and social preferences in an irrational manner into absolute expectations about themselves, others and the world around them. Such reasoning can lead to serious emotional suffering and impairment and, consequently, unfit, clearly absurd and self-harming behaviour. Four core types of irrational beliefs are defined: demandingness, awfulizing, human-worth ratings, low-frustration tolerance. *[S. Lenzi, C. Caramalli]*

REFERENCES. Ellis A., *Reason and emotion in psychotherapy*, 1962; Id., *The biological basis of human irrationality*, in« Journal of Individual Psychology», 32, 1976; Walen S.R., DiGiuseppe R., Dryden W., *A practitioner's guide to rational-emotive therapy*, 1980.

IRRATIONAL THOUGHTS

In Ellis' vision (principal author of rational emotive therapy), pathological (dysfunctional) emotional states depend mainly on dysfunctional cognitive processes. According to this theory, the underlying thought processes have a fundamental role in the genesis and the development of psychological problems. The fundamental belief is that the "functioning" of human beings is guided by a complex fundamental system – feelings, movement, thoughts, emotions – that carry out their functions in an integrated manner. Starting from the sensory experience of an internal or external stimulus, the first phenomenon that takes place is the perception of the stimulus, immediately followed by the establishment of cognitive processes of a descriptive or evaluative nature. These cognitive processes will then be accompanied by an emotional reaction and will consequently produce behaviour.

According to Ellis, the majority of irrational beliefs can be ascribed to one of four principal categories: → must-urbation: expectations of oneself, of others or of events that are not realistic (for example "I must behave well and be approved by all the people I love", "Others must treat me well and behave in the right way", "Everything must easy and pleasant, otherwise life is unbearable"; awfulizing (→ awfulizing of events): exaggeration of the negative consequences of a situation (for example "If I fail this exam it is the end, I will never graduate, I will be a failure for the rest of my life"); poor tolerance of frustration: ("I cannot handle it, I cannot tolerate something that happens or someone who behaves in a way that I decide that they should not"); devilifying: "demonization", making value judgements towards oneself or others ("Because I – or another person – have made this awful mistake, and in view of the fact that these mistakes should not be made, therefore I – or this other person - should be condemned because I am worthless").

Irrational beliefs are rational beliefs that have taken the form of expectations, needs, obligations, duties: the rational belief "I would like to pass this exam" becomes the irrational idea of "I must not fail this exam!". Irrational beliefs can be changed; the process of → change requires an active and persistent effort to recognize, challenge and reformulate the irrational aspects of one's thoughts (→ disputing), as well as working directly on containing one's emotions. These sort of dysfunctional thoughts (→ functional, equilibrium), are also cited by Beck in the standard type of cognitive therapy. According to Beck, there is an automatic but conscious connection between an external event and a particular emotional reaction.

Dysfunctional beliefs are the fundamental components that are the most superficial of the dysfunctional → mental scheme (relatively stable representations of knowledge stored in the system of memory that include beliefs and convictions) that cause the emotional and psychological suffering of the individual. Examples of how dysfunctional beliefs play a role in causing and maintaining a pathology can be found in Wells, with regard to anxiety disorders: in the case of panic attacks, for example, panic arises in the moment in which every feeling, whether related to anxiety or not, is interpreted as a sign of an imminent physical, mental or social catastrophe. Irrational beliefs also play a role in the genesis and maintenance of obsessive-compulsive disorder: in this case, the individual's behaviour is guided by the adoption of a behavioural repertoire aimed at, in particular, the prevention of an eventual → sense of guilt associated with one's actions or omissions. *[C.Petracca, M.Procacci]*

REFERENCES. Beck A.T., *Cognitive therapy and the emotional disorders*, 1975; De Silvestri C., *I fondamenti teorici e clinici della psicoterapia razionale-emotiva*, 1981; Ellis A., *Reason and emotion in psychotherapy*, 1962; Mancini F., *Un modello cognitivo del disturbo ossessivo-compulsivo*, in «Psicoterapia», 2001, 22, 23; Wells A., *Trattamento cognitivo dei disturbi d'ansia*, 1999.

ISOLATION OF AFFECT → DEFENCE MECHANISMS

K

KID'S SKILLS

Kid's Skills is a method developed by → brief solution-focused therapy aiming at helping children overcome behavioural and emotional problems. The method has been developed through the cooperation of Helsinki Brief Therapy Institute and the Keula daycare centre for children with special needs. In Kid's Skills the focus is not on problems but on skills that children need to acquire in order to overcome their problems. The process appeals to children and to parents. There is no parent blaming, and learning skills is designed in a way that is fun and rewarding for the child. Kid's Skills appears to be child-centred but, as the people in the child's environment are actively involved in the process, the method has positive effects not only on the child but also on the child's entire environment. *[B. Furman]*

KNOWLEDGE

Prevalent form of functional adaptation of complex organisms, actively built through → cognition and useful to the organization of the world of experience. In the traditional conception of knowledge, individuals know the features of an external reality through an empirical-inductive process by identifying only existing "facts" through their own senses and their own rationality. In this conception of "naive realism", reality is considered as something objective and existing independently from the subject that knows it, and only one true and objective knowledge is considered possible. On the contrary, in an advanced constructivist view (→ constructivism), it is claimed that knowledge does not provide a reproduction of an independent ontological world, but only a map of what can be done in the environment as it is perceived, and it shows itself in pragmatic efficacy. Therefore, actions must be evaluated for how they work in the world of experience and for their coherence: if an experience works according to what was previously assumed, it is called "practicable" (operational efficacy). Thus, not only senses become sources of knowledge but also the reflection of mind itself on its own actions through the concepts of difference and equivalence. As effectively expressed by J. Piaget in his genetic → epistemology, knowledge involves a methodological, constitutive-deductive process, based on the interaction between the subject and the phenomenon (reality) to be known, where the only possible realities are the ones generated by the operations of distinction of the observer. In other words, we know through experience: it is not things or relationships of a world that exists as it is to be observed and described, but the results of distinctions made by the observer through reflections. Subjects generate their ability to think by seeing themselves as an operating, observant, reflecting object. Therefore, in a constructive conception, there is no objective system but numerous distinctions made by different observers. According to the concept of knowledge adopted, each psychotherapeutic perspective changes its cognitive tools and methods of research and uses different diagnostic and intervention instruments, but these are always coherent with the chosen epistemological conception. *[R.]*

REFERENCES. Salvini A., *Pluralismo teorico e pragmatismo conoscitivo: assunti metateorici in psicologia della personalità*, in E. Fiora, L. Pedrabissi, A. Salvini, *Pluralismo teorico e pragmatismo conoscitivo in psicologia della personalità*, 1988.

L

LABELLING THEORY

Labeling theory has its theoretical background in → symbolic interactionism and considers deviant actions within the complex relationship between the definition of norms and the means aiming at controlling transgressions. According to this approach → deviance does not lie in a way of being or acting, but in a social process of interpretation and meaning. According to labelling theorists, in their most extreme formulation, the deviant is the one who is labelled as such (Becker, 1963). The "secondary" deviance, resulting from social attribution, may be even heavier than "primary" deviance, which is related to individual problems or behaviour. Ryan argued that a social system that creates an imbalance of power and resources, and then acts on the "fault" attributed to the individual, does nothing more than "blame the victim" for the situation. Matza also stated that the attribution of responsibility of deviance to those who are labelled as different is often linked to a form of correctional intervention. Acting on phenomena in order to correct them and bring them back to normality can hinder understanding, as the sole aim is to "get rid" of them. Moreover, there is a risk to cause – through a → self-fulfilling prophecy – the individual's adaptation to the attributed → stereotype. The process originates in the performed action and in its social stigma, and then it becomes a "chronic" deviant career through formal sanctions applied until the individual accepts them and internalizes the social role of deviant. *[P. Meringolo]*

REFERENCES Becker H.S., *Outsiders: Studies in the sociology of deviance*, 1963; Lemert E.M., *Human deviance, social problems, and social control*, 1981; Matza D., *Becoming deviant*, 1976.

LANGUAGE

A set of sounds (paraverbal) associated with conventional signs (verbal) through which man expresses himself. By extension, also defined as language is the set of physical movements (nonverbal, or "body language") that, along with paraverbal language, conveys the → relationships between interlocutors. The verbal component of language is studied from different perspectives. These include linguistics, etymology, grammar, rhetoric, etc. The paraverbal component is characterized by volume, or intensity of the voice, by its tone, speed and by the rhythm with which words and pauses come in succession. By combining these four elements in different ways, different "colours of voice" can be obtained, with different pragmatic effects on the interlocutor. Finally, the nonverbal component of language is characterized by: facial expressions (associated with a limited number of → emotions); look and eye- contact (it is one of the most powerful nonverbal signals and it is regulated in a discreet way based on gender, status, intimacy and nature of relationships); body posture (theoretically a high number of postures are possible, but in practice, many of them are inhibited by social conventions and congruence with the context); spatial orientation, proxemics or interpersonal distance (it varies depending on the type of interaction, which can be intimate, personal, casual, social, public); movements and gestures (of the arms and hands, nods of the head, leg and feet movements, etc., or actions produced intentionally to communicate information); haptic, or physical, contact (shaking hands, hugging, patting on the back, etc.). All three types of language – verbal, paraverbal and nonverbal – have a syntax, semantics and pragmatics. The syntactic aspect of language indicates its structure in sequences from which can be extracted recurring rules (for example, the grammatical rules); the semantic aspect indicates its being characterized by sense or by a socially shared meaning; finally, the pragmatic aspect indicates the effect that the union of semantics and syntax has on one's relationships with oneself and with others. From the point of view of human interaction, the combined use of verbal, paraverbal and nonverbal language is essential because, if taken individually, the first one is not provided with a proper semantics, whereas the other two are not provided with a proper syntax. Among the many functions and typologies of language described by psychologists, linguists and philosophers, the following have a direct application in psychotherapy: → injunctive language is used to directly prescribe behaviours that need to be performed (for example, this is used in → Ericksonian hypnotherapy to prescribe behaviours to patient with a low tone of voice and constant eye-contact); performative language, which "creates" a reality when pronounced ("I now pronounce you man and wife"), is used to induce an action without prescribing it (for example: "Pay attention to positive exceptions that will occur during the day", instead of: "You must look for positive exceptions during the day"; by implying that there will be positive exceptions, this sentence will work as → self-fulfilling prophecy); evocative language, typical of influence, is metaphorical (→ metaphorization) and analogical –

it allows the therapist to raise the attention of the interlocutor through evocative images and to ensure the content of communication is more easily accepted. Language, meant as communication between therapist and patient, is essential in all forms of psychotherapy, although it is used with methods and objectives that vary depending on the paradigm and of the reference model used. *[R]*

▷ In Lacanian psychoanalysis, language is the foundation of the psychic life of human beings; it is what precedes them and generates them as → *parlêtre*, because if man speaks it "is because the symbol has made him man". From structural linguistics studies (F. de Saussure and Jakobson), Lacan draws contributions that allow him, starting from Freudian texts, to formulate the hypothesis of a close link between language and the unconscious; the central thesis of this perspective is the idea that the unconscious is structured like a language. Language appears to be the very condition of the unconscious. In fact, as its laws make a radical distinction between signifier and signified, it places the speaking being in the irreducible position of non-coincidence between the level of the statement (what is said) and that of the enunciation (the repressed meaning). J. Lacan also assimilates the metaphoric and metonymic mechanisms. According to Jakobson, these mechanisms underlie the action of language and the concepts of displacement and condensation detected by Freud in unconscious primary processes. *[S. Guido]*

REFERENCES. Austin J.L., *How to do things with words*, 1962; Brown G.S., *Laws of form*, 1969; Di Ciaccia A., Recalcati M., *Jacques Lacan: Un insegnamento sul sapere dell'inconscio*, 2000; Ekman P., Friesen W.V., Ellsworth P., *Emotion in the human face*, 1972; Hall E.T., *The hidden dimension*, 1966; Hewes G., *The anthropology of posture*, in «Scientific American», 1957, 196; Imparato C., *La tua voce può cambiarti la vita*, 2009; Jakobson R., *Linguistics and poetics*, 1960; Rifflet-Lemaire A., *Lacan*, 1971.

LATENT LEARNING

In the behavioural paradigm, latent learning, investigated by E. Tolman, consists of structuring cognitive maps of the environment that, when settling in the person, can translate, at any time, into an effective mental guidance for any behavioural performance. In fact, when a new situation requires it, due to the occurrence of specific subjective needs or due to the presence of desirable environmental stimuli, individuals will unconsciously go back to their cognitive maps, trying to choose the most appropriate means to achieve the final result. It is a form of learning that characterizes finalized behaviour and that adopts three essential criteria: the → goal-objects, or aims, represent what the behaviour tends towards or flees from; means-goals are elements that can facilitate the achievement of the meta-goals; the cognitive map is the underlying array of learnings that supports the intentional process. For example, a rat tends to the meta-goal "food"; it will reach it faster if it uses the means-goal "shortest route" outlined by its internal cognitive maps. *[A. Tamburello, E. De Monte]*

REFERENCES. De Monte E., Tamburello A., *Storia del pensiero psicologico*, 2008; Tolman E.C., *Purposive behaviour in animals and men*, I–II, 1932; Id., *Cognitive maps in rats and men*, in «Psychological Review», 1948, 55 (4).

LAW OF EFFECT

The law of effect was discovered in laboratory experiments by E.L. Thorndike. It refers to operant conditioning processes (→ behavioural model of operant conditioning) and it can be applied both to human and animal behaviour. When a subject expresses any type of behaviour, this will have consequences on the environment and therefore on the same subject that expressed the behaviour. At this point, the subject will assess whether such consequences represent an advantage (gratification) or a disadvantage (a frustration or something not useful). Then, the subject who expressed the behaviour will tend, depending on the effect, to repeat the behaviours that brought him an advantage and to avoid repeating those that were either useless or source of frustration. *[F. Fois]*

LEARNING

Learning is a long-term modification of one's behaviour derived from experience, acquisition of some knowledge, competences or specific capabilities through studying or being taught. The ability to learn allows an organism to adapt to the environment. Any new learning can, thus, be seen as an efficient → response to a sizeable change (→ stimulus) in the environmental conditions. It follows that the process of learning implies a change in the interaction between the → behaviour of an organism and the environmental events. Two main perspectives are usually found in the study of learning processes: conditioning (→ classical conditioning, → operant conditioning), which can be classical or operant (I.P. Pavlov and F.B. Skinner); and problem-solving, which may happen by trial and error or by → insight (W. Koehler). In human beings, learning is mostly an intentional and conscious process, aimed towards problem-solving through complex cognitive strategies. J. Piaget showed that the acquisition of new notions occurs with a process that goes from action to experience to cognition (→ development stages (Jean Piaget's)). Only after a change, or new learning, has occurred, cognition allows it to be repeated. Vygotskij showed that the acquisition of new learning occurs through language, as the carrier of the interaction with the environment. J. Bruner interpreted the process of learning as a creative action, through which new ways and styles of thinking are formed. *[R.]*

LIBIDINAL DEVELOPMENT STAGES

In Freudian psychoanalysis, → libido is defined as the energy created by sex drive, present as its dynamic manifestation in psychic life. It has a quantitative value (amount of energy invested), a source (erogenous zones) and an aim (object, sublimation). During growth from childhood to adulthood, psychosexual organization develops in stages characterized by the investment of libido in specific erogenous zones, that is, the mouth, the anus and the penis. The first stage is the "oral" stage (up to the age of about two years), and has the double meaning of eating and being eaten; it is also subdivided into two activities: sucking (early oral stage, whose aim is incorporation and introjection), and biting (oral-sadistic stage, which implies a destructive attitude). The second stage is the "anal" stage (at the age of about two to four years) characterized by active–passive polarity, in two forms: sadistic–anal–expulsive, associated with evacuation and destruction, and erotic–anal–retentive, associated with control and the desire for possession; the latter polarity gives rise to the famous triad of orderly–parsimonious–obstinate traits, described by Freud in *Character and anal Erotism* (1908). The third stage is the "phallic" stage (from about three to five years) characterized by phallic–castrated polarity, but not yet male–female polarity; this stage applies to both boys and girls (the source for girls is the clitoris, equivalent to the glans in boys), and leads to castration anxiety in boys and penis envy in girls. This stage is closely linked to the "Oedipus complex", characterized by feelings of love and hate for their parents, in a triangular situation of conflict; the term "phallus" (and not penis) takes on, above all, an allegorical meaning, in a symbolic sense. Due to the fear of → castration (in boys) or the lack of a penis (in girls), the phallic stage plays a decisive role in an individual's ability to overcome the → Oedipus complex. The previous psychosexual organizations are known as pre-oedipal or pre-genital. The "Oedipus stage" takes place at the height of the phallic stage, at the age of about five years, and its decline leads into the subsequent stage, called the "latency stage". This stage lasts from the age of five or six years to puberty; it is accompanied by defence mechanisms of repression and sublimation. The last stage of libido development, after puberty, is the "genital stage", in which the individual, through the lessons learned during the pregenital stages, overcomes autoerotism and the polymorphous perversity of the partial sexual drives of childhood. The supremacy of the genital area and the choice of the love object imply an adult attitude (probably somewhat utopian, or socially determined), that includes: mutual orgasm, with a single companion of the opposite sex, with whom to share mutual trust, work, procreation, leisure, and thus ensure a satisfactory development for their children. *[M.A. Caponeri]*

REFERENCES. Freud S. (1901–1905), *A case of hysteria, Three essays on sexuality and other works*, in *The Standard Edition*, VII, 1953–1974; Id. (1908), *Character and anal eroticism*, in *The Standard Edition*, IX, 1953–1974; Id. (1908), *On the sexual theories of children*, in *The Standard Edition*, IX, 1953–1974.

LIBIDO

In the context of Freudian psychoanalysis, it is the energy that governs the transformation of sexual drive. The theory of libido has been subjected to several developments, in line with the different stages of development of Freud's → drive theory. Therefore, it is difficult to provide an unambiguous definition. However, it can be said that two aspects of this concept have remained constant: the libido is always linked to sexual drive and it is a quantitative concept, capable of measuring processes and transformations within sexual excitement. Libidinal energy follows the transformation of sexual drive mainly in relation to three aspects: the object of the drive satisfaction (through the psychological mechanism of "displacement"); the goal of the drive (through "sublimation"); the source of excitement, with the distinct mapping of erogenous zones and the connected stages of sexual development. If drives are the somato-psychological representative of sexuality, libido represents its psychological side. Freud formulated an evolutionary hypothesis about libidinal investment that assumes an initial investment on the Ego (primary → narcissism) and only later an investment on external objects. Although some of the libidinal energy is then released for objectual investments, primary narcissism remains always fundamentally active. The psychopathological hypothesis turns around a shift and a perversion of libido that cannot access the object investment phase but remains attached on the Ego, creating the psychopatological manifestations of secondary narcissism, such as can be observed in delusional psychosis. In this sense, the psychotherapy derived from the classical Freudian approach retraces the development stages to correct and rebalance the two aspects of the libidinal investment of the Ego and of the external object. This is mostly done by using → transference and → interpretation. In analytical psychology, the concept of libido, utilized by Jung as a synonym of energy, is instead detached from a fixed reference-point and represents a "tendency towards", that is, a form of intentionality. Jung points out that his view is not a metaphysical hypostasis but a purely psychological assumption, and he tends to assimilate the concept of libido/energy to the more general concept of "interest", considering it "*en fonction du réel*" (P. Janet), that is, a psychic organizer of the relationship between a subject and external reality. This flexibility in considering libido highlights clearly Jung's anti-naturalistic intent and opens up the possibility to understand the phenomena from an exclusively psychological perspective. The libido is distinct from the concept of (phenomenal) psychic force because it represents the indisputable and unexplainable inner part that supports the concept of the psychic; it eludes any representation but it expresses its visible strength in every manifestation of reality. Its main feature is the possibility of transforming, and the ability to take, different forms through the symbolic function. In analytical psychology, libido is the driving force of psychic life and presides over the possibility of existence of the manifestations of reality. It is expressed in the theory of → feeling-toned complex, the smallest psychic unity, where affection (very close to the concept of libido) represents the associative link between the individual elements of sensation, thoughts and representation. The libido is expressed in the individuation process through two movements: progression and regression. In relation to psychological types it defines the introverted and extroverted type: in the first, the libido turns inwards, weakening the object; in the second, it turns outward, and it becomes objectual. The originality of Jungian therapy consists mainly in interpreting the libidinous events without adopting a fixed grid of interpretation but by adapting them to the personality of the patient and also by taking mainly finalistic perspectives and not only a causalistic points of view. *[A. Iapoce]*

REFERENCES. Freud S. (1901–1905), *A case of hysteria, Three essays on sexuality and other works*, in *The Standard Edition*, VII, 1953–1974; Jung C.G. (1912), *Symbols of transformation*, in *Collected Works*, V, 1967.

LIE

A deliberate and conscious alteration or falsification of reality in its narrative or description. It becomes an object of interest in psychotherapy when it is a symptom of psychological disorders (for example in some personality disorders) or therapeutic boycott. However, the ability to lie also represents a confirmation of the abilities of the subject and highlights the non-alteration of their intellectual faculties and communication skills. *[R.]*

LIFE PLANS

In Individual Psychology, "ideal projects" about oneself and the environment; personal, compensatory inventions finalized to a future and more positive integration. They are the push-effect towards self-improvement of every creative person. Such perceptions of oneself and the world organize ameliorative plans of the "Self in the world", that Adler has variously defined as "life plan", "pattern of life" and finally "style of life". A life plan is therefore a creatively self-built fiction, a work of art where everybody is the author and, if dogmatized, the victim. It is the "masterpiece" and the personal "sense of life" of every child, which arises "from the constant repetition of encountered difficulties, both real and unreal "and that gradually turns into a specific and sole way (style) of "being in the world". *[L. Cerioli]*

REFERENCES. Adler A., *Social interest: A challenge to mankind*, 1938; Dreikurs R., *Fundamentals of Adlerian Psychology*, 1950.

LIFESTYLE

In individual psychology, lifestyle is a set of opinions that individuals have of themselves, the world and life problems, their perceptive and cognitive schema and the interpretations that are articulated and serve prevalent goals. Lifestyle refers to the concepts of Self, personality, individuality and creativity. It is formed in early childhood and is composed of conscious and unconscious aspects. Together with goals, it comprises the individual's only way of striving to achieve them. Lifestyle originates through a gradual process of selection and dynamic adjustment. In psychotherapy, lifestyles are reoriented by modulating the valences of → social feeling and striving for power (→ individual psychology) in a more creative and authentic life project. *[A. Bianconi, S. Fassina]*

REFERENCES. Adler A., (1935). *The fundamental views of individual psychology*, in «International Journal of Individual Psychology», 1, 1, 5–8.

LOGIC

In psychotherapy, a discipline concerning the planning of actions to achieve a purpose and also the study of criteria by which the result of an utterance is produced. Logical reasoning can follow two paths: hypothetical-deductive and constitutive-deductive. In the first case, it is based on assumptions formulated on the basis of one's theory of reference and, through applications and results, it reaches the correct definition. In the second case, the deduction is the result of interventions based on the objective to be achieved rather than on the theory of reference, and the process is gradually adjusted to adapt to the effects. The application of these two logical models to psychotherapy brings different approaches. On the one hand, some paradigms and models start from data collection and diagnostic observation based on the theories of reference and then perform the expected therapeutic intervention according to these theories; other paradigms and models start from the action-research (→ intervention-research) construct or cybernetic feedback. In this case, a change in the observed system is introduced to identify the possible effects and, on this basis, to know how the system works: in this way, it would be possible to progressively adjust the therapeutic intervention and to tailor it to the reality with which the therapist interacts rather than to the theory and method of reference. Similarly, the analysis of the reasoning can follow two paths: linear and ordinary logic and non-ordinary-logic. Starting from Aristotle, to Descartes up to I. Kant and the modern thinkers, linear and ordinary logic have given rise to a model based on the criteria of non-contradiction, excluded middle, consistency and congruence. The purpose of these procedures is the elimination of logical contradictions and ambivalence. Instead, non-ordinary logic contemplates → ambivalence and its way of expressing itself in contradiction (→ logic of contradiction), in paradoxes (→ logic of paradox), in beliefs (→ logic of belief) and self-deception (→ logic of self-deception) as a tool to be used for the achievement of purposes. Within the field of psychotherapy, all rationalist therapies refer to linear and ordinary logic, whereas suggestive and evocative therapies refer to non-ordinary logic. Among these, a few of them, as systemic and strategic approaches, have developed special therapeutic techniques based on ambivalent logic. *[R.]*

LOGIC OF BELIEF

A logical criterion that is expressed in two directions. In the first, a thought informs behaviours that, once implemented, confirm the initial thought, which in turn becomes a belief. For example: I believe my partner is betraying me; I question him constantly; he defends himself; whoever defends themselves, is guilty: therefore, he betrays me. In the second case, behaviours are structured on the basis of a → perception. These behaviours give rise to a belief that activates actions aiming at confirming it. For example: I fear the worst for my loved ones; I begin to pray; what I fear does not happen: therefore, it works. Prayers become a propitiatory ritual that, when repeated, builds a belief informing my actions; I will have to continue to pray, otherwise what I fear will come true. A dysfunctional belief starts from incorrect assumptions and, following a compelling logic, leads to wrong conclusions. If the initial belief is changed – by introducing a new belief or a change in behaviours, which induce a new belief – the system is subverted, and the initial belief is replaced by a functional belief (→ functional balance). This type of logic underlies both some forms of pathology and some therapeutic techniques (→ counter-ritual technique; → miracle prescription; → "as if" technique). *[R.]*

LOGIC OF CONTRADICTION

A type of → ambivalence expressed within a timeline, with a contradictory "before" and "after". A contradiction can be "logic" when the premise, in its effects, turns into its opposite or it can be "linguistic" when the statement evolves and becomes contradictory. Contradiction is different from paradox (→ logic of paradox), for its characteristic of temporal evolution and of non-unison coexistence of ambivalence. This type of → logic can be observed in all those disorders in which a person acts in a way that at first relieves the discomfort, but then increases it. The same mechanism underlies the formulation of therapeutic techniques that apparently follow the structure of the disorder, but that aim at taking it to its extinction (→ strategic reframing technique; → contradictory confirmation prescription). *[R.]*

LOGIC OF PARADOX

A logical criterion expressed in the simultaneous presence of ambivalent statements (→ ambivalence). One of the best-known paradoxes is the affirmation of the liar: "I lie"; another popular paradox is: "Be spontaneous" (→ be spontaneous paradox), which suppresses spontaneity at the very moment when this is imposed. The logic of paradox underlies several types of disorders, and as many types of therapeutic technique. In family psychotherapy (by M. Selvini Palazzli, J. Haley and others), in brief therapy MRI model and in brief strategic therapy Nardone's model, paradox has played an essential role in the development of therapeutic strategies. V.E. Frankl had already adopted it, with a therapeutic purpose, in → logotherapy. The use of paradoxical strategies appears to be of great importance to treat phobic disorders (→ symptom prescription; → worst-fantasy technique; → counter-ritual technique). *[R.]*

REFERENCES. Nardone G., *Brief strategic solution-oriented therapy of phobic and obsessive disorders*, 1996; Wilson R.R., *Don't panic*, 1986.

LOGIC OF SELF-DECEPTION

In the process of formation of beliefs, J. Elster, a logician and scholar of social dynamics, defines self-deception as the tendency to "identify reality with one's own desires". This definition distances itself from traditional assumptions, which consider self-deception as the effect of weakness of will or a lack of impulse control. It overturns the historical perspective by considering self-deception as the cause of origin and maintenance of beliefs and related behaviours. Self-deception logic refers to the common tendency to bring reality close to one's established pattern of perception and reaction. In this view, each person alters reality according to their redundant perceptive-reactive predispositions (→ perceptive-reactive system), which are built and consolidated by virtue of one's past significant experiences. This happens both in the event that such perceptions are pleasant ("I am a very desirable person and everybody wants me") and when they are clearly unpleasant ("All refuse and avoid me because I am not good enough"). Because of these characteristics, self-deception logic pervades every dimension of our existence and it represents a powerful tool that can both cause difficulties and problems to be solved and provide solutions and possibilities of change. In this perspective, a "truthful" perception of reality, that is, a perception that it is not a self-deception, is not possible. Therefore, the only notable difference is assessing whether or not the way self-deception is implemented is functional (→ functional balance), that is, if it allows people to be effective in their relationship with themselves, others and the world, or if it is dysfunctional in one or more of these three interdependent relationships. All this has considerable operative implications for experts working with → change in general, and psychotherapy in particular. In fact, any personal or → interpersonal work aiming at change, implies guiding a person to transform their dysfunctional self-deceptions into functional ones. *[R.]*

LOGOS → WILL TO MEANING

LOGOTHERAPY AND EXISTENTIAL ANALYSIS

A psychological and psychotherapeutic approach that sees the search for meaning as the fundamental reason of existence and indicates detailed rules to intervene in the solution of existential malaise. It was founded by the Austrian psychiatrist Frankl, who presented his theory on the "meaning of life" in his work *Logotherapy and Existential Analysis*. He offered an original interpretation of the origins of neurotic disorders, which he identified not in repressed sexuality, but in existential emptiness and lack of sense of meaning in life. Frankl discovered the importance of having a task, an ideal, a reason to live, in the concentration camps of Theresienstadt, Auschwitz, Kaufering III and Türkheim, where he was interned for three years; only those who were able to identify a task to accomplish, could find the strength to overcome that hell. For this reason, his theoretical system, which in previous years had taken shape around the theme of search for meaning, found the most noble and significant confirmation in that experience. The anthropological vision of logotherapy and existential analysis has three starting assumptions: the first states that man is basically free, not because he is not exposed to any biological, psychological, sociological, cultural religious conditioning, but because man always retains the radical possibility of assuming an attitude against conditioning. The second assumption affirms that man does not seek, as a primary motivation of his actions, the satisfaction of pleasure (as stated by Freudian psychoanalysis) or power (as claimed by Adler's individual psychology). Instead, man is driven by a "will of meaning" (and in this context the Greek word *logos* is interpreted as meaning of life), which manifests itself in a continuous tension between the existential reality in which man lives and the world of values that is presented to him as a challenge. The third assumption states that man's life always retains its own meaning, despite the limitations of age, health, suffering, emotional failures and professional failures. Consequently, man needs to respond to the calls of life not only by implementing "creation values" (work, activity, political commitment) or "experiential values" (love, music, art), but especially "attitudinal values" in extreme situations such as inevitable suffering, guilt, death. Therefore, "an unconditional faith in an unconditional meaning of life" represents the core of logotherapy and existential analysis. This was strengthened both by Frankl's tragic experience in Nazi concentration camps, and from the contact with patients suffering from existential disorders, diagnosed as "noogenic" neurosis. According to Frankl's vision, conceiving existence as a unique and original assignment, which must be identified and realized with full responsibility, involves a threefold attitude: accepting and living the dialectic between "to be" and "have-to-be", between everyday life and the world of values, between concrete achievements and countless potentialities; being fundamentally oriented outside themselves (with regard to this, Frankl coined the word "self-transcendence"), and then overcoming the easy temptation of seeking only the immediacy of pleasure, or the illusion of success; being able to take a proper distance from the situations of difficulty and extreme situations (in this case the word used is "self-detachment") by leveraging "the defiant power of the human spirit". Next to three tragic phenomena (suicide, aggression and drug abuse), which are eloquent expressions of lack of values and the existential vacuum, logotherapy and existential analysis identifies other neurotic forms widely present in the contemporary social fabric: "mechanic" neurosis is the result of the increase in free time, which is filled with escapades leading to deviant behaviour; "Sunday neurosis" shows itself in mass, alienating behaviours in discos, in stadiums, in places where there is an exasperated search for pleasure; "unemployment neurosis" concerns both young people looking for jobs and elderly people who, at the end of a hard-working life, feel excluded from the productive process as a consequence of retirement. It should also be noted that Frankl's theory emphasizes a therapeutic relationship based on the identification and implementation of unique and original personal tasks, corresponding to the uniqueness and originality of individuals. Similarly, it is important to stress the fundamental role of freedom, responsibility and conscience, which are needed to identify the "ten thousand commandments arising from the ten thousand unique situations of which [t]his life consists". And since no one can "give" a meaning to someone else's life, nor can recipes be provided for what others should do, the psychotherapeutic encounter can be represented as an equation with two unknowns. The first unknown factor is the therapist's personality and the second is the individuality of the patient. Both are unique and original and both aim at: overcoming every sense of dependence on thinking and action; discovering the unpredictable qualities of daily life; identifying a hierarchy of values that assign to pleasure and control, self-affirmation and satisfaction of instincts, their true place as side-effects of a proper accomplishment of one's sense of existence. *[E. Fizzotti]*

REFERENCES. Frankl V.E., *Man's search for meaning. An introduction to logotherapy*, 1946; Id., *Homo patiens*, 1950.

LOSS

Life event of a person that entails the end of something – or someone – that is an important part of his life: for example, the loss of a loved one as a result of death, the loss of a partner as a result of abandonment, the loss of a physical function. Generally speaking, one can say that the experience of loss tests the psychological capacity of the individual to accept what has happened, tolerate the suffering and change the points of reference in his life. For these reasons, in psychotherapy, loss is frequently treated in association with the grieving process. *[R]*

LOVING

In Fromm's thought, an attitude or productive orientation of human beings towards the world and not exclusively towards an object of love. Fromm distinguishes between mature love and symbiotic partnerships. Mature love is an active experience achieved with the act of giving to the Other, by offering one's own vital expressions within a relationship that creates reciprocity (not in a childish and immature vision of impoverishment or sacrifice). In this exchange lies also a mature answer to overcoming human existential loneliness. The characteristics of mature love are: caring, responsibility, respect and knowledge. The symbiotic partnership, a passive experience focused on being loved, has the mother–baby relationship as its model and expresses itself in two forms – active (sadism) and passive (masochism). *[C. Benelli, E. Benelli]*

REFERENCES. Fromm E., *The art of loving*, 1956; Id., *For the love of life*, 1986.

M

MANA

Term of Polynesian origin, used to express a "supernatural impersonal force" and "what is extraordinarily effective." Mana is considered as a healing magic energy, universally widespread, which can invest human beings, animals, plants, objects. A great power depends on its acquisition. Jung argues that the mana expresses the primitive idea of psychic → energy, and highlights its affinity with the concept of → libido. He also uses the term "mana personality" to define the individual (shaman, magician, hero, king or doctor) who possesses hidden extraordinary capabilities of influencing and curing. The projection of the mana personality operated by the patient, that is, the unconditional trust in the alleged omnipotence of the psychotherapist, may represent a formidable obstacle to the process of understanding and block the analytical dialectic. *[G. Antonelli, B. Rinaldi]*

REFERENCES. Jung C.G. *The relation between the ego and the unconscious*, in *Collected Works*, VII, 1928; Id. (1934–1954), *The archetypes and the collective unconscious*, in *Collected Works*, vol. IX/ I.

MANDALA

In ancient Eastern traditions, mandalas are circular representations of the cosmos. In Tibetan Buddhism they map the meditative path leading to the depths of being. In Western culture, Jung was among the first to use the mandala as a study and therapeutic tool. While exploring his own → unconscious, as well as the unconscious of his patients, the Swiss psychologist found that, in periods of stress, disorientation or psychic dissociation, mandala-like images emerge spontaneously in dreams, fantasies or pictorial and even choral expressions of the individual, showing the possibility of a new inner order. These individual mandalas express the integration of conscious and unconscious, which is the → Self in Jung's language, centre and wholeness of being, landmark of the inner depths of the psyche. According to Jung, the order imposed from the concentric mandala – where everything is exactly "centred" – acts as a compensatory factor for disorder and inner division and promotes the integration of the multitude of unconscious contents and opposites, combining what appears incompatible to the → Ego. Jung called this fundamental pattern of human nature "the archetype of wholeness". The "quaternity as a complete whole", symbol at the same time of differentiation and integration – present in mandalas, which were studied by Jung, as well as in Gnosticism and alchemy – is, at a deeper level, the very essence, the divine spark within each person, and the principle characterizing the image of God. *[G. Antonelli, V. Salles]*

REFERENCES. Jung C.G., *Concerning mandala symbolism*, in *Collected Works*, IX/I, 1950; Id. (1955), *Appendix: Mandalas*, in *Collected Works*, IX/I.

MANIFEST BEHAVIOUR

Within the behavioural paradigm, an objective behavioural response, scientifically observable and assessable, and, therefore, suitable for use as a verification tool during an experiment, studied by → behaviourism. Researchers observe and record the subject's behaviour and relate it to previous stimuli and to the immediate consequences of the manifest phenomenon observable in the surrounding environment. Cognitive-behavioural psychotherapy used manifest behaviour as a tool to identify the connections between thoughts, emotions and behaviour. Identifying the connections between those levels through manifest behaviour and understanding their mutual influence, has always been, according to cognitive-behavioural theory, a constant pathway to formulate, develop and disprove theories. *[M. Balbo]*

MANIPULATION

In Gestalt therapy, a tendency to shape the outside world according to one's own needs. *Homo faber* is, by his very nature, capable of manipulating the external environment and even the internal one, through representative and symbolic functions. Therefore, according to an interactionist (individual–environment) perspective, his ability to adapt can develop in an autoplastic or an alloplastic direction, depending on situational and/or character tendency, to adapt himself to the environment or to adapt the environment to his needs. In psychology, the persistence of manipulative attitudes that have been structured at an early age is of interest, as these attitudes often create a negative interference instead of being useful to creative adaptation. In the words of Perls: "I call neurotic any man who uses his potential to manipulate others instead of growing up himself". In Gestalt therapy, manipulation is an existential attitude and a mode of → contact directed to receiving support from the environment for the satisfaction of one's own needs, to the detriment of an autonomous activation. Perls wrote: "We stay immature, we go on manipulating the world, rather than to suffer the pains of growing up". *[R. Zerbetto, I. Corti]*

REFERENCES. Naranjo C., *Character and neurosis*, 1994; Perls F., *Gestalt therapy verbatim*, 1969; Id., *Here and now*, 1979.

MASCULINE

In Jung's analytical psychology, it is identified with the → animus and closely linked to its female counterpart, the → anima. The term animus, like its counterpart anima, is not to be considered from a Christian or spiritual perspective, but rather as a peculiar completion that the → feminine and its opposite, the masculine, already possess to some extent aspects of the other, and/or acquire and/or integrate it during the lifespan in order to balance their gender identity. Jung identifies in the animus the archetype of the eternal masculine (*logos*, or rationality). Similarly, the anima embodies the eternal feminine (*eros*, or psychic relatedness). In the course of a Jungian analysis anima and animus often emerge, particularly in the dreams of the patient, who gradually learns to recognize and integrate them, thus enriching his/her personality. *[G. Antonelli, A. Caruso]*

REFERENCES. Falcolini L., *Animus e anima*, in A. Carotenuto (ed.), *Trattato di Psicologia Analitica*, 1992; Jung C.G. (1951), *The syzygy: Anima and animus*, in Id., *Aion: Researches into the phenomenology of the self* (1951), in *Collected Works*, IX/II, 1959.

MEANING → WILL TO MEANING

MECHANOMORPHISM → ANTHROPOMORPHISM

MEDICAL DIAGNOSIS

The medical diagnostic method is a type of reasoning that allows experts to recognize signs as clues of evaluation of a pathological situation. Diagnosing a disease means deciding into which classes of a pre-existing classification system, composed of disease categories, symptomatological and objective data, collected by a medical doctor, *have* to be collocated. In this perspective, diagnosis represents a logical process of comprehension of → symptoms, which are turned into "signs" able to compose the global picture of a "disease". It is defined as medical diagnosis not just diagnostic reasoning, but also its product, the definition of which represents the basis of a prognosis and a process of therapy and treatment. The elements that, logically and correctly in a methodological sense, are part of the scientific reasoning promoted by the medical doctor have to show themselves as empirically reliable: it is not possible to perform a diagnosis just through "subjective" symptoms; the doctor has to identify "objective" signs, the "observability in principle" of which confers them scientific features. The expression "observability in principle" is used to indicate the possibility to record, with instruments of different kinds, a specific object or the existence of phenomenon, in order to measure them. Nevertheless, a diagnostic process with different presuppositions with regard to "observability in principle" is used not only in medicine but even in the clinical sciences of the psyche: → psychiatric diagnosis, → psychological diagnosis or clinical/psychological → assessment and → neuropsychological diagnosis are examples of this. *[R.]*

MEDICAL MODEL IN PSYCHOTHERAPY

It is the theoretical framework of disciplines that deal with health and illness at an organic level. As pointed out by A. Salvini, the medical model applied to psychotherapy interprets psychological problems in analogy to physical illnesses of organic origin. This model goes as far as to claim the existence of nosological entities – mental illnesses – whose etiology, course and outcome is similar to other pathogenic processes of organic nature. According to this perspective, a mental *illness* must be inferred from the symptoms, but it cannot be cured through their modification, since it assumes a biochemical or anatomical substrate as responsible for the pathogenic process. Consistent with these assumptions, the medical model considers the essential process of mental illness as universal and not as culturally specific. *[R.]*

MEDITATION

Meditation is considered a form of therapy thanks to its original definition as a practice to release human beings from suffering. Meditation can be defined as a mental presence training: by bringing the mind to a quiescent mode and a deeper level of awareness, it acts on the body as well as on the energetic, mental and spiritual components, thus contributing to → healing and preserving health. Meditation can also be seen as a practice to awaken a very subtle level of consciousness, allowing the mind to abandon all the conditions of interference and discomfort, and to go beyond the individual dimension of the Self. As is well-known, the first scientific study on the efficacy of meditation dates back to 1935 and was carried out by the French cardiologist T. Brosset. However, it was not until the mid-1960s that, for the first time in the world of Western science, the studies by H. Benson, of Harvard Medical School in Boston, demonstrated the → efficacy of meditation in the treatment of → anxiety and → stress – alongside the treatment of hypertension, digestive disorders, cardiovascular diseases and some types of headache. As regards the efficacy of meditation in the treatment of psychological diseases such as anxious-depressive disorders, depression, panic attacks and insomnia, the studies carried out by Goleman, J. Gordon, R. Wallace, R. Davidson and J. Kabat-Zinn are particularly interesting. In oncology, L. Leshan's and C. Simonton's pioneering studies have demonstrated that meditation – associated with medical treatments and cognitive strategies – is effective in treating some types of tumour, strengthening the immune-system response and improving the response to surgery and medication. In Italy, an important experience is being carried out in Bologna by the clinical psychology unit at the department of oncology of the local health organization (AUSL). *[G. Pagliaro]*

▷ In the area of psychosynthesis, meditation is a psychological practice, used in psychotherapy but also widely employed in personal growth, which aims at free Self-expression: a vital, existential need going beyond the "moment" of therapy, which, however, is its starting point. Meditation consists in the conscious, deliberate, creative use of mind and thought to reach a specific goal. The three main forms of meditation are: reflective, receptive and creative. Meditation actively connects the internal and the external world; physical relaxation, emotional tranquility and concentration are the three phases preparing the individual to move from outward-oriented, ordinary life to internal action. It also implies evoking dynamizing, positive qualities such as joy, courage, love, friendship, sense of humour, peacefulness, wellbeing, kindness, unselfishness: not only does meditation mean "to wait for", but it is also "an action towards". According to psychosynthesis, meditation involves the human being as a whole, not being limited to the conscious part alone. *[A.G. Tallerini]*

REFERENCES. Assagioli R., *Psychosynthesis: A manual of principles and techniques*, 1965; Eastcott M.J., *The silent path: An introduction to meditation*, 1969; Goleman D., *Healing emotions*, 1998; Pagliaro G, Salvini A., *Mente e Psicoterapia*, 2007.

MEMORY

An affective-cognitive function dedicated to acquisition, preservation and recalling of information coming from the outer and inner worlds. Memory is not a faithful reproduction of perceived reality or of events lived in the past, but a reconstruction and an active reworking of experience. The → re-evocation may not be free from distortion, and it is strongly influenced by emotional and motivational elements. Memory can be divided into short-term memory (STM) – which includes sensory memory and working memory – and long-term memory (LTM), which includes episodic, semantic and procedural memory. Phenomenologically, three categories of mnestic activities can be identified: *recollection*, which includes the reproduction of what was previously acquired (for example, a poem) and narration (the account of an event experienced); *recognition*, namely the identification in the environment of an object that was previously perceived; *relearning*, that is, the process of reacquiring some information previously memorized, which appeared to be forgotten. The decay of a mnestic trace is called *oblivion*. In psychotherapy, remembering, reconstructing or narrating one's own story is one of the most frequent and classic techniques and therapeutic interventions. Memory is particularly involved in post-traumatic disorders. In these cases, individuals feel invaded by images, recollections and intrusive, unpleasant and recurrent memories related to unpleasant experiences lived in the past. Finally, it is important to mention a mnestic phenomenon that is widely studied in therapeutic → settings, especially in relation to the theoretical views that emphasize the therapeutic research of real or alleged childhood trauma. This approach has been criticized because it can potentially generate false childhood memories, usually related to episodes of incest or violence, never having occurred in reality but imagined and then "mnestically rebuilt" due to the therapist's suggestion. *[R.]*

MENTAL RESEARCH INSTITUTE (MRI)

Founded in 1959 by Donald D. Avila Jackson, the Mental Research Institute established today in Palo Alto, California, acquired important funds to study human interaction, communication and psychotherapy. The first team was composed of Jules Riskin, a psychiatrist interested in schizophrenia and Virginia Satir, a social worker and great pioneer in systemic therapy. Bateson's research team (John Weakland and Jay Haley) collaborated with them until 1962, when Bateson left California. The rest of the group moved to MRI, joining Paul Watzlawick who had arrived in 1961, interested in exploring the pragmatics of communication. Richard Fisch joined the group later, and convinced Jackson to sponsor the now-famous Brief Therapy Center (BTC), where they saw clients in therapy using the systemic approach of Bateson's group and Milton H. Erickson's strategies. Since 1967, Watzlawick, Wealkland and Fisch have remained active members at the BTC, until each has retired. Taping and debriefing treatments with individual clients and/or their families permitted them to create and develop the Brief Therapy model. Their breakthrough assumption is the cybernetically inspired notion of "attempted solutions". In all problematic situations, the solution put into practice by the client either solves the problem or maintains, or even increases, the problem. So, therapist's first responsibility is to help all clients stop sustaining their "more of the same solutions". Their research, formalization and therapeutic work has inspired hundreds of articles and books, and has lit the way for their followers (Milwaukee Group, Institut Gregory Bateson and Circé, and CTS of Giorgio Nardone). MRI has hosted more than 45 researchers, among them Arthur Bodin, Carlos E. Sluzki, James C. Coyne. MRI has received funding to complete 60 research projects, such as Soteria (putting into practice Laing and Cooper's inspired work with young schizophrenics) and the Emergency Treatment Center (where the Everstines developed a model for crisis intervention in collaboration with the authorities). More than 800 articles and books have been published by MRI team members. Since Ms Satir's first training, concerning couples and family therapy, MRI has been a world-renowned training institute, hosting thousands of participants while broadening its scope to encompass different models of interactional therapy training, including brief therapy. *[T. Garcia-Rivera]*

REFERENCES. Ray W. (ed.), *Don D. Jackson: Interactional Theory in clinical practice*, in *Selected Essays*, ii, 2005; Watzlawick P., Weakland J.H., Fisch R., *Change: Principles of problem formation and problem resolution*, 1974. Fisch R., Weakland J.H., Segal L., *The tactics of change: Doing therapy briefly*, 1982.

MENTAL SCHEME

Human knowledge is clearly made up of more than the spurious sum of information regarding individual concepts or the relationship between different concepts. The most commonly used theoretical construct used to explain the organization of complex knowledge is that of a "scheme". A scheme is a structured group of concepts, usually based on general knowledge, which can be used to represent events, sequences of events, rules of behaviour, situations, relationships, objects. The scheme refers, in particular, to the attributes of certain phenomena and to the interconnecting relationships between these attributes. I. Kant had originally proposed the idea of mental schemes as being innate structures according to which the perception of the world is organized; in his innativist theory, that of the *a priori* structure of the mind permits the understanding of the concept of time, of three-dimensional space and of geometry. From F. Bartlett to J. Piaget to Gestalt theory, and above all with the affirmation of the cognitive sciences in the 1970s, the concept of a mental scheme was recaptured and developed in a modern sense. Schemes develop according to a process of extraction of general knowledge and of patterns departing from the single observation and variations in the environment. At the foundation of scheme theory is the assumption that the perception of the world is not objective, but reflects a dynamic interaction between the mind and what is situated in the outside world. This interactive and reconstructive property of the mind is not conscious or voluntary and for this reason it appears to us that our mental representations are photographs or faithful reproductions of what we perceive. Mental schemes guide the categorization and the understanding of reality, influencing three important cognitive processes: the encoding of new information (that is, the schemes determine, from the very first moments of perception, the objects towards which attention is directed, and therefore determine the selection of the information entering the brain); the memory of the information stored (as a result of which we tend to better remember information that is relevant to the scheme and to forget that that is irrelevant or somewhat incoherent); and finally, inferences regarding missing information (the application of a scheme ensures that from a stimulus one can deduct the presence of typical characteristics, which are not immediately available, departing from those that are instead available). When a scheme is coherent and well-structured it gives the individual utilizing it a feeling of understanding himself and the world around him, and of managing to control and predict the environment. Mental schemes can also be transmitted socially, both in interpersonal relationships as well as through mass media of communication. It would therefore be useful to consider them as being a product of the cognitive activity of the individual as much as of the construction and social sharing of reality. *[A. Meluzzi, R.S. Pecorara]*

REFERENCES. Barale F., Bertani M., Gallese V., Mistura S., Zamperini A. (ed.), *Psiche: Dizionario storico di psicologia, psichiatria, psicoanalisi, neuroscienze*, 2006; Eysenck M.W., Keane M.T., *Cognitive psychology*, 1973.

MENTALISM

A tendency to relate every aspect of behaviour to mental processes or states that are considered accessible through self-reflection and able to explain the behaviour of an individual. This term is often used synonymously with *psychologism*, meant as a philosophical attitude expressing the tendency to seek the understanding of reality in consciousness and in the description of phenomena appearing to consciousness.

The word "mentalist" was also used by behaviourists to criticize the non-scientific attitude of the psychological models that make extensive use of unobservable terms indicating intrapsychic processes. In this regard, the cognitive tradition claims the status of mentalism, affirming that a scientific discipline does not need directly observable entities to be defined as scientific. Moreover, this tradition claims that not only mental entities exist regardless of behaviours, but they may also cause these. *[R.]*

MESSAGE

In transactional analysis, a transactional exchange occurring between the → Ego-states of two or more individuals. Transactional analysis began as a revision of the Freudian psychoanalytic doctrine with an interpersonal base. In this, therefore, the concept of message assumes a central role, although with different interpretations. In sum, a message can be considered from the following points of view: within communication theory (it can be explicit, or social, or also implicit, or psychological); within intrapsychic theory (it is the "internal dialogue" between the three Ego states); within the theory of the psychological script (there are different parental messages that influence the development of the child: counter-injunction [→ counter-script] and → injunction); within the therapeutic relationship (the eight → "therapeutic operations" described by Berne, with which he illustrates the various communications between the therapist and the patient). A special therapeutic message is provided by → permission, a specific transaction through which the therapist supports the patient in relieving him from the conditioning of his → script. *[M. Novellino]*

REFERENCES. Berne E., *Transactional analysis in psychotherapy*, 1961; Novellino M., *Psicoanalisi transazionale*, 2004.

MESSIANIC IDEA

According to Bion, a creative and new idea brought by an individual member to the institution or group to which he belongs, which challenges, enlivens and threatens the status quo of the group. The institution then has two tasks: how to make the messianic idea available to the group for purposes of growth and mental development; and how to keep it under control so that it does not disrupt and destroy the institution. If the institution is unsuccessful in these tasks, either the idea is restricted to the point of destruction or the institution itself is destroyed by the idea. This is an example of a parasitic container–contained relationship. In a successful containment of the messianic idea, both the institution and the idea would grow and flourish, generating a symbiotic relationship. *[J. Symington]*

REFERENCES. Bion W.R., *Attention and interpretation*, 1970.

META-MODEL

In neuro-linguistic programming, it is a set of questions designed to collect useful information from a person with whom one is communicating. The meta-model was developed in 1975 by R. Bandler and J. Grinder and helps to learn how to listen effectively and how to identify communication patterns in other people's languages. Bandler and Grinder created this model by studying V. Satir and F. Perls and by analyzing the type of questions asked: questions aimed at exploring → deletions, → generalizations and → distortions and the language patterns creating lack of precision in communication – with oneself or with other people – and tending to eliminate, hide or alter information. Through meta-model questions, it is possible to eliminate ambiguity from a person's language and help them to define the missing parts in their expression (deletions), to specify general terms (generalizations) and clarify undefined parts of their speech (distortions). The application of the meta-model leads people to enrich their subjective experience – getting them closer to a more complete representation of reality – and to open up their model of the world, enabling them to face alternative ways of thinking about their experience. A few examples of meta-model challenges are: "They don't listen to me": "Who specifically doesn't listen to you?"; "People around me don't understand me": "All people?", "What do you mean by 'don't understand'?", "What would need to happen for you to feel understood by these people?"; "When he smiles at me, I feel that he doesn't value me": "How do you know?"; "Research shows that . . .": "Which research specifically? According to which model was it made, by whom exactly, and when?". *[A. Roberti]*

REFERENCES. Bandler R., Grinder J., *The structure of magic Vol. 1,* 2007.

META-PROGRAMS

In neuro-linguistic programming, a meta-program is a mental way of sorting information, based on which a person takes decisions or acts. Meta-programs are the selection and perception rules that direct people's thoughts, feelings and, consequently, actions. They identify mental predispositions that govern, mostly unconsciously, how each person tends to behave in specific contexts. Meta-programs are also known as "decision styles", because they represent the mental strategies behind reactions and choices. *[A. Roberti]*

REFERENCES. Knight S., *NLP at work,* 1995.

METAPHOR

A figure of speech based on the transposition of a meaning to a narrative or poetic, figurative context to enhance its evocative power. In the *Poetics*, Aristotle defines metaphor as "the transfer of the name of a thing to another thing", but this second thing needs to be presented in the form of an evocative and not of a descriptive language to be metaphorical. In psychotherapy, the use of metaphorical language is a fundamental technique in many different approaches. In fact, outside of those forms of psychotherapy that are based on a rationalist and explanatory language, the use of metaphors can be found in various ways, in all the different languages of psychotherapy. Some models, such as hypnotics and strategic approaches, have formalized several therapeutic uses of metaphor. In these cases, the focused use of metaphors is aimed at achieving specific therapeutic effects. In demonstrative and rationalist therapies, metaphor can be used after the logical description of a concept, to facilitate its understanding. *[R.]*

METAPHORIZATIONS

A linguistic form and a communicative mode widely used in psychotherapy, either explicitly or implicitly. It can include → metaphors, similes, comparisons, analogies, metonymies, assonances, discursive genres and registers, apologues, allegories. The client/patient may use them with descriptive purposes aimed at communicating an experience, whereas the therapist can use them to induce performative effects or to create restructuring interpretive modes (→ strategic reframing technique). Therefore, metaphorizing means using a linguistic medium to transfer a meaning from a conceptual domain to another. In this regard, the protolinguistic forms, typical of the sensory experience, can be mentioned: for example, the proprioceptive form ("I have a lump in my throat") or the olfactory form ("I smell a rat"). The metaphorizations used by the client/patient may reflect resistances, entrapments, pervasive theories about oneself and the world; whereas those used by the therapist are meant to be disassociating, restructuring, interpreting, consolidating a change. Also, psychological terms are metaphorical forms designed to define a certain psychological state. If metaphorizations are considered real (→ reification), they can facilitate → self-fulfilling prophecies. *[R.]*

MILAN SCHOOL OF FAMILY THERAPY

Within the systemic-relational paradigm, the school of psychotherapy born in Milan, also known to international literature as the Milan Approach, or with reference to the group that founded it, the Milan Associates. Towards the end of the 1960s, Selvini Palazzoli, a psychoanalyst from Milan, feeling disappointed by the poor results of lengthy, individual psychotherapy in treating anorexia, studied new models of intervention for eating disorders and for psychosis. Together with Boscolo, Cecchin and Prata, she experimented with a psychoanalytic approach to family therapy. The group then worked on a systemic-strategic model under the guidance of Watzlawick, who, with other researchers, developed in Palo Alto (California) a model inspired by the studies of G. Bateson on the types of logic in → communication and on the → cybernetics of homeostatic systems. In 1975, the four researchers published a paper in which they described a model of therapy of not more than ten sessions, carried out by two therapists (a male and a female) assisted by two colleagues acting as supervisors who would follow the conversation from an adjacent room through a one-way mirror. Each session took place in five stages: the pre-session, in which the team formulated an initial hypothesis; the session with the family, during which the supervisors could interject in the session by talking to the therapists; the discussion by the therapeutic team; the conclusion of the sessions, with an intervention that consisted of communicating a final message to the family; the final discussion on the → feedback of the family about the intervention. The distancing from psychoanalysis took place in the attention given to the relational configurations instead of the mental processes (the → "black box", useless because they cannot be known): if the therapy intervenes at the level of these configurations (for example, by positively connoting and prescribing behavioural symptoms rather than opposing them, with the paradoxical effect of instantly modifying the framework within which they have been working), change can be macroscopic and already observable in the first sessions. At the heart of the "silent revolution of Milan" (to quote Hoffman) there was the idea that psychosis is born within a family dynamic in which, in an "absurd game", each member of the family fights for power and control in their relationships with each other but in which, paradoxically no one can prevail, because this would mean abandoning the game. One of them becomes the → "designated patient": his mad behaviour – given that the effect of this kind of environment is that of generating a strong sense of confusion about oneself and about one's role in life – guarantees the → homeostasis of the nucleus and the continuation of the conflict. But he is simply the bearer of the symptom: in reality the whole family system is captive to this hubris that imposes itself on them the need to persevere. In their last paper, the group (by now very popular in Anglo-Saxon countries), outlined the guidelines for a systemic conversation. Their hypothesis substituted what, within the framework of individual thought, is the diagnosis: it is the process of connecting the information available by formulating a hypothesis (that is systemic, that is, that includes all the components of the nucleus) on the global relational functioning of the family. The circularity is an attitude of the therapist that, in conducting the session and in asking questions, allows himself to be led by the feedback of the family. Additionally, it translates itself into a complex questioning technique: the circular interview. As a result of the position of → neutrality adopted, inherited from the psychoanalytic background of the members of the group, the therapist, observing the system at a different level from that of the members of the family, manages to avoid aligning himself with any single member of the family (in this the help of the supervising colleagues is crucial).

The group split up in 1980, at the same time as the publication of work that contains some of the themes on which the divergence of opinion between the individual members proved to be unsurmountable. For example, the hypothesis of the group refers to a scientific language: but for Boscolo and Cecchin it would increasingly connote as a process that is continually developing, that does not stop once the hypothesis is verified; on the contrary it proceeds in a constant generation of points of view. Increasingly, Selvini Palazzoli was involved in a project of systematic research on the pathogenesis of schizophrenia and of anorexia, whilst the two men in the group appeared to be more interested in therapy as a creative conversation guided by a therapist who is never external to the reality he is observing.

In 1982, Selvini, together with Prata and M. Viaro, gave life to the New Centre for the Study of the Family, whilst Boscolo and Cecchin looked for an evolution of the model primarily through discussion with numerous professionals, both Italian and foreign. In a paper written in 1987, Cecchin proposed substituting the concept of neutrality with that of "curiosity" as a position that, differently to the framework of "true/false", is able to generate descriptions that are polyphonic. Boscolo was increasingly interested in the language of therapy and in the use of → metaphor as a door that allows the therapist to access the emotions of the clients. In other words, on both ends of the Milan model, the password remained the → relationship and the → context: but Boscolo and Cecchin continued to study in greater depth Bateson's work and to establish closer relationships with the constructivist epistemologists H. von Foerster and H. Maturana; Selvini Palazzoli reconstructed the group with Cirillo, Selvini and Sorrentino in order to continue the study of the relational determinants of schizophrenia and of eating disorders.

Whilst Selvini's group worked within the walls of its own centre in order to provide consistency in their research, the other two psychotherapists invested in the training of new therapists and in building a therapeutic model inspired by the epistemology of complexity and by the theory of the observer.

In their own words, the ongoing relationship with students and professionals in training would be a fundamental element in the evolution of their model. This stimulus towards self-reflection would contribute to the explicit movement towards second-order cybernetics, that is, towards a school of thought that places the observer within the system and that looks at how his descriptions contribute towards the construction of reality. The focal point of therapy was no longer the change in the family being observed with the presumption of objectivity, but the recursive relationship between the therapist's position and the reality that he is observing.

An enthusiastic witness to the exchange between clinicians from all around the world was the book titled *Clinica Sistemica* (translation by Milan Systemic Family Therapy, 1987), in which the Italian masters dialogued with two American therapists regarding the Milan Approach. The following year, the Selvini group illustrated the method of the "invariable prescription ", an ingenious intervention through which the therapeutic team defied the system of co-dependence of the families of psychotic patients by prescribing that the parents "disappear" from the family for progressively longer periods of time (from one evening, up to a whole month), this being agreed upon without the knowledge of the son or daughter who were the bearer of the symptoms: the invariability of the prescription was coherent with the prerequisite of repeatability in the context of a research that is scientific.

From the 1990s onwards, the Selvini group submitted its own → model to rigorous revision, and, to a prolonged period of → follow-up of the therapies of the previous years, and also revisited psychoanalysis – especially with reference to attachment theory – and to the concept of individual diagnosis. Boscolo and Cecchin's group moved towards social constructivism and the narrative approach (→ narrative, therapy) and developed their vocation towards education by dedicating themselves to the training of students, many of whom would go on to distinguish themselves by following their own lines of personal research, demonstrating the capacity of the work of Boscolo and Cecchin to hybridize and produce new ideas. Together with Bertrando, Boscolo celebrated the overcoming of the dogma of the 'black box" and the recovered interest in the internal world; he would also revisit psychoanalytic concepts in his clinical work within a framework that, however, continued to be coherently systemic: however, with an increased awareness of the fact that new models and new ideas do not cancel out preceding ones, but that they can be epigenetically connected with those ideas that have in the past proved to be useful. Purism is a position necessary to the student in training: but it is equally necessary that the trained clinician allows himself to be touched by and to experience other models and other ideas with which they come into contact, even in an unconscious manner, and that he cultivates a vision of reality that is multiverse and contextual. In 2004 Cecchin died, leaving behind an inheritance to the systemic movement of his irreverent work of deconstruction of the prejudices of the therapist. Those were the days of dialogue between family therapy and postmodern thought. *[M. Giuliani]*

REFERENCES. Boscolo L., Bertrando P., *The times of time: A new perspective in systemic therapy and consultation*, 1993; Id., *Systemic therapy with individuals*, 1996; Boscolo L., Cecchin G., Hoffman L., Penn P., *Milan systemic family therapy*, 1987; Cecchin G., *Hypothesizing, circularity and neutrality revisited: An invitation to curiosity*, in «Family Process», 1987, 26, 4; Selvini Palazzoli M., Boscolo L., Cecchin G., Prata G., *Paradox and counter paradox*, 1978; Id., *Hypothesizing-circularity-neutrality: Three guidelines for the conductor of the session*, in «Family process», 1980, 19(1); Selvini Palazzoli M., Cirillo S., Selvini M., Sorrentino A.M., *Family games*, 1989; Id., *Ragazze anoressiche e bulimiche*, 1998; Watzlawick P., Beavin J.H., Jackson Don D., *Pragmatics of human communication*, 1967.

MIND–BODY MODEL

According to F. Bacon's and R. Descartes' theories, body and mind are two separate entities, which are defined, by psychosomatic studies, as interplaying between each other. The mind–body model is radically different from this interpretation, since it is founded on completely different theoretical premises: mind and body are the same entity; the mind is not generated by the brain but is both present all over the body and spreads outside. This model derives from concepts and experiences originated in different environments: B. Spinoza's philosophy, which considers mind and body a single entity; G. Bateson's interactionist and ecosystemic theories (→ interactionist model and therapy), which interpret it as a circular interaction process between the individual, others and the surrounding reality; the scientific evidence that what happens in the body also happens in the mind, and vice versa. This process is clearly dominated by the system of beliefs (→ logic of belief), personal opinions, cognitive elaborations and emotions; for instance, emotions – through their energy, their cognitive elaborations and the biochemical processes they trigger – reverberate on the biological level, thus contributing to preserving a state of wellbeing or causing disease. Other origins of the mind–body model lie in some of the principles of quantum physics. These principles consider mind and body as the expression of two different forms of the energy density of the same entity; also, neurobiology considers the body as the rough objectification of the mind in physical space. Therefore, the mind of the individual is described as having two dimensions: one is body-related, the other is extended and is present both inside and outside the body; this latter dimension, according to quantum physics, is considered an intelligent, interconnecting tissue which unites and generates everything. *[G. Pagliaro]*

REFERENCES. Capra F., *The turning point*, 1982; Pert C., *Molecules of emotion*, 1997; Pagliaro G., *Mente, meditazione e benessere*, 2004.

MINDFULNESS

The term "mindfulness" is the English version of the word "*sati*", which in the Pali of ancient scriptures refers to "mindful attention" and "mindfulness meditation", concepts that are typical of the oldest of Buddhist meditation practices, known as *vipassana*, which stands for "clear vision" (similar to English → "insight"). This form of "mindfulness meditation" can be defined, according to Montano, as the ability to acquire knowledge that possesses the quality of seeing, an act of perception unmediated by thoughts of the mind, able to generate over time an intuitive, deep, non-conceptual understanding of what is happening when it happens. Thus, mindfulness refers to a state of mind in which people listen to and observe their emotions, physical sensations and thoughts, accepting them as they are, without thinking about them, without changing anything, without judging, without trying to change them or block them. This leads to a full understanding of the present moment and to letting in and out the negative aspects of common everyday experience, without triggering negative lasting emotional states and behavioural counterproductive reactions. Mindfulness helps both to recognize, and not get involved in, ruminating habits – which, as agravating negative emotions, are ineffective – and to not react impulsively. The practice of mindfulness is useful to reach the understanding that thoughts and feelings are transient events of the mind and not necessarily self-reflections or true readings of reality. Being able to pay attention to our inner experiences, becoming aware of them, also leads to distancing oneself from them (as in the classical procedure of "distancing", widely used in cognitive-behavioural therapy). So, through mindfulness it is possible to disidentify from one's mental contents, which are only internal experiences and not our full being. As Kabat-Zinn says, thoughts are just thoughts, not facts, not reality. The awareness that we are not our thoughts leads to distancing ourselves from them and to the possibility of entering into a relationship with them for what they really are: mere mental events, regardless of their content or their emotional charge. Through the practice of mindfulness, we simply bring awareness to our own internal experience and thus strengthen the "willingness" (in the terminology of → Acceptance and Commitment Therapy) of our mind to accept the same experience. Being willing to experience the wide range of thoughts and emotions as they emerge in life does not coincide with the desire to experience these internal experiences, or with judging them to be to our liking. Assuming an attitude of willingness means simply accepting, tolerating, negative internal experiences as a means to achieve our values, what is really important to us. Consider the case of obsessive-compulsive disorder (OCD). As we know from the literature, the element at the base of a great part of OCD phenomenology is represented by a hyper-control of specific aspects of self and/or environment with intolerance of uncertainty. In relation to certain domains, the obsessive patient has an absolute need to do everything in his power to avoid any possible threat. Moreover, as obsessive patients are well aware, any attempt to prevent a threat opens, inexorably, further concerns in an endless loop. So, any behaviour aimed at finding security creates uncertainty with a consequent negative emotional state. The total elimination of risk, so desired by the patient, represents a physically impossible target. Life, in fact, is inherently risky and therefore it is only when the patient comes to accept that a risk quota exists, beyond his power, can he abandon the attempt to do everything possible to avoid it: uncertainty is connatural with existence. In the face of any threat, we learn how to have the thought "I cannot be sure" or "Something can always happen" or "I cannot exclude the possibility."

This technique, designed to accept uncertainty, is something completely different from "thought stopping", consisting in interrupting an unwanted thought. The idea behind the "thought stopping" technique is that you cannot tolerate having a certain type of thought. The exercises in which we let ourselves be submerged by thoughts of uncertainty, without doing anything to acquire certainty, help us to become aware that we can live with the uncertainty itself. And so change occurs. Thus, the energy spent in taking the slightest precaution at this point can be available in order to live a life that is more productive and more responsive to our values. The practice of mindfulness to achieve awareness and acceptance in order to produce therapeutically useful changes was introduced into the West for the first time by Jon Kabat-Zinn at the Stress Reduction Clinic of the University of Massachusetts during the late 1970s. Its Mindfulness-Based Stress Reduction (MBSR) protocol, derived from ancient Buddhist practices of meditation, has been successfully applied, with evidence-based efficacy studies, in subjects with physical illnesses and severe and debilitating disabilities, who through this approach succeeded in avoiding those automatic mental reactions leading to increased → stress. Subsequently, the conceptualization and procedures of mindfulness have been incorporated within a broader set of structured and therapeutic methods and techniques, basically almost all belonging to the so-called "third generation of cognitive-behavioural therapy": Dialectical Behavioural Therapy (DBT), by Marsha Linehan, which is considered one of the treatments of choice and more evidence-based for → borderline personality disorder; the Four Steps treatment programme for obsessive-compulsive disorder; Acceptance and Commitment Therapy (ACT) developed by Hayes, Strosahl and Wilson, which aims to help patients to accept their thoughts and emotions and live in a consistent manner with their values; Mindfulness-Based Cognitive Therapy (MBCT), by Segal, Williams and Teasdale, demonstrated as empirically valid for relapse prevention in the treatment of depression; Compassion-focused Therapy (CFT) by Gilbert, aimed at activating in patients a "compassionate" and accepting attitude towards themselves (see related item). Without any doubt we can say that mindfulness has been and is an important new concept, which introduced fertile developments in psychotherapy, particularly of a cognitive-behavioural orientation. In fact, in addition to the broader therapeutic proposals outlined above, other authors have proposed the use of this practice in cognitive and behavioural treatments for generalized anxiety disorder, post-traumatic stress disorder, substance dependence, eating disorders, attention deficit disorder/hyperactivity, psychosis, treatment of family problems and marital therapy. It is, however, still a new intervention proposal, which, although promising in relation to future developments in its application, requires new evidence-based efficacy studies, capable of confirming its scientific bases and to better specify the utility and conditions of employment in specific cases and disorders. *[D. Dèttore]*

REFERENCES. Dèttore D., *Il disturbo ossessivo compulsivo*, 2003; Didonna F. (ed.), *Clinical handbook of mindfulness*, 2008. Gilbert P., *Compassion: Conceptualisations, research and use in psychotherapy*, 2005; Gilbert P., *Compassion-focused therapy: Distinctive features*, 2009; Gilbert P., Irons C., *Focused therapies and compassionate mind training for shame and self-attacking*, in P. Gilbert (ed.), *Compassion: Conceptualisations, research and use in psychotherapy* (263–325), 2005; Hayes S.C., Strosahl K.D., Wilson K.G., *Acceptance and commitment therapy: An experiential approach to behaviour change*, 1999; Kabat-Zinn J., *Full catastrophe living: Using the wisdom of your body and mind to face stress, pain, an illness*, 1990; Kabat-Zinn J., *Coming to our senses: Healing ourselves and the world through mindfulness*, 2005; Linehan M.M., *Cognitive behavioural treatment for borderline personality disorder*, 1993; Linehan M.M., Skills training manual for treating borderline personality disorder,1993; Montano A., *Mindfulness*, 2007; Segal Z.V., Williams J.M., Teasdale J.D., *Mindfulness-based cognitive therapy for depression: A new approach to preventing relapse*, 2002; Schwartz J.M., *Brain lock: Free yourself from obsessive-compulsive behaviour. A four-step treatment method to change your brain chemistry*, 1996.

MIRACLE PRESCRIPTION

A solution-oriented technique, formulated within the brief strategic therapy Nardone's model to define the objective to be reached in therapy. The prescription is formulated by the psychotherapist in the following manner:

> This task is a fantasy that you have to imagine every morning, from now until our next meeting. Whilst you are washing, getting ready, getting dressed, I would like you to imagine yourself going out of this room, in the same way as you are going out of this room today, that you are closing the door behind you, as you are going to close the door behind you today, and as soon as you go out of here, suddenly, by miracle, your problem has disappeared, does not exist anymore. What would change in your life? What other problems would arise once you have solved this one? I would like you to imagine this fantasy every morning, imagining that you have managed to overcome your problem.

This prescription is derived from a reorganization of the → "as if" technique formulated by P. Watzlawick and from the → miracle-question technique of S. Shazer, but with a slight variation in the content, and differs from the latter in that it is prescribed as a question the patient needs to ask himself between one therapeutic session and the next, and not as one to be explored with the therapist within the therapeutic session itself.

The prescription of the miracle is firstly a therapeutic manoeuvre aimed at the induction of a positive form of self-deceit (→ logic of self-deception). By introducing a positive suggestion, in fact, this manoeuvre exploits the logic of the → self-fulfilling prophecy, suggesting that the "miracle" can happen, and diverting the patient's attention from his or her current difficulties onto a future without these difficulties. This shifting of the patient's perspective through the use of hypnotic suggestion, is in itself therapeutic, in that it opens new horizons and enables the patient to see beyond his or her problem. This often produces a "magical" effect by causing an unexpected resolution of the symptoms from the very first session to the second. In addition, by means of this technique, the patient is able to analyze not only the advantages of the imagined change, but also the possible negative consequences of this change, such as side-effects or the possible → secondary gain of the problem. This will also allow the adjustment of the therapeutic goals in the process of change, by also taking into consideration, in addition to the benefits, the possible risks and the difficulties the individual and/or the system have to overcome. As a result of its efficacy and flexibility, the prescription of the miracle can be applied to a wide range of situations not only in the clinical field, with patients who are particularly easily influenced and who are not completely "blocked" by their problem, but also in an organizational context (educational, sporting). In the latter, it is used in a variation called "the technique of the scenario beyond the problem", where the type of language used is a logic that is no longer tied to the fairy tale image of a "miracle", that would not be welcomed by managers, headmasters and athletes. *[G. Nardone]*

REFERENCES. Nardone G., *Problem solving strategico da tasca*, 2009; Nardone, G., Watzlawick, P., *The art of change*, 1993; Nardone G., Mariotti R., Milanese R., Fiorenza A., *La terapia dell'azienda malata*, 2000.

MIRACLE QUESTION TECHNIQUE

It is the main manoeuvre of the → brief solution-focused therapy. It is aimed to help clients to project themselves beyond the problem, providing useful descriptive information to clients and therapist to be followed in order to reach the solution of a problem. This technique was born accidentally thanks to I.K. Berg, who first tested this kind of intervention in response to a client who, in the grip of desperation, said: "Perhaps only a miracle could save me". Berg and his colleagues immediately realized the usefulness of this concept. They started to invite clients to imagine what their lives would be like once they had eliminated the problem. The question, formulated at a later time by de Shazer, is: "Suppose tonight, while you are at home asleep, a miracle happens and your problem is solved. How would you notice it? How would you know that the miracle has happened? What would be different? How would the people around you notice it?". Thanks to this question, the patient and the therapist start a joint research into the daily life of the patient to discover all those signals that would indicate that the miracle had happened and the problem had disappeared. The effect of the "miracle question" is not based on the therapist's opinion about how patients should live their lives, but on that of the patient, which results from their knowledge and personal abilities. Although it appears to be a simple question, the therapeutic use of this manoeuvre is not immediately obvious nor easy to implement. First, the conversation that leads to the question requires great discipline and self-control by the solution-oriented therapist. The therapist needs to abstain from giving interpretations and unsolicited advice and should remain attentive to every client's verbal and nonverbal nuance, while exploring their "miraculous" scenario. Moreover, the question requires a change in the way of thinking in both the client and the therapist and in their ability to focus on the solution rather than the problem. Starting from this manoeuvre, G. Nardone has developed one of the fundamental prescriptions of → brief strategic therapy Nardone's model, namely the → miracle prescription. *[G. Nardone]*

REFERENCES. De Shazer S., *Clues: Investigating solutions in brief therapy*, 1988.

MIRRORING

In psychodrama, this term can refer to a mental function or to a technique. One speaks of the function of mirroring when an individual captures aspects of himself in the images related to his person built by others, and presented to him. It is an event – recurring within a group where the behaviour of each expresses perceptions related to the other members – that contributes to the construction of self-image. One speaks instead of the technique of mirroring when there is a protagonist: he sees, from outside, a scene just performed by himself and now acted out again by an alter-ego placed in *his* own role. The protagonist, observing from outside, can usefully take advantage of any dissonance between this self-perception, while acting out the scene, and the alter-ego's performance. *[G. Boria]*

REFERENCES Boria G. (2005), *Psicoterapia psicodrammatica. Sviluppi del modello moreniano nel lavoro terapeutico con gruppi di adulti*, 2005. Boria G., Muzzarelli F., *Incontri sulla scena*, 2009; Moreno J.L., *Psychodrama first volume*, 1946. Moreno J.L., *Who shall survive?*, 1953.

MIRROR STAGE

In Lacanian psychoanalysis, a child's development stage, when the six-month-old infant recognizes his own image in the mirror. Starting from his identification with the mirror image, the infant sets himself as an "I", as a unit. An observation of this phenomenon was Jacques Lacan's first contribution to psychoanalytic theory, even though he always considered that the only true innovation he brought to psychoanalysis was the object little *a*: the cause of unconscious desire. Lacan starts from an empirical experience that comes from James Mark Baldwin. It deals with the interest that the infant

(6 to 18 months old) shows in front of the mirror. The baby, physiologically premature, exults in recognizing himself in the mirror. In the reflected image he sees himself as an entirety that he really does not yet possess. He sees an image that is both his own image and that of someone else: the other one is an image that seduces him and with which he identifies. "On such occasions, the child anticipates at the mental level the conquest of his own body's functional unity, which is still incomplete at the level of volitional motricity at that point in time". Hence Lacan derives the idea that imaginary alienation is constitutive of the Ego (*moi*) and that its human development is marked by ideal identifications. This principle accounts for the human being's ambivalent aggressiveness with regard to his peers, for his fundamentally paranoid relationship with the object and for the hysterical character of his desire, which is always a "desire of the other". For Lacan, the Ego of a human person, consisting of a bunch of imaginary identifications, and which is the one that we believe it to be, is not to be confused with the I (*je*): the subject of a sentence, and the subject of the unconscious desire, which is revealed by the symptoms and formations of the unconscious (dreams, lapses, faulty acts, etc.). *[A. di Ciaccia]*

REFERENCES. Lacan J. (2006). *The mirror stage as formative of the I function as revealed in psychoanalytic experience*, in *Écrits*, 1936–1949; Id., (2006), *Aggressiveness in psychoanalysis*, 1948, in *Écrits*, 1936–1949.

MOBBING

A workplace relationship aiming at invalidating, oppressing, discriminating, persecuting a colleague, irrespective of his/her being in a subordinate position. Mobbing can negatively affect the personal and professional identity of the individuals suffering it, jeopardize their social adaptation to the workplace, undermine their → self-esteem, their sense of self-efficacy and their professional status. From the point of view of the law, mobbing is an illegal behaviour, which offends the right and the dignity of a person and his/her work reputation; for this reason, if verified by evidence, mobbing may be subject to damage compensation. Mobbing may cause biological, moral and existential damage. The psychological evaluation of mobbing requires the demonstration that it actually occurred (description and modalities of occurrence, frequency and duration, evidence of persecutory episodes and intentions). It also requires the verification of the effects on the job position, the tasks and the working potential of the victim, and the consequences on his/her psychological balance. Evident damage is similar to the consequences of a reaction to chronic stressing events (→ stress), causing disorders in the cognitive, emotional, relational and psychosomatic spheres. Besides damage evaluation, mobbing may require two types of intervention: one involving workplace organization (work environment, the management of competition and conflict), the other consisting in recovering the damaged resources of the victim through relevant psychotherapy. *[R.]*

MODEL

In psychotherapy, a coherent system of constructs aimed at organizing, analogically, interpretation, evaluation and forms of intervention in relation to certain problematic or dysfunctional events (such as actions, beliefs, feelings and perceptions), addressed with the intention of curing or creating a change. In regard to this, two superordinate models, or meta-models, have established themselves in the history of psychotherapy. Their semantic and representational field refers to the constructs of "disease/cure" borrowed from the medical field, or "problem/change" typical of social and behavioural sciences. Their paradigms of reference are positivism on the one side and → pragmatism on the other: the first is realist, the second is constructivist.

In clinical practice, the emphasis on the causes rather than the effects leads to distinguishing between determinist and finalist models (→ anthropomorphism). The epistemology behind these models implies that the therapist, when affiliating to either meta-model, steps into a different way of acting, perceiving and thinking. Therefore, the affiliation to a model implies, for a therapist, different ways of configuring the therapeutic relationship, its objectives and the semantic and narrative system in which the person is involved during the therapy. *[R.]*

MODELLING

Within the behavioural paradigm, modelling represents the third learning model – in addition to classical and operant conditioning (→ behavioural model of classic conditioning; → behavioural model of operant conditioning) – born from the observation that many behaviours are indeed learned by imitating a model. Modelling helps the learning of → adaptive behaviours such as social skills, but also the acquisition of pathological behaviours when exposed to inadequate models. In cognitive-behavioural therapy, modelling can help improve the behaviour of a patient when, for example, the therapist tackles, along with him, a feared or difficult situation. It can also be used outside the classic therapeutic → setting, as in mutual support groups, where the model is a recovered alcoholic or drug addict rather than an expert. Modelling is particularly used in emotional disorders, conduct disorders, learning disorders (where it is used primarily to facilitate self-training processes) and autistic-spectrum disorders in addition to addictions, mental retardation and many forms of schizophrenia. *[F. Celi]*

REFERENCES. Bandura A., *Social Learning theory*, 1977; Galeazzi A., Meazzini P., *Mente e comportamento: Trattato italiano di psicoterapia cognitivo-comportamentale*, 2004; Miller N.E., Dollard J., *Social learning and imitation*, 1941.

▷ In the field of neuro-linguistic programming, it is a process of observation and mapping of behaviours and of effective thinking strategies used by people who excel in any specific activity. In practice, modelling consists in analyzing the ways that allow an individual to perform a task with very positive outcomes and then in systematizing them, so that they can become communicable. In this way, other people are able to achieve the same results by following these rules. In this process, the behaviour to replicate is broken up into single elements concerning the different levels of experience (mental representations, beliefs and values, skills, actions, linguistic schemas, etc.). Then, these elements are structured in a "map", which is a pragmatic model of behaviour that can be used by third parties to reproduce the same results. Modelling was first used by R. Bandler and J. Grinder, the co-creators of neuro-linguistic programming, in order to achieve, with patients, the same results of some exceptional psychotherapists, such as F. Perls, M.H. Erickson, V. Satir, and it was later applied to many other areas. *[A. Roberti]*

REFERENCES. Dilts R.B., *Modelling with NLP*, 1998.

MONOTHEISM

Jung indicates in monotheism a non-defensive psychic tendency that grows beyond polytheism in each individual who is open towards the sacred and the quest for the truth. Such dynamics shows an emerging need for unity. According to analytical psychology, Hebraism, Christianity, Islam, Buddhism can be considered as parts of a millenary developmental process, characterized by the primacy of the → anima and of the mother, of the paternal figure, of the birth of the son, of the emerging prophet, until the becoming of an "enlightened spirit", the Buddha. The psychic process typical of monotheism involves conflict, sacrifice, transformation. Monotheism must be compared with a state of psychic equilibrium, which arises from containment of beliefs, illusions, dogmatism. In Jung's thought the dogma appears as a strong expansion, but also as a limit of the vitality underlying any monotheistic attitude. *[A. Vitolo]*

REFERENCES. Jung C.G. (1928–1954), *Psychology and religion: West and East*, in *Collected Works*, 11, 1958.

MOTHER (GOOD MOTHER – BAD MOTHER)

According to Sullivan's thinking, good mother and bad mother are personifications created by the infant's mind as a consequence of the interpersonal experiences within the relationship with his caregiver, usually the mother. Right from his early interaction with the mother, through bodily contact, the infant discriminates the latter's affection and even unconscious hostility and he is able to detect in her facial expressions and voice tone those elements of acceptance and disapproval that will be associated to pleasant (→ wellbeing) and unpleasant (→ anguish) experiences. When the mother is able to accept and hold the infant's anxiety, this will lead to a positive and empathic relationship; should this not be the case, her behaviour will increase the infant's anxiety and cause a snowball effect. The discrimination between anxiety-based and non–anxiety-based states will result in the first couple of personifications: the "good mother" and the "bad mother". However, given that they are composite personifications originating from both anxiety-free and tender experiences as well as from anxiety-ridden and frustrating ones, these personifications do not adhere perfectly to the image of the "real mother". Thus, the good mother rushes to soothe the infant's distress by signifying herself as the source of immediate satisfaction, whilst the "bad mother" – either because of her own anxiety or for other reasons – is unable to dispel the infant's needy tension deriving from the emergency of needs and this will cause anxiety and growing distress in the infant. *[A. Cresti, S. Brizzi]*

REFERENCES. Sullivan H.S., *The Interpersonal theory of psychiatry*, 1953.

MOTIVATION

A set of psychological factors that lead an individual to achieve a specific goal. This construct refers to the activation, direction and persistence of human → behaviour. At the basis of motivation there is an activation of the organism, a drive to action and a search in the environment for what it takes to meet one's own needs or desires. The study of motivation is one of the main topics investigated by psychology. It is also essential for psychotherapy, since understanding the motivation of a behaviour means that this can be predicted and influenced. The research in this field is intertwined with the research on → needs. However, the latter describes what states of need can be activated in human being, whereas research on motivation is mainly on explaining some of the "how and why": how and why a state of necessity in people can become active, how and why people do what they do, how and why people continue to do what they do. *[R.]*

MOTIVATIONAL SYSTEM

The psychological regulation of physiological needs, the attachment-affiliation system, the exploration-assertiveness system, aversion and the pleasure of sexual sensual-excitation constitute fundamental needs and are defined as being motivational systems. The satisfaction and regulation of these takes place according to different but interconnected modalities that form the motivational system of the individual, and that participate in the development, maintenance and reintegration of the cohesive Self. This in turn constitutes the organizer and the functional integrator of the motivational systems.

In classical psychoanalytic theory, the causation, the activation and the motivation of behaviour depends on energy drives that activate the apparatus of the psyche, and that tend to discharge by taking the shortest possible path, the primary process (→ primary and secondary processes) and the → pleasure principle, or according to a more articulated path, that of the secondary process or the reality principle. Although these meta-psychological concepts hinge on the economic principle permeated throughout psychoanalytic theory, to the latter is added → drive theory, according to a biological interpretation that is flanked by the psychophysical one of drive theory. In the face of contemporary criticism to meta-psychological explanation, Lichtenberg and Lachmann proposed a new model to explain the numerous phenomena that are observable in psychoanalysis, according to a perspective-based on → systems theory. According to them, the concept of motivational systems should replace the classical metapsychological concepts and take the place of drive theory and that of the binomy of the life instinct and death drive in a way that allows it to be integrated with Self psychology, recapturing the methodological indications from the work of Klein in the context of a perspective that is systemic, autopoietic and evolutionistic.

Every motivational system can be activated both from within as well as from outside of the individual and, in evolution and interaction with all the others, determines the behaviour, the thoughts and the emotions of the individual. In every moment of life, the activity of each motivational system can intensify itself so much that it can constitute the prevailing motivational aspect of the self; a fixed hierarchical order does not exist: every system can become dominant over the others. The final aim of the motivational systems is that of recreating a pleasurable characteristic emotion for every motivational system, previously experimented, giving or restoring the cohesion and integration of the Self whose autopoietic equilibrium (→ autopoiesis) remains the ultimate goal of every motivational regulation. The only exception appears to be the aversive motivational system, whose objective is that of alleviating suffering, that can produce itself in the action of every single one of the other systems, through signals that are recalled and activated by the caregiver, facilitating the satisfaction of needs and the regulation of the wishes of the other systems.

PSYCHIC REGULATION OF THE PHYSIOLOGICAL NEEDS. From the first day of life the child passes through progressive changes in states, dictated by physiological needs, to which the caregiver responds in a way that is more or less synchronic and empathetic, functioning as a pad that mutes the excessive variations of emotional activation both in an upwards and in a downwards direction. This combination creates a system characterized by a sensitivity that is mutually regulated, by a level of coherence, by a rhythm that allows both partners to experiment a positive affectionate relationship in which small moments of discomfort are inserted as well as their relief, and from which the first and prototypical experience of the → Self-object is derived. This event is registered in the memory of the child as a procedural experience and as part of a series of correlated events in a chain of episodes.

The capacity of the person taking care of the child to correctly recognize, in an empathic manner, the information regarding the state of need that the child perceives internally will give confirmation to the child's sense of the physical reality of his own body. The repetition of the pattern of the physiological need and its satisfaction, together with the perception of being able to recreate continuity, establishes and permits the experimentation with familiar states through which the child recognizes himself. For example, in the case of hunger, a successful reciprocal caregiver–child regulation contributes to the creation of a model of the perceptive action of hunger-nourishment and creates a definition of hunger as motivation. The reality of a state of the Self as hunger-satiety derives from a combination of an internal perception and of a consistent confirmation of a response and an external acknowledgement of an empathic nature, the result of which is a combination of an attachment having a positive tonality and of the differentiation of the Self as a source of motivation that is internally recognized.

ATTACHMENT-AFFILIATION. The motivational system of attachment (→ attachment theory) develops around the desire of the pleasure of intimacy and starts with innate models of perceptive–affective action that are described by J. Bowlby. These models give rise to a request of responsivity, indicated as need. The readiness with which the attachment figure responds to the requests of the child, as well as the desire to help the child to initiate the request are in equal measure a part of the attachment process and derive from the motivational system of the caregiver. Therefore, each one contributes to that modelling, tone and intensity that characterize the child–attachment-figure couple in a mutual regulation that originates from the activation of motivations and functions that are relevant to both. Successively, the child starts to become motivated to affiliate himself to groups characterized by the sharing of an emotional bond, of a relational goal, of a belief or of an ideal. The model of affiliation starts when the child perceives his parents and siblings not only as individuals but also as a united entity, and is able to derive the pleasure of intimacy and a sense of belonging also from the family group. The first behaviour presents itself during the age of "latency" in groups of team play. It requires an awareness of the rules and the desire to share the pleasure of intimacy with a variable number of individuals whose personal characteristics are less meaningful, in that it is not the being in the blue team or in the green one. Experience of attachment with individuals and of affiliation with groups can fulfil similar functions: reduce feelings of anguish and of discomfort and receive an evaluation of one's abilities or of one's opinions. With respect to the attachment, affiliation provides another resource so that the individual will calm down, and will find affirmation and confirmation of his own worth.

EXPLORATION-ASSERTIVENESS. In all motivational systems, exploration and assertiveness are components of every activity and the success achieved by the different motivational efforts is increased by the pleasure of efficiency. For example, when a parent is successful in making a child smile or obtains a response in a social exchange, the child has successfully employed his assertiveness and it is likely that he will experience a sense of Self as being competent in the attainment of intimacy. Exploration and assertiveness also constitute a separate motivational system, of such width as to allow self-organization and to establish itself in an adaptive manner. Sander has observed that from birth, children in a state of alertness have moments of relative equilibrium, in which neither their physiological needs nor their attachment needs are in the forefront. This makes possible a temporal space in which the child and the caregiver can experiment a relative sense of disengagement. For example, when the child focuses on an object that is in movement, the organization of the attention (exploration) and the consequent organization of his activity (assertiveness), represent an activity that takes place when the attachment needs or the need for physiological regulation or the need to react in an aversive manner do not occupy a central position in the attention of the child. In these moments the child is able to discover his own personal life rather than a "life built on reactions to external stimuli". The affective tone lies in the pleasure of competence and of efficacy that derive from the ability, learnt by the child, to reproduce a new experience of a desired state, in which the novelty and the discovery of associated feelings prolong the state of attentive excitement.

ADVERSITY. The aversive system is reactive to stimuli perceived as being threatening or that induce discomfort. In infancy, behavioural signs of an aversive experience, for example crying, function as signs to solicit the action of the person who takes care of the child. The capacity of this person to respond to signs of discomfort, fear, frustration or anger by eliminating its source or by reducing it, consoling or offering a solution, is probably the most important factor in ensuring the strength of the attachment. In the relationship with the caregiver, the child seeks not only the direct pleasure of intimacy but also relief from aversive experiences. During early infancy, the expression of feelings continue to function as a sign, but the functioning of the aversive system becomes, in an increasingly complex manner, tied to the → problem-solving situation. Whilst in the other systems, positive feelings, deriving from an efficient functioning, provide a motivation to recreate the experience, the feelings triggered by the aversive system do not become organized as intrinsically self-reproducing. The infant does not seek situations in which to re-experiment with crying, disgust, fear or shame, but the function of these dystonic and unpleasant feelings consists of the search of relief from the suffering caused by these feelings that can present itself in each of the other systems. The aversive system has to provide moments of motivational domination that organizes itself around two feelings: anger, which by increasing the capacity to seek efficiency and competence allows the overcoming of frustration and obstacles and provides a sense of strength (antagonism); and fear, which allows the activation of escape from situations perceived as being dangerous (withdrawal).

SENSUAL PLEASURE – SEXUAL EXCITATION. Whilst sensual pleasure is the result of an innate programme of newborns and becomes a regular event of daily experience, sexual excitation appears to start to form part of the everyday experience of daily life only relatively late in childhood. Initially, sexual excitation represents a model of physiological response strictly correlated to the state of the REM phase of sleep, but that occasionally takes place when the child is awake. The innate programme is very easily triggered by feelings of sexual pleasure that arise during the normal interactions between the child and the person taking care of him (breastfeeding, touching, stroking, bouncing, rocking). Normally, the activation of the sensual-sexual motivational system is assured by the receptivity of the innate programme associated to areas of the body that provide feelings of significant tension and their stimulation in the normal exchanges between child and caregiver in the course of feeding, excretion, bathing, when the baby is stroked. The sensual motivation is stabilized when children seek to obtain the repetition of sensual pleasure from the person taking care of them but also by their own actions. Only gradually do the genitals take on a prominent role in providing sensual pleasure and, even later, sexual excitation. Touching the genitals triggers sensual pleasure and plays a prominent role in ensuring the integration of the bodily Self, in the same way as it is responsible for the consolidation, both of gender identity and of role identity, of the image and the function of the genitals in infants of both sexes. *[M. Casonato, M. Gaffuri, S. Sagliaschi]*

REFERENCES. Klein G.S., *Psychoanalytic theory: An exploration of essentials*, 1976; Lichtenberg J.D., Lachmann F. M., *Psychoanalysis and motivational systems: A new look*, 1992; Lichtenberg J.D., Lachmann F.M., Fosshage J.L., *Self and motivational systems*, 1992; Sander L., *The event structure of regulation in the neonate-caregive system as a biological background for early organization of psychic structure*, in A. Goldberg (ed.), *Frontiers in Self Psychology*, vol. III, 1988.

MRI → MENTAL RESEARCH INSTITUTE

MULTIPLE CODE THEORY

A theory developed in the 1990s by Bucci, an American researcher and psychoanalyst, with the aim of combining Freudian assumptions concerning mental functioning (according to primary and secondary process) with the context of cognitive psychology. This consolidates, with empirical evidence, a clinic intuition of psychoanalysis: the presence of different registers of mental functioning in processing information. Bucci suggests the existence of three different levels of coding that work simultaneously and that are connected to each other by referential activity: 1) a sensory and visceral processing level (non-symbolic and nonverbal), which includes emotions and operates synchronously without the participation of subjective attention; 2) the level of processing through images (nonverbal and symbolic), which operates sequentially and compacts experience through sensory, motor or somatic representations, according to the different sensory channels; 3) the level of processing through language (verbal and symbolic), which operates sequentially with different levels of abstraction and with the possibility of creating new symbolic forms at any time through the combination of words and the construction of sentences. These three levels are linked together by referential activity, which creates the links that are necessary for symbolization by connecting the non-symbolic level with the nonverbal symbolic level and the latter with the verbal symbolic level. This theory interprets psychopathology as the result of the dissociation between emotional patterns and explicit or declarative memory (level 2 or 3). This prevents the person accessing further processing of emotional experience through images and words and it leaves the dissociated patterns active only in the implicit memory (level 1). This dissociation depends on the deactivation of the connecting functions of referential activity. Psychotherapy (defined by Freud as "talking cure"), operates a gradual reconnection of previously dissociated emotional *patterns* through verbal exchanges produced during the therapeutic relationship marked by expectations and affective responses. These patterns are reconnected to the totality of the emotional patterns in interpersonal interactions and stimulate the referential activity of the patient through autobiographical narratives and the therapist's interventions.

Together with her collaborators, Bucci has developed a method, based on this theory, to evaluate processes in the context of psychotherapy research to monitor the efficacy of the therapeutic work during its progress and to evaluate the changes occurring between therapy sessions or periods. This method involves the evaluation of oscillations in Referential Activity (RA) both in the patient's narratives and in those of the therapist, by studying the transcripts of the sessions, recorded with the patient's consent. In the first version, the method was applied by segmenting the texts of the sessions in ideative units and by rating them (from 0 to 10) on four scales for each ideative unit: "concreteness" (which measures how much the language used contains words that refer to sensory characteristics and/or intense emotional experiences); "specificity" (which measures the amount of detail contained in a narrative); "clarity" (which measures the logical organization and understandability of thought in the language used by the patient); and "imagination" (which measures how much the language of that unit is able to recall vivid images in the mind of the listener, through the use of metaphors or other narrative stratagems). The RA values correspond to the average of the values of the four variables. Subsequently, computerized measures were built that evaluate variations in referential activity, emotional tone, reflection and disfluency of speech of patient and therapist, thanks to a software that assigns specific weights to words considering the linguistic context in which each word is included.

Thanks to the research conducted on various protocols of psychoanalytic-oriented therapies, the comparison between the clinician's judgement of transcribed sessions and computerized dictionaries of referential activity has allowed researchers to support the hypothesis that a "good hour", that is, a session that promotes symbolization and therapeutic change in the patient, is characterized by a "four-step" referential cycle: the first phase, where an emotional dissociated pattern is activated, is characterized by low RA, low reflection, high affect and high disfluency. This is followed by a second phase, in which the increase of imaginative processes (for example, through the description of a dream or a memory) is characterized by high RA, low fluctuating values, low disfluency and oscillating values of affective tone. This is followed by a third phase, characterized by emotional reflection processes, with lower values of RA, high reflection, high affect and oscillations in fluency values. Finally, in the fourth phase, reflection and RA diminish and then increase again, while affect and fluency remain high: in this phase, the risk of disassociation would present itself again, with new solutions that lead to the consolidation of the integration process started in the two previous phases. The referential cycle can be repeated several times within the same session, but there can also be an alternation between phases with a good referential cycle and less productive phases from a change perspective. Similarly, in successful therapies, some sessions can be generally identified as ineffective, with few oscillations in referential activity, high disfluency and low values both in affect and reflection. Studies based on the multiple-code theory also allowed researchers to identify specific relations between referential activity in the patient and the therapist's interventions: in particular, it was found that therapists tend to intervene more often when the patient makes reflections (in the presence of low values of RA). However, when the patient describes episodes, and their language shows high values of referential activity, the therapist's interventions are rarer but they tend to be more interpretative. *[A. De Coro]*

REFERENCES. Bucci W., *Psicoanalisi e scienza cognitiva*, 1997; Id., *La ricerca sul processo*, in E.S. Person, A.M. Cooper, G.O. Gabbard (eds.), *Textbook of psychoanalysis*, 2005; De Coro A., Mariani R., *L'attività referenziale*, in N. Dazzi, V. Lingiardi, A. Colli (eds.), *La ricerca in psicoterapia: Modelli e strumenti*, 2006.

MUST-URBATION

A neologism formed from the verb *must* and the noun *masturbation*, invented by Albert Ellis in his psychotherapy framework to represent the pervasive manner in which a subject uses the concept of *must* (duty) in internal dialogue. This way of thinking is characterized by judgements and expectations in relation to perceived events in personal life, expressed in the form of rigid and absolute imperatives ("I must have everyone's approval", "Things must happen in a way that gives me what I want"). Since this exposes the person to negative results and failure, must-urbation is placed within → irrational thoughts that increase the subject's vulnerability to psychological disorders. *[S. Lenzi, C. Caramalli]*

REFERENCES. Ellis A., *Reason and emotion in psychotherapy*, 1962; Walen S.R., Di-Giuseppe R., Dryden W., *A practitioner's guide to Rational-Emotive Therapy*, 1980.

MUTATIVE PSYCHOANALYTIC PROCESS

Mutative Psychoanalytic Process (MPP), a psychotherapeutic method inspired by the theoretical psychoanalytic model, uses a technique that is distinctly transformative of psychic functioning right from the first meeting.

The theoretical reference model starts out from the Freudian theory of drives from a genetic-developmental perspective (oral, anal, phallic, genital phase) and particularly from the concept of support on the object; this is associated with the action of the appropriation drive, in turn closely related to the compulsion to repeat, and explains the type of relationship that the patient tends to establish immediately with the psychotherapist, evidently because in her/his life s/he has already sought to maintain her/his own psychological equilibrium. The patient's behaviour from the very first contact, even if it is just on the telephone, thus allows for deductions to be made about the organization of his or his/her intrapsychic world and way of functioning. The MPP therefore integrates the contribution of object relations theory into its theoretical model with its development of the mental representations of the object, which are the result of creative building processes shared with the environment. The enhancement of intersubjectivism, a further aspect characterising the theory from which the MPP is inspired, had already been carried out by Ferenczi, to whom we owe much, not only on the technical level but also on the theoretical level, because of the heuristic importance attributed to countertransference, which, as one knows, entails the full involvement of the psychotherapist in the analytical relationship. More recent psychoanalysis has thus stated that mutual influence between patient and psychotherapist at the intrapsychic and interpsychic level is therefore unavoidable. Drawing on the Bolognini theory on the interpsychic level, which is to be understood as the basis of fusional and transformative movements of the two internal worlds, the MPP places renewed emphasis on the preconscious concept of the first Freudian topic, listening to which would facilitate access to one's internal world.

Making the subconscious conscious has always been the primary objective of classical psychoanalysis, whereby this can be achieved only through the psychoanalyst being capable of advancing along the main ways that allow him/her to enter the subconscious itself. In this regard, the Mutative Psychoanalytic Process does not come into line with classical psychoanalysis, because it does not share the idea of transformation understood in the Freudian sense, as overcoming repression, through the analysis of transference and the so-called transference neuroses, but neither in the Kleinian sense as resolution of the action of primitive defence mechanisms. Based on the MPP, at any time in the therapeutic process a field of influence is created on the therapist by the patient who is internally threatened by distress and therefore activates mechanisms of projective and introjective identification. His distress is always related to the emergence of parts of the Self which s/he does not manage to integrate, resulting in the establishment of a therapeutic relationship based on the appropriation drive that reinforces the dissociative tendency and inaccessibility to mentalization; it is not to be excluded but, rather, transformed. In other words, it is impossible to avoid meeting/conflict between the pre-objects of the patient and the therapist, which have developed to a threefold level – imaginary, symbolic and real.

The MPP, instead, is inspired in its use of transformation by the mathematical theories of the infinite and limits; furthermore, it focuses on the space that exists between *from* and *to*, which is made up of so many possible points. Thus the patient can free herself/himself from a fixed, axiomatic, defensive way of thinking in order to attain flexible, moveable, open-minded, processing thinking. Each problematic situation in life, which was previously experienced dramatically, becomes an opportunity to express parts of the Self, which are unexpressed and truer. It helps the patient to cross or pierce (transform, from the Latin "*transformare*") her/his representation of the crisis as a catastrophic event and enables her/him to transform it into a developmental opportunity, as well as self-representation, built up within primary relationships, to avoid the awareness of vexation, humiliation and limits placed on herself/himself. The dissociation of the true part, subjugated to secondary benefits of relational nature, thus evolves dramatically as a spin-off.

In the MPP, it is assumed that the transformations take place continuously, regardless of how they occur, and that in order to avoid a "standstill" it is essential to accept the coexistence of opposites; hence each point of equilibrium is always and, fortunately, unstable.

Psychopathology develops every time an individual needs to keep her/his point of equilibrium fixed and immobile or to make it perpetually unstable.

Good mental functioning, on the other hand, is based on endorsing acceptance of the coexistence of opposite representations, which allow and ensure oscillation and movement of the point of equilibrium in all directions in space, without however being decentralized. In other words, a person succeeds in being sufficiently balanced the more he facilitates the transfer from the true Self to states of obfuscation of herself/himself required to maintain relationships.

Transformation in itself, as understood by the MPP, is comparable to a limit concept, because between "*from* and *to*" there are an infinite number of transformations, each smaller than the other, in which there is ideally only one fixed and basically static point of equilibrium, which is the point one starts again from.

Transformation, therefore, is also that which deals with the paradox of change: to change there must already have occurred a change in one's life, which prevents the person from returning to the static, fixed point, which nevertheless, at a closer look, is never completely static and fixed, because it is always a point in which propulsive thrusts, both forward and backward, both progressive and regressive, eventually converge.

Therefore, the crisis of "psychic equilibrium", to be understood not as static, but always as dynamic, does not occur when something changes in one of the aspects on which the construction of our self-images in relation to the surrounding reality rests. The crisis is always linked to an irruption in the conscience of evidence relegated to a preconscious level, because it is feared and experienced as a threat to the guarantee of one's own narcissism. The psychic defences adopted with the intention of not seeing what would distress us if we had been made aware of it, are no longer sufficient or adequate. The subject in crisis attempts initially, with his usual means of defence, to recover the point of equilibrium that we could conventionally identify as the point *from* in the sequence "*from . . . to*"; he even tries to do it with the figure of the therapist during the first meeting, thinking that he can get back to the past. Based on the MPP, as long as a person in crisis tends to focus on explaining it to herself/himself with the future less of a biopsychosocial support, s/he will never be really ready for a transformation, but only for an internal oscillation to the preceding point of equilibrium identifiable with the point *from*.

Therefore, as early as the first meeting, the MPP offers a method that, focusing on the relationship between object representations and experiences of the here-and-now, confronts the patient with the precariousness of the equilibrium reached with her/his own psychic functioning, crumbling under the action of a change.

In the Mutative Initiative Interpretation addressed by Gillièron in the IPB (Investigazione Psicodinamica Breve – Brief Psychodynamic Investigation), which is already at the end of the first meeting in the MPP, th e therapist starts the transfer *from . . . to*, proposing herself/himself as a subject initially attuned to the support on the object the patient desires and then reporting to the patient not only countertransference experiences and their development displayed as personalized and hypothetical observations with regard to the relational past, but much more besides. Thus the therapist proposes to the other subject of the relationship, i.e. the patient, to transform the relationship patterns acted out perpetually in ways thought of as defensive in order to not completely see the visible, demonstrating to her/him how misleading it can be to consider the image that one has constructed of oneself to be protective. A transforming moment certainly consists in demonstrating to the patient that the act of seeing clearly or of reaching a hyperconscious state with regard to what one has tried to not see for a lifetime, is the only chance to no longer oscillate internally around the same point of "equilibrium", "*from*", but to achieve a real transforming transfer *from . . . to*.

The transformation can therefore be speeded up on just one condition, i.e. that the therapist fully enters into it, not only in the sense of going along with any investment made by the patient but also any transfer of elements of the preconscious of these to one's own Self and from one form/representation to another of a different approach.

Each time that a person enters into a deep relationship with someone else – and the psychotherapeutic relationship set up as psychoanalysis is certainly this – s/he knows that there will be a transformation within herself/himself in what s/he believes of herself/himself *from . . . to*, with inevitable consequences also regarding behaviours going from less functional to more functional.

In order for the therapeutic relationship to become a means of transformation, the therapist needs to be inspired by a mental functioning model of the genital type; therefore significant representations are constructed of the hoped-for change for the patient and focused interpretative actions put in place, and not only that. *[P. Petrini, A. Mandese, A. Casadei]*

MYSTICAL

According to Bion, the apprehension of truths beyond understanding. Everything goes beyond what we see or understand with our senses. There is an underlying ultimate reality or truth, independent of us which we cannot know but which we can have experiences of being at one with – Bion's "O", also named the infinite, Godhead, infinity, the psychoanalytic object or group. The importance of O is that, for mental growth to occur, there have to be experiences of being at one with it. It is not enough to understand new facts about ourselves, we have to become ourselves. It is the difference between knowing about psychoanalysis and being psychoanalyzed. The mystic is one who can apprehend or experience ultimate reality directly and bring this experience to the institution to which he belongs. *[J. Symington]*

REFERENCES. Bion W.R., *Transformations*, 1965; Bion W.R., *Attention and interpretation* 1970.

MYTH

In anthropology, it is the common attitude of several individuals that defines the collective consciousness of a specific culture. The term derives from the Greek word *mythos* ("word", "news"). It was subsequently conjugated with *logos* ("narrative") and it acquired the character of fabulation and legend (mythology). The narrative of myths often expresses sacredness and their protagonists are gods and heroes, anthropomorphic, immortals and omnipotent supernatural beings. The supernatural world described by myths comes from the need to give a causal explanation and a logical sense to the unintelligible or inconsistent events of reality. A myth conveys knowledge through sentiment by means of analogic language, therefore a story can become truth and vice versa. People are able to decode it subjectively and intuitively. The need of mystique participation, typical of primitive thinking, would be at the basis of myths. This type of thinking does not distinguish between real and imaginary worlds; therefore the existence of the supernatural is not deduced but given. Myths are transcultural and the existence of similar myths in different cultures could be due to the fact that sensations, perceptions, thoughts and needs of man shape similar images in → experience. The tense of a narrative is the past, the "once upon a time", but it evokes feelings that involve present and future. In sociology, myths would be the retrospective justification of group life; they feed the cultural force and regenerate themselves continuously in every historical change. This process consists of precedents, moral rules and sanctions: all elements common to religions and societies. In → phenomenology, myths have the features of historic events and of ahistorical exemplary models. S. Freud talks about myths as a projection of the contents of the unconscious. According to Jung, myths are an expression of an atemporal structure of the unconscious, which does not have to be explained but understood. The concept of myth does not distinguish between word and being, as myths border on the state of dreams and not on that of reality; myths does not require nor include demonstration of the truth. As stated by G.B. Vico, myths have no wisdom to reveal, they express their conception in primitive humanity and belong to the emotional and sentimental world. Myths are full of subjectivity that becomes illusory objectivity, an immediate reality that calls into question what reality itself is. If a subjective psychological reality is shared by multiple individuals who have the same attitude, that reality is objectified and becomes a reality within a system of beliefs (→ logic of belief). It becomes a logical model that can be used to resolve contradictions (→ logic of contradiction) and a semantic frame for individual, family and collective schemes. For this reason, the concept of myth can be crystallized by placing a person in a narrative pattern that constrains them to the myth of themselves, of their family or to a forced social adjustment (brief strategic therapy, systemic-relational paradigm). This is a concept with a broad-spectrum use for psychoanalysis, which puts it in the psychological and psychotherapeutic dimension of the collective manifestations of human thinking and adds the anthropological dimension through the concept of → archetype. *[R.]*

▷ In classic psychodynamic, myths are the dream of populations and, conversely, dreams are the myth of individuals, a middle ground between normal and pathological psychology. According to Jung and his followers – Neumann and Hillman above all the images of the deeper unconscious have a clear mythical character and they point to an encounter with the archetype. Through the myth, the psyche generates a discourse of itself. It shows itself both psychopathologically – therefore Jung can state that gods have returned in the form of diseases, or that Wotan (Odin) prefigures the coming of Nazism – and in relation to the potentialities of individuals, that is, the act of "becoming aware" that he believes is everyone's task. Thus, myths do not only regard the collective sphere, but they penetrate the existence of individuals and even claim, through this way, a radical redefinition of how therapy should be performed. Consequently, Jung speaks of "personal myth" and explains its nature in *Transformations and Symbols of the Libido*, the work that marks its detachment from Freud. Ultimately, myths need to be met, lived and removed from their mere coercive happening, from their being a metaphor of eternal, unconscious archetypal returns. *[G. Antonelli]*

REFERENCES. Jung C.G. (1912), *Symbols of transformation*, in *Collected Works*, V, 1967; Neumann E., *The origins and history of consciousness*, 1954.

N

NARCISSISM

In Freud's first theoretical formulation, this term refers to the investment of the libido towards oneself, and deals with all the processes related to the love directed towards one's own image. The concept of narcissism allowed Freud to redefine some forms of pathology in terms of his drive theory, the earliest stages of the development of the psyche, and some problems of a technical-therapeutic nature. Consistently with his → drive theory, from a developmental point of view, the earliest stages of the development of the psyche, in which there is no distinction between external objects of gratification and internal objects of gratification (auto-erotic phase), are followed by a phase in development whereby a distinction starts to be made between the self and the external world and in which the → libido is directed towards oneself (primary narcissism); this is therefore the phase in which the libido may be invested in external objects (object-libido) which can then be redirected to the self (secondary narcissism). The prevalence of the narcissistic investment does not therefore allow the investment of the libido in external objects, and therefore does not allow → transference with the psychoanalyst to be established. For this reason, neuroses are also defined as "transference neurosis", and are treatable by means of the therapeutic relationship, whereas psychoses, initially defined by Freud as being "narcissistic neurosis", are not considered as being treatable through psychoanalysis. Freud also talks about the "choice of narcissistic objects" that are aimed at satisfying the need for validation; therefore, the investment of love towards oneself, through the relationship with an external object that possesses characteristics that have been lost or that are desired by the person. The concept of "narcissistic transference" could therefore at first appear to be a kind of contradiction in terms, but clinical experience showed that these types of patients could establish a kind of transference that was structured in such a way as to exhibit also that need for the validation of the self that we define as narcissism.

As a result of this, some writers have conceived the possibility of the establishment of transference also in those pathologies that Freud had believed to be an unsurmountable obstacle to the establishment of a therapeutic relationship with the therapist. The most prominent exponents of this theory are Kohut and Kernberg.

Kernberg compares normal narcissism, which he describes as being the libidinal investment of the Self, and the foundation on which a healthy degree of self-esteem can develop, to a pathological narcissism, defined as a form of primitive defence mechanism, that acts in conjunction with other, more archaic → defence mechanisms. This leads to the development of a "grandiose self", that is able to express both an attitude of contempt and a tendency toward belittling others, as well as a tendency towards idealization of others, obtained through a projection of their own illusions of grandeur, so that the self does not develop a level of self-esteem that is based on reality, but is an integral part of a defensive process. Kernberg hypothesized that pathological narcissism is, in actual fact, a reaction to feelings of frustration and hatred, and that it is therefore necessary to continuously interpret the defensive purposive of the narcissistic attitudes, which are in reality expressing, within the transference relationship, the painful conflicts from which they have developed.

For Kohut, instead, the development of a healthy sense of self develops from the "experiences of the Self-Object": mirroring Self-Objects, idealized Self-Object and twinship Self-Object (→ Self-object; → Self-object transference); the absence of these kind of experiences results in the establishment, within the therapeutic relationship, of transference that reproduces with the therapist the need for gratification in order to compensate for the lack thereof experienced by the patient; as a result the transference thus formed is based on mirroring, idealization and twinship. The analyst, therefore, does not have to interpret this kind of transference, but has to satisfy the needs that it is expressing, whilst at the same time, clarifying its meaning and therefore allowing the gradual development of a realistic sense of self.

The two points of view express positions that are in some ways symmetrical: for each of them the therapeutic approach of the other is based on a lack of understanding of the psychological needs underlying the excessive narcissistic demands. For Kernberg, the narcissistic pathology is a defensive reaction to archaic sources of anguish and does not express the need to compensate for the absence of gratification; for Kohut, it is the result of a failure in the development of the self that is the result of a lack of gratification for which the therapeutic relationship has to compensate. As is demonstrated by the comparison of these two therapeutic approaches, the therapy for narcissistic pathologies and the understanding of their etiology are amongst the most relevant and controversial topics in the contemporary debate on psychotherapy, and one of the contexts in which the most intense future research will take place. *[P. Cruciani]*

REFERENCES. Freud S., *On narcissism: An introduction*, 1914; Kernberg O.F., *Borderline conditions and pathological narcissism*, 1975; Kohut H., *The analysis of the Self*, 1971.

NARRATIVE THERAPY

The narrative approach is an epistemic position (→ epistemology) according to which people understand their experiences in the form of → stories. In this sense, personal roles and definitions ("male", "depressed", "anorexic", etc.) does not match reified "objects", but rather stories. People confer a meaning on facts and actions through the stories that they tell in their therapy; as they change the stories that have assigned meaning to events, the meanings of those same events will change. From this point of view, it is clear that there is a substantial impossibility of formulating any theory of general validity beyond the patients' individual story, or rather, beyond the specific relationship between a specific patient and his specific therapist. To better understand this position, it is necessary to refer to the psychologist Jerome Bruner, who has identified two parameters to assess whether a certain assumption can be considered "true".

A statement can be considered true when it can be demonstrated as such through objective proofs: in this sense of truth, the reference is to what Bruner defines as paradigmatic thinking, which is the pursuit of formal and mathematical descriptive and explanatory systems. According to the second parameter, a statement can be considered true because it provides the personal impression that it is a story with meaning: because it connects memories into a frame of significance; because it supplies explanations for experiences and feelings; in other words, because it is intimately perceived as plausible. This is truth according to *narrative* thinking. Therefore, the Self is a product of our storytelling and not some kind of essence that we can find by digging through the bottom of subjectivity. Mair even goes to the length of stating that psychology as a whole knows through narration, with a cross-reference from the epistemic perspective to the object of the discipline – cognitive functioning – in accordance with the vision that calls for an internal observer and implies their crucial role in observation. The correspondence between reality and the object of knowledge is a condition of paradigmatic thinking. The mind processes information that is found in the real world and organizes it into a corresponding logical system. Instead, a narrative approach considers that only perturbations exist. The latter are lacking informational and significance content, which are granted in relation to the structure of the person who knows, based on the dissonant details that they observe. It is non-linear, analogic, image-related thinking. The two thinking modalities cannot be reduced to one another, as they are independent from one another and different. This premise has a transversal influence on many psychotherapeutic approaches. In psychoanalysis, it is used by the hermeneutic approach, which dominated Europe and the United States in the 1960s and 1970s. In particular, J. Harbermas and P. Ricoeur facilitated the positioning of psychoanalysis among *Spiritual* Sciences (or Human Sciences) – as opposed to *Natural* Sciences (according to Dilthey's distinction) – given that it does not conform to proof, replication and rebuttal criteria, but is rather characterized as a discipline of significance, to the extent that Hillman states that psychotherapy should not be considered in any relation to medicine, but rather to literature. One of the founders of the approach is psychoanalyst Spence, who suggested that psychoanalysis contained less "consolidated theory" then one could imagine, although Freud did see it as exposing truths in a traditional sense. There are two consequences: one is that the analyst "is busy in an artistic struggle with the patient and with all colleagues"; the other is that findings are to be intended in a situational sense and in relation to their immediate context. The narrative paradigm also influences cognitive psychotherapy with equal force. The works of Guidano, although more strongly related to the constructivism of H. Maturana and F. Varela, show how the narrative plot is connected to the topic of change and human identity. One key point of his elaboration is the vision of a developmental and ontological Self, holder of meanings that emerge through interaction. The significance that is produced in the narrative plot of conversations represents the way the Self organizes its experience.

The evolution of the individual undergoes phases of disorientation: there are events that cause such emotional perturbations that they cannot be integrated into the life story of the individual. Therapy represents the occasion to build a dynamic reorganization, where the therapist is not concerned in providing their own direction, but rather in respecting the peculiarities and knowledge already possessed by the person. The sense of oneself corresponds to the internal coherence of the unique life story; it is a self-aware act of creation of significance, through the encounter between the historic and linguistic dimensions. Experience acquires meaning when it is viewed in a historical perspective. Systemic therapy (in particular the one originating from the Milan School) winds up being notably affected by narrativism, as the therapy itself is an activity of construction and deconstruction of hypotheses. L. Boscolo and G. Cecchin will eventually show great interest in the topics of stories, of metaphors and of construction of reality through language, mindful of the fact that the very same Gregory Bateson had cleared out his idea that human thinking is of a narrative type: men think through stories. In reading the authors who have introduced narrative thinking in systemic and family therapy, one may have the impression that it gave rise to two interpretations: a strictly narrative one that we may define as "rewriting", meaning that it tends to replace narrations that generate suffering with new stories that better adjust to the needs of the individuals; a second one, which could be defined "multiplicative", that considers the possibility of observing and describing reality from multiple perspectives, in order to produce narrations that may be conflicting but can coexist. In this case, therapy is not the frame for building and learning new descriptions of the world that can replace the previous ones: it is rather a context of deutero-learning, that encourages people to construct and deconstruct stories and to pursue a multiple and hypertexted vision of themselves. The connection is clear between narrative and postmodernity in therapy, which is also underlined by the fact that if actual substantiating criteria are no longer the only ones that are used to judge "truths", then the "expert" voice loses its exclusive power, to become a voice among others, alongside "popular psychology" and the client's storytelling. An important chapter of narrative therapy was mainly developed by White, at the Dulwich Centre of Adelaide, Australia: his personal and professional relationship with Epston generated original and prolific theories. Even though White's background is not in family therapy, his narrative approach has dialogued with systemic therapists. White has ruled out any reference to psychiatric categories from his theory, and preferred to engage with the ways dominance-relations in families and groups are defined by master narratives; his reference is the analysis on the relationship between knowledge and power by Michel Foucault. According to White, people reach therapy with a problem-saturated story, a problem-saturated vision of themselves, which becomes a dominant family story. Therapy identifies marginal and neglected aspects of experience, the client's resources and unique outcome, and inserts them into a new story. Reference is to those episodes that are usually considered irrelevant, where the person was stronger than the problem. In his work with encopretic children (children with stool "accidents") for instance, the symptom becomes a grotesque character and the child is invited – through a series of questions on mutual influence – to discover how he can act upon the "little monster" and not only be influenced by it. Such externalization of the problem implies that the problem is not the child (as the shared master narratives by families and school may indicate): the problem is the problem. White is not the only one who explored the political implications of a narrative vision. Mary Olson can be pointed out: in the interview with a fasting woman, she explores the topic of "having a say in the matter" from a feminist point of view; by acting as "external witness", the researcher encourages self-narration, which allows the individual to experiment themselves in their own fullness and not only as an anorexic patient. In a non-clinical setting, Demetrio envisions the use of narrative thinking as *epimeleia heautou* (self-concern, care of the self) in the autobiography. Through memory, individuals recover traces of meaning that can be recomposed into new figures: they therefore reach "re-identification" and confer a new meaning on their own story. It is granted dignity, for the mere fact that it can be narrated. Through narration it acquires the possibility of transforming itself, thanks to a short circuit on the narrative level: the narrator is the leading actor of the story, the past becomes present and it becomes a tool to understand oneself. *[G. Ganda, M. Giuliani]*

REFERENCES. Balbi J., *La mente narrativa*, 2009; Barbetta P., Naclerio R., Benini P., *Ascoltando le voci dell'anoressia. Il ricercatore come testimone esterno*, 2003; Boscolo L., Bertrando P., *Systemic therapy with individuals*, 1996; Bruner J., *Actual mind, possible worlds*, 1986; Id., *The narrative creation of self*, in L.E. Angus, J. McLeod (eds.), *The handbook of narrative and psychotherapy*, 2004; Demetrio D., *Raccontarsi*, 1995; Guidano V.F., *The self in process*, 1991; Hillman J., *Healing fiction*, 1983; Mair M., *Psychology as story telling*, 1988; Migone P., *Terapia psicoanalitica*, 1995; Polkinghorne D.E., Narrative therapy and postmodernism, 2004; Spence D.P., *Narrative and historical truth*, 1982; White M., *Narrative means to therapeutic ends*, 1992.

NARRATIVE TRUTH

In psychoanalysis, it is the truth built during therapeutic sessions, which is expressed as a well-constructed story, able to seize the psychic reality of an experience by considering the coherence, continuity and completeness of accounts as something relevant and meaningful for the process of therapeutic → change, independently from its correspondence with historical elements of the patient's past. Hermeneutical perspective in psychoanalysis, represented for example by Spence's contribution, considers that historical truth cannot be known as such, and anyhow it is less relevant than the narrative truth of an → interpretation or construction. The latter, although it cannot be verified through fragments of the past, assumes a meaningful impact on clinical processes. Therefore, narrative truth is built on therapeutic work and it is an important part of the analytical process. *[A.M. Speranza]*

REFERENCES. Spence D.P., *Narrative and historical truth*, 1982.

NECROPHILIA

According to Fromm, the "love for death" represents a tendency towards loving 'that which is dead', and also "the ultimate answer to life that is the completely opposed to life". The necrophiliac is immersed in his past, is controlling and hates life because he experiences it as chaotic and uncontrollable, he is attracted to obscurity and the night because he wants to return to the "obscurity of the womb", and finally because he perceives strength not as a transitory attitude but as a moment to be experienced. In contrast with → biophilia, necrophilia is believed by Fromm to be a secondary potentiality of human nature, that finds fertile ground in those who have grown in the absence of stimulation, in people who "love death", in environmental conditions that consist of a routine that is lacking in interest and submerged in a mechanical order, characterized by poverty, instead of making of it an environment characterized by economical and psychological abundance. According to Fromm, the absence of even a minimum guaranteed income instils in human beings the fear of dying of hunger, making them dependent on economical blackmail. *[A. Barabuffi, E. Benelli]*

REFERENCES. Fromm E., *The Heart of Man: Its genius for good and evil*, 1964.

NEED

A state of deprivation or deficiency that activates the body, directing it towards the search for an object able to alleviate or eliminate such tension, that can be tangible or intangible, like a pleasant feeling. The concept of need is investigated within the framework of personality psychology by Murray and Maslow. The first, the inventor of "personology", distinguished between "viscerogenic" needs, referred to as organic necessities, and "psychogenic" needs of a purely psychological-motivational nature, whereas Maslow, at the turn of the 1950s, formulated the "hierarchical theory of needs." According to this theory, needs are arranged in a pyramid. At the base of the pyramid lie the physiological needs (hunger, thirst, etc.), followed in order by the needs for security, belonging, love and esteem, and → self-actualization. According to this distribution, people can dedicate themselves to satisfying higher needs only when those at lower levels have been satisfied. Needs can be classified as primary (when their satisfaction is essential for the survival of the individual) and secondary (when their satisfaction improves the standard of living). They can also be defined as: subjective (since they vary from individual to individual); resurgent (when, once satisfied, they tend to arise again in variable degrees); satiable (when their strength and intensity decrease progressively once satisfied); unlimited (according to some authors, the "number" of needs increases in relation to the degree of economic and social development of the environment). In the most recent social theories, they have been also defined as individual needs (when they are experienced by single individuals) or collective needs (when they express the need of more individuals belonging to the same group). It is clear that what leads to the request of therapeutic intervention is the need to move from suffering to → wellbeing or from dissatisfaction to satisfaction. *[R.]*

REFERENCES. Maslow A., *Motivation and personality*, 1954; Murray H.A., *Exploration in personality*, 1938.

NEGATIVE REINFORCEMENT

In the behaviourist paradigm, this can be defined as the elimination of an environmental stimulus that is unpleasant or aversive to the individual; this removal will increase the probability of a future incidence of the associated behaviour. This term, in fact, unites the concept of "reinforcement", which always denotes an increase in the frequency of the behaviour that is activated, with the concept of "negative", which can be at first glance deceiving in that it can lead one to think of something similar to → punishment; this term indicates, however, the loss, or to be precise, the elimination of an environmental stimulus. In fact, if an individual experiences an unpleasant situation (for example a headache) that he is able to eliminate by activating one or more behaviours (for example, by taking a pill), then those same behaviours will be reinforced, with a high probability of their repetition in future when faced with similar situations. *[A. Tamburello, E. De Monte]*

REFERENCES. Hill W.F., *Learning: A survey of psychological interpretations*, 1963; Skinner F.B., *Science and human behavior*, 1953.

NEGATIVE THERAPEUTIC REACTION

A form of psychological → resistance to change in the course of psychoanalytic treatment. This takes place by means of a strong opposition to the analytic process that is experienced as being an ulterior source of suffering. Freud describes this phenomenon for the first time in 1922, attributing the attachment to suffering of the negative therapeutic response to an "unconscious feeling of guilt". In 1924 he proposes the existence of a strong relationship between the negative therapeutic response and "primary masochism" connected to the "cruel" Superego with respect to the Ego. Finally, in 1937, he considers it as being an expression of the death drive. For Rousillon, the negative therapeutic reaction can be tied to the activation in the analytic process of traces that reactivate the anguish without a name of the "primitive agonies" described by Winnicott. *[M. La Scala]*

REFERENCES. Freud S. (1922), *The Ego and the Id*, in *The Standard Edition*, XIX, 1953–1974; Id. (1924), *The economic problem of masochism*, in *The Standard Edition*, XIX, 1953–1974; Id. (1937), *Analysis terminable and interminable*, in *The Standard Edition*, XXIII, 1953–1974; Roussillon R., *Paradoxes et situations limites de la psychoanalyse*, 1991; Winnicott D.W., *Fear of breakdown*, 1964.

NEGATIVE VIEW

A totality of perceptions, emotions and cognitions that provide a negative representation of oneself (→ self-concept) and the world. Negative view indicates a person's subjective way of assimilating and explaining experience, which is reordered in terms of personal meaning. Because of the invariant patterns developed during growth in a person's organization, any negative experience can be referred to by oneself in terms of threat, constraint, loss of control, carelessness and solitude in subjects operating an *inward* focus; alternatively it can be experienced in terms of disapproval, inadequacy, imperfection, and guilt in subjects operating an *outward* focus. Depending on individual adaptive skills, a negative view of life can be observed both in existential physiological depression of the mood (i.e. sadness, pessimism), and in clinical depressive disorders. *[B. Nardi]*

REFERENCES. Guidano V.F., *Complexity of the Self*, 1997; Nardi B., *Costruirsi: Sviluppo e adattamento del sé nella normalità e nella patologia*, 2007.

NEO-BEHAVIOURAL MODEL

The 1930s witnessed the spreading of what is called neo-behaviourism. It encompasses all the behavioural theories that broke away from J.B. Watson's radical and molecular behaviourism. Among the various representatives of this psychological movement, Tolman is undoubtedly the greatest figure, but C.L. Hull, D.O. Hebb and others are worth remembering. Tolman's neo-behavioural model recognized the role of subjectivity and consciousness through the attribution of purpose to the behaviour of the living organism, giving the human mind a more active role in the exploration of the environment and the development of knowledge, unlike Watson's molecular behaviourism, which ignored the contents of the mind and reduced everything to the → stimulus–response relationship. Tolman introduced a new element compared to Watson's reductionism, by which the Watsonian stimulus–response (S–R) relationship is modified with the S–O–R relationship, where the intermediate variable is what happens inside the body (O) and causes a certain response as a reaction to a given stimulus. In fact, the neo-behavioural model refers to the internal states of the individual, as well as to → stimuli and → responses, expressed as objective aspects of behaviour. While accepting the basic principles of classic behaviourism, i.e. basing the analysis of the psychic experience not on introspection but on the observation of external reactions, and using experimental work on animals, Tolman highlighted the intentionality of the acting subject. For the first time, the concept of the intervention of cognitive factors that affect the purely environmental stimulus–response relationship was introduced into the behavioural sphere. Through several experimental studies performed on rats using labyrinths, Tolman developed a type of behaviourism, which he called finalized or purposive, in which purpose and cognition are objective aspects of behaviour that are not separable. Laboratory mice placed inside a maze learn to associate a series of stimuli and responses and, by doing so, learn the way out of the maze. According to Watson's hypothesis, by introducing water into the maze, the process would have to start from scratch because the movements for swimming are different from those for running. In fact, Tolman's observations revealed the contrary: the mice swam straight for the exit, guided by a mind map of the shape of the maze, that is, a "cognitive map", not directly observable, but inferred by observing the behaviour itself. This behaviour led Tolman to infer that the mice did not learn specific movements needed to reach a place, but formed cognitive maps, i.e. the memories organized according to the spatial relationships between components of the environment. The concept of cognitive map was a precursor for the development of models on spatial memory and spatial thinking. These experiments led to the development of the theory of latent learning, which describes learning that takes place in the absence of a foreseeable and not immediately observable reward. In his model, Tolman introduced the concept of "purpose", according to which each behaviour is directed to a purpose or → goal-object, and that of → cognition: any behaviour aimed at a goal is "cognitive", as it is supported by cognitive maps. All of these factors, the cognitive map as well as other variables, which fit in the S–R relationship between the stimulus and the response, are defined intervening variables. An intervening variable is a hypothetical construct that is neither real nor measurable, yet still capable of altering the relationship between stimulus and response, and corresponds to internal processes that connect the "initial stimulus" situation with the observable response. It can be simply inferred from overt behaviour. It is thanks to these internal processes that it is possible to understand the extreme differences in individual responses to identical conditions of stimulation. Tolman identified three categories of intervening variables: need systems, related to the deprivation of a certain physiological state at a given time; the reasons relating to the → beliefs and values that refer to the degree of desirability of certain goal objects and their relative value in gratifying needs; behavioural spaces, which the body is attracted to, if they have a positive value, or rejects, if they have a negative value. An original mind whose thought diverged from radical behaviourism in its heyday, Tolman can be considered a pioneer of the cognitive-behavioural approach and a precursor of cognitive theory. His theory of cognitive maps is still extremely valuable and fruitful. *[G. Lo Savio, G. Papale]*

REFERENCES. Tolman E.C., *Purposive behaviour in animals and men*, 1932; Id., *Cognitive maps in rats and men*, in «Psychological Review», 1948, 55; Id., *Behaviour and psychological man: Essays in motivation and learning*, 1951.

NEO-FUNCTIONALISM → BODILY FUNCTIONALISM

NEOPSYCHE

In transactional analysis, an elaborative system related to the idea–affect analysis of the → here-and-now that manifests itself through the state of the adult Ego (→ Ego-state). It integrates, moment by moment, the experiences coming from the → archeopsyche, from the → exteropsyche and from the → environment, synthesizing a reaction based on the evaluation of the possible consequences. *[F. Guglielmotti, R. Leone Guglielmotti]*

REFERENCES. Berne E., *Transactional analysis in psychotherapy*, 1961; Liverano A., Piermartini B., *Il concetto di Adulto integrante e le sue implicazioni nella relazione terapeutica*, in «Psicologia, Psicoterapia e Salute», 2010, XVI, 1; Tudor K., *The neopsyche: The integrating adult Ego state*, in C. Sills, H. Hargaden (eds.), *Ego states*, 2003.

NEURO-LINGUISTIC PROGRAMMING

Neuro-linguistic programming (NLP) was originally developed in the early 1970s by Richard Bandler, a mathematician, and John Grinder, a linguist. What they had in common were skills in detecting → patterns of behaviour and response, in contrast to content. They originally studied the work of Fritz Perls and Virginia Satir, and a bit later, Milton H. Erickson. The question "What is NLP?" is a bit like asking, "What is Physics?", because there are so many possible ways to answer it. One answer is that NLP is able to accomplish much of what the beginnings of psychology promised a hundred years ago, and never quite delivered – a practical way of understanding our thinking and our behaviour that can be used to make rapid and useful changes in our lives. Another answer is that it is the study of the structure of subjective experience, the inner workings of our minds, and how to use that knowledge to enrich our choices. Much of this structure is typically unconscious, or preconscious. However, much of it can become conscious, altered, and then allowed to become unconscious and automatic again. Someone once described NLP as "cognitive behavioural therapy on steroids" because although it is fundamentally similar in orientation, NLP makes more and finer distinctions and has many specific processes, principles and presuppositions that make → change much faster. Someone once joked that "[t]he human brain is the only self-maintaining, general purpose computer that can be manufactured by unskilled labour." It is also the only computer that is only partially programmed at the factory, and does not come with an operating manual. A child's brain does not have the kinds of programmes that we have as adults, and there are no instructions about the operating system, or how to programme it well.

Although there is still some disagreement about exactly what kind of computer the brain is, it is clear that we: *input* information through our five senses; *process* it in a variety of ways, using our ability to remember, forecast; connect different experiences and generalize about them; and then *output* behaviour and responses – which become additional inputs to be processed, in a never-ending cybernetic process. Since we have no operating manual – and no keyboard or mouse – each of us essentially had to programme ourselves, with some help from our parents and others. Despite their best efforts, much of our programming was somewhat random, and was often the result of accidental events, some supportive and some traumatic. Much of our programming operates reasonably well, while other parts usually don't work well at all. So another definition of NLP is that it is an operating manual for the human brain, providing "software for wetware", which can be used to reprogramme ourselves when we are less than fully satisfied with our responses. Every discipline has three aspects: technology, methodology and epistemology.

TECHNOLOGY. NLP has a large number of different specific patterns: sets of instructions that can be used to help people reach specific outcomes. It does this by making changes in our experience – in our perceptions, our thinking, our actions and our feeling responses to events. Psychotherapeutic applications include how to transform unpleasant feelings, change unwanted habits such as smoking, overeating or nail-biting, how to cure phobias, fears and anxieties, resolve grief, shame, guilt and other internal conflicts, eliminate addictions, compulsions, PTSD, etc.

METHODOLOGY. NLP has a coherent set of ideas or understandings that can be used to understand the wide-ranging applications of the technology. One basic understanding in NLP is that *all* our experience consists of either sensory-based experience in the moment, or internal representations of sensory-based experience that are remembered from the past or forecast into the future. We can only know the world indirectly, through the *representations* of the world that we build out of what we receive through our senses. These representations will always include one or more of the following five sense modalities: *visual* images, *auditory* sounds, *kinaesthetic* feelings, *olfactory* smells and *gustatory* tastes. Most of our thinking and responding is some combination of the three major sense modalities – visual, auditory and kinaesthetic. These sensory modalities are the building blocks, or the "atoms", of *all* our experience. Even our most abstract words and conceptualizations are composed of some combination of images, sounds or feelings. These different modalities can be combined simultaneously in a moment in time, or they can be combined in a sequence, rather like a linear computer programme, in which, for instance, an image of a goal is followed by some words suggesting what to do to reach it, followed by a feeling of certainty in response to those sounds. We can rearrange these "atoms" of experience in order to resolve problems, and reach the outcomes that we want.

A further development of NLP methodology is the realization that each of the primary sensory modalities can be subdivided into smaller parameters or elements, called *submodalities*, each of which can also be changed to alter our experience. If modalities are the "atoms" of our experience, submodalities are the "subatomic particles" of experience that alter the properties of the atoms of experience. For instance, a *visual* image can vary in distance from the observer, location in space and size. It can be flat (2-D) or 3-D (holographic), framed or panoramic, bright or dim, moving or still, colour or black-and-white. You can be *inside* a memory as if an event were happening again, or you can see it as if you are an *outside* observer watching someone else experience that event; the same is true of your images of the future – you can be in them, or you can see yourself in them. A visual memory that is a large, close, 3-D, colour panoramic movie will be much more emotionally impactful than one that is a small, distant, two-dimensional, framed, black-and-white still photograph. You can easily confirm this in your own experience by representing the same memory in those two different ways. An *auditory* sound can also vary in distance from the listener, location in physical space and loudness. It can be monaural or stereo, vary widely in tempo, tone, timbre and frequency range, and you can hear it by being inside that panoramic experience, or being *outside* it, as if you were hearing it coming from a tape recorder or CD player. A sound that is loud, close, full and panoramic will be much more emotionally impactful than one that is faint, distant and coming from a point source. Again you can easily verify this in your experience by recalling a piece of music in both ways, and notice the difference. A *kinaesthetic* feeling can vary in intensity, duration and location. It can vary in temperature, pressure, texture and extent. It can be still or moving – spreading from one location to another. It can be a surface, tactile feeling or an inner, emotional feeling. A remembered feeling that is intense, moving and involving the whole body will be much more impactful than one that is weak, still and involves only a very small part of your body. Modalities offer three alternative ways to represent experience, offering choice. Submodalities offer hundreds of different alternatives, which can be combined in various ways to create hundreds of thousands of alternatives, for even more choice.

APPLYING THE METHODOLOGY OF SUBMODALITIES TO TECHNOLOGY. Someone who has a phobia – or any other trauma, abuse, PTSD flashback, etc. – remembers a terrible experience by being *inside* it, as if they were experiencing it all over again. As a result, they have all the awful feelings that they had in the original experience. Others, who have had equally horrible experiences, can recall them comfortably because they see them as an observer watching a movie on a movie screen, as if it were happening to someone else. Since they are *outside* the experience, they don't have any of the feelings of being *inside* it. Either they feel neutral, or they have the feelings that a compassionate *observer* might have. It is easy to teach someone with a phobia to take their memories of a terrible event and project them onto a movie screen, so that they can respond to them neutrally – totally independent of content.

The structure of grief is exactly the *reverse* of a phobia or trauma. In a phobia, someone remembers a *horrible* experience by being *inside* it, so they have all the awful feelings again. In grief, someone remembers a *wonderful* experience by being *outside* it, so they can't feel the treasured feelings that they previously had with the dead person, leaving them with only an empty feeling. Since the structure of grief is the reverse of a phobia, the resolution for grief is also the reverse – to remember being with the dead person by being *inside* their special memories of them, so that they can easily re-experience all the good feelings that they once had with them.

Epistemology is how we know what we know, a way of deciding what evidence to use to determine what is true or valid as we test both the technology and methodology. The epistemology of NLP is fundamentally the same as that of all science. We discover what is true through experimentation and testing. Every pattern or method in NLP includes ways to test whether each step has been successful or not, using nonverbal response from the client as the primary feedback, along with verbal report. Most of NLP has been tested "clinically" in the experience of those who have made changes in their lives, but has not been tested well in rigorously controlled experiments – which is true of most therapies. *[S. Andreas]*

REFERENCES. Andreas, C., Andreas S., *Heart of the mind*, 1989. Andreas S., Faulkner, C., *NLP: The new technology of achievement*, 1994.

NEUROPSYCHOLOGICAL COGNITIVE PSYCHOTHERAPY

Theory and practice that brings together scientific contributions of biological and psycho-phenomenological aspects within one single framework. This involves a psychotherapeutic approach whose rationale is based upon an "embodied" and "embedded" vision of the human being and his ways of experiencing. Assuming that the human being is basically "embodied" and "embedded" means being part of the Heideggerian and post-Heideggerian hermeneutic-phenomenological tradition according to which the individual is, above all, a "*dasein*" (being-there) and a "who?", a subject of action and passion, whose ways-of-being cannot be isolated from his bodily dimension, life story or particular existential plan. Having overcome the old diatribe between the dualist and materialist reductionist approaches, this psychotherapeutic model adopts a form of "semantic dualism", a perspective that realizes dialogue between specialized disciplines that, in their own language, "try" to say the same thing, a phenomenon that in reality is single: the ways in which individuals act and feel. Neuropsychology has the responsibility of performing an adequate interdisciplinary translation, with the aim of promoting a complex but coherent biopsychosocial vision of the individual, of his ways of being healthy and ill, as well as appropriate psychotherapeutic treatment. Cognitive psychotherapy makes two assumptions that have animated the story of cognitivism: interdisciplinarity and attention to empirical verifiability. Instead, in regard to the traditions of orthodox cognitivism (standard cognitivism) and in agreement with recent neuroscientific research, the "mentalist" and cogito-centric vision (the mental models) of the human being have been rejected, along with the rigid abstract modelling and categorizing of his ways of being-in the-world. *[D. Liccione]*

REFERENCES. Arciero G., Liccione D., *Vittorio Guidano a dieci anni dalla scomparsa: riflessioni sul passato e sul futuro del post-razionalismo*, in «Quaderni di Psicoterapia Cognitiva», 2009, 25; Jervolino D., *Ricoeur: la fenomenologia della memoria*, in M. Cappuccio, *Neurofenomenologia. Le scienze della mente e la sfida dell'esperienza cosciente*, 2006; Liccione D., *Psicoterapia cognitiva neuropsicologica*, 2011.

NEUROPSYCHOLOGICAL DIAGNOSIS

A diagnostic process that links the presence of lesions, deficits and brain diseases to the functioning of basic psychological processes such as memory, learning, language, attention, recognition, visual-spatial and imaginative abilities, movement. Neuropsychology uses the contribution of various diagnostic interdisciplinary instruments, taken in particular from neurosciences and experimental psychology: bio-image methods (computerized tomography, nuclear magnetic resonance, methods of nuclear medicine), electro-physiologic methods (electroencephalography, myography, etc.), neurological methods based on clinical observation, methods concerning behaviour studies (psychological experimental paradigms about the study of human behaviour; stimuli, measures and study techniques of mental performance; cognitive models of mind functioning). Diagnostic activity aims, then, to the study of neural correlates of mental activity. A careful and preliminary neuropsychological assessment may have important repercussions in leading the psychotherapeutic intervention, as for example for language disorder treatment in developmental age or in case of a humour disorder developed after brain damages caused by ictus or neoplasia. *[R.]*

NEUROSIS

A term coined by W. Cullen in 1769 to describe a psychological disorder caused by a general affliction of the nervous system. This included neurasthenia, (lack of energy), and in more popular terms, a nervous breakdown. At the beginning of the twentieth century, with the advent of psychoanalysis, the term was used to indicate a psychological disorder caused by the unconscious repression of instinctual drives and the failure to overcome the oedipal phase of infantile development (→ Oedipus complex; → libidinal development stages), with a dysfunctional management of its immediate consequences. According to Freudian theory, the origin of every neurosis lies in an unresolved conflict related to the sphere of sexuality; nevertheless, neuroses are interpreted differently and treated differently according to the respective psychological theories and therapeutic models. These were subdivided mainly into phobic neurosis, hysterical neurosis, obsessive neurosis and anxiety-related neurosis. Neurosis is distinguished from → psychosis by means of reality testing, that is, the capacity to keep in touch with reality in accordance with the beliefs and interpretation of the social context in which the person lives. Neurosis translates into more various disorders at a clinical level and the different subcategories depend on the nature of the symptoms; in the most recent psychiatric classification of the *Diagnostic and Statistical Manual of Mental Disorders* (→ diagnostic manuals), this term has been eliminated and disorders that were previously considered as being "neurotic" have presently been redefined and substituted by a different series of clinical frameworks. The old categories of neurosis have in this way been redistributed in new and more accurate diagnostic categories. The term, now obsolete, continues to be used in everyday language to describe an individual exhibiting bizarre behaviour. *[R.]*

NEUTRAL STIMULUS

The behavioural paradigm provides two definitions of neutral stimulus. In the model of operant conditioning (→ behavioural model of operant conditioning) a neutral stimulus for each event (or all events), environment or context, at a given time, has no effect on → behaviour and therefore does not induce any response. Instead, in the model of classical conditioning (→ behavioural model of classical conditioning), a neutral stimulus is any stimulus that, by its nature, does not induce any response, but it can become a → conditioned stimulus. *[A. Pedon].*

REFERENCES. Carlson N.R., Heth C.D., Miller H., Buskist W., Martin G.N., *Psychology the science of behaviour,* 7th ed., 2010.

NEUTRALITY

One of the main principles of psychoanalytic theory that requires the analyst to avoid becoming directly involved in the events recounted by the patient but to listen in a way that is non-directive. It constitutes an important therapeutic factor. This term – which was first used by Freud in his essay *Observations on Transference-Love* in 1915 – outlines an attitude of the analyst that aims at limiting the analyst's reactions related to → countertransference and involvement with the patient, in order to avoid the imposition of one's own moral, religious and social values onto the patient, and in order to ensure that the free associations (→ free associations technique) are not guided by the desires of the analyst but by those of the patient's unconscious. The psychoanalyst should avoid extreme detachment and being emotionally cold, but also avoid getting too involved, with the aim of reducing the distortions that would be introduced in the relationship if the analyst tried to teach and impose values on the patient that are based on his own countertransference and his own personal values.

According to the structural hypothesis (→ topographical model of the mind), neutrality refers to the placing of oneself in a position that is equidistant from the needs of the Id, Ego and Superego. In spite of this, the values of the analyst (especially those regarding the search for truth, for understanding, for knowledge and those oriented towards change and growth) are always operative and influence the therapeutic process as a sort of guideline. Freud's assertions on this topic are rather ambiguous: in some cases, he advises the adoption of an attitude that is emotionally cold; in others, an attitude of empathic understanding or the attitude of a constructive ally. In fact, these concepts would later evolve into other notions: → empathy and → therapeutic alliance. From a historical point of view, one finds that the very idea of the possible existence of "neutrality" had already been superseded by the philosophy of science as early as the 1920s and then, progressively, also by psychoanalysis. The notion of a cognitive and clinical strategy was then introduced "as if" neutrality was possible. It is therefore a fiction that is integrated into psychoanalytic theory rather than a state that is truly achievable. For clinicians who believe in → interpretation, in → insight, in object relations or those of the → Self-object, the therapeutic alliance as a therapeutic factor typical of and specific to psychoanalysis (factors that contribute to therapeutic change), the concept of psychoanalytic neutrality assumes the value of a heuristic attitude. *[S. Sagliaschi, M. Casonato]*

▷ Within the Milan School of Psychotherapy, the family therapist aims at achieving an equal relational distance from each member of the → family. The therapist must neutralize every attempt made by a member of the family to establish a privileged relationship with him; although this remains a fundamental tenet of the therapy, it is justifiably disputed as a therapeutic philosophy when working with families where there are clear injustices and acts of violence. In addition, this concept advocates for a therapeutic relationship that is too disengaged; at present, one aspires more to a therapeutic attitude of benevolent intensity when taking charge of plural and parallel relationships in family therapy, as advocated by Selvini Palazzoli in an article that has been cited for many years in the international literature of systemic therapy. *[M. Selvini]*

REFERENCES. Freud S. (1911–1913), *Further recommendations on the technique of psychoanalysis I,* in *The Standard Edition,* XII, 1953–1974; Id. (1938), *An outline of psycho-analysis,* in *The Standard Edition,* XXIII, 1953–1974; Selvini-Palazzoli M., Boscolo L., Cecchin G., Prata G., *Hypothesizing-circularity-neutrality: Three guidelines for the conductor of the session,* in «Family process», 1980, 19(1).

NEUTRALIZATION

In Ego psychology, the process by means of which libidinal and aggressive drives are transformed from being instinctual to being non-instinctual. The neutralization of aggressiveness is particularly important because it gives man the possibility of overcoming the tragic choice between destroying himself and destroying the object. It is useful to hypothesize different phases or degrees of neutralization, stages of transition between drive energy and neutralized energy. One can also theorize that the optimal functioning of the different activities of the Ego depends on different modalities and degrees of neutralization. The degree of the neutralization seems to be correlated to the stages of transition in the attempt to substitute primary processes with secondary processes. Neutralization is a process that is more or less permanent. Finally, according to Hartmann, one can define

> neutralization as being the transformation of energy, both libidinal and aggressive, by means of which it is able to distance itself from instinctual form and become more non-instinctual in mode. The process of neutralization is fundamental to what we call sublimation.

Later on, Hartmann writes that

> situations from which the process of neutralization originates or the genetic determinants of its contents, or the mechanisms that are in the majority of cases connected with it, have not always been clearly isolated from the process in itself, a carelessness that has frequently produced ambiguity

[L. Longhin]

REFERENCES. Hartmann H., *Essays on Ego psychology*, 1947.

NON-ADAPTIVE THOUGHTS

Thought, when it is formulated as a "rule", (for example: when . . ., then . . .), can substitute direct learning experiences in regulating and in managing behaviour (both motor and emotional). It is however "maladaptive" if it controls dysfunctional behaviour or behaviour that causes emotional suffering, in spite of the direct experience that it is replacing. Non-adaptive thought is reinforced (→ reinforcement) and maintained, not by being realistic or rational, but by the fact that it is socially accepted by the individual's cultural environment. In functional analytic psychotherapy, the intervention changes the function of thoughts without needing to reject their content; analogously, in Acceptance and Commitment Therapy the technique of "de-literalization" – a specific verbal technique – the individual is taught how to perceive his own thoughts as being just that, and not as the cause of his behaviour. *[R. Mosticoni]*

REFERENCES. Hayes S.C., Strosahl K.D., Wilson K.G., *Acceptance and Commitment therapy: An experiential approach to behaviour change*, 1999; Kohlenberg R.J., Tsai M., *Functional analytic psychotherapy: Creating intense and curative therapeutic relationships*, 1991; Schlinger H.D., Blakely E., *Rules: Function-altering contingency-specifying stimuli*, in «The Behaviour Analyst», 1987, 10.

NORM

Psychology correlates the process of internalizations of norms according to the way in which a person perceives and re-elaborates his/her social context, creating criteria to predict another's behaviour. Using a statistical meaning, "normal" is the behaviour that the majority of people adopt (Gaussian curve). An abstract model is defined on the basis of a valuable criterion (ethical, social, juridical) that considers everything that approaches this model within certain qualitative and quantitative limits as normal.

Normality, like → deviance, is affected by semantic modifications, such as those caused by change of habit, society, political and territorial contexts. However there are ambiguous bordering territories, where norm and deviance are confused and superimposed. Indeed, as Bergeret states:

> The person that does well is the person that has conflicting fixations within that prompt him/her to become a sick person like many others, but who hasn't found difficulties concerning his/her discretion of defence and adaptation and who can flexibly modify their instinctual needs, primary and secondary processes, in a personal and social context, taking into account the reality.

If the norm coincides with the ability to evaluate reality with others, to side with a common convergent opinion, then this is of no significant value, but the result of a convention shared on a social level. *[P. Meringolo, M. Chiodini]*

REFERENCES. Amerio O., *Fondamenti teorici di psicologia sociale*, 1973; Bergeret J., *La personnalité normale et pathologique*, 1974.

NORMALITY → NORM

NOSOGRAPHY → NOSOLOGY

NOSOLOGY

In medicine, the study of the classification of the different forms of disease. The term nosology in the stricter sense of the word refers to the logic of classification used to arrive at a description, or nosography, of the pathological entity being dealt with. The two terms are frequently used as synonyms of diagnostic classification. Applied to psychotherapy, the nosological approach is affected negatively by its profoundly medical and psychiatric approach, according to which it is desirable to operate a distinction between the various forms of afflictions in discrete diagnostic categories similar to those used to describe forms of illness in medicine. The application of a nosographic approach to psychotherapy also hides a second etiological assumption, according to which, every nosographic entity should have a corresponding organic – neurobiological and neurochemical – framework of reference, analogous to the medical anatomical–pathological model of disease. Typical examples of the nosographic approach in psychotherapy are the psychiatric classifications of mental illnesses, of which the best-known at a global level is that produced by the American Psychiatric Association (APA) with the publication of the *Diagnostic and Statistical Manual of Mental Disorders* (DSM), published in 2000 in its fourth edition Text Revision (TR). Other well-known → diagnostic manuals are that of the World Health Organization and that of the Chinese Society of Psychiatry, published both in Chinese and English, which, in terms of distribution and demographic importance is acquiring an increasing recognition at an international level. In the field of psychotherapy, a dimensional and functional approach, in which psychological suffering is conceptualized not as a category of what is healthy and what is not healthy (disease), but as an expression of a dysfunctional → adaptation (→ functional balance) within the life context of the individual, has been historically preferred to the nosographic-descriptive approach.

The impossibility of psychiatric research translating into reality the hypothesized correspondence between symptom and anatomy has led psychiatric nosography to develop classification criteria that are increasingly detailed and multi-dimensional, which, however, have rendered even more artificial and conventional the symptomatological frameworks that it is proposing. *[R.]*

NOT-KNOWING

In narrative psychotherapy, H. Anderson considers the "not-knowing" attitude to be the root of any psychotherapy. The therapist, freed from the role of expert and from any prejudice that might forcefully frame the patient's story within a rigidly prearranged matrix, will be able to ask questions inspired by pure "curiosity": this will enable the development of peer conversation capable of inducing therapeutic → changes in the patient. *[G. Manfrida, E. Giachi]*.

REFERENCES. Anderson H., Goolishian H., *The client is the expert: A not-knowing approach to therapy*. In. S. McNamee, J.K. Gergen (eds.), *Social construction and the therapeutic process*, 1992; Cecchin G., *Revisione dei concetti di Ipotizzazione, Circolarità, Neutralità: un Invito alla Curiosità*, 1988, 5.

NOT-ME → GOOD-ME - BAD ME - NOT-ME

NOVEL OF THE TRAUMA TECHNIQUE

In the field of → brief strategic therapy Nardone model, a therapeutic → prescription for the treatment of post-traumatic stress disorder. The therapist asks the patient to write down the story, in as detailed a manner as possible and to do so on a daily basis, in which he has to include all the memories of the trauma he has experienced: images, feelings, reminiscences and thoughts. Every day, the patient will have to go through those terrible events experienced through writing, until he feels that he has written down everything that there is to say. Once written down, he will avoid rereading what he has written, put it into an envelope and in the next session, give all that he has written to the therapist. By means of this instruction, some important effects are obtained. First of all, the patient is guided to externalize all the memories, images, the flashbacks that are continuously assailing him, transfering them onto paper and, in this way, gradually freeing himself from them. The fact that he has to go over the trauma on a daily basis triggers a sort of "habituation" effect with respect to the traumatic memories, that will be retrieved actively and on a daily basis, and will no longer be experienced as being intrusive and uncontrollable. Over the course of days, the re-experiencing in writing of the tragic events will also allow the patient to gradually acquire distance from the fear, from the pain and from the anger that this has provoked, triggering in this way a fourth important effect, that is, the allocation of the past in the past. The past, reallocated in its proper place, will in this way cease to continually invade the present of the individual and to limit the construction of his future. Lastly, the handing over of the story of his past to the therapist, represents a sort of → rite of passage, of the overcoming of the traumatic event that amplifies in a suggestive manner the effect produced by the carrying out of the therapeutic prescription. The novel of the trauma can be considered to be the principal and distinctive therapeutic manoeuvre of the strategic treatment of post-traumatic stress disorder, and has proved to be extremely effective in producing an initial unblocking between the first and the second session of treatment. *[R. Milanese]*

REFERENCES. Cagnoni F., Milanese R., *Cambiare il passato*, 2009.

NUMINOSUM

It is an obscurity of an unknowable origin and of any later psychic irruption. According to Greek and Latin culture, anthropology (L. Lévy Bruhl, E. Durkheim), history of the religions (R. Otto) and philosophy (A. Schopenhauer, F. Nietzsche), C. G. Jung's idea of the unconscious psyche is near to that of the *numen*. *Numinosum* can be any impersonal force that is superior to the human level. As index of complexity, the *numinosum* works, between normal and pathological states, in rites, myths, dreams, in the transcendent function, in symbols. In oneiric activity, the *numinosum* is above all "the great dream", whose extraordinary intensity can overflow into the subjective psyche, promoting a psychotic state. *Numinosum* goes through images, words, numbers, time, that is, through the basic factors of an individual's passage across the transformative phases of the psychic life, of the → transference, of individuation. *[A. Vitolo]*

REFERENCES. Jung C.G. (1916–1952), *The structure and dynamics of the psyche*, in *Collected Works*, VIII, 1969; Id., (1934–1955), *The Archetypes and the collective unconscious*, 9, I, II, 1959.

O

OBJECT

In psychology and psychotherapy, term that has three different meanings. In the first it designates an individual, or part of an individual who is on the receiving end of an action, in this case in direct contrast to the term → subject, which instead implies the presence of a sense of initiative and freedom. The second meaning of this term is used to refer to a specific field of research or psychological phenomenon that is being experimented upon, observed or being subjected to therapy. The last meaning in which this term is used refers to a goal, an ending or an objective towards which one is aiming; this third meaning acquires direct importance when used in relation to behaviour with a high degree of emotional value, for which the individual is configured as an object with which to establish meaningful psychological relationships. The latter use of this term is frequently used in psychoanalytic theory (→ drive; → object relations; → relational psychoanalysis; → libido; → Self-object). *[R.]*

OBJECT CHOICE

In the triangular scheme of the → Oedipus complex, S. Freud believed that the choice of the love object had to be necessarily heterosexual, and the choice of the gender identification be with the caregiver of the same sex. Nature and culture acted together in determining this outcome. Following the line of reasoning with regard to the object of identification alongside that of the love object, as outlined by J. Benjamin, the possibilities become more diverse and more complex: the outcome of these choices depend on the value of the individual subject and object: an attachment object (heterosexual) can become an object of identification and vice versa. *[S. Panizza]*

OBJECT RELATION → RELATIONAL PSYCHOTHERAPY

OBJECTIFICATION OF A PROBLEM

Within narrative psychotherapy, a technique developed by White aiming at defining a problem before externalizing it and outlining its impact on clients' lives and relationships. People coming to therapy have "problem-saturated stories"; only by distancing themselves from them, may they become authors of their own lives again. The objectification of a problem appears as a "counter-practice" of the normal cultural process of objectification: according to M. Foucault, people, having focused on the normative ideas (the dominant discourse), are urged to adhere to them and to take action to ensure compliance. People are structured as objects, they submit themselves to the rules of organizations, then develop problems that appear subjective and personal to them rather than dictated by the conflict between their freedom and the normativity to which they spontaneously submit. Once the problem has been identified, clients can take steps to redefine their actions. According to White, the description of a problem may evolve in the course of therapy: it can take a more general form (from a sleep problem to a problem of insecurity); it can be of "common sense" rather than specialist (from a person with schizophrenia to a person "without direction"); and it can be shared with the members of the system to cooperate to counter its effects. *[G. Ganda]*

REFERENCES. White M., *La terapia come narrazione*, 1992.

OBSERVATION

The process of visual acquisition of knowledge regarding a given → object or phenomenon. Experimental psychology and clinical psychology have taken behaviour in all its various aspects as their object of study (behaviour, perception, physical movement, communication, nonverbal behaviour, etc.), as an observable manifestation of the underlying psychological processes. According to this perspective, by means of a systematic process of collection of data, one can find patterns in every type of behaviour (→ empiricism). In this sense, observation can be considered to be a method within a continuum that goes from the qualitative analysis of phenomenon to their quantitative measurement, according to the degree of structure in the clinical or experimental → setting. The laboratory observation, both clinical and experimental, is characterized by the presence of a highly structured setting, by the control of the variables being studied. Vice versa, the naturalistic observation is characterized by a lesser degree of control over the independent variables, that is, a lesser degree of manipulation by the clinician/experimenter. In the clinical field, observation is aimed at the quantification or measurement of symptoms and of behaviours, or at the construction of meaning from the individual's → experiences and life story. *[R.]*

OEDIPUS COMPLEX

A concept developed within the context of Freudian psychoanalysis and inspired by the Greek myth of Oedipus. Oedipus is the mythological character who killed his father and married his mother without knowing their identities. It represents the most famous theme of Freudian psychoanalysis: male children (from 4 to 7 years of age) develop erotic fantasies towards their mother and enter into competition with their father. Conscious of their own inadequacy and fearing the father's punishment (→ castration) they renounce the mother as sexual object, they identify themselves with the father and develop the → Superego. The Oedipus complex is a speculation that replaces the real → trauma of incest with a fantasy. To make this theoretical advance possible, Freud was obliged to "discover" infantile sexuality and to claim that the unconscious is unable to differentiate reality from fantasy. Further theoretical formulations gave more importance to castration anxiety (up to making castration a concrete event in the so-called "primitive horde"), to traumas taking place in the pre-oedipal stages of the formation of libido (oral, anal, phallic) and to possible maternal pathologies. M. Klein appeared to overcome all the theoretical controversies by introducing the concept of the death instinct; a positive quality ascribed to libidinal energy followed this theoretical innovation, while the neurosis-inducing function of the Oedipus complex lost importance (→ libidinal development stages). *[G. Fossi]*

REFERENCES. Freud S. (1886–1889), *Extracts from the Fliess papers*, 1950; Id. (1900), *The interpretation of dreams*, in *The Standard Edition*, IV–V, 1953–1974.

OK-NESS

A term (composed of *ok* and of the suffix *-ness*) which has contributed to transactional analysis becoming popularly widespread. It refers to the potential presence in each human being of an availability for authentic relationships, based on respect for the other. This can be understood by an accepted, popularized explanation, introduced by T. Harris, with his → existential positions, but above all, as the most profound expression of the humanistic philosophy of Berne's vision. OK-ness is availability to grow with others through → transactions and the exchange of → strokes, which derives from these. It is not to be understood, therefore, as a magical and illusory position of unconditional acceptance by others, but as an acknowledgement of oneself and of others in the common difficulty of living, as autonomy in one's decisions, spontaneity in one's emotional life, intimacy in the sharing of one's internal world with the other. OK-ness presents as a potential seed at the birth of each individual, it becomes modulated with balance in a welcoming and protective paternal environment, but also debased and distorted in a neurotic environment: the consequence of the latter is the → script of the adult individual, in which the person loses faith in his own OK-ness and that of others. The profound aim of transactional analysis (non-medicalized psychotherapy) is to favour the recovery of the patient's lost capacity of OK-ness, in a realistic opening of his world towards that of others. [*M. Novellino*]

REFERENCES. Berne E., *"Hello!" . . . and then what?*, 1972; Novellino M., *Seminari clinici. La cassetta degli attrezzi dell'analista transazionale*, 2010.

OMNIPOTENCE → DEFENCE MECHANISMS

ONESIDENESS

In analytical psychology, the tendency to exclude or inhibit contrasting contents with the conscious attitude of the → Ego. The directionality of consciousness, Jung writes, is an important achievement of civilization, culminating in the ability to discriminate → opposites. Normally the one-sidedness of consciousness is compensated by the fact that the inhibited or excluded psychic elements continue to be present in the unconscious, maintaining their "energy charge", so that the dialogue between the Ego and the → unconscious remains open and allows the changes that are necessary to the flow of life. The risk is that this process becomes so rigid as to generate a sharp division between opposites, a real disjunctive operation, judging just one of them as valid or "true". It follows that not only no "otherness" can get into this monotheistic building, but also that the individual's basic needs are threatened by the exclusion of the many aspects of → personality. The pathological event that follows can manifest itself in a → neurosis, where the conflict presents itself as violent, as in a → psychosis, where the energy-charge accumulated in the unconscious ends up overwhelming the consciousness, or even in certain → borderline situations, where the two extremes of the conflict appear alternately, from one to the other, but with no relationship between them. The aim of treatment is to restore the → compensation. *[A. Benvenuti]*

REFERENCES. Jung C.G. (1917–1943), *On the psychology of the unconscious*, in *Collected Works*, VII, 1982–1993; Id. (1947–1954), *On the nature of the psyche*, in *Collected Works*, VIII, 1969.

OPERANT CONDITIONING

Within the behaviourist model, it refers to the investigation of an experimentally replicable aspect of the → learning process, where a class of behaviours is selected based on their consequences. Operant conditioning, also known as instrumental conditioning, is the analysis model of learning developed by B. Skinner: behaviour is shaped by the consequences produced by behaviour itself in terms of → reinforcement or → punishment of a spontaneous response (as opposed to an elicited response as in the → behavioural model of classical conditioning). Any behavioural change can be modified or lost, it can be generalized to new situations or placed under the control of special events: that is, it can be subjected to the processes of extinction, discrimination and generalization. *[P. Moderato]*

REFERENCES. Moderato P., *Interazioni umane*, 2005; Skinner F.B., *Science and human bevavior*, 1953.

OPERATIVE DIAGNOSIS

In the context of the strategic models, a diagnostic method that focuses on how a problem works and how it dynamically maintains itself in the present. As with → diagnosis-intervention, operative diagnosis stands in contrast to the prevailing descriptive-categorical diagnostic method (→ psychological diagnosis; → psychiatric diagnosis), which focuses on the description of symptoms and their placement into categories based on symptom similarity. The typical psychological and psychiatric diagnosis consists of a mere descriptive compilation of symptoms and it does not allow the therapist to obtain any kind of information on "how" to solve the problem presented by the client. Instead, operational diagnosis has not only the advantage of defining the characteristics of the problem that needs to be solved but also the specific treatment goals, since it allows the therapist to identify the mechanisms that keep the problem in the "here-and-now". Therefore, once the problem has been operationally diagnosed, the focus of the intervention will naturally proceed towards the unlocking of the mechanisms of persistence of the problem that was identified through the operational diagnosis process. While the categorical-descriptive diagnosis process is separate from the therapy, operational diagnosis is an integral part of the treatment, as the diagnostic process itself indicates the direction that the treatment should take to unlock the problem. In particular, this type of diagnosis is used by the → brief strategic therapy Nardone's model, where it led to the formulation of effective and efficient treatment protocols for the main psychological disorders. *[C. Hybarger]*

REFERENCES. Nardone G., Portelli C., *Knowing Through Changing*, 2005.

OPPOSITES

Conflicting psychic elements connected by a high-tension dynamic. Although Jung started from a monistic conception of the → libido, he based analytical psychology on relativity and on otherness, and he placed the opposites within this framework Some examples of the composite variety of the opposites are: "directed" and "non-directed" thinking; the typological categories of "introversion" and "extraversion"; the "inferior function" and the "superior function"; "causality" and "acausality" in the field of the psychic timing; the "subjective" and the "objective" level of the interpretation of dreams; the themes of light and shadow, of energy and of entropy. The Jungian idea of a bipolar psyche (consciousness–unconscious, → animus–anima, → *puer–senex*) enlightens the *coincidentia oppositorum* and the *coniunctio*, which are the prominent levels of the opposites. Both create a psychic harmony, where the process and the goal are a valid metaphor of the analytical work. *[A. Vitolo]*

REFERENCES. Jung C.G. (1944), *Psychology and alchemy*, in *Collected Works*, XII, 1968; Jung C.G., *Mysterium coniunctionis*, in *Collected Works*, XIV, 1970.

ORDEAL

In strategic family therapy, a strategy (→ therapeutic strategy) developed by the therapist to generate a situation where the cost of maintaining the symptom is more than the benefit of the symptom itself. To this purpose, in the presence of the symptom, the patient is asked to implement an unpleasant or even hated behavior which, however, could entail gains, especially in interpersonal relationships.

Haley first provided an account of the theoretical basis of this technique, illustrating how it builds on the work of M.H. Erikson. This therapeutic strategy is especially useful when applied to a relational and interactive context. For example, every time a spouse puts to use a symptomatic behaviour considered dysfunctional, the ordeal would be to make a gift to the other (action deemed demanding and difficult), or doing housework (action deemed heavy and tough). This prescription implies a sure "win": if the problem occurs, there will be an improvement for what concerns significant relations, since an action useful within a family is performed (even if obtained using unwelcome means for the patient, such as commitment or additional tasks); if the problematic behaviour is blocked, the therapeutic → change will be promoted successfully. *[E. Molinari, F. Pagnini, G. Pietrabissa, G. Castelnuovo]*

REFERENCES. Haley J., *Ordeal therapy: Unusual ways to change behaviour*, 1984.

P

PACING TECHNIQUE

In → neuro-linguistic programming, it is the direct application of the principle of → utilization developed by Erickson, who is considered the greatest clinical hypnotherapist (→ Ericksonian hypnotherapy) of all time. "Pacing" somebody means mirroring some of his or her behaviours on a verbal, paralinguistic, and body-language level. A typical form of verbal pacing consists in using the same "sensorial predicates" (in neuro-linguistic programming these are verbs, adverbs and adjectives) of the interlocutor. If he or she says: "I want to understand this clearly", one could reply: "Let's see if we can clarify it". Regarding body-language, one could adopt the same posture; while on the paralinguistic level, one could imitate his or her voice tone, high or low. It is also possible to verbally pace unperceived behaviour, provided that one speaks in abstract terms, such as: "You are doing/thinking/listening to something". Whereas → therapeutic alliance is directed to the patient's awareness, pacing involves what Erickson defines "unconscious mind" and it is necessary to establish a rapport with the patient, which determines his or her availability to be "led". To be able to pace somebody, it is necessary to be perceptually focused on him or her, while to be able to guide them, it is necessary to adopt a flexible behaviour. *[S. Boschi]*

REFERENCES. Bandler R., Grinder J., *The structure of magic*, 1975; Id., *Neurolinguistic programming: The study of the structure of subjective experience*, 1979; Erickson M.H., *Advanced techniques of hypnosis and therapy*, 1967.

PAIN

An unpleasant physiological-sensory and emotional experience usually associated with harm in our body, which can be in progress or just potential. Pain can also be defined as a sensation of suffering linked to a subjective response in relation to a stimulus or event interpreted as harmful or reducing one's → wellbeing. More specifically, pain is considered as a complex psychosensory phenomenon resulting from the presence of at least two components. The first is a perceptual part (nociception), which represents the sensory modality through which the central nervous system receives and sends potentially harmful stimuli to the body. The second is an experiential part (the subjective experience of pain), which is the psychological state linked to the perception of a sensation experienced as unpleasant. Therefore, the experience of pain is modulated by the emotional and cognitive dimension, from past experiences, from → personality and socio-cultural factors. Pain itself is a physiological reaction, a defence system and alarm, essential for the biological survival of the organism. Pain becomes pathological when, if persisting for a long time, it loses its initial protective role and becomes a disease in itself, up to a point where, in some cases, it becomes a "pain syndrome". In addition to physical pain with a psychological component, there is a pain whose source is exclusively psychological. S. Freud stressed that psychological pain, related to the frustration due to the loss of a beloved object, is essential for the formation of the Ego and personal growth. In psychotherapy, there is no specific treatment for pain, as psychological and physical suffering situations occur in almost all psychopathological conditions. An increasing number of clinical psychological practices support the medical treatment of acute or chronic organic diseases. In these cases, psychotherapy does not heal from pain, but it enables a better management and treatment of issues and experiences related to the situation of pain. *[R.]*

PALO ALTO SCHOOL

A systemic-strategic interactional approach first launched based upon the studies of the MRI (→ Mental Research Institute); subsequently it evolved into a substantially wider concept of psychotherapy as a method based on the → pragmatics of human communication, both as a foundation of the understanding of the origin of pathology and as an instrument for the development and application of therapies (Watzlawick, Nardone, S. de Shazer, C.E. Sluzki, J.C. Coyne, Wittezaele, Garcia, L. Boscolo, G. Cecchin, M. Selvini Palazzoli, H. Stierlin). *[R.]*

REFERENCES. Garcia T., Wittezaele J.J., *À la recherche de l'école de Palo Alto*, 1992; Nardone G., Watzlawick P., *Brief Strategic Therapy*, 2005; Watzlawick P., Beavin J.H., Jackson Don D., *Pragmatics of human communication*, 1967.

Paradigm → Please refer to the "Introduction" and the opening chapter, "The eight paradigms and their respective theoretical-applicative models".

PARADOXICAL CHANGE

In Gestalt therapy, a change that is not mechanically caused, according to a cause–effect relationship, but facilitated by behaviours not directly related to the problem. For example, a contradictory command can lead the interlocutor to behave autonomously, as this would be the only way to avoid satisfying any part of the injunction. Also, describing one's own intrapsychic conflicts, without judging them, could facilitate a spontaneous change and obtain an effect similar to paradoxical communication, in which the person is unable to relate to the usual behavioural parameters. The paradox eliminates mechanical influences and stimulates a change consisting of "becoming what you are". The therapeutic work of Gestalt therapy develops on this fabric: the possibility of operating in this direction is due to the work with the patient on that *limen* or → contact boundary border, whose paradoxical nature (contact as distance–proximity) contains and opens to opposing and connecting forces of one's own existence. To avoid becoming what you "are not", it is necessary to abandon the impersonal preconditions on which one's own need for change are usually based. *[P. Quattrini]*

▷ In → brief strategic therapy – Nardone's model, a paradoxical change is a therapeutic change induced in the patient as a result of a request or a communication by the therapist patently opposite to the patient's expectations of improvement. For example, the request to maintain a symptomatic behaviour or to avoid any voluntary change in the achieved balance (→ symptom prescription; → be spontaneous paradox), may lead the patient to "take position" against the therapist's request and activate personal resources promoting improvements. Or again, the request to recall, rather than dismiss, feelings of fear (→ worst-fantasy technique) or the request to think and focus on ways to worsen one's own condition instead of improving it (→ how-to-worsen technique) can produce the same kind of paradoxical therapeutic effect, bringing, in the first case, the patient to overcome their fears by facing them and, in the second case, to identify and block their own dysfunctional behaviour (→ functional balance). *[A. Bartoletti]*

REFERENCES. Bateson G., *Steps to an ecology of mind: Collected essays in anthropology, psychiatry, evolution, and epistemology*, 1972; Friedlaender S., *Schöpferische Indifferenz*, 1918; Nardone G., Balbi E., *The logic of therapeutic change*, 2015; Quattrini P., *Per una psicoterapia fenomenologico-esistenziale*, 2011; Watzlawick P., Beavin J.H., Jackson Don D., *Pragmatics of human communication*, 1967; Watzlawick P., Weakland J.H., Fisch R., *Change: Principles of problem formation and problem resoultion*, 1974.

PARADOXICAL DIET

An expression coined by Nardone in the context of →brief strategic therapy Nardone's model to indicate a particular type of diet (meant in its original meaning of "lifestyle") based on pleasure and not on forced control. By observing that the majority of diets fail to maintain the achieved results, it was found that the reason for the failure lies in the fact that these are all based on the idea of control, limitation and sacrifice. This makes them sooner or later unbearable, because they heavily interfere with the fundamental feeling on which man's relationship with food is based: pleasure. Paradoxical diet allows people to escape from this trap by putting the feeling of pleasure at the base of the food programme, making it effective and persistent in its balance. This dietary organization is divided into several steps. The first of them, "pleasant fantasies", guides the person to orientate their fantasies in the direction of the most desired foods, evoking the feelings, before choosing what to eat during the day. This is a suggestive self-induction in which food temptations become a possible voluntary choice and no longer a loss of control. The second step is to allow oneself to eat, during the three main meals, only what one likes the most, taking care about all the details of mealtimes to make them as pleasant as possible. By virtue of this, starting from an initial choice of "forbidden" foods, the person discovers that once these are allowed, they are no longer so desirable. In the long run, paradoxical diet becomes a revival of the most natural dispositions towards food. In this way, needs orientate the choices and what pleases coincides with what is healthy. The last essential step of this organization is to integrate physical activity into one's life, also chosen by adopting the criterion of pleasantness. Only in this way will the physical activity make the person experience sensations, emotions and activate thoughts, stimulating the whole psychology of the subject and not just their musculoskeletal system. *[R. Milanese]*

REFERENCES. Nardone G., *La dieta paradossale*, 2007.

PARADOXICAL INTENTION

In logotherapy and existential analysis, psychotherapeutic technique invented in 1929 by Frankl and published in 1939. In relation to → dimensional ontology and to the human capacity of' → self-distancing, it aims to promote a humorous and self-ironic approach towards people, guiding them to desire what they fear and avoid, according to the logic of the → symptom prescription. This technique has proved particularly effective in phobic and obsessive-compulsive disorders, anticipating the use of paradoxes by the cognitive-behavioural approach and by the strategic approach of the Palo Alto School and its systemic-family derivations. *[D. Bellantoni]*

REFERENCES. Bellantoni D., *L'analisi esistenziale di Viktor E. Frank*, 2011; Frankl V.E., *Man's search for meaning: An introduction to logotherapy*, 1946; Id., *The will to meaning*, 2003.

PARANOID–SCHIZOID POSITION

The description Melanie Klein made of the development of the infant in the first year of life distinguishes two modalities of mental functioning and of object relations (originally represented by the maternal breast), defined as being the paranoid– schizoid position and the depressive position. The former, characteristic of the first three months of life, is characterized by the difficulty the infant experiences in tolerating the ambivalence caused by the presence of both libidinal impulses and aggressive impulses together with the experiencing of an intense persecutory anxiety.

The fundamental defence mechanisms utilized by the infant in this phase are the defences of splitting and projective identification. The object (mother, breast) is experienced as being good (→ good object) when the baby experiences feelings of gratification and projection of libidinal impulses; on the other hand, the object is experienced as being bad (→ bad object) in the absence of gratification and the projection of aggressive impulses. This results in the infant perceiving his world as being made up of → partial objects, good and bad. The Ego itself is split and the overall experience of the self and the external world tends to be one of fragmentation.

As the infant develops further (depressive position), he acquires an increasing capacity for perceiving the mother (or the breast) as a whole object, possessing both good characteristics and bad characteristics simultaneously (ambivalence); as the object becomes more integrated, so does the Ego of the child. With the acquisition of a more holistic vision of the mother, who is therefore invested with as much love as it is hate, feelings of depressive anxiety and guilt, connected with the possibility of having damaged, destroyed or lost in an unredeemable manner the object on which he depends, start to emerge.

Although these fundamental modes of functioning characteristically take place in a developmental sequence, the choice of the term "position" and not "phase" or "stage" highlights the characteristic mobility and oscillation from one position to another. Described by Klein as a constellation of relationships, fantasies, anxieties and defences, the two positions not only correspond to developmental phases, but represent conditions that can be present throughout adult life; the positive development of personality is, however, related to the successful passage from the paranoid–schizoid position to the depressive position, and to the degree to which the latter is also overcome.

Bion reconnects to the Kleinian conceptualization of the development of the Self, highlighting the aspect of ubiquity and oscillation from one position to another and referring to this as being a general model of functioning of the mind. With the expression Ps ↔ D, characterized by the substitution of the abbreviations at the ends and the introduction of the double arrow, Bion indicates, in fact, a process of thinking that includes moments of disintegration, fragmentation and chaos, as well as moments of integration, self-awareness and order. In this sense, neither one nor the other of these two positions is preferable; the development of thought is essentially linked to the alternation from one state to another. Therefore, if D represents moments in which it is possible to grasp the connections between different elements, identify an organizing principle (chosen fact) and build an integrated mental representation, Ps corresponds to moments in which the given meanings are questioned in order to discover new ones. *[C. Neri, L. Selvaggi]*

REFERENCES. Bion W.R., *Learning from experience*, 1962; Klein M. (1946), *Notes on some schizoid mechanisms*, in Id., *The writings of Melanie Klein, III*, 1975.

PARENT

In the area of transactional analysis, name given by Berne to one of the three → Ego-states, in particular to that organic entirety of ways of thinking, feeling and behaving that the individual, in the course of development, borrows from the parental figures of reference. These ways lead the subject to face the environment following, unawares, the defensive ways learned, which can be both of a directive value (normative Parent) and a protective one (emotional Parent). These modalities can exist in a constructive comparison with the environment (positive Parent), or otherwise reactivate the → script constructed unconsciously in childhood (negative Parent). Berne hypothesized a biological structure underlying the Parent, called → exteropsyche, seen as an organ with the aim of developing a protective system from primitive impulsiveness. In the individual, the intrapsychic comparison between Parent and → Child leads to a conflict, called *impasse*, where, in the → here-and-now, contrasts between needs for archaeopsychic drives and exteropsychic needs not mediated by the Adult Ego state are reactivated. In contrast to the Freudian → Superego, the Parent is diagnosed in an inductive way and not just in a deductive one. In the undercurrent of transactional psychoanalysis, the Parent is analyzed as an area of parental experiences and images projected in the → transference on the therapist. The latter helps the patient to recognize and to elaborate the ancient images that he tends to project both onto the therapist and onto extra-analytic emotional ties. *[M. Novellino]*

REFERENCES. Berne E., *Transactional Analysis in psychotherapy*, 1961; Novellino M., *Psicoanalisi transazionale*, 2004.

PARENT TRAINING

Model of intervention arising from the field of cognitive-behavioural therapy that views the parents as being agents of primary importance in the relationship with their children and that aims at helping them become more competent and more effective in their affective and educational relationships with them, whether the child is developing normally or abnormally. The Italian model of parent training has a particular interest in the management and sustainability of the interventions, to be carried out in a "naturalistic" environment. *[F. Pergolizzi]*

REFERENCES. Pergolizzi F., *Parenting style come sorgente di interazioni normali e patologiche*, in F. Rovetto, P. Moderato (eds.), *Progetti di intervento psicologico*, 2006.

PARLÊTRE

In the Lacanian vocabulary, this term refers to the talking being, in other words, man. This term indicates the intrinsic inseparability of human nature from → language, based on the hypothesis that language is not a property or a psychological faculty of man acquired in the course of evolution, through experience and memory; rather, language is perceived as being a net into which the human being is permeated, in a fundamental synchronicity, even before being born. Lacan's theory was that it is not man who learns how to talk, but that he is established as being subject to language, or in other words, that it is language that "speaks" to man. *Parlêtre* is a "mode of expression of the unconscious"; it, therefore, defines the position that man, as a being who speaks, takes in his relationship with the dimension of language that, far from being seen as a simple instrument of communication, constitutes a structure on which man depends and by which he is governed. *[S. Guido]*

REFERENCES. Di Ciaccia A., Recalcati M., *Jacques Lacan. Un insegnamento sul sapere dell'inconscio*, 2000; Lacan J. (1953), *The function and field of speech and language in psychoanalysis*, in *Écrits: A selection*, 1977.

PARTIAL OBJECT

In the context of psychoanalysis, a partial object is defined by Abraham as a part of the body representing the whole object. A baby first relates to the breast. The → good breast has all the needed qualities; the bad breast is not available and therefore is depriving. Thus, the good or the bad breast is a partial or part-object representing the mother in a non-ambivalent way (Klein). Similarly, in manic states, the erect penis, standing for the father, is felt to be able to magically repair the damaged mother. Bick says a new mother might relate to her baby in a part-object way, not able to think about him but relying on the baby to make use of her lap, hands and voice as part-objects. Bion emphasizes that the part-object relationship is not with anatomical structures but with the function they represent, not with the breast but with feeding, poisoning, loving, hating. *[J. Symington]*

REFERENCES. Abraham K., *Selected papers on psycho-analysis*, in "International Psychoanalytical Library", 1927; Klein M. (1921–1945), *The writings of Melanie Klein* Vol 1, 1992; Bick, E. *Notes on infant observation in psycho-analytic training*, in «International Journal of psycho analysis», 45, 1964; Bion W.R., *Second thoughts*, 1967; Segal H., *Introduction to the work of Melanie Klein*, 1964.

PASSIVE AGGRESSION → DEFENCE MECHANISMS

PATHOGENIC BELIEFS

They constitute the psychopathology of the patient's reasoning that is addressed as part of the treatment. In the → control-mastery theory, Weiss argues that the patient's problems arise from unconscious pathogenic beliefs (learned in childhood and resulting from traumatic experiences lived in the family context), which adversely affect self-esteem and prevent the achievement of adaptive goals. On the therapeutic path, the patient brings an unconscious plan with him, that he actively pursues in the attempt to test the pathogenic unconscious beliefs in order to disconfirm them. The continuous effort of the patient to translate their childhood experiences into the current context of therapy, finds an answer in the therapist's activity. The therapist's task is to understand the patients' pathogenic beliefs and goals and help them to disconfirm the first and to pursue the latter. The unconscious plan, linked to the patient's life project and oriented towards adaptive purposes, should be supported by the therapist through appropriate interpretations and behaviours for the plan. On the one hand, the unconscious mental activity is aimed at research into safety and mastery in interpersonal relationships. On the other hand, it is able to discriminate between pathogenic beliefs and current favourable experiences in the therapeutic relationship. The essence of mental activity would not be energy discharge, achievement of drive goals or repetition of past experiences, but adaptation to the environment and an active search for new situations that could disconfirm the pathogenic beliefs that make people suffer and that cause them difficulties in human relations. The patient's unconscious plans represent the driving force of the therapeutic process: emotions, motivations, goals and their evaluation become focal points to give meaning to the clinical intervention. The patient's childhood traumas may have different causes and appear in different forms. *Survivor's guilt*: when patients believe they are more privileged by destiny than their parents or their siblings. It may be present during childhood in the "replacement child" that acts as a substitute for a dead or handicapped sibling, etc. Patients will expect a misfortune that could balance their success or they will feel compelled to give something back to others to "balance" fate. *Separation guilt*: this can be typically observed in widowers' children who give up relational experiences and career opportunities to avoid leaving the surviving parent alone. *Omnipotent responsibility guilt*: the patient may have been the victim of a traumatic shock in childhood (mourning, disaster, disease, violence, etc.). In this case the child will tend to experience the event as a punishment for something they did or wanted. This brings the dual implication of feeling guilty or omnipotently responsible or capable of things beyond children's abilities and the idea that something serious, sudden, frightening can happen at any time, so that they must be always ready and alert. *[S. Sagliaschi]*

REFERENCES. Weiss J., *How psychotherapy works: Process and technique*, 1993; Weiss J., Sampson H., *The role of pathogenic beliefs in psychic reality*, 1997; Weiss J., Sampson H., Mount Zion Psychotherapy Research Group, *The psychoanalytic process: Theory, clinical observation, and empirical research*, 1986.

PATHOLOGY

A term used in psychotherapy indicating a situation of psychologically uncomfortable feeling and suffering. The construct of pathology (or psychopathology) represents the complex of the → disorder that the patient wants to alleviate or extinguish. According to the paradigms of reference (see the opening chapter, "The eight paradigms and the respective theoretical-applicative models"), there are different representations and definitions of psychic and behavioural pathologies, some of which have been expressed in diagnostic classifications (→ diagnostic manuals). This meaning of pathology should not be confused with the one used in medicine, which indicates an organic affection and the study of the biological mechanisms that lead to it. The medical concept of pathology has widely influenced psychiatry, but only marginally psychology and psychotherapy, which have kept their own non-reductionist identities (→ reductionism). For example, until 1975, in Italy, there existed, in medical faculties, the teaching of "neuronal and mental diseases clinic", where the organicist concept of mental disease was substantially affirmed. This is due to the fact that psychiatry was considered common to neurology and, practically, it was contaminated by the same diagnostic and therapeutic mechanisms. Still today, the main part of psychopharmacological therapies is given and managed by medical doctors specialised in neurology, with nosological criterion equivalent to diseases of medical and neurological interest. The similarity between mental disease and diabetes is still much used. As in diabetes, the therapy consists in the pharmacological administration of insulin for a person's entire life, so, equally, for mental diseases, is it necessary to administer neurotransmitters, which equilibrate encephalon neurochemistry, for a person's entire life. On the contrary, in psychotherapy, the concept of pathology derives from the etymology of the term, which does not contain any direct link to medicine. It comes from the Greek word *pathos* (an intense sensation that is felt physically and mentally, an upset state of mind, passion, emotion, suffering) and *logos* (speech), and it is referred more to emotive tensions and individual discomfort than to diseases, states that need a psychological and not medical-psychiatric treatment. *[R.]*

PATIENT

The person who is unwell or who has a problem. In therapy, in the majority of cases, the patient is the person who contacts the therapist and who asks for help in order to be able to resolve a problem; but the term "patient" can also refer to a couple, a family or a small group of people (group therapy). Finally, the patient can be a third person (usually a relative, a colleague, a partner) who has a relationship with the individual who contacts the specialist; in these cases one talks of "indirect" therapy, because the objective is that of changing a person who is not directly present in the clinical → setting; this goal is achieved through changing the nature of the relationship of the person who has requested the intervention of the specialist with the person not directly present. Common examples of indirect therapy are situations in which parents ask for help in order to deal with the oppositional and defiant behaviour of their children, or in order to understand better how to behave with their daughters who have an eating disorder. Independently of whether the therapy is direct or indirect, in psychotherapy the person who has directly asked for help is considered as being the patient, because in both cases the aim of the intervention is that of improving the relationship that the individual has with himself and with others, and therefore his or her wellbeing. *[R.]*

PDM

Acronym of the *Psychodynamic Diagnostic Manual,* a manual written in 2006 as a result of the work of a task force composed of the principal international psychoanalytic associations, as well as the collaboration of the American Psychological Association. The PDM represents the first example of a psychodiagnostic manual that organizes the many different theoretical models within the psychodynamic paradigm in a systematic manner. Its structure, unlike that of the medico-psychiatric manuals such as the → DSM and the → ICD-10, is based on the grouping of the different classes of pathology not on the basis of the syndromes (cluster of co-morbid symptoms), but rather on the basis of prototypes: the syndromes described are intended to represent a Gestalt or "ideal type" with which the patients can relate to a greater or lesser degree. The degree of similarity between the prototype of a pathology and the clinical presentation of a patient will indicate the degree to which the patient can be considered as presenting the particular pathology.

The PDM has a multi-axial organization based on three principal axes: personality disorders (axis P), which describes the different organizations of personality based on seven basic functions of personality (identity, object relations, tolerance of affect, impulse and emotional regulation, integration of the Superego, Ego-Ideal and Ideal Ego, reality-testing, Ego strength and resilience); mental functioning (M axis), which evaluates nine specific functions of adaptation; and the subjective experience of the pattern of symptoms (axis S), which reformulates the different syndromes present in Axis 1 of the DSM in terms of the subjective experience of the individual.

A characteristic of the PDM is that of considering the patterns of symptoms not as separate syndromes, but as an expression of the comprehensive structure of the personality of a patient and of the profile of his or her mental functioning, therefore presenting the diagnosis as an integration of the evaluations obtained based on the three axes. Finally, as had already happened in the DSM and ICD-10, the PDM distinguishes between adult disorders, childhood disorders and adolescent disorders. The PDM has, undoubtedly, the advantage of offering for the first time a collection of diagnostic frameworks that can serve as a point of reference for all psychodynamically oriented psychotherapists, providing at the same time some general indications on the therapeutic approaches to be used with patients according to the different types of personality structures. *[A.Bartoletti]*

PERCEPTION

A psychological process that allows the integration and synthesis of sensorial data in emerging forms endowed with meaning. → Sensations can be circumscribed essentially to the (psycho)physical environment since it is mainly connected to the activation of sensorial receptors thanks to a peripheral stimulation. In contrast, perceptions represent a first incursion into a mainly psychological level. This is achieved by transforming and organizing elementary signals into an experience meaningful to the individual. Several theories have contributed to the scientific study of perception. Some theories have suggested an associationist conception of the perceptive action, according to which the identified object is defined inductively (*bottom-up* processing) and corresponds to the sum of the most elementary stimuli. Other theories (e.g. Gestalt psychology) have started to underline the deductive character of perception (*top-down* processing). These latter theories show how the global reorganization of the elements occurs through composition laws that produce forms that are more complex than the mere sum of the single parts. Nowadays, more advanced explanatory models tend to consider the perceptive action as a more articulate process, where the two processes are integrated and interchangeable, instead of opposed and mutually excluding. Most of these models, however, converge in considering perception as a process that gives human experience not only the possibility of registering empirical objects, but also the capacity to build and synthesize a-sensorial "objects". These are reality-free and have a purely ideating origin, as is the case of → illusion, hallucination and delirium. In cognitive and constructivist psychology, the perceptive action is taken on as the process at the basis of meaning construction and attribution. This is a process that evolves as the comparison of two elements that are similar to one another but, simultaneously, different from a third one. Owing to the fact that this process can assume several forms, (psychological) meaning emerges as a distinction of conceptually and socially defined entities rather than simply relying on perceiving concrete elements. Although there can be similarities in the way individuals perceive entities, perception remains an individual and subjective process, as it is the product of senses, mind organization and personal experiences. Thus, the study of perception goes through the idea of the → perceptive-reactive system which, in turn, organizes its perception and reaction of the organism accordingly. In general, the aim of psychotherapy consists in changing dysfunctional perceptions (→ functional balance) of the client. *[R.]*

PERCEPTIVE-REACTIVE SYSTEM

In → brief strategic therapy Nardone's model, a redundant modality of perception and reaction of the individual in relation to reality, that is expressed in the functioning of the three fundamental interdependent types of relationships: the relationship between Self and Self; the relationship between Self and others; and the relationship between Self and the world. According to this perspective, psychological and behavioural disorders are determined by the modalities with which the individual perceives reality, a reality towards which he reacts with dysfunctional behaviour (considered, however, by the individual as being the best possible reaction to the situation). The redundant repetition of the failed attempted solutions of the problem (the so-called → attempted solutions), in fact, instead of leading to the resolution of the problem, tend to actually feed it, determining the formation of a veritable → system that is able to maintain itself and build itself (→ cybernetics, → autopoiesis) between the attempted solutions and the persistence of the problem. This circular dynamic of → feedbacks tends to maintain the stability and the equilibrium of this system, even if it proves to be dysfunctional (→ functional balance) to the individual. In this way, what the brief strategic therapy Nardone's model defines as being a pathological perceptive-reactive system is established, that is expressed in the obstinate perseverance in utilizing a strategy that is apparently productive, or that has functioned in the past in a similar situation, but that in the current situation functions as a reverberator of the problem itself. *[F. Cagnoni]*

REFERENCES. Nardone G., *Suggestione → ristrutturazione = cambiamento*, 1991; Nardone G., Watzlawick P., *The art of change*, 1993; Nardone G., Portelli C., *Knowing through changing*, 2005.

PERCEPTUAL POSITION

In neuro-linguistic programming, a possible allocation of awareness at a sensorial level. Perceptual positions are different points of view, of listening, of tactile perception of the external world and visceral perception of the inner one. Initially, neuro-linguistic programming identified three perceptual positions; a fourth was added later. In the first, awareness is located inside our own body, which allows us to get in touch with our needs and emotions. In the second, awareness is located inside the person with whom we are talking, which allows us to step into his or her shoes. In the third, we can acquire an expanded state of consciousness, which is shared among ourselves and the others who are present in the scene. In some contexts, such as the religious and political ones, using "us" develops a sense of membership. Every perceptual position represents an important source of information about ourselves and other people, even though each of us have the tendency to focus on one and disregard the others. *[S. Boschi]*

REFERENCES. Dilts R., *Modelling with NLP*, 1998.

PERMISSION

One of the milestones of the transactional analysis methodology, which refers to two conceptual levels. On the first level, permission is part of a triad, together with → potency and → protection, and it describes the "presence" that the therapist has to have to help the patient in his effort to leave his → script: in this sense, it refers to the attitude of constant authorization that maintains a strong therapeutic alliance. The second conceptual level is that of a specific "permission transaction", through which the therapist, at specific moments in the course of therapy, supports the patient and "authorizes" him to rebel against a specific → injunction of his script. It needs to be carefully considered that permission is not to be understood as a sort of "parentalization", in which the movement towards the patient's autonomy would be damaged, but, on the contrary, as a constant transmission to the patient of faith in his capacity to recuperate his "healthy" potential. *[M. Novellino]*

REFERENCES. Novellino M., *Psicoanalisi transazionale*, 2004; Id., *Seminari clinici. La cassetta degli attrezzi dell'analista transazionale*, 2010.

PERSISTENCE

The ability of a → system to maintain its equilibrium as a result of interactive modalities that operate within the system or in between the system and the environment. In psychotherapy, persistence is an important concept that refers to those approaches that work on the present and not the past, in that it is what one observes that becomes the system that is the point of reference for the formulation of → therapeutic strategies. Within these theoretical frameworks, the concept of the formation of a pathology over the course of time is replaced by the concept of the persistence of a pathology as an operative diagnostic construct, based on the concept of circular causality (that answers the question: "How does the system work?") that will substitute that of linear causality (that answers the question: "Why does it exist?"). *[R.]*

PERSONA

In the field of analytical psychology, the point of contact between the Ego and society. Jung (1921) wrote: "With the term *persona* I am referring to the attitude towards the exterior, the exterior character, with the term *anima* the attitude towards the interior". This juxtaposition is central to Jungian analytical psychology, according to which all psychological dynamics are governed by the tension between opposite polarities. It is necessary to mediate between → anima and persona, they are two entities that are inseparable: the psychological equilibrium of the individual depends on their interaction or conflict. If the anima is the carrier of all that is related to the interior of the individual, if it constitutes its deepest and most subjective propensity, it can only find its expression in the world by means of the persona, that is, according to modes of functioning that are shared, understood and accepted by the social context of the individual. This term is used with reference to the masks used in ancient Latin comedies – usually having a fixed expression that would render the character of the actor immediately identifiable; "persona" is the term that Jung uses to indicate the recognizability and credibility that are necessary for an individual to be accepted in his relationships with others.

It is necessary to wear a social mask in order to be accepted socially, but conformity and the desire to emerge will lead to the subjugation of the individual characteristics of the anima, so that an individual may have great difficulty in not betraying the multiplicity of his interior world with respect to the judgemental expectations of the collective. Every individual has to resolve the tension between his anima and his persona: from this will result the completion or failure of his process of individuation (→ individuation), that is, the ultimate goal that gives meaning to our existential journey. *[B. Meroni, A.Benvenuti]*

REFERENCES. Jung C.G. (1921), *Psychological types*, in *Collected Works*, VI, 1971; Meroni B., *La maschera inevitabile. Attualità dell'archetipo della maschera*, 2005.

PERSONAL CONSTRUCTS PSYCHOTHERAPY

Application of G.A. Kelly's personal construct theory to psychological disorders and their psychotherapeutic treatment. Elaborated in the 1950s, this psychotherapy is considered to be the first constructivist theory of personality, and it is among the most advanced within the panorama of contemporary therapies definable as constructivist. Personal construct psychotherapy is a complex and rigorous theory, structured in a "fundamental postulate" and eleven corollaries, and based on a philosophical assumption that Kelly defines as "constructive alternativism". Questioning the traditional view – defined as "accumulative fragmentalism" – according to which scientific knowledge evolves through the accumulation of fragments of truths, Kelly assumes that "all of our present interpretations of the universe are subject to revision or replacement". Hence knowledge is an interpretation, a personal construction, not the representation nor, least of all, the mirroring of a given and independent reality; as such, it can always be reconstructed. The roots of personal construct psychotherapy in American pragmatism have been pointed out (particularly Dewey and Mead), and its affinity with European phenomenology has been suggested. Personal construct theory was elaborated by Kelly with a view to its application to psychotherapy, defined as "the psychological reconstruction of life". The assumption from which Kelly chooses to derive all the theory is defined by the fundamental postulate: "a person's processes are psychologically channelized by the ways in which he anticipates events". Therefore, the person is not determined by environmental stimuli, inner drives, or past experiences. Regarded as sets of processes, it is not necessary to suppose motivational forces that set people in motion: they are already "forms of motion", and it is their anticipation of events to give a direction and "canalize" their processes. It is also important to consider that Kelly does not speak of psychological processes, but of "psychologically channelized" processes, where the adverb stands for "from a psychological viewpoint", "according to a psychological interpretation". In fact, consistently with the philosophical assumption of constructive alternativism, the processes are not recognized as endowed with intrinsically psychological (physiological, physical, or chemical, etc.) properties; it is the way in which the events are construed to attribute to them specific properties (and it is this view that has important implications in the conceptualization of emotions). Anticipation is narrowly connected to the personal interpretation of experience deriving from the construction of regularities. Thus, knowledge is supposedly based on bipolar "personal constructs", definable as "a way in which at least two elements are similar and contrast with a third". Personal constructs are part of a system within which they are hierarchically ordered, and any construct is applicable to a certain number of elements among those composing personal experience. The change of knowledge that people have of themselves, of other people and the world consists in a reconstruction (a reinterpretation) of experience, which in turn is constrained (permitted and limited) by the possibility that the new interpretation is assimilated into the constructs at the top of hierarchy. Therefore, the process of knowledge is recursive, any change being inevitably based on existing knowledge (a point of contact with Piaget). Kelly refers to the metaphor of "man as scientist" to explain his view: any person, like a professional scientist, puts forward hypotheses, puts them to the test and revises his or her theories in the light of the outcome. In other words, people act on the basis of the predictions deriving from their theories about themselves, other people and the world, and therefore behaviour (action) has the function of an experiment. It appears particularly easy to substitute this metaphor with the more present one of the "person as storyteller", peculiar to the narrative approaches (in psychology and psychotherapy) of which Kelly is considered a forerunner. In the light of such a perspective, what is a psychological disorder? In fact, the constructivist perspective is not compatible with the idea – peculiar in particular to the rationalist cognitive therapies (Beck, Ellis) – that the disorder corresponds to an error in the structure or the content of personal knowledge. Instead, a disorder is a halt in the continuous process of elaboration of knowledge in a particularly central area of the system: in Kelly's definition, "any personal construction which is used repeatedly in spite of consistent invalidation". The psychotherapeutic process is carried out on two levels at the same time: the level of the therapist's understanding of the client's personal knowledge, and that of the professional construction of such understanding. For a better understanding of their clients, therapists strive to put themselves into their shoes, to see the world through their eyes, thus adopting a "credulous approach" consisting in an attitude of openness and acceptance (that is, the information provided by the clients is presumed to be experientially true). Besides conversation as a means of understanding the client, the clinician can make use of some tools specifically devised by Kelly, such as the repertory grid and self-characterization. The professional construction of such understanding makes inevitable use of constructs (consistent with the epistemological assumption of the theory): the so-called "diagnostic" or "professional constructs", that is, constructs that the clinical psychologist or the psychotherapist can apply to the clients' personal constructs or to particular processes in their construction systems. For instance, the personal constructs leading to unvarying predictions are called "tight", whereas those leading to varying and flexible predictions are said to be "loose"; and still, the "core" constructs are those specifically involved in the conservation of the person's identity and existence, in contrast with those defined as "peripheral. Particularly important in relation to diagnostic purposes are the professional constructs relating to "transition", a term that refers to experiential processes that replace the entities defined as emotions by traditional psychologies. For example, the therapist defines "guilt" not as an entity/emotion that can afflict a person, but the clients' awareness of their dislodgment from the way they believe things to be. In a similar manner, the therapist construes as "threat" what he/she supposes the clients experience as an imminent comprehensive change in their core structures. The use of these professional constructs (and of many more that have been described) is the basis of the diagnostic process. Rather than pigeonholing clients within nosological categories belonging to systems of classification such as the *Diagnostic and Statistical Manual of Mental Disorders* (→ diagnostic manuals), the diagnostic characteristic of personal construct psychotherapy is defined as "transitive diagnosis", that is, aimed at change, and consists in the use of diagnostic dimensions (professional constructs) capable of suggesting the paths of change regarded as viable to the clients, so as to allow them to overcome the block of elaboration implied in the disorder. On the basis of such diagnosis the psychotherapist tries to help clients reconstruct their experience, by means of conversational techniques that can favour the elaboration of the complaint and, starting from that, the elaboration of the construction clients have of themselves, aiming to favour a change in the way they tend to relate to other people. It is actually this "core role" that is implied, in the final analysis, in the psychological disorders of greater clinical importance. This is why particular attention is given to the therapeutic relationship, which in itself can represent the social environment in which the client can experiment alternative relational modalities. After being confined for a long time to an inner circle of specialists, personal construct psychotherapy has spread widely in recent years thanks to the success of constructivist (→ constructivism) and narrative (→ narrative therapy) psychotherapies *[G. Chiari]*

REFERENCES Armezzani M., Grimaldi F., Pezzullo L., *Tecniche costruttiviste per l'indagine della personalità [Constructivist techniques for the investigation of personality]*, 2003; Bannister D., Fransella F., *Inquiring man: The psychology of personal constructs* (3rd ed.), 1986; Butt T., Kelly G., *The psychology of personal constructs*, 2008; Chiari G., Nuzzo M. L., *Psychological constructivisms: A metatheoretical differentiation*, in «Journal of Constructivist Psychology», 1996, 9; Id., *Kelly's philosophy of constructive alternativism*, in F. Fransella (ed.), *International handbook of personal construct psychology*, 2003; Id., *Constructivist psychotherapy: A narrative hermeneutic approach*, 2010; Epting F.R., *Personal construct counselling and psychotherapy*, 1984; Kelly G.A., *The psychology of personal constructs*, 1955, reprinted 1991) ; Mancuso J.C., *Constructionism, personal construct psychology and narrative psychology: Theory & psychology*, 1996, 6. Winter D.A., *Personal construct psychology in clinical practice: Theory, research and applications*, 1992.

PERSONAL EQUATION

A subjective factor interfering with observation and psychological knowledge. Only what one's individuality allows can be known; this already selects and organizes data, according to its own perspective and to its abstractive processes. The expression is borrowed from the German astronomer F. Bessel, who used it to indicate inter-individual differences in the analysis of time based on the observation of stars by different astronomers. Similarly, in psychology, individuals enter into the field of investigation both through their own perspective and through the → archetype that organizes and structures, more or less unconsciously, their specific position. The personal equation needs to be recognized and known by therapists, who has to be aware of their own history, typology, cultural tendencies and their own emotional ups and downs. *[M. Gay]*

REFERENCES. Jung C.G. (1921), *Psychological types*, in *Collected Works*, VI, 1971; Id., (1934–1954), *Archetypes and the collective unconscious*, in *Collected Works*, IX, 1969.

PERSONAL IDENTITY

The problems related to personal identity are part of human history: this is attested to by fragments that take us back to the thought of Parmenides and Heraclitus or by the Platonic dialogues, which take us back to the Socratic "know thyself". The problem of identity has stimulated philosophers' speculations for centuries. However, the problem was tackled in a comprehensive way mainly by English empiricists. In particular, Locke defined identity as a "reflection of the Self" over time. Locke emphasized both mnemonic mechanisms and relationality, which he considered a reflection between "present self" and "past self". Locke's definition is a psychological definition because it is based on the dynamics of psychic life and it is still valid because, nowadays, identity can be defined as an active representation of the self (what individuals thinks of themselves over time), which is implemented to meet the continuous disturbances imposed by changeable external contingencies. This representation develops together with an individual's development, which may be more or less stable and structured or diversified (that is, characterized by multiple roles derived from various belongings) or positive (that is, characterized by a sense of the Self as more or less positive). However, this representation is always dynamic, as personal identity is based on continuous adaptations to face new situations throughout the whole life cycle. These are essential adaptations to prevent malaise and discomfort and sometimes even extreme behaviour. Identity is subject to an uninterrupted dynamism, but if it mutates without maintaining some continuity during changes, unbalances become inevitable. In this case, one's sense of identity can be filled with distress, sadness, depersonalization, panic and depression. Reactions may be more or less severe and vary according to: individual characteristics, the sense of identity that was in place before the environmental triggering events, and the culture of belonging. In fact, in addition to a personal identity there is also a cultural identity, which contributes to shape one's sense of personal identity, which is built during a person's development thanks to the continuous interactions between individuals and their → environment. Personal identity is based on knowledge and on the representation of one's body, a long process that involves the individual from birth and continues throughout the life cycle. Initially, a progressive motor, perceptual and cognitive maturation, enables a gradual differentiation between Self and others. Certainly, this is not an easy path, and this becomes clear starting from the eighth month of life, when children begin to distinguish themselves from others and to give an identity to people. At this age, the disturbance is substantial, as evidenced by the appearance of fear of everything that is new, which is overcome only by an increased cognitive maturity. Around two years of age, the opposition of one's Self to other people's Self enables a greater differentiation, which is expressed through the understanding that everything other than the Self may also exist outside one's own visual and perceptive space. Next to the acquisition of an initial body identity, also gender identity makes its appearance, and a major role is assumed by the processes of → identification and by interactions with significant people, who are the first model contributing to construction of one's identity. Thanks to the identification processes, the skills and values of the culture of belonging are acquired; people become what they are and realize their "continuity", which is defined through change, or rather through continuous adaptation to change. Especially in adolescence, identity is subjected to great changes, as emancipation from family and the realization of life projects starts. As mentioned above, in addition to personal identity there is also a cultural identity: they form an inseparable combination, as also the construction of cultural identity begins very early, first with the acquisition of family rules and subsequently with the introjection of behavioural patterns, lifestyles and contexts that represent the culture of the society of belonging. Until last century, when "social mobility" was rarely allowed (he who was born a farmer could hardly change his social status and culture), family identity overshadowed individual identity. The possibility of being identified as "sons of" could give individual identity a higher or lower value: in fact, it was kinship and family membership that provided identity to the individual. In this way, one's identity was marked since birth and individual inclinations needed to be silenced if they were not appropriate to their social condition. Today, however, change is the norm and it can take place both in the social and working sphere (where it is encouraged or made necessary) and in the affective sphere. Change can be superficial or deep, or rather refer to a change of attitude towards reality or towards oneself or to a changed self-image. If these changes result in intense emotional fluctuations, which are not or cannot be integrated into one's sense of identity, and if this state persists too long without this change being integrated into one's system, this can determine an inability to explain one's own emotional fluctuations, which are experienced negatively as → symptoms. To keep the balance, a person must maintain some continuity through change or change through progressive adjustments. Unfamiliar patterns, sudden changes from the usual to other new, strange, unusual situations, can determine alterations of our sense of identity, causing more or less mild and transitory experiences of depersonalization. Identity is based on different roles, arising not only from the culture of belonging, but also from other cultures, and this is particularly true nowadays. Various mechanisms are put in place to reconcile culture and different values, to cope with the sense of exclusion, marginalization or diversity: some people minimize cultural diversities, some isolate themselves, some emphasize their own culture of origin, some create a barrier between themselves and others, some adapt to a new culture and take distance from the culture of origin and from their fellow countrymen. In summary, some people accentuate, some reduce and some oppose cultural diversities to maintain their own identity, but the goal is not always reached. Several interacting factors, concerning environment and personality, define the type of psychic disorder that occurs.

However, the construction of identity never stops, it continues its path, which started at birth and ends only with the end of one's life. *[M.F. Pilleri, M.A. Reda]*

REFERENCES. Erikson E.H., *Childhood and society*, 1950; Locke J., *An essay concerning human understanding*, 1690; Reda M.A., *Sistemi cognitivi complessi e psicoterapia*, 1986; Reda M.A., Canestri L., Pilleri M.F. (eds.), *Continuità e cambiamento in psicoterapia*, in «Atti del Convegno di Psicologia e Psicopatologia Post-Razionalista», 2001, III.

PERSONAL MEANING ORGANIZATION (PMO)

PMOs are specific modes gradually shaping the course of individual development, with which each person organizes his/her own knowledge, relates to the Self, to the Other and the world, due to a recursive process of meaning attribution. According to the constructivist perspective (→ constructivism) the subject is conceptualized as an autopoietic system (→ autopoiesis) constantly evolving into a dynamic balance between the preservation of → personal identity and the adaptation to physical and relational perturbation, arising from the environment. Therefore, psychopathology becomes situated on a continuum with normality as an outcome of difficult situations concerning the maintenance of self-coherence by facing an emotional perturbation that the system is not able to integrate. Four different styles of organizational closure have been identified, defined as: obsessive-prone (or analytical/principles-oriented); depressive-prone (or responsible/detached); psychogenic-eating-disorders–prone (or imaginative/contextualized); and phobic-prone (or volitive/controller); these styles are based on particular themes around which the individual organizes his/her own personal meaning. Personal change occurs in the intersubjective dimension, by increasing self-awareness and modifying meaning attribution, but by maintaining the personal coherence of the Self. *[G. Rezzonico, M. Bani]*

REFERENCES. Guidano V.F., *The Self in process*, 1991; Nardi B. (2007). *CostruirSi. Sviluppo e Adattamento del Sé nella Normalità e nella Patologia [Self construction. Development and adaptation of the Self in normality and pathology].*

PERSONAL SOCIAL NETWORK

Within the systemic-relational paradigm, our personal social network envelops us throughout life and has a crucial impact on our experience of self and of social relevance, and our health and wellbeing. The personal social network is composed of four interconnected sectors, → family, friends, work and school relations and community relations. Each sector includes relations that are intimate and close to our heart, social connections that are friendly but not intimate; and distant acquaintances – those with whom we connect superficially but who are distinct from the world of those whom we do not know and who do not know us. Placing the informant at the centre, these distinctions configure a map with four quadrants and three concentric circles that allows visualization of a personal social network, and the evaluation of its attributes (e.g. distribution, density, accessibility) and its evolution over time. Prospective studies show increased risk of disease and death among persons with a poor quantity/quality of social relationships, while a robust social network is protective against disease and functional decline. These processes are mediated by virtuous cycles by which social networks promote health among their members, which facilitate the maintenance of an active social network, and vicious cycles where the presence of disease negatively affects networks availability, which in turn makes recovery more difficult. Network-oriented therapy has been a part of family therapy since early in its conception, and proves powerful during crises as well as severe psychopathology. *[C. E. Sluzki]*

REFERENCES. Berkman L. F., *Assessing the physical health effects of social networks and social support*, in «Annual Review of Public Health», 5, 1984; Berkman L.F., Syme S.L., *Social networks, host resistance, and mortality: A nine-year follow-up study of Alameda County residents*, 1979, 109 (2), 186–204; Berkman L.F., Kawachi I., (eds.), *Social Epidemiology*, 2000; Blazer D.G., *Social support and mortality in an elderly community population*, 1982, 115(5); Cohen S., Doyle W.J., Skonner D.P., Rabin B.S., Gwaltney J.M., *Social ties and susceptibility to the common cold*, 1997, 277, 1940–1944; House J.S., Robbins C., Metzner H.L., *The association of social relationships and activities with mortality: Prospective evidence from the Tecumseh community health study*, 1982, 116; Kawachi T., Colditz G.A., Ascherio A., Rimm E.B., Giovannuci E., Stampfer M.J., Willett W.C., *A prospective study of social networks in relation to total mortality and cardiovascular disease in men in the USA*, in «J. Epidemiol. Community Health», 1996, 50, 245–251; Seikkula J., Arnkil T.E., *Dialogical meetings in social networks*, 2006; Sluzki C.E., *La Red Social: Frontera de la Terapia Sistemica*, 1996; Sluzki C.E., *Migration and the disruption of the social network* in McGoldrick M., (ed.), *Re-visioning family therapy: race, culture and gender in clinical practice*, 1998; Sluzki C.E., *Social networks and the elderly: Conceptual and clinical issues, and a family consultation*, in «Family Process», 2000, 39(3); Speck R., Attneave C., *Family networks*, 1973; Unger J. B., McAvay G., *et al.*, *Variation in the impact of social network characteristics on physical functioning in elderly persons: MacArthur studies of successful aging*, in «Journals of Gerontology», Series B: Psychological Sciences and Social Sciences, 1999, 51.

PERSONAL UNCONSCIOUS

In the structure of the psyche, Jung distinguishes between personal and → collective unconscious. He considers the first a surface layer of the psyche, as it is more easily accessible to consciousness. In the personal unconscious, Jung places all the acquisitions of the individual existence, "everything which, involuntarily and without paying attention to it, I feel, think, remember, want, and do; all the future things that are taking shape in me", and not only, as thought by S. Freud, repressed materials considered morally unacceptable by society. It also includes what could not become conscious and that, in becoming so, would contribute to the extension of the personality of an individual. In this view, the unconscious has a function of → compensation in respect of consciousness as well as its own autonomous and creative activity. Finally, the contents of the personal unconscious are the → feeling-toned complexes: as these are self-sufficient, they elude the control of the Ego and affect its daily life. If they are brought to consciousness, they can be corrected and modified. The "dark side" of an individual, the → shadow, is largely derived from the contents of the personal unconscious and this can facilitate the process of making it conscious. *[A. Benvenuti]*

REFERENCES. Jung C.G. (1947–1954), *On the nature of the psyche*, in *Collected Works*, VIII, 1969.

PERSONALITY

On a metatheoretical level, the concept of personality can be defined as a "polysemic, hypothetical construction": through a predefined theory of personality and the knowing process related to it, it is possible to attribute psychological predicates to a person in order to hypothetically explain his/her behaviour or a specific mental state. The various descriptive, interpretive and explicative constructions related to personality may concern different dimensions – intrapsychic, interpersonal, relational, expressive, pathological, etc. Descriptive and interpretive data can be gathered in different, homogeneous classes (diagnostic categorization). The best-known, most traditional theories are the so-called "dispositional psychologies" or psychologies of "personality traits", which can employ psychometric, psychodynamic and nosographic (→ nosology) instruments for the purpose of evaluation and diagnosis. The classic instruments used to analyze normal or pathological personality traits are psychometric tests and personality projective tests. These theories, however, have turned out to be unreliable for three reasons: their insufficient correlation between personality traits and behaviour, several mistakes in attributing causality and meaning, and the → reification "effect". Due to these and other reasons – such as its predictive weakness (→ predictability) – the concept of personality has lost significance and reliability on an explicative level. Released from the positivist epistemology that provided its justification, it is partially revitalized by new, little-known, theoretical models of research adopted in a clinical environment. Dispositional theories are being substituted by cognitive, constructivist and relational models (person–situation) on the one hand, and investigations on temperamental or psychobiological dimensions on the other. The models traditionally stressing the objective, predictive, psychodiagnostic features are set against the different approach of some psychotherapy models: what is conventionally called "personality" is the recurring way for a person to give meaning and continuity to the world of his/her experiences; at the same time, the expected meaning is kept stable and coherent, both with respect to the observers and according to the person's goals, social episodes, the roles he/she plays and his/her narrative contexts. *[A. Salvini]*

▷ In general, within Jungian analytical psychology, the term indicates a set of features constituting psychic individuality, both in a historic and dynamic sense, and in a structural and functional sense. Starting by referring the concept of psyche to conscious and unconscious psychic processes as a whole – i.e. to "total personality" – Jung distinguishes conscious (or external) personality and unconscious (or internal) personality. On the one hand, the former designates all those aspects that are functional to adapting to environmental conditions; such aspects are enacted by the individual on the basis of conscious intentions that, explicitly or implicitly, take the others' expectations into account. Jung observes that external personality is a mask and, consequently, represents the way in which a person "wishes to be" and "wishes to appear". On the other, interior personality includes all subliminal aspects of "total personality" that are incompatible with the full functionality of external personality and are denied (or suppressed) during autoplastic adaptation processes. Psyche, therefore, is conceived as a functional activity whose dynamics are based on pairs of opposites: conscience and unconscious, → Ego and → shadow, → *persona* and → anima, Ego and → Self, etc. Accordingly, "total personality" cannot be exhaustively described, since its traits are continuously affected by the permanent interaction between the conscious psychic process and the unconscious one. *[E. V. Trapanese]*

REFERENCES. Fiora E., Pedrabissi L., Salvini A., *Pluralismo teorico e pragmatismo conoscitivo in psicologia della personalità*, 1988; Salvini A., *Psicologia clinica*, 2004; Salvini A., Dondoni M. (eds.), *Psicologia clinica dell'interazione e psicoterapia*, 2011.

PERSONALITY INTEGRATION

In psychosynthesis, structuring of the parts within a system where unity has greater relevance than its single components. The definition applies perfectly to → personality: a whole, made up of components and characteristics that structurally represent man's biopsychosocial totality. This implies an integration between the parts, allowing functioning, relating the environment and individual uniqueness, aiming at stability and transformative and developmental possibilities.

In the personality models, all the various psychological schools have in common the aim of integration, even in the differences of the various therapeutic processes. The emphasis laid on the dynamic and interactive aspect of the constituents of personality or on the integration of unity and multiplicity can vary. *[M. Rosselli]*

REFERENCES. Ferrucci P., *What we may be: Techniques for psychological and spiritual growth through psychosynthesis*, 2009; Firman J., Gila A., *The primal wound: A transpersonal view of trauma, addiction, and growth*, 1997.

PERSONALITY TESTS

Personality tests represent one of the instruments used to meet the need for a scientific study of → personality. Since its origin, the central and most fascinating aspect of psychology has been the possibility of acquiring instruments and methods to "understand others", or rather to study their mental and behavioural processes. In the process of evolution of modern psychology, the need to identify methodologies for the acquisition of interpersonal knowledge characterized by validity and scientific rigour has increased. Even though the use of tests originated thousands of years ago (the first rudimentary forms can be traced to 2,200 BC in ancient imperial China and to 450 BC with Hippocrates), in the scientific literature it is only in 1890 that the expression "mental test" appears, in the psychological studies of J. McKeen Cattell. The etymology traces back this word to the Latin term "*testum*", in its meaning of "earthenware jar", that is, a receptacle into which the medieval alchemists used to place metals and, by means of the chemical reactions taking place in it, would verify the eventual presence of gold.

As in any good scientific experiment, the objective of a test is that of providing the individual being tested with a series of standardized stimuli, in other words, stimuli that will remain the same in different administrations and with different subjects, in order to generate in them reactions that constitute an objective "measure" of their psychological characteristics. In psychology, measuring means transforming an empirical system (a collection of observable characteristics) into a numeric system, according to specific rules, in such a way as to ensure that the specific relationships between these numbers correspond to the relationship between the characteristics being measured. The necessary prerequisites of a valid psychological test are the degree of precision and accuracy with which it measures what it proposes to measure, and the capacity, through the use of such measures, to make inferences possible and consequently decisions based on the results of the test. *[F. Vincelli]*

REFERENCES. Dobson K.S., *Handbook of cognitive-behavioural therapies*, 1988; Pedrabissi L., Santinello M., *I test psicologici*, 1997.

PERSONIFICATIONS

In interpersonal psychoanalysis, the images that a person has of himself, or of significant others. The personifications are made up of a collection of feelings, attitudes and emotions that originate from the experiences connected to the satisfaction of needs or with painful experiences, and for this reason do not coincide exactly with the "real" persons that are being personified. *[A. Cresti, S. Brizzi]*

REFERENCES. Sullivan H.S., *The interpersonal theory of psychiatry*, 1962.

PERSUASION

Process of communication aimed at changing the attitude of an individual, inducing adherence (previously absent) to the ideas contained in the message. In a meaning that is even more pertinent to psychotherapy and with reference to the pragmatic effects of communication, persuasion is aimed at increasing the probability that a subject will behave in a certain way. Persuasion does not only utilize purely rational means of convincing the person (in other words, demonstration, as is used in the pure sciences), but also argumentative, rhetorical and oratorical procedures that act on the emotional and instinctive level, by means of the use of linguistic techniques and specific modes of communication.

If one takes this term literally, avoiding ideological connotations, one could assert that all psychotherapeutic processes are fundamentally a process of persuasion, so much so, that a good number of psychotherapies deliberately adopt the use of linguistic techniques of persuasion, whilst others, whilst trying to avoid using them in a direct manner, cannot altogether avoid it. *[R.]*

PERVERSE TRIANGLE

Within systemic interactional psychotherapy, a term coined by Haley that identifies the coalition between two persons against a third. The two persons involved in the coalition are usually not in an egalitarian relationship, or rather they belong to different levels of the hierarchy of power: for example, in a → family, one of the children enters into a coalition with one parent against the other parent (intergenerational coalition), or, in an organization, a superior with one subaltern against another, at his same level. Such a coalition, however, remains latent or is denied or disqualified at a metacommunicative level.

The perverse triangle generates violence, breakdown of a system and symptomatic behaviours. In a family where this kind of configuration exists, the separation between generations is overcome in ways that are hidden: the authority of the parental dyad is weakened and the son or daughter may find him or herself experiencing a conflict of loyalties. Through the study of these behaviours in schizophrenic families, Haley hypothesized therefore that within these families there is not only confusion at the level of communication but also confusion between the levels of a system of relationships. [*M. Genchi]*

REFERENCES. Haley J., *The family of the schizophrenic: A model system*, 1959; Id., *Toward a theory of pathological systems*, in P. Watzlawick, J. Weakland (eds.), *The interactional view*, 1977.

PHALLUS

It is the symbol of → libido in both sexes. This term generates confusion between sexuality and procreation and becomes, in this way, the disturbing element in the relationship between man and woman. According to S. Freud, the phallus is the object of desire of the mother, who is the woman forbidden to the father's son. In fact, → castration is what connects sex and word, a prohibition that regulates the enjoyment of sexuality. Therefore, according to Freud, the phallus is not a ghost, not an → object (partial, internal, good, bad, etc.) and even less is it a real organ, penis or clitoris. According to Lacan, the → signifier phallus is accountable for the loss caused by the taking of sexuality in language. In Lacan's opinion, the phallus is the signifier of sexual enjoyment, it expresses the assumption by man of his own sex, which explains its symbolic importance in the unconscious. *[M. Drazien, C. Fanelli]*

REFERENCES. Lacan J. (1966), *The signification of the phallus*, in *Écrits: A selection*, 1972; Id. (1969-1970), *The seminar of Jacques Lacan XVII, The other side of psychoanalysis*, 1969–1970.

PHENOMENOLOGICAL METHOD

Process that, through *epoché* (abstention from judgment), enables the essence of phenomena to be grasped. It does not coincide with → introspection (based on a naive separation of the Ego and the world), but is a way of relearning to see the world, a rediscovered ability to feel amazement when faced with the world. The relationship between the phenomenological method and Gestalt therapy is complex and diverse. With Jaspers, the therapist aims at understanding the patient's experiences through identification, without seeking naturalistic explanations; to this is added attention to countertransferal and co-constructed experiences. In agreement with the teaching of Merleau-Ponty, bodily experiences (constitutively in relationship) are the place that puts patient and therapist in contact with the flow of the "world-of-life" from which sensations, emotions, thoughts emerge and hence the direction of therapy. The essence of the Gestalt method is to support, in the therapeutic encounter, the emergence of a figure that is co-created, starting from the "experienced-world". In order to accede to this level of experience, it is necessary to experience what Husserl called "phenomenological conversion" by means of *epoché*: this is the suspension of the ingenuous attitude whereby one generally interacts with the world through the Ego. The concentration in the → here-and-now through the contact with the body-experienced is the application of the phenomenological *epoché* to the psychotherapeutic process: it is the presence at the → contact boundary, a "no man's land" in which experience springs forth in a nascent state, even before being constituted as belonging to the I or to the You. In Gestalt therapy, at the beginning of the session, the therapist is focused on the "*Id* of the situation" (i.e. the ability to be in contact through the implicit bodily, nonverbal and pre-reflective processes), tolerating the chaotic movement at the boundary and supporting the encounter with the emerging novelty in the patient. Presence, in this sense, becomes the therapeutic tool and the experience gone through becomes the relational nourishment that has no need of interpretation, but of awareness. This method is also used for qualitative research in Gestalt therapy. *[M. Spagnuolo Lobb, G. Francesetti]*

REFERENCES. Bloom D.J., *The phenomenological method of Gestalt therapy: Revisiting Husserl to find the "essence" of Gestalt therapy*, in «Gestalt Review», 2009, III, 9; Borgna E., *I conflitti del conoscere*, 1988; Cavaleri P.A., *Vivere con l'altro: per una cultura della relazione*, 2007; Fergnani F. (ed.), *Merleau-Ponty, il corpo vissuto*, 1979; Fleming Crocker S., *Phenomenology in Husserl and Gestalt Therapy*, in «British Gestalt Journal», 2009, 18, 1; Galimberti U., *Psichiatria e fenomenologia*, 1979; Husserl E., *Logical investigations*, 1900–1901; Id., *Ideas pertaining to a pure phenomenology and to a phenomenological philosophy*, 1913; Id., *The crisis of European sciences and transcendental phenomenology*, 1954; Jaspers K., *General psychopathology*, 1913; Merleau-Ponty M., *Phenomenology of perception*, 1945; Minkowski E., *Lived time*, 1933; Perls F., Hefferline R.F., Goodman P., *Gestalt therapy: Excitement and growth in the human personality*, 1951; Philippson P., *The emergent self*, 2009; Polster E., Polster M., *Gestalt therapy integrated*, 1973; Robine J.M., *Plis et deplis du self*, 1977; Wysong J., Rosenfeld E., (eds.), *An oral history of Gestalt therapy*, 1982; Spagnuolo Lobb M. (ed.), *Psicoterapia della Gestalt. Ermeneutica e Clinica*, 2001; Id., *L'awareness dans la pratique post-moderne de la gestalt-therapie*, in «Gestalt», XV, 27, 2004; Id., *Therapeutic meeting as improvisional co-creation*, in M. Spagnuolo Lobb, N. Amendt-Lyon (eds.), *Creative license: The art of Gestalt therapy*, 2003.

PHENOMENOLOGY

In Gestalt therapy, according to Husserl's definition, it is the study of the essences, a transcendental philosophy that relocates the essences in existence, a method by which the world is "already always there" before reflection, an attempt to provide a description of our experience as it is. The philosophical area that goes back to phenomenology has been a source and a fundamental reference for Gestalt theory from its birth. Husserl's concept of intentionality and the worldliness of the Ego (hence embodied in and inseparable from the world) is the epistemological territory by which the subject becomes constituently relational and founds a totally new concept of the self as function of the organism–environment field. The separation of subject–object becomes a secondary dichotomy with regard to an underlying reality that is the "world-of-life" perceptible by means of the experienced body. The therapist's interest is directed to understanding the patient's experiences as they are offered to the listener, according to Jaspers' lesson, to which is added the indispensable relational dimension because the human condition is constituently "being-with". The meaning of the experiences is to be found in this dimension, the place of treatment of the disorder, which is none other than an appeal to the relationship itself. The therapist, thus, goes back to Heidegger's "things themselves" and to the interest in what exists as it emerges in the present situation, thus bringing about another epistemological leap: the passage from a model that is extrinsic to health to an aesthetic evaluation that grasps the emerging beauty of the encounter. Therapy is the place of authentic contact that leads to the original co-construction of new creative adaptations. Interpretation is no longer necessary: it is the emergence of the world-of-life itself, in the → here-and-now of the encounter, and directed towards the approaching nascent temporality, which constitutes the itinerary of growth that the therapist specifically supports. *[M. Spagnuolo Lobb, G. Francesetti]*

REFERENCES. Francesetti G., *La sofferenza della Zwischenheit. Una lettura gestaltica di "Colpa e sensi di colpa" di Martin Buber*, in L. Bertolino (ed.), *Colpa e sensi di colpa*, 2008; Galimberti U., *Psichiatria e fenomenologia*, 1979; Heidegger M., *Being and time*, 1962; Husserl E., *Logical investigations*, 1900–1901; Id., *Ideas pertaining to a pure phenomenology and to a phenomenological philosophy*, 1913; Id., *The crisis of European sciences and transcendental phenomenology*, 1954; Jaspers K., *General psychopathology*, 1913; Perls F., Hefferline R.F., Goodman P., *Gestalt therapy: Excitement and growth in the human personality*, 1951; Sichera A., *Un confronto con Gadamer: per una epistemologia ermeneutica della Gestalt*, in M. Spagnuolo Lobb (ed.), *Psicoterapia della Gestalt. Ermeneutica e Clinica, 2001*; Spagnuolo Lobb M., *Therapeutic meeting as improvisional co-creation*, in M. Spagnuolo Lobb, N. Amendt-Lyon (eds.), *Creative license: The art of Gestalt therapy*, 2003.

PHILOSOPHICAL COUNSELLING

A discipline born in Germany in 1981, when the philosopher Achenbach began receiving "consultants" (or, in his language, guests) in his study to answer their questions and talk about their problems. This is not a form of psychotherapy and, in fact, it is not intended for people suffering from mental disorders, but only for people concerned with existential problems: a separation, dismay in the face of death, questions about the meaning of life, a particular moral dilemma, difficulty in accepting or handling the → alienation caused by work, more or less cynical or romantic questions about love. Philosophical counselling does not investigate the past, plumb the unconscious or use techniques; it does not teach how to overcome blocks or difficulties: it simply helps the consultant, through an equal dialogue with the counsellor, to reflect on their worldview in a critical manner. Differently from a psychotherapist, a philosophical counsellor does not need a specific professional qualification. The "method" used by Achenbach – which, however, denies having a method – is based on an open meeting overtly free from preconceptions or prejudices, resulting in a philosophical dialogue oriented by the discursive tools and techniques used. Some important elements of this approach are: welcoming, respect of thought and experience of others, acceptance of others, sincerity and equal dignity of the discourses of the people involved, love and the search for truth. Moving from Achenbach's approach, the new "philosophical practice" has developed quite quickly in all Western countries, reaching China and India. The distinctive features of the discipline, beyond the aforementioned traits of the Achenbachian dialogue, are quite controversial. For example, S. Schuster, although he shares with Achenbach a very negative view on psychotherapies, defines philosophical counselling as a "philosophical cure of the Self", able to induce wellbeing and solve mental discomfort. Instead, according to R. Lahav, philosophical counselling is basically a reflection and reconfiguration of people's "worldviews" that can induce therapeutic effects, without having the intention. Moreover, many counsellors claim an effect or a move similar to the husserlian *epoché* (suspension) that facilitates a kind of "lifting" or disconnection from the "identification with the problem", "according to an expression used by A. Prins-Bakker. Even though many counsellors distance themselves from psychotherapy (particularly from therapeutic "intentionality"), some of them do not hesitate to consider philosophical counselling as close to and intertwined with psychotherapy. For example, L. Marinoff, emphasizes the orientation to problem solving and Chung-ying Cheng claims that his practice has a strong psychoanalytic connotation. Similar differences concern also other aspects, such as the degree of neutrality of the consultant, the importance of education to philosophize and the orientation to search for wisdom, only to mention a few. However, beyond the differences, it is possible to identify some elements common to all the practices put in place by the various philosophical counsellors. The first element is a complete absence of prejudices, which, on the one hand, underpins most part of Achenbach's work and, on the other, represents the very soul of philosophy. In fact, philosophizing means examining, questioning everything, including the discourse itself; the choice to avoid putting limits on meta-discourse is probably a defining characteristic, powerful enough to separate philosophical counselling (and philosophy) from any other scientific or non-scientific discourse, psychotherapy included. Another feature, generally shared by all philosophical consultants is a clarifying intentionality, or in stronger terms, a regulative ideal that gives value to truth as a norm of belief and action (it should also be mentioned that the idea or the concept of truth are not considered obvious but, indeed, always problematic). This clarifying intention is generally valued and seen as a way to broaden one's horizons and potential, as a liberation, as something good after all (a strong philosophical concept and consubstantial with philosophy itself). This seems to imply a connection, or a relationship of mutual implication between epistemology and ethics. Also, it is important to underline the work on concepts and on productive thinking: the path of philosophical counselling is in general cognitive and the work on the emotions and perceptions can take place only through reasoning and speech. The practical-operative orientation of philosophical counselling has considerable consequences on the importance that the particular has on the discipline – in contrast to the focus on the universal typical of much of traditional philosophy – and indeed the process is always activated starting from a single case, a narrative, a fact, an example, a request or an emotion. This is the reason why philosophical counselling seems always focused on new ways of thinking in order to create new concepts, as if the understanding of existence and experience had value only when these are included in broader, deeper and more powerful conceptual frames. *[P. Cervari]*

REFERENCES. Achenbach G., *Philosophische Praxis*, 2004; Lahav R., *Essays on philosophical counselling*, 1995; Raabe P.B., *Philosophical counselling: theory and practice*, 2006.

PLACEBO

A substance or psychological procedure that is considered as not having specific curative effects on a given disorder or disease. Placebo is typically applied in "double-blind" studies to test the efficacy of a drug by comparing it to a pharmacologically inactive or non-specific substance. In these studies, the therapeutic effects are measured in two groups. One group is treated with the medication and the other with the placebo; neither the doctor nor the patient knows in advance which of the two substances is provided. Research carried out using double-blind trials has shown that significant therapeutic changes may occur even in placebo-taking groups. The expression "placebo effect" originates from this observation and it indicates the occurrence of therapeutic effects that are not caused by chemical-pharmacological interactions of the substance in the patient's body or by the principles underpinning a psychotherapeutic intervention, but by the attributions, beliefs or auto-suggestions of the patient following the intervention. Instead, when the suggestion leads to a harmful reaction in the organism, the term used is "nocebo effect". In order to explain such effects, it is hypothesized that the attribution of therapeutic efficacy to a treatment or to a non-specific/inactive substance by the patient can generate a sequence of neurovegetative or psychological changes. These can lead to concrete improvements of the symptoms or to visible changes in the experience and behaviour of the patient. Research claims that the placebo effect consists of a series of psychological elements: the efficacy expectation attributed to the placebo medication or the therapeutic procedure, the competency ascribed to the therapist (or doctor), the symbolic context in which the intervention takes place, the unique relationship that is created between therapist and patient, the communicative and persuasive skills of the therapist. *[R.]*

PLANNING

In individual psychology a shared definition of a plan and its concerning strategies for the gradual changing of one's own style of life. After the stages of exploration and disclosure of the fictions and of the neurotic projects that hold the lifestyle of the patient, the therapeutic procedure reaches the delicate phase of settlement of the possible and desirable → changes. "The project of transforming the personality can only be a work of the patient himself," A. Adler says, "whose recovery calls for the transformation of the subject thanks to a pedagogic action". In fact, the → secondary gains of the symptom and the acquired habits represent generally powerful restrictions to that change, which, instead, the therapist can encourage (as if he were an experienced friend) by sharing with the patient his new projects and realistic existential "texts". *[L. Cerioli]*

REFERENCES. Adler A., *The practice and theory of individual psychology*, 1920.

PLAY TECHNIQUE

Between 1918 and 1923, Klein, encouraged by S. Ferenczi, her first analyst, turned her attention to the psychoanalysis of children and developed a technique consisting in the creation of a → setting that includes, besides the analyst, also toys, pets and real objects. Inside such a setting, the analyst develops a meticulous interpretation of the unconscious, where the contents of play assume their symbolic meaning and are treated as elements of a dream, comparable to adults' free associations (→ free associations technique). By using the technique of play, Klein was able to analyze children under 3 years of age. In fact, she realized, ingeniously, that playing could become an instrument of communication in the analysis and permitted the exploration of anguish and the contents of the internal world of her little patients as a whole. In Kleinian theory, playing is considered "work", a way to give relief to inner persecutory states by the external projection of aggressive and disruptive phantasies; such presuppositions opened the way to future theoretic evolutions, concerning the role, in psychoanalysis, of the analysis of the negative → transference and of the → interpretation of deep anguish. *[A. Voltolin, M.L. Ricci]*

REFERENCES. Klein M., *The psychoanalytic play technique*, 1953; Klein M., *Personification in the play of children*, 1929.

PLEASURE

A term that designates an experience and, at the same time, a general category, in which one can find emotions – such as joy, love, interest, happiness, excitement – or else sensory perceptions – such as the taste of good food or the experiencing of an orgasm during sexual relations. Pleasure is connoted as being essential for the survival of the individual and for → adaptation, and is construed as being a fundamental motivational factor.

S. Freud asserted that the seeking of pleasure, and the consequent avoidance of pain are the fundamental motivational factors underlying all human behaviour (→ pleasure principle and reality principle). Frequently, people go to therapy complaining of lack of pleasure in one or more areas of their lives, or of an inability to experience it fully; nevertheless, pleasure is frequently underestimated, as some forms of pathology originate precisely from the spasmodic, exaggerated or distorted seeking of this sensation: some eating disorders such as bulimia and → vomiting, manias, addiction to drugs or to the use of the internet, the compulsion to shop or to gamble and sexual perversions can be considered as falling under this category. These pathologies, in common with obsessive rituals and compulsions, have in common the inability of the individual to resist acting upon these behaviours. However, contrary to the latter, which are characterized as being an attempt to control → fear, these pathologies are maintained by the pleasure that one experiences in enacting them. *[R.]*

PLEASURE PRINCIPLE AND REALITY PRINCIPLE

This term refers to one of the two main principles that govern the functioning of the psyche, according to Freud; the other is the reality principle. The pleasure principle is manifested as the tendency to seek to avoid painful experiences at all costs, independently of their cause, and, in this way, it governs all the activities of the psyche.

The reality principle is found at the level of the preconscious and the conscious and it regulates the functioning of the secondary processes. Even when it enters into conflict with the demands of the pleasure principle, they are not in opposition, but it acts by evaluating the conditions imposed by reality that will allow the pleasure principle to achieve its aims in the most effective way possible. This will allow for the identification and definition of the adaptive functions of the Ego, through which the reality principle can exert its influence by organizing the psychic processes, regulating them according to rational and realistic criteria. *[P. Cruciani]*

REFERENCES. Freud S. (1900–1901), *The interpretation of dreams*, in *The Standard Edition*, IV–V, 1953–1974; Id. (1911), *Formulations on the two principles of mental functioning*, in *The Standard Edition*, XII, 1953–1974.

POLARITIES → TOPDOG VS UNDERDOG

POSITIVE AND UNCONDITIONAL ACCEPTANCE

In the context of client-centred therapy, a concept outlined by Rogers that identifies a → need, in the sense described by Maslow. The malfunctioning of personality can depend on the dissatisfaction of this need, due to the absence of "unconditional love" from one's parents. The Rogersian therapist is "accepting" when, having a sincere interest towards the client, is able to open up to him with respect and availability, facilitating the exploration of any thought and feeling in the client. The acceptance ability of a therapist – not as a mere intellectual action, but as the ability to create a deep relationship – facilitates acceptance and the subsequent change in the client if the therapist is also capable of → empathy and → congruence. *[A. Zucconi]*

REFERENCES. Lietaer G., *Unconditional positive regard: A controversial basic attitude in client-centred therapy*, in R.F. Levant, J.M. Shlien (eds.), *Client-centred therapy and the person-centred approach*, 1984; Maslow A., *Toward a psychology of being*, 1962; Rogers C.R., *Client-centered therapy*, 1951.

POSITIVE CONNOTATION

Within the systemic approach of the Milan school (→ Milan School of Family Therapy), it concerns assigning a positive effect and function both to the patient's symptom and to all the family behaviours related to the symptom. M. Selvini Palazzoli invented this concept in the early 1970s when he abandoned his psychoanalytic practice to join the pioneers of family therapy. In the first family sessions, the classic psychodynamic explanations were experienced as highly judgemental and caused immediate withdrawal from psychotherapy. Interpretive or educational techniques were abandoned in favour of provocative or paradoxical actions (→ logic of paradox) that provided a positive connotation of patients' symptoms as self-sacrificial behaviours to promote wellbeing in the other family members (this was adopted, for example, to keep the pair of parents together, to give a mission to a mother and fill her existential emptiness, to give a father a good example of how to behave). Selvini Palazzoli and his school have understood the positive connotation of the symptom as a provocation aimed at triggering change. Other systemic therapists believe that the patient really makes sacrifices for the family's balance/wellbeing (systemic functionalism). Today Selvini's school considers the concept of positive connotation as outdated because, although it highlights the mutual protection bonds in the family, it emphasizes, excessively, altruism as a primary motivation. However, some implicit aspects of the concept remain essential: emphasizing the active role of the patient as a protagonist and creating a positive atmosphere of goodwill between the psychotherapist and all family members. *[M. Selvini]*

REFERENCES. Selvini M., *Reinventare la psicoterapia*, 2004.

POSITIVE PSYCHOLOGY

Positive psychology can be defined as the scientific study of individual experiences and positive traits, and of the structures and social organizations that facilitate their development. It tends to promote individual and collective → wellbeing, valuing the individual resources and the social context. For a structured plan of this approach it is necessary to refer to Seligman's (1998) contribution, at the time of his appointment as the president of the American Psychological Association (APA). On this occasion, he demonstrated the opportunity to direct research towards the factors that promote wellbeing and personal development, and the psychological interventions aimed at improving the living conditions of the individual and the community. In the introduction to the special issue of *American Psychologist*, published in 2000 with Csikszentmihalyi, Seligman identifies the positive qualities that make life worth living and outlines their relationship with happiness, health and self-actualization. The considerable interest among researchers and practitioners has led to the establishment of various scientific societies. *[S. Sirigatti, B. Giangrasso].*

REFERENCES. Peterson C., Ruch W., Beermann U., Park N., Seligman M.E.P., *Strengths of character, orientations to happiness, and life satisfaction*, in «The Journal of Positive Psychology», 2007, 2, 3; Schueller S.M., Seligman M.E.P., *Pursuit of pleasure, engagement, and meaning: Relationships to subjective and objective measures of well-being*, in «The Journal of Positive Psychology», 2010, 5, 4; Seligman M.E.P., Csikszentmihalyi M., *Positive psychology: An introduction*, in «American Psychologist», 2000, 55, 1.

POSITIVE PSYCHOTHERAPY

According to this approach, the promotion of positive experiences and emotions will be more beneficial for patients than an intervention aimed primarily at changing cognitions and behaviours. Positive psychotherapy aims, therefore, to stimulate and promote positive aspects – such as optimism, happiness, self-determination, individual optimal functioning – in order to achieve an improvement in quality of life and greater personal satisfaction. Sometimes, the concept of positive psychotherapy is comparable to wellbeing psychotherapy. *[S. Sirigatti, B. Giangrasso]*

REFERENCES. Seligman M.E., Rashid T., Parks A.C., *Positive psychotherapy*, in «American Psychologist», 2006, 61.

POSITIVE REINFORCEMENT

Within the behavioural paradigm, positive reinforcement is defined as being any event that, when presented in a consistent manner following a behaviour, increases the → frequency of its incidence. The behaviours that one wants to maintain can be reinforced (→ reinforcement) by arranging for events to occur in a systematic manner following the incidence of these behaviours. The reinforcements used in the different behavioural schedules can vary in nature (real or symbolic rewards, social praise, etc.). An example of an intervention based on positive reinforcement is the treatment of stammering in preschool children. In these programmes, the children receive positive reinforcement of a social nature (appreciation or praise by the parents, recognition of a good performance) when they speak in a fluent manner. *[M. D'Ambrosio]*

REFERENCES. D'Ambrosio M., *Balbuzie. Percorsi teorici e clinici integrati*, 2005; Dobson K.S., *Handbook of cognitive-behavioural therapies*, 1988.

POST-RATIONALIST COGNITIVE DEVELOPMENT THERAPY

According to the post-rationalist cognitive approach (→ post-rationalist cognitive therapy), each individual is a complex system able to actively assimilate experience and organize it for the construction of the self. Thus, psychotherapy is an exploration of these subjective abilities, which are unique in each individual. V.F. Guidano defined such abilities as depending on the → personal meaning organization (PMO), i.e. the specific individual ability to maintain the sense of uniqueness and temporal continuity, despite changes during the lifespan. Continuity and change are interdependent: their balance is assured by stabilization ("closure") of some basic organizational processes concerning emotional management. These processes, allowing a coherent and consistent sense of the self, unique for each individual, provide many flexible evolutionary possibilities of change with respect to personal manners of perceiving and assimilating new experiences. According to Nardi, each PMO develops providing the subject with better adaptive behavioural responses in the environment in which s/he is growing (first of all, his/her caregivers). Subjects developing "inward focus" construct emotional reciprocity patterns that are overlapping in the same conditions; further, they perceive any change moving from their internal activations. Repetitiveness of caregiver's manners, recognized and memorized during situations of protection/sureness or of desertion/danger, allows them to decode precociously basic feelings (fear, anger, sadness, joy); the ability to recognize internal activations allows them to move to decode environmental characteristics, to look for available points of reference and to explore new environmental aspects. Communication is based on physical reciprocity, depending on caregivers' availability (i.e. presence or absence, nearness or remoteness), in terms of protection when reciprocity is high, in terms of detachment when reciprocity is low. Therefore, in inward developments, when physical reciprocity is high, detachment and exploring the environment is perceived as possible when the subject feels him/herself safe (i.e. able to control the situation): these conditions are possible both directly, when the caregiver is actually present, and indirectly, when the caregiver encourages and reassures the subject to learn how he/she can solve problems and overcome difficulties. In all these cases, when physical reciprocity is high, "controller" PMOs become stable. In inward developments, when physical reciprocity is instead low (the caregiver seems fragile, impotent, not available, unsympathetic, cold, refusing or is missing), the child defines the sense of the self (→ self-schema) from his/her ability to manage detachment and loneliness, perceived as the usual conditions of life. Thus, moving from low availability of help, the subject looks for adaptive answers to his/her internal needs. In all these cases, when physical reciprocity is low, "detached" PMOs become stable. The subject is centred on loneliness control, early awareness of his/her responsibility, self-resolution to cope with problems in the lifespan, and being sensitive to him/herself and others (when the subject is not afraid to lose them). Subjects developing the "outward focus" perceive that his/her caregiver is not predictable, as he/she is not focused on his/her own internal activations but, on the contrary, on external messages. In these cases, the child decodes later, and more vaguely, basic feelings and he/she mostly perceives self-evaluating emotions (i.e. shame, guilt, satisfaction and pride). Environmental signals seem full of judgement and guidelines, focused on by the subject, who tries to catch them, tuning in with them and taking possession of them. Thus, they are employed to read and verify internal activations, which are recognized and accepted only if they seem to be in line with caregivers' messages. The complexity and variability of environmental signals make them unpredictable and not storable during overlapping situations; thus, construction of personal meaning organization is made with continuous attention to these signals (both verbal and nonverbal), by which information on the self is obtained. Communication is centred not on physical reciprocity (as distance regulation between protection and desertion) but on semantic reciprocity, in terms of approval and corroboration when reciprocity is high, in terms of norms, rules, precepts and values to be respected and possessed. In outward developments, when semantic reciprocity is high, the child constructs the sense of the self on signals received by the caregiver, who seems very present (positively or negatively); these signals are updated based on whether the child feels appreciated or not. In particular, when reciprocity is high, the continuous signals received drive the individual adaptive strategies to court approval or disapproval, in order to verify results obtained and to match them with those obtained by others. In all these cases, when semantic reciprocity is high, contextualized PMO become stable. They are centred to update internal activations according to environmental responses and confrontation with significant other persons. The sense of the self, related to approval or disapproval, drives future behaviour, constricting or widening expectations towards the goals perceived as possible to reach. In outward developments, when semantic reciprocity is instead low, "principle-oriented" PMOs become stable. From the caregiver (who seems present but emotively measured) the child learns mainly rules, criteria and instructions on what he/she can do or not do, first by practice, then also morally. In particular, when semantic reciprocity is low, the caregiver seems more rationally than empathetically engaged; thus, the child drives his/her adaptive strategies to look for rules and behaviours useful (i.e. right and effective) to being approved of and nurtured. He/she must internalize rules and values by which it is possible to reach the necessary certainties to stabilize the sense of the self and of the world, defining a universe of positive thoughts and behaviours to promote, and excluding the categories of thoughts and behaviours that appear negative. Criteria, rules and values sufficiently available are employed to construct a coherent representation of the internal and external world, looking for more and more complex, integrated and generalized theories and models; the possibility of explaining experience in a satisfying, definite and undoubted manner allows the exceeding of the possible contradictory and opposing aspects that can produce anxiety. Personal commitment, more than results obtained, is used by the subject to verify his/her own behaviour. Adaptation is developed, looking for caregiver's approval through common rules and values. Rational control of emotions promotes the prevalence of the self-evaluating ones (i.e. pride, guilt) that are explained and justified; in this manner they do not appear as an expression of weakness and do not destabilize the internal balance. Thus, psychic processes are strongly logical and analytical, focused on details, on opposite aspects of life (i.e. if one is or is not friendly, righteous, good, and correct), and on reaching an integrated view of reality. In the cognitive post-rationalist psychotherapy, the therapist is a "strategically oriented perturber", who reconstructs experience, focusing it during significant episodes analyzed/reviewed in slow-motion ("moviola setting"); using different interventions depending on each personal meaning organization, the therapist reorders psychopathological disorders as subjective modalities in self-referring experience. Any symptom must not be simply eliminated, but it is a useful tool to explore personal functioning. Thus, also in severe mental disorders, the adaptive abilities on which the individual is operating ("therapeutic alliance") can be focused in order to reach more mature and adequate competencies. In this manner it is possible to broaden the subject's managing range, discovering new manners in self-referring experience, thus increasing flexibility, and abstractive, integrative and generative abilities of the system of personal-meaning organization *[B. Nardi]*

REFERENCES. Guidano V.F., *Complexity of the Self,* 1997; Nardi B., *CostruirSi. Sviluppo e Adattamento del Sé nella Normalità e nella Patologia,* 2007; Nardi B., Guidelines on the construction of a post-rationalist therapeutic approach, in «European Psychotherapy», 9 (1), 57–67, 2010; Nardi B., Arimatea E., Vernice M., Bellantuono C., *How subjectivity can be investigated in the post-rationalist cognitive approach: Clinical and psychodiagnostic tools,* in «International Journal of Psychological Studies», 4(2), 2012.

POST-RATIONALIST COGNITIVE THERAPY

THE ORIGINS. The term post-rationalism was coined by Guidano at the end of the 1980s to indicate a new way of thinking about psychology characterized by the recognition of the individual as irreducible generator of meaning. The appearance of this term defines a movement that had its roots in the cognitive revolution in the 1970s and which had been characterized by the particular emphasis on epistemology. This was considered as the basic discipline on which both the theoretical and clinical programmes of scientific psychology should be based. When psychology was preparing to study the mind – that sort of "black box" always banished by behaviourist research programmes – the problem of ensuring the scientific value in those studies was resolved by the emerging cognitive psychology in two ways: the first, characterized by an empirical approach, considered cognition as a belief system hierarchically ordered, which, as a computational programme, guides both the actions and the emotions of an individual; the second, in which Guidano was one of the prominent figures, looked at cognition as a dimension corresponding to the "interiority" of an individual and considered the active role played by the subject in the construction of their own reality. However, this posed a fundamental problem for those claiming to provide a scientific study of the mind: the need to "objectively" investigate interiority through the rigour of the scientific method. For this reason, the path of Popperian epistemology, also called evolutionary epistemology by Campbell, was followed. This perspective considered man as an organism actively organizing their own reality through the generation of theories, whose preservation or elimination was regulated by natural selection. In this way, the scientific value of research on the human mind was ensured, without renouncing the study of people's interiority. From this perspective, knowledge corresponds to an active, adaptive and historical process that produces structures – that is, theories – that individuals generate during their relationship with the environment. In this way, the cognitive sphere could be marked in terms of stable configurations that are maintained throughout individual history. The recognition of those cognitive structures in the patient would guide the intervention strategy.

THE DEVELOPMENT. The transition from post-structuralist to rationalist cognitivism was generated by a change that has its roots in evolutionary epistemology. Campbell underlined how the internalization of the processes of selection and conservation of theories was characterized by self-regulation. But his analysis of the autonomy of the subject was still heavily dependent on the neo-Darwinian perspective. In fact, the traditional approach to the problem considered natural selection as specifying the structural changes of the organism and considered evolution as the optimization of adaptation to the environment. This view was completely overturned in the early 1980s by Maturana and Varela, who changed the evolutionary explanation concerning the internal dynamics of each animal group, and consequently the history of structural changes of lineage in relation to environmental changes. The fundamental aspect is that an organism and the environment vary independently. The focus on the autonomy of living beings leads to an analysis of the autonomous unit as a self-referential system: a system that, while it is continuously shaping its own order within a fluid flow of stimuli, at the same time distinguishes the domain of meaningful environmental disturbances in order to maintain their identity as a system. The metaphor of the scientist who generates theories, dear to Popper's followers, was replaced by the metaphor of the observer who, through their observations, constructs a self-referential reality order. Another important aspect, driven by studies on self-organized systems, is the introduction, in the field of cognitive sciences, of a new methodological perspective. To account for the generation of a certain meaning, the new epistemological approach consisted in building a mechanism able to generate a particular behaviour, defined as a mental state, as a result of the internal coherence of its operations. This approach, called constructivist, distinguished itself from that of physical sciences, which was methodologically based on anticipation and prediction according to rational principles. Hence the term post-rationalism. For example, it makes little sense to elaborate a theory, as required by the predictive approach, to make predictions about the mental acts generated at a given time by a person and to understand why that individual behaves in a certain way in a particular situation. It is much more interesting to reconstruct the semantic coherence through which that person gives meaning to a series of occurring events. Therefore, the constructivist method is about reconstruction of system operations and their internal cohesion. Starting from this way of conceiving how meaning is generated, Guidano distinguished between different categories of organization of semantic consistency. He spoke of "organizations of personal meaning" to indicate a unitary process of organization whose internal continuity and consistency are to be found in the specificity of the formal and structural properties used to process knowledge (i.e. flexibility, creativity, abstraction level, etc.). Directed by the same differentiation of invariants, which a decade earlier he had called "cognitive structures", Guidano based his distinction of categories on various attachment modes that take shape during a person's development. On the one hand, the maintenance of organizational patterns of attachment in a person's lifespan would ensure the continuity of their internal consistency and, on the other, an increasingly articulated self-referentiality. As it had ten years earlier, the therapeutic strategy resulting from this concept of individual cognitive system focused on the recognition of those patterns and on the conscious integration of experiential disturbances within the organization of those invariants of personal meaning.

THE CURRENT PERSPECTIVE. The most important aspect of this formulation is that, through focusing on the internal dynamics of the system, accompanied by the simultaneous suspension of "reality", the lived experience is matched to the configuration of the internal processes of the organism. This act, made to scientifically grasp the knowledge organization of an individual, introduces another unknowingly made act that eliminates the concept of person. That is, the "being mine" of actions and feelings, the occasional singularization of acts, is deleted in the name of internal consistency. Through the act of putting people's actual experiences "in brackets", the history of a person – their identity – is reduced to a portrait that, like a zodiac sign, governs the fate of the subjects from the first stages of their life until death. This way of describing the cognitive sphere assumes, as a matter of fact, the ontological categories of interiority, continuity and unity through which modernity had conceptualized the first-hand experience. Therefore, inevitably, this approach ignores the fact that this view was rooted in an ontology that, from Plato through to Descartes and up to I. Kant and cybernetics, considered subjectivity as a thing, using the same ontological categories adopted to conceptualize objects. Existence was understood as the way of being of a thing, which belongs to that thing just because it was produced; the Self, as the demiurge's box, is what, through the multiplicity of acts, remains identical through time. But what happens if, instead of considering the Self as a thing it is considered as a "who"? Herein lies the phenomenological hermeneutic turn of the current post-rationalism. Inevitably, this consideration changes the perspective of the problem; it is a matter of accounting for the uniqueness of a person, starting from their ways of being, which are no longer reducible or related to the internal dynamics of a system. If there are no longer attributed properties to the being of the subject (like to something that is produced), but ways of being, that, from time to time, the person living in the world feels in this or that way, then there is an ontological difference between the being of a star, the being of a rose, the being of an ape and of a human being. Being a man is thus characterized by possible ways of being, by ways of feeling life: the experience is personal. The single individual is involved each time in their unique possibility of existing, in their projects, in their expectations, in their meetings, in their choices! It is no longer about grasping the Self through an act of reflection, but to grab how "being oneself" is self-aware, is pre-reflexively conscious in its everyday life, in its actual experience, in dealing with this and with that. This new perspective, emerging from the ontological necessity of seizing the person from their ways of being, subtends the big theme of identity, which reintroduces the theme of "who" into actions and feelings in an individual's personal life story. Therefore, telling who a person is implies that each individual's passion and action are understood in a temporal dimension characterized by the permanence of the person, designated by their name, as the same over time. Narrative is here understood as the act under which pre-reflexive experience is reconfigured through language in a plot that, connecting events in a narrative, forms, at the same time, personal identity. Therefore, if the narrative allows a person to recognize their experiences as personal, making self-identification possible, the different variations of a narrative reflect different ways of experiencing life. From these considerations on the relationship between the pre-reflexive dimension and its narrative configuration, a psychological personality typification can be made according to the possible emotional tendencies that settle during a person's life and that are reflected in the construction of one's personal life story. This opens a dialogue with neuroscience research. On the other hand, a therapeutic intervention concerns the appropriation and reconfiguration of one's own experience in a renewed narrative. *[G. Arciero]*

REFERENCES. Arciero G., *Sulle tracce di sé*, 2006; Arciero G., Bondolfi G., *Selfhood, identity and personality styles*, 2009; Bertolino A., Arciero G., Rubino V., Latorre V., De Candia M., Mazzola V. *et al.*, *Variation of human amygdala response during threatening stimuli as a function of 5'HTTLPR genotype and personality style*, in «Biol. Psychiatry», 2005, 57; Campbell D.T., *Evolutionary Epistemology*, in P.A. Schlipp (ed.), *The philosophy of Karl Popper*, 1973; Guidano V.F., *Il sé nel suo divenire*, 1991; Maturana H., Varela F.J., *Autopoiesis and cognition*, 1980; Mazzola V., Latorre V., Petito A., Gentili N. *et al.*, *Affective response to a loved one's pain: Insula activity as function of individual differences*, in «PLoS ONE», 2010, 16; Ricoeur P., *Oneself as another*, 1992; Rubino V., Blasi G., Latorre V., Fazio L., *et al.*, *Activity in medial prefrontal cortex during cognitive evaluation of threatening stimuli as a function of personality style*, in «Brain Res. Bulletin», 2007, 74; Varela F.J., *Principles of biological autonomy*, 1979.

POSTPONING PLEASURABLE COMPULSIONS

This term refers to a technique formulated by G. Nardone in the field of → brief strategic therapy in order to intervene on compulsions based on pleasure, which, differently from those based on fear, are extremely resistant to change and therefore require particular modes of intervention. Amongst these types of compulsions, the most common is that of → vomiting, an evolution of an eating disorder based on the pleasure derived from the ritual of eating in order to vomit. Usually the most common → attempted solution of individuals that are suffering from this disorder is that of trying to control the binges and the vomiting, with the resulting effect of increasing the desire to perform this ritual. As any type of intervention aimed at controlling or repressing the compulsion will generally only serve to increase the strength of the compulsion to eat and then vomit, the technique developed is oriented towards having a direct effect on the pleasurable nature of the ritual. The patient is asked to avoid trying to control the desire to binge, but instead to insert an interval of an hour between the end of the binge and the vomiting, without eating anything else in this time. This prescription interrupts the temporal sequence of the ritual and alters the uncontrollable nature of the pleasure of vomiting. In this way, the therapist will take charge of the symptom through the use of a therapeutic manoeuvre that retains its structure but inverts its meaning, leading it towards self-destruction, thanks to a → change that is geometric-exponential in nature. The interval of time will then be increased to an hour and a half, two hours, until, having reached an interval time of three to four hours, the individual, having already gradually reduced the frequency of the ritual, will gradually cease altogether. By altering the spontaneity of the sequence of eating and vomiting, this technique reduces the pleasure of the liberating act of vomiting, usually experienced as having an urgency that is almost orgasmic in nature, that with the increasing of the interval of time makes it increasingly tiring and unpleasant, transforming it into a form of torture. Besides, in the moment in which the individual stops vomiting, his relationship with food becomes more normal, in the sense that, for fear of putting on weight, the patient ceases to binge and consumes enormous amounts of food. The therapist can in this way proceed, in the course of therapy, to guide the individual towards substituting the void left by the cessation of the ritual with more "healthy" sources of pleasure. *[R. Milanese]*

REFERENCES. Nardone G., Verbitz T., Milanese R., *Prison of food,* 2005; Nardone G., Selekman M.D., *Uscire dalla trappola*, 2011.

POTENCY

In transactional analysis, a verbal and nonverbal communication intervention by the therapist in the relational care process for change aimed at protecting the healthy part of the client – the → Child – from negative intrapsychic parental interference. The effective therapist forms an alliance with the Child of the client to allow him or her to disobey the provocations and injunctions of the introjected → Parent. Together with → protection and → permission, potency is an effective form of modelling for change. *[F. Guglielmotti, R. Leone Guglielmotti]*

REFERENCES. Crossman P., *Permission and protection*, in «Transactional Analysis Bullettin», 1966, 5, 19; Lister-Ford C., *Skill in Transactional analysis: Counselling & psychotherapy*, 2002.

PRAGMATICS OF CHANGE

In the history of psychotherapy, the term "pragmatics" is mostly associated with the landmark contribution of the book *Pragmatics of Human Communication: A Study of Interactional Patterns, Pathologies, and Paradoxes,* authored by Paul Watzlawick, Janet Beavin Bavelas, and Donald D. Jackson. Using semiotics, information theory, and cybernetics, with an emphasis upon the theoretical contributions of anthropologist Gregory Bateson, this work helped define how communication could provide a basis for understanding therapeutic interaction. Here "meaning" (the semantics of communication) is depicted as arising out of (and secondary to) the relations and social interaction of a communicational situation. Though pragmatics is often formally regarded as a subfield of linguistics that addresses the context of the utterance, the brief therapists from the Palo Alto-based → Mental Research Institute broadened its meaning to such an extent that it became a way of emphasizing the nuts-and-bolts practicalities of therapeutic interaction. This emphasis upon the "how" rather than the "why" of transformative communication was later described by Keeney and Ross as the difference between political and semantic frames of communication. Whereas semantics concerns linguistic meaning, politics points to the who-is-doing-what-to-whom-when-where-and-how. The pragmatics of change can be said to address "empirical pragmatics", which is defined by the circumstances of a situation, as distinct from what Habermas calls "formal pragmatics", a reference to the intuitive linguistic knowledge of competent communicative practice.

The pragmatics of change is a call to underscore the communicative performance of a therapist and client. Rather than emphasize interpretation, understanding and narrative – which characterized the originating historical schools of psychotherapy – a pragmatic orientation to therapeutic change aims to bring forth evocations and interactions that facilitate transformation. This shift in perspective – from narrative to drama, or from meaning to performance – was a paradigmatic shift in the organization of therapeutic conduct. Arguably best exemplified by the practical, present-focused clinical strategies of Milton H. Erickson and of the therapists of the Brief Therapy Center (→ Brief Therapy Project; → Mental Research Institute), the pragmatic approach to therapeutic change spawned numerous brief therapeutic approaches (→ brief solution-focused therapy; brief therapy MRI's model; brief strategic therapy Nardone's model) to human problem-solving and conflict resolution. Though it is impossible to have a pragmatics of interaction without inherent contexts of meaning, the early proponents of a pragmatics of therapeutic change often voiced their theoretical presentations in a way that minimized and sometimes overlooked the importance of the reciprocal and recursive relation between meaning and action. This led to decades of dispute between therapy orientations that took sides between emphasizing either interpretative narratives or performed scenarios for inducing change. The dominant perspective of a "pragmatics of change" was challenged by the more encompassing view of systemic aesthetics, an alternative meta-frame for change, that includes pragmatics, first suggested by Gregory Bateson and followed up with Keeney's *Aesthetics of Change*. Here semantics and pragmatics (and their other analogues: meaning and politics, narrative and performance, art and technique) are depicted as a complementary yin–yang-like relationship. The introduction of an aesthetics of change initiated a heated debate in the field of family therapy that arguably resulted in more polarization rather than dialogue among the major schools of therapy. More recently, → creative therapy invites the importance of both aesthetic and pragmatic frames for therapeutic change. *[B. Keeney]*

REFERENCES. Bateson G., *Steps to an ecology of mind: Collected essays in anthropology, psychiatry, evolution, and epistemology*, 1972; Habermas J., *On the pragmatics of communication*, 1998; Keeney B., *Aesthetics of change*, 1983; Keeney B., Ross J., *Mind in therapy: Constructing systemic family therapies*, 1985; Watzlawick P., Beavin J., Jackson D.D., *Pragmatics of human communication: A study of interactional patterns, pathologies, and paradoxes*, 1967.

PRAGMATICS OF HUMAN COMMUNICATION

The application of the field of pragmatics derived from formal linguistics to the field of human interaction. In 1967, Watzlawick, Beavin and Jackson formulated the concept of the "pragmatics of human communication"; this has become a key construct for such a large number of therapeutic approaches that it is not possible to list them all. Based on the contributions of semiotics, of information theory and of → cybernetics, this formulation has led us to better understand the therapeutic process and has made fundamental contributions to the study of therapeutic communication. It deals with an attentive and detailed study of the pragmatic level of human communication, in fact, after having identified the three areas in which human communication takes place: syntax (dealing with all the difficulties related to the encoding and decoding, to channels, to repetition); semantics (dealing with the meaning of the communication for the communicators); and pragmatics (dealing with the behavioural effects of the communication), the study continues by demonstrating how pathological behaviours (psychopathology) do not exist internally to the individual in isolation, but are the result of pathological → interactions between persons. The demonstration of this is based on the following five axioms that have been identified as being fundamental: 1) "One cannot not communicate": a non-behaviour does not exist, and all behaviour that takes place within an interaction contains in itself a communicative message; 2) "Every communication has a content and a → relationship aspect such that the latter classifies the former and is therefore a meta-communication"; in other words, every communicative exchange in transmitting information also establishes a form of relationship defined by the nature of the command (→ injunction); 3) "The nature of a relationship is dependent on the → punctuation of the partners' communication procedures"; in other words the punctuation organizes the behaviour and is fundamental for the interaction; 4)

> Human communication involves both digital and analogic modalities; the numeric → language (in other words digital) has a logical syntax that is very complex and extremely effective, but is lacking in an adequate syntax in the area of relationships, whilst analogic language (in other words using images) has the semantics but does not have an adequate syntax to define in an unambiguous way the nature of relationships:

this would indicate that the numeric aspect of language alone can be insufficient in understanding a communication when there is a problem at a relational level, and that therefore the same message can contain two levels of communication at the same time; 5) "Inter-human communication procedures are either symmetric or complementary, depending on whether the relationship of the partners is based on differences or parity." In the first case the speaker tends to speak at the same level as the other; in the second the behaviour of the speaker complements that of the other such that one will assume a *one-up position* and the other a *one-down position* (→ complementarity; → symmetry). *[F. Cagnoni, J.J. Wittezaele]*

REFERENCES. Watzlawick P., Beavin J.H., Jackson Don D., Watzlawick P., Beavin J.H., Jackson Don D., *Pragmatics of human communication*, 1967.

PRAGMATISM

In psychotherapy, a group of therapeutic models sharing the same metatheoretical framework; these models are coherent with the analogous philosophical tradition – which may be ascribed to Protagoras – established in the United States at the end of the nineteenth century (Ch.S. Peirce, W. James, J. Dewey, G.H. Mead) and continued in twentieth-century Europe by philosophers such as J. Ortega y Gasset, H. Vaihinger, G. Vailati. An important contribution to pragmatic psychotherapies also comes from semiotics, as regards people's interaction mediated by a system of signs (Ch. Morris) and the relation between linguistic acts (J. Austin). The metatheoretical assumptions of pragmatism have also been transferred to some approaches to social sciences – anthropology, sociology, linguistics – through communication theory and action theory. From this wide, coherent metatheoretical framework, pragmatic psychotherapies borrow important theoretical and applicative assumptions, whose core lies in the idea that – socially meaningful – human thought is not restricted to registering reality and facts; on the contrary, it tends to build them through the goal-oriented action of the people involved in personal relationships and the contexts they generate. The statement that "it is the nature of human beings that explains their actions" is substituted by the idea that "it is action that constitutes and explains the nature of human beings. For example, acted roles generate the perception of the world and the correlated feelings". This position is the opposite of the psychological-personological-diagnostic tradition. Another assumption derived from pragmatism is the idea that communication – intended as performative languages, i.e. representational, rhetorical, persuasive and prescriptive utterances – creates the medium that builds the perceptive interpretation of events, that is, the way people attribute sense and meaning to the world. Pragmatism in psychotherapy is a theoretical-applicative perspective that, coherently with its assumptions, diverges from the position of positivism, typical of the academic, behavioural, psychiatric and psychoanalytical tradition of psychology. A feature of this position is the emphasis on linear determinism, etiopathogenesis, observee–observer separation, the ontological realism of psychic entities and diagnostic constructions, the naturalism of rules and norms, the idea that psychic "data" are independent of the "actor-situation" relationship. The position of pragmatism is non-normative, relativistic, conventional, interactionist and constructivist, oriented to problem-solving rather than searching for a cause. Adopted by most recent postmodern perspectives, the individuals postulated by pragmatism are active, semantically interacting, and experience the effects of the realities they produce, which may sometimes turn out to be dysfunctional, or → attempted solutions. The work of P. Watzlawick and his continuers (G. Nardone, J.J. Wittezaele, T. Garcia, etc.) represents the turning point in the transition between positivist psychotherapies and pragmatic psychotherapies, whose central role is played by the communication process: through appropriate guidance, it allows patients to change how they configure the way they emotionally perceive their relationship with themselves, the others and the world. *[A. Salvini]*

PREDICTABILITY

A concept borrowed from the pure sciences to indicate the capacity of a psychotherapeutic model to anticipate the effects or the results of a particular therapeutic intervention on the → patient. If a therapeutic model is structured on the foundation of its predictability, it must be able to predict the outcomes not only between the beginning and the end of therapy, but also for every single technique applied within the therapeutic process. This allows, even in the field of psychotherapy, the formulation of intervention → protocols specific to different types of problems, structured in a sequence of actions the effects of which are predictable. This characteristic, typical of technology, connotes those models of psychotherapy that are more rigorously scientific. *[R.]*

PRESCRIPTION

A therapeutic indication consisting in asking patients to perform specific behaviours and actions towards themselves and/or others, or to implement specific methods of managing emotions and thoughts. Usually, prescriptions are suggested during the session with the therapist and they can be performed during the session itself, or during the interval between sessions as → "homework". The objectives of prescriptions and their various forms can differ depending on the theoretical guidelines followed by the therapist. However, these share the aim of producing a → change at the level of behaviour, emotions and cognition (→ reframing; → corrective emotional experience), which could lead to improvements and the cessation of suffering, and to developing new repertoires of personal skills. *[R]*

▷ In cognitive-behavioural therapy (CBT), a prescription represents an ongoing, systematic, empirical effort to identify specific therapeutic principles and strategies (→ therapeutic strategy) tailored to the unique needs of individual patients. When prescribed appropriately, these principles increase the likelihood of positive change and the magnitude of positive change. CBT is well-suited to the application of an empirically supported prescriptive model. For example, depending upon patient presentation and coping style, CBT may assume a symptom-focused stance (prescribed for externalizers, targeting the most problematic, destabilizing, symptoms) or an insight-focused schema perspective (indicated for internalizers). Patient reactance levels, functional impairment and problem complexity and chronicity are other examples of prescriptive patient dimensions. *[M. Harwood]*

REFERENCES. Baldini F., *Homework: Un'antologia di prescrizioni terapeutiche*, 2004; Dobson K.S., *Handbook of cognitive-behavioural therapies*, 1988.

PRESENT (EXPERIENCE OF)

In the field of Gestalt psychotherapy, attitude towards the focusing of one's awareness on the → here-and-now. It is a fact that we exist, we "are" in the present, at the very least in the experience of seeking greater awareness of oneself and our own → Being-there (*dasein*) in relation to the world. According to Perls

> What exists, exists in the here-and-now; the past exists now only as memory, nostalgia, regret, resentment, fantasy, legend or history. The future exists here and now as anticipation, planning, rehearsal, expectation, and hope or dread and despair. Gestalt psychotherapy is based on the assumption that the present exists only in the here-and-now, not in how it used to be or how it might have been. It is a phenomenological-existential focus to the degree to which it is experience.

Focusing on the here-and-now represents, therefore, the taking back of one's own story, taking on in a responsible way one's own subjectivity and one's own destiny beyond the projections (frequently convenient) with which we like to see ourselves as the victims of others. Quoting Perls once again: "For me nothing exists except the present. Now = experience = awareness = reality. The past is no more and the future is not yet". The focus on the present in Gestalt therapy is aimed at increasing one's awareness as part of the present reality, exploring one's environment and taking the risk of changing one's → behavioural patterns, which have originated in the past and have now become redundant. *[R. Zerbetto, L. Bianchi]*

REFERENCES. Perls F., Hefferline R.F., Goodman P., *Gestalt therapy: Excitement and growth in the human personality*, 1951; Perls L., *Living at the boundary*, 1992.

PRESENT MOMENT

In Gestalt therapy, it is the minimum amount of time required for an → experience to acquire meaning on an existential level. The existential approach is based on the view that "to exist" means to live in the moment, and do it "with meaning": in Gestalt therapy, time is the central theme of human existence. Past, present and future are very different from each other: if the past is gone and the future is not yet present, the → here-and-now is the only time that can influence the direction of one's life, it is the bridge between the past and the future, between motivation and purpose, and it is the only real moment of experience. The present time is the only field of action of free will, the faculty according to which a person may decide, follow a direction and give up the others. As it flows incessantly between past and future, the present time seems to have no measurable dimensions: despite this aspect, it is the only real time, the time of events and the origin of all meaning and value. It is in the present moment that emotions and feelings can be recognized, as they run away with the passing of time: the Gestalt practice brings attention to the → here-and-now to operate therapeutic transformations that open doors to future possibilities. *[P. Quattrini]*

REFERENCES. Heidegger M., *Being and time*, 1962; Lévinas E., *Totality and infinity*, 1961; Naranjo C., *Techniques of gestalt therapy*, 1973; Sini C., *Il silenzio e la parola*, 1989.

PRETEND TECHNIQUE

In family-strategic psychotherapy, a strategic-structural technique proposed by Madanes consisting in inviting a family to accentuate its usual interaction. With this paradoxical method (→logic of paradox) children are encouraged to pretend, acting out their →symptoms, and parents are invited to do the same things they do for them at home. An "acting", without emphasis, is performed, which leads to a *reductio ad absurdum* of the symptoms. Madanes believes that children develop their symptoms to protect parents from their personal concerns and to create a situation in which affection can be expressed: symptoms make parents skillful. The technique of simulating the symptom aims at changing this incongruous family organization. The problem can also be solved without the family being aware of it, without them knowing how and why. *[G. Ganda]*

REFERENCES. Madanes C., *Protection, paradox, and pretending*, 1980; Id., *The prevention of rehospitalization of adolescents and young adults*, 1980; Telfener U., *Le mille vite di Jay Haley: un percorso polifonico*, 2002.

PRIMAL SCENE

Term introduced by Freud to refer to the scene of the sexual relations between parents that the child observes or reconstructs in his fantasy, and which he interprets as an act of violence by the father towards the mother. For the child, this remains enigmatic and incomprehensible, provoking in him anguish and at the same time sexual excitation. Freud started to reason about the primary scene as a result of his investigations into the phenomenon of hysteria. He wanted to show that this derived not from a degeneration, but from a traumatic experience created and preserved as a separate entity; the scope of the investigation is therefore that of "aiming at the primary scenes" that preserve it. At times, the primary scene is arrived at directly, in others only by indirect means, through fantasy, simple "psychological facades of these memories". With the discovery of infantile sexuality, these fantasies acquired the consistency of a psychological process based on the first infantile experiences that are sexual in nature. The objective reality of these experiences is never in doubt, but equally real is the internal psychological processing of this experience. The sexual scene regarding intercourse between the parents is the product of this process; this takes place in two phases – in the moment in which the scene is observed and when, years later, it is reproduced in a dream. The content of the dream reflects the issues related to sexuality and the identity of the infant and the scene described as the original scene takes on an exemplary value of the questioning of oneself. *[P.L. Rossi]*

REFERENCES. Dayan M., *Inconscient et réalité*, 1985; Freud S., *Project for a scientific psychology*, in *The Standard Edition*, I, 1953–1974; Id. (1914), *From the history of an infantile neurosis*, in *The Standard Edition*, XVII, 1953–1974.

PRIMARY AND SECONDARY PROCESSES

In Freudian psychotherapy, the two fundamental modes of the functioning of the psyche. Primary processes characterize the mode of functioning of the mind in the → unconscious and are directed towards the immediate "fulfilment of desire". In the primary process, a mental image representing the fulfilment of the desires of the Id – through the activation of specific psychological processes such as "displacement" and "condensation" – is formed. The functioning of these mechanisms is rendered possible due to the ability of this part of the apparatus of the psyche, psychic energy – also defined as "free energy" – to flow easily from one memory trace to another, in such a way as to highlight those elements that are most adequate for representing any object that appears suited to the → discharge of the accumulated stimulation. The transition from one representation to another follows only associated connections that satisfy the need for the fulfilment of the desire without being limited by considerations relative to the criteria of logic or correspondence to reality, with the exclusive aim of "the repetition of the fulfilment of the first fulfilment experienced".

Primary processes influence the way the → defence mechanisms work in the production of symptoms and are the instruments of the "dream work" in the formation of dreams.

Secondary processes, active in the preconscious and the conscious, connect the libidinal energy to their representations in a stable manner, making it possible to create connections between thoughts and images that correspond to reality and coherent logic. The energy found in this system is defined as "bound energy". In this part of the apparatus of the psyche – that Freud described as the "second system" – over the evolution of time, and with evident advantages in terms of adaptation – the capacity to control the primitive tendency towards the immediate discharge of accumulated energy has developed. This is accomplished through the creation of obstacles to this flow in order, making this energy available for the development of thought and the control of one's actions. Secondary processes therefore allow the activity of the mental functioning that characterizes the conscious level of psychic functioning and that are organized according to the → reality principle: attention, reasoning, judgement and the control of "voluntary movement". These faculties allow the regulation of the individual's activity in the external world and in external relationships, in this way enabling the individual to engage in behaviour that is effective in achieving the desired form of gratification.

The terms "primary" and "secondary" can also be regarded from a genetic perspective, because primary processes are the first to appear during the lifespan of the psyche, preceding the emergence of secondary processes, that are more complex and more stable. As Freud observed: "it is a fact that primary processes are present [. . .] from the beginning, whilst secondary processes only develop gradually [. . .] these inhibit and take over the primary processes, and will fully dominate them, perhaps only with the advent of maturity". *[P. Cruciani]*

REFERENCES. Freud S. (1900–1901), *The interpretation of dreams*, in *The Standard Edition*, IV–V, 1953–1974.

PRIMARY GAIN → SECONDARY GAIN

PRIMING

Term that indicates the facilitation of the responses to a 'target' stimulus, when another stimulus is presented, called prime, that is correlated to it. This phenomenon depends on the setting in motion of an automatic diffuse activation of a semantic net that can take place even when the subject is not aware of the semantic connections that that are present between the "prime" stimulus and the "target" stimulus. *[R.]*

REFERENCES. Làdavas E., Berti A., *Neuropsicologia*, 1995.

PROBLEM SOLVING

This term refers to an English expression that defines those sets of procedures aimed at the solution of problems. There are various models of problem solving that refer to different traditions of the → logic of intervention. Particularly well-known are the cognitive model of problem solving and the strategic model of problem solving. The application of these models of problem-solving techniques to psychotherapy redefines the psychotherapeutic intervention from being viewed as a process of "healing" a disease, typical of the medical model, to a process of resolution and overcoming of psychological suffering, in which the → pathology is viewed as being a problem to be resolved rather than as a disease. *[R.]*

REFERENCES. Haley J., *Problem-solving therapy*, 1976; Meazzini P., *Problemi quotidiani*, 2009; Nardone G., *Problem solving strategico da tasca*, 2009.

PROFLECTION

In Gestalt psychotherapy, this term refers to a manoeuvre in which a person does to another person what he would like to be done to himself. From the perspective of the functions of the self, it can be defined as the opposite of → retroflection in that it describes the presence of excessive "outwards permeability" between the inner and outer worlds. In its dysfunctional aspect it is reminiscent of the pathology of the loss of impulse control. In its positive connotation, it highlights the drive that is necessary to achieve one's goals. *[R. Zerbetto, M. Parmeggiani]*

REFERENCES. Perls F., Hefferline R.F., Goodman P., *Gestalt therapy: Excitement and growth in the human personality*, 1951; Zerbetto R., *Gestalt: la terapia della consapevolezza*, 1998.

PROJECTION

In Gestalt therapy, tendency of the individual to project parts of the self (internal world) onto his environment (external world). Perls defines it a "the tendency to attribute responsibility to the external world of everything that originates from the self". Projection, when it is not a → defence mechanism, allows individuals to develop → empathy, the ability to put themselves into another person's shoes and to be able to predict their behaviour; it becomes a dysfunctional defence mechanism when the individual disregards his own emotions, ideas or parts of the self, alienating himself from them.

This process of disowning parts of the self generally originates from the conscious or unconscious disapproval of them. *[R. Zerbetto, I. Veronesi]*

REFERENCES. Perls F., Hefferline R.F., Goodman P., *Gestalt therapy: Excitement and growth in the human personality*, 1951; Zerbetto R., *Gestalt: la terapia della consapevolezza*, 1998.

PROJECTIVE IDENTIFICATION → DEFENCE MECHANISMS

PROJECTIVE TESTS

A particular type of → personality test, based on the theory that individuals attribute meaning in relation to their own subjective experiences, to the characteristics of their personality and to their own defensive dynamics in situations that are open or ambiguous. Projective techniques consist of stimuli that are not structured (for example an ink blot, as in the Rorschach, or an ambiguous/incomplete situation, as in the Thematic Apperception Test of Murray) that the individual is asked to interpret, complete or restructure. The variable that is being measured through the use of these stimuli cannot be known to the subject, who has to operate in the conviction that there are no right or wrong answers to the questions of the evaluator. *[R.]*

PROTAGONIST

In psychodrama, a person in charge – at certain stages of the session – of the work of the whole group. The protagonist, accompanied by the therapist, with the collaboration of his companions in the role of → auxiliary egos and under the observation of the audience, explores through his action on stage some areas of his inner world, clarifying and correcting the modes of mental functioning that prevent a satisfactory interaction with others. The therapist, at the beginning of the representation, already knows some critical aspects of the protagonist, that need to be submitted to the psychodramatic work; additional elements emerge as the action develops, until the end, when the protagonist will return to the group as an equal member. *[G. Boria]*

REFERENCES. Boria G., *Psicoterapia psicodrammatica. Sviluppi del modello moreniano nel lavoro terapeutico con gruppi di adulti*, 2005; Boria G., Muzzarelli F., *Incontri sulla scena*, 2009; Moreno J.L., *Psychodrama First Volume*, 1946; Id., *Who shall survive?*, 1953.

PROTECTION

In transactional analysis, an empathetic relational modality offered by the therapist to support the change and liberation of the patient from the catastrophic fantasies deriving from transgression and/or parting from the internalized parent. Through the care process, the client is confident that the protection, → potency and → permission of the therapist are more powerful and will protect him from his inner fantasies. *[F. Guglielmotti, R. Leone Guglielmotti]*

REFERENCES. Crossman P., *Permission and protection*, in «Transactional Analysis Bullettin», 1966, 5, 19; Lister-Ford C., *Skill in transactional analysis: Counselling & Psychotherapy*, 2002; Stewart I., Joines V., *T.A. today: A new introduction to transactional analysis*, 1987.

PROTOCOL

In transactional analysis, *locus* where the very first, fundamental unconscious relational experiences of → attachment, prior to language development, are programmed. Implicit memory of nonverbal intersubjective emotional experiences, of a traumatic nature too. It conditions the emotional, cognitive and social life of a person, by colouring the affective quality of his or her future relations. *[F. Guglielmotti, R. Leone Guglielmotti]*

REFERENCES. Berne E., *"Hello!» . . . and then what?*, 1972; Berne E., *What do you say after you say hello?*, 1972.

PSYCHIATRIC DIAGNOSIS

Diagnostic method of *syndromic* type. Since psychiatry has developed using traditional medicine model and praxis, psychiatric diagnosis uses conceptualizations that link psychical disturbances to physical diseases, presuming a hypothetical morphological dysfunction (that is, that symptoms are caused by a bad functioning of the encephalic organ and/or of the central nervous system). It avails itself, then, of a characteristic complex of → symptoms, of which, though, rarely is it possible to individuate a known cause, in a different way to → medical diagnosis, in which the cause of the clinical forms is generally known. For the definition of its syndromic accounts, psychiatry adopts different models: *nosological classifying model*, which divides syndromes in discrete and separated forms; *nosographic describing model*, in which symptoms referring to the whole of syndromes are described (for example in → DSM or in → ICD); *nosographic structural model*, oriented to the analysis of the structural bases of different disturbances, a model used prevalently by psychoanalytical psychiatry, in which diagnosis is functional to psychotherapeutic process. Within all models, nosographic categories have been modified over time. Through psychiatric diagnosis, the methodology of which comes from medical diagnosis, psychiatrists classify and frame symptoms referred by the patient in a diagnostic category, prearranged from the model adopted. From this, the → cure has as its purpose to remove the symptom, although etiology is uncertain and unknown, with the use of drugs, admissions and staying in hospital, trying to recreate a good neurochemical functioning for restoring to health the normal physiology of the organ that is thought to be damaged. Psychiatrists does not cure with psychotherapy, unless they are also psychotherapists. Due to the impossibility of defining objectively the etiology of psychiatric symptoms, psychiatrists do not just execute these peculiar praxes of medicine, but they can perform a diagnosis also using instruments as tests, which are proper to clinical psychology. *[R.]*

PSYCHIATRIZATION

This term refers, on the one hand, to the act of classifying and dealing with psychic suffering and discomfort according to the medical/psychiatric approach; on the other hand, it refers to the related psychological and psychosocial negative effects produced on the subject by this act. The process of assessment of a "mental disease", in accordance with a medical model and a model of diagnostic labelling (→ labelling theory), relates psychological suffering and psychological pain to organic diseases, becoming in this way a tool of social control, which defines the border between normal and pathologic. Throughout an exclusively individual interpretation of disorders, problems are contained at the social level, a mechanism that is behind the process of the blaming of the patient, for example in cases of violation of social and legal regulations, in which the behaviour is encoded as disease or pathology. Psychiatrization can lead to further reductionism, in which the pathology is defined according to the effects of the drugs given for the treatment. The field of psychotherapy has often been subjected to the attempt of psychiatrization of its own action: an example is the attempt to adopt the psychiatric diagnostic *tout court* (→ DSM; → diagnostic manuals) to psychopathology, and the sponsorship and mass distribution of psychopharmacological drugs for any kind of psychological disorder by the pharmaceutical industries. *[R.]*

PSYCHIC INSTANCES → TOPOGRAPHICAL MODEL OF THE MIND → ID → EGO → SUPEREGO

PSYCHIC ORGAN

A biological metaphor used in transactional analysis to describe aspects of human mental activity. Each psychic organ is organized according to two independent functions: inner and phenomenological influences. The following are considered psychic organs: → archeopsyche, → exteropsyche and → neopsyche. An → Ego-state is the phenomenological and behavioural manifestation of a given psychic organ. *[F. Guglielmotti, R. Leone Guglielmotti]*

REFERENCES. Berne E., *Transactional analysis in psychotherapy*, 1961; Holloway W.H., *Transactional analysis: An integrative view*, in P. Scilligo, M.S. Barreca, *Gestalt e Analisi Transazionale*, 1977; Oller-Vallejo J., *Freudian agencies, psychic organs, and ego states*, in «Transactional Analysis Journal», 2006, 36, 1.

PSYCHIC ORGANIZER

A concept elaborated by Spitz to indicate a structure that allows the different components of development to become integrated into the different areas of personality. This is present during critical periods of the development of the infant away from the mother. The restructuring of the psychic system is the result of this integration. Spitz applied new methods of observation and new theoretical perspectives to systems of regulation. The baby is studied, not as an isolated individual, but in his interactions with the mother. A new theory of the Self of the infant was developed by Spitz, who described the serious, at times even fatal, consequences of the lack of an adequate level of mothering care in the early phases of an infant's development. *[L. Longhin]*

REFERENCES. Spitz R.A., *The first year of life*, 1965.

PSYCHIC POLARITIES

In the field of analytical psychology, this term refers to psychological → opposites that are in contrast with one another. Jung considers the psychological tension between opposites as characteristic of the antimony of the human psyche, that finds its equilibrium in its dialectic relationship with opposites. If there is a lack of tension between opposites, there will be no circulation of energy.

> Every psychological extreme has hidden in itself its opposite or is in some way in an intimate and an essential relationship with it. Not only, but it is from the tension inherent in this antithesis that it will derive its particular dynamism.

When the irreconcilable pairs of opposites are experienced as being constantly at the mercy of either one or the other force, and the tension becomes intolerable, then it becomes likely that the individual will experience an → enantiodromia, that is, falling into the polarity that is opposite to the one that is predominant. If the Ego is able to endure the tension caused by the conflict between two opposing forces, a reorganization that is the result of the transcendental function of the symbol becomes possible. This will allow the passage to a different psychological state in which the opposites re-establish a dialectic relationship. The attainment of this reorganization is the objective of therapy. *[A. Benvenuti]*

REFERENCES. Jung C.G. (1912), *Symbols of transformation*, in *Collected Works*, V, 1967; Id. (1916), *The transcendent function*, in *Collected Works*, VIII, 1958.

PSYCHOANALYSIS (FREUD'S)

Form of psychotherapy developed by Freud, and the theoretical framework on which it is based, inspiring its objectives and dictating its mode of application.

> Psychoanalysis is the name of a process of investigation into psychic processes which it would be otherwise impossible to access; of a therapeutic method (based on this investigation) for the treatment of neurotic disorders, the systematic acquisition of knowledge regarding the psyche acquired by means of this method that will gradually assimilate and converge to form a new scientific discipline:
>
> this definition is the one given by Freud himself in 1922 and illustrates the interdependent nature of the relationship between the application of this theory (psychoanalytic technique); the method of investigation on which it is based (psychoanalytic method) ideal for exploring psychic phenomena that would otherwise prove to be inaccessible in that they are unconscious; and the sum total of the empirical knowledge and the theoretical constructs, that are at the same time the result of this investigative process and foundation of the clinical work (psychoanalytic theory).

THE THEORY. The theory and practice of psychoanalysis is based on a number of fundamental assumptions, in particular, the role played by unconscious processes in the life of the psyche of an individual. Basing his thinking on the initial experiences of treating patients suffering from hysteria and other neurotic disorders using → hypnosis, Freud realized that psychopathological symptoms originated from the effects of early infantile trauma that persisted into adulthood, active at an unconscious level and not accessible to memory. He dedicated his monumental work to demonstrating the presence of an unconscious psychological life, towards identifying the way in which these processes take place at an unconscious level, and towards the way in which the products of these unconscious processes, themselves inaccessible to the conscious mind, can be identified in their mental and behavioural manifestations. He postulated that → dreams were the "royal road" to accessing the unconscious, the contents of which ("latent content" of the dream) are manifested – even if in a disguised form – can therefore be decoded through a process of → interpretation of the images of the dream retained in the memory ("manifest content" of the dream). Involuntary errors of language (*lapsus*) and of behaviour *(parapraxis)* were also individuated by Freud as being the outward manifestations of the normal functioning of the psyche, that reveal the workings of the unconscious mind. Psychopathological symptoms are also to be considered in analogous manner, as being the outward manifestations of obscure and deep-rooted manifestation of a compromise made between unconscious tendencies and forces that act against their expression. In fact, psychological disorders (for example, unmotivated fears or phobias, compulsive behaviour, disorders of sexual behaviour and eating disorders, psychosomatic symptoms, etc.) are not considered by him as being bizarre and incomprehensible behaviour or the result of distorted learning processes, but as being the final expression of a compromise that the individual makes, at an unconscious level, in order to avoid the anguish generated by the presence of inner conflicts that also take place at an unconscious level – between the different components of his personality, from the opposition between impulses experienced as being unacceptable (→ Id, in the Freudian sense), and moral prohibition (→ Superego) or aspiration towards achieving idealized models of the self (Ego-Ideals), or conflicts between incompatible representations of the self.

The dynamic and conflictual nature of the psyche is universal, but the presence of a particularly bitter conflict generates anguish, from which the → Ego of the individual, that is, that aspect of the psyche that allows us to adapt to reality and to maintain an intrapsychic equilibrium, defends itself using various unconscious strategies (→ defence mechanisms), by means of which it tries to re-establish a cohabitation that is more balanced between the different forces at work in the unconscious life of the individual. Freud gave primary importance to sexual impulses (→ drive), intended, however, in a wider sense and not corresponding only to genital sexuality, that constitute the forces that, from birth, animate the life of the psyche and the relationship with reality. Other conflicts can be related to aggressive impulses, to the need for security, to the need for dependence and autonomy, to those related to competition and rivalry with others, but also to the simultaneous presence of diverse representations of the Self that are incompatible, and to representations of significant figures of childhood, internalized during the early stages of psychological development. The objective of psychoanalytic treatment is that of understanding, dissolving or attenuating these unconscious conflicts that are at the basis of the different psychopathological manifestations. This objective is achieved by means of specific therapeutic techniques devised by Freud towards the end of the nineteenth century, initially aimed at curing neurotic disorders, but subsequently extended to the treatment of other forms of psychological disturbances, in adulthood and in childhood, by means of therapeutic interventions that are aimed at exploring the unconscious, deep-rooted and archaic causes of the psychological disorder.

THERAPEUTIC TECHNIQUE. Psychoanalytic therapeutic technique takes place by producing a → change in the psychodynamic structure of the individual, who can only reach self-actualization through the acquisition of a better understanding of the nature and meaning of his unconscious psychological processes, made up of impulses, of prohibitions and of aspirations, of self-representations, of his fears and their origins, etc. The psychoanalytic treatment is in practice the research for the truth regarding one's own emotional life that leads to an increase in awareness and interior freedom, the recovery of increased resources on an adaptive level (→ adaptation) and on that of creativity, to the modification of pathological personality traits, as well as the attenuation or disappearance of → symptoms. The process of increased understanding and subsequent change that follow are favoured by → interpretations, or rather by the suggestions and explicative hypotheses given by the psychoanalyst based on what the patient expresses freely during the session (→ free associations technique); the patient is in fact asked, as a fundamental rule of the treatment, to express his thoughts freely and without any reservations, so that, through the connections made whilst the patient is talking freely, elements of the patient's unconscious thoughts and feelings can emerge.

However, the most efficient and powerful means of acquiring knowledge is above all the understanding of the dynamics of the therapeutic relationship that develops between the patient and his therapist. In fact, in psychoanalytic therapy, the interpretations that the therapist makes with reference to the emotional attitudes – in the majority of cases determined by the unconscious – that the patient develops with respect to the therapist and the therapeutic relationship, which reproduce within the relationship the expectations, motivations and ancient conflicts tied to the relationship with significant figures from childhood – above all those with the parents – that make up the deep roots of the present pathology, are considered to be most effective and incisive. This is the phenomenon of → transference, that is, the transfer into the present of relational models of the past. Freud asserted that "no-one can be beaten in *absentia* or from a *picture*", meaning that a substantial and effective change can only be obtained if one acts on what is actually happening in the session. This is done by picking up on the unconscious attitudes of the patient that are the source of maladjustment, involving the figure of the psychoanalyst in their presence during the treatment and by then tracing them back to their ancient origins.

The analytic work, however, aiming at challenging the psychological make-up that the individual has managed to construct for himself, even if this is at the cost of symptoms that are limiting and unpleasant, frequently generates in the patient the fear of being once again exposed to painful experiences; because of this, although at a conscious level he wishes to get rid of these symptomatic manifestations with the help of the psychoanalyst, on an unconscious level the patient will tend to resist the cure in various ways; the psychoanalyst, therefore, has to help the patient to confront his → resistance to change, induced and supported in doing so by the new awareness that the treatment is trying to achieve.

The analysis of the resistances and interpretation of the transference are among the defining characteristics of psychoanalysis, a therapy that is meant to be aimed at achieving a profound change in the structure of the psyche of the individual. Other forms of therapy, although they work within the framework of Freudian theory, and are therefore defined as being psychoanalytic or psychodynamic, tend to try to help the patient primarily through the provision of → support and strengthening of his resources and of his capacity to adapt, whilst seeking to avoid resistance and using the positive collaboration of the patient, without insisting on the analysis of the transference.

The transference, or rather the displacement of the internal world of the patient onto the therapist, is favoured above all by the rules of treatment and by the manner in which the psychoanalyst presents himself and the way he works with the patient (therapeutic → setting): the patient is required to lie down on a couch with the psychoanalyst seated behind him. During the session, the patient is asked to speak freely about everything or anything that comes to his mind without censoring it or having reservations; the psychoanalytic treatment is generally very long (usually lasting a few years) with sessions taking place very frequently (three to five sessions a week); in therapy, the psychoanalyst does not give concrete responses to the patient, such as advice, reassurance, reprimands, and so on. The therapist must instead adopt an attitude of attentive listening and of openness to receiving the communications of the patient, adopting a position of → neutrality. This does not signify a lack of participation and a refusal to be involved but rather a respectful acceptance of all the different parts of the personality of the patient that emerge in the course of treatment. The psychoanalyst, therefore, is present to a very limited extent as a real interlocutor, but works above all by helping the patient to become more aware of the underlying meaning of his behaviour and emotional experiences, in particular those related to transference and that can be traced back to the dynamic of the therapeutic relationship.

In this delicate work, the understanding and elaboration by the therapist of his own emotional reactions generated from his relationship with the patient, (what is usually defined as being → countertransference) plays a very important role in helping him to understand what is happening in the therapeutic relationship and, consequently, acquire a better understanding of the internal world of the patient. However, the correct use by the psychoanalyst of his own emotional responses – this involves making them become an instrument of understanding and not an impulse to act in an uncontrolled manner, as happens usually in real life – is facilitated through the acquisition of a good level of self-awareness about one's own internal world, that can be acquired and developed through a personal experience of psychoanalysis. The practice of psychoanalysis, in fact, requires a long period of training, characterized not only by a long period of theoretical preparation as well as a prolonged period of training in the practice of the therapeutic techniques under the guidance of expert psychoanalysts, but also by a long period of personal psychoanalytic treatment (→ didactic analysis). This in-depth and demanding training, is necessary in order to guarantee not only the acquisition of technical abilities but also of an adequate capacity to handle the emotional dynamics of therapy, at times particularly intense, that take place in a relationship that is as engrossing as the psychoanalytic one. This kind of training takes place at the different training institutes of the Society of Psychoanalysis, found in various countries, that are all affiliated to the International Psychoanalytic Association, founded by Freud himself in 1910. *[N.Rossi]*

REFERENCES. Di Chiara G., *Curare con la psicoanalisi. Percorsi e strategie*, 2003; Etchegoyen R.H., *The fundamentals of psychoanalytic technique*, 1990; Freud S., *The Standard Edition*, I–XXIV, 1953–1974; Id. (1912), *The dynamics of transference*, in *The Standard Edition*, XII, 1953–1974; Id. (1923), *Two encyclopaedia articles*, in *The standard Edition*, XVIII, 1953–1974; Laplance J., Pontalis J-B., *The language of psychoanalysis*, 1988; Musatti C.L., *Trattato di Psicoanalisi*, 1950; Id., *Freud. Con antologia freudiana*, 1964; Semi A.A. (ed.), *Trattato di Psicoanalisi*, 1988–1989.

PSYCHOANALYSIS (KLEIN AND BION'S)

Psychoanalytic theories by M. Klein and W.R. Bion are commonly associated because they converge on three basic points: the centrality of anguish in the development of the inner world; the primary splitting of the objects and of the Ego in the → paranoid–schizoid position; and the process of integration between good and bad breast (→ good breast/bad breast) that brings one to the second position, the depressive one. It is important to remember, anyway, that Klein, differently from S. Freud, places earlier – in child development – the mental representation of the Oedipus scenery and, consequently, the development of the Superego. It is on the role of the projective identification (→ defence mechanism) – one of the cornerstones of the Kleinian clinic – that the work of Bion proposes a more articulated development than the former one by Klein. In fact, according to Klein, projective identification is the mechanism allowing a person to project the paranoid–schizoid anguish into external objects, so that one can be free from them and control and attack them in an external object. Instead, Bion notices that the first object onto which the breast-fed baby projects his anguish is the mother's mind, which is therefore destined to elaborate the received projections and to offer them back to the child in the form of tolerable objects. The passage to the depressive position can take place if there is a motherly function, capable of tolerating the instinctual dimension of the breast-fed baby and gradually giving suitable answers. So, if for Klein, the passage takes place with the integration of the split parts, for Bion it is possible only by an oscillation between the first and the second position, indicated by the symbol Ps↔D. Also, for Klein, the word "position" is destined to indicate a type of status that is not in evolution, but which is qualitative; nevertheless, Bion focuses his attention on this datum and considers the oscillation not only possible, but necessary for the elaboration of a thought. Therefore, in the relationship between mother and child, a relation between "a content" and a "container" is outlined: this represents a fundamental feature of Bion's way of thinking. Such a relationship may take different shapes (symbiotic, convivial, parasitical), but it will be, anyway, possible, unless an overwhelming dominance by the container or the content occurs; this would lead to the destruction of the relationship itself. Furthermore, the relationship is only possible if continuous modification/destruction of the previous setting is tolerable. The psychoanalytic work, performed by the couple analysand–analyst (even in this case we have an enlargement and a modification of the Kleinian conception concerning transference and its employment in the therapeutic job), largely coincides with the capacity of tolerating the anguish coming from the necessity of facing objects and relationships that had not been observed in advance, without the feelings connected to are immediately acted out or expelled. If Kleinian theory appears as non-developmental, for Bion the progressive passages leading to awareness are always the result of a difficulty that can be overcome or not. The difficulty, rooted in everyday life, represents for Bion, a continuous challenge to the functioning of the human mind, which, for definition, escapes from the fatigue of "thinking" painful experiences. The demonstrations of violence, intolerance, disruptive aggressiveness, for instance, show simplified and reassuring solutions, when one is face-to-face with complexity: they are a way to free oneself from a problem through an action. In this sense, Bion sees behaviour turned to an immediate solution as psychotic mental functioning. A problem can be faced and, in this way, it is possible to modify the profile of the problem itself: If this were possible, the "solution" would be the leasing of a projective functioning. If a patient, Bion states, sees the room where therapy is set, full of blood, it is useless to tell him that it is not true; it is necessary to assume his point of view and try to understand why that room is full of blood for him. What stands at the origin of anguish is never reachable, since it is the mark, according to Kleinian theory, of the original separation from the breast; such an event establishes human existence. What produces the anguish can be thought of as an ultimate origin, O. Such a symbol, adopted by Bion, may be read both as the initial letter of the word Origin, or as the number zero at the origin of Cartesian axes. The concept of O, that is analogous to the "thing-in-self" by I. Kant, also represents something constantly attracting and which is able to overcome every barrier: anyway, O is destined to be transformed, but never reached. With O and its transformation, Bion, on the same line traced by Klein, proposes again the decisive importance of the death drive, that is intended, as Freud did, as a state of serenity preceding life, compared to which the latter is a temporary solution of continuity. The transformations of O are necessary, as they make it intelligible and tolerable: of course, the transformation distorts O, but this is the only way one has of tolerating anguish. The transformation of O would be a "catastrophic change" that would precipitate the subject into a psychosis, in case the symbol T (indicating the processes of transformation) were absent. Such an occurrence would cause the impossibility of distinguishing oneself from O, that is, from an original situation of anguish. On the contrary, the transformation of O is different: this, just to give an example, is the same as the painter who when, wanting to represent – in perspective – a round lake, would paint an ellipse, as a matter of fact. Hence, O coincides with a "truth" too difficult to be tolerated and that requires a certain degree of distortion (the neurosis) to be held up. The process is similar, Bion states, to the establishing of the atmosphere surrounding the Earth: it distorts solar rays (that would otherwise burn us) and makes them not only tolerable but even beneficial. The mother who cures the baby, notices Bion, "elaborates" (or she accomplishes a T) the feeling of anguish of the baby, and gives it back to him in a tolerable form. Such a capacity of cleaning something unknown and menacing – indicated by Bion as elements – so that it can be made tolerable, is defined by him as a function. In agreement with Klein, Bion does not ignore that the cleaning function of the breast can give rise to feelings of gratitude, even of envy. The "constant conjunction" that determines the relationship between a container and a contained brings into action the feelings deriving from the drive, that may be ties of L (love) and H (hate). In the commensal relationship between container and contained, both of them are oriented towards learning and this establishes a knowledge link, that is, K (knowledge), indicating the capacity of apprehending and of understanding the links L and H. If the envy towards the breast prevails, the links L, H and K become the negative of themselves, but for instance, -L does not become H and vice versa. As suggested by Melzer, what happens is the "disassembly" of the constant conjunctions. Such an occurrence, might bring to behaviour – Bion does not give precise examples on this matter – such as puritan conventionality (-L), the pretence of harmony (hypocrisy) (- H), and finally the imperviousness to what is new, as it occurs with philistinism (-K). Along the path of the transformation, that is, during the analytic work, O may become, in an incessant process, knowledge (K), even its destruction, that is H. The disciple of Klein, H. Segal, has shown in an emblematic way, how some patients destroy the interpretation made by the analyst just to remain in a feeling of triumph over the analyst himself: this is precisely the destructive role that envy has in the Kleinian theory. The transformation of O requires that something belonging to O or to the feeling that O evokes, or to a preceding transformation, is maintained (according to the lexicon used by Bion, these are the "invariants") both in a direct form (in this case we have the so-called transformations "in rigid movement"), or in more complex ways: in this case we have the so-called "projective" transformations. Bion here proposes, again, the dialectic model of Heraclitus and K. Marx, according to which the repetition is never exactly the same; even in the most linear transformation into a rigid movement, something is conserved and something else is destroyed. Hence, we have not only the possibility of a "catastrophic change", but one can easily evince that every transformation causes the fading of what existed before: Bion, in fact, distinguishes between T1, T2 . . . Tn transformations. In the original Greek meaning, *katastrophè* means "upheaval", or "overturning", and only in a transference way; it has also the meaning of "disaster" or "radical destruction". What follows is that the only possibility there is to face what is unknown (the Freudian *Unheimlich*) is to transform it progressively (we can think that transformations for Bion are the equivalent of the activity of symbolization for Klein), but, to do it, it is necessary, in the meantime, to overcome and save (as happens in the *Aufhebung* of the dialectics in Hegel) the preceding transformation. During the transformation in analysis, O may produce knowledge (overturning), but the transformation may cause the destruction of the relationship container–contained, bringing it to complete annihilation (transformation into O). The transformations into knowledge appear as elaborations of something that existed before, the O or the previous transformations, that Bion – ingeniously – indicates are thoughts waiting for a thinker or "thoughts not yet thought". So far, mind is definable as an "apparatus to think thoughts", which can elaborate the truth, or can fail in this painful and difficult work. Synthesizing his own thought, Bion writes, in *Memory of the Future*, that the analytic work is the best we make of a bad job. *[A. Voltolin]*

REFERENCES. Anderson R. (ed.), *Clinical lectures on Klein and Bion*, 1992; Grinberg L., Sor D., Tabak de Bianchedi E. *Introduccion a las ideas de Bion* 1972; Grotstein J., *A beam of intense darkness*, 2007; Meltzer D. *The Kleinian development, 3*, 1978; Meltzer D. *Studies in extended metapsychology*, 1986.

PSYCHOANALYSIS (INDEPENDENT OR MIDDLE GROUP OF BRITISH ANALYSTS)

Initially called the "Middle Group" (that is, situated between the Kleinians and the Freudians), the school of thought of the Independents was born in the British Psychoanalytic Association during the "Controversial Discussions" of 1942 (with the British Society on the verge of internal division), but was officially inaugurated only two years later, with the introduction of the new statute. The birth of the Independent school of thought can be traced to a letter by J. Strachey to E. Glover, where Strachey expresses his preoccupation regarding the conflict that was taking place: the so-called "war of the two dames" (Anna Freud and Melanie Klein). Alarmed by the doctrinal extremism of both parties that was more a religious war than a scientific debate, Strachey, in the tradition of British Empiricism, called for a free discussion at a theoretical level and a reasonable compromise between gentlemen on the practical level. Various psychoanalysts such as S. Payne, E. Freeman Sharpe, Balint, Bowlby and others, sympathetic to his concerns, intervened in the discussion in a very balanced manner. They argued that it was possible to "partly" uphold Klein's theory and "partly" Freud's theory, without the necessity of defining oneself as being "Kleinian" on the one hand or as being "Orthodox" on the other, and that one could be free to propose further elaboration and integration of these theories, based on reason and experience. Having avoided an internal division, the statute instituted three different schools of thought, resulting in three different training programmes: Kleinian (A), (Anna) Freudian (B) and the so-called "middle group" (C). For the purposes of training, it was agreed that every trainee from group A or B would have one of the two supervisors that were from group (C). The name Middle Group was then substituted for Independents, in order to avoid defining themselves in relation to others, but also to assert the intellectual independence, not only of the group but also of the individual members. The Independents played an important role in the Tavistock Clinic of London, presided over by J.D Sutherland (1948–1968).

THE INDEPENDENT MIND. A "doctrine" of the Independents does not exist. However, this school of thought did have convergent ideas and a common mentality (Rayner called it "Independent Mind"), that were not wholly the "object relations theory", but that lay at its roots. In particular, all members of this school of thought agreed on Fairburn's revision of the concept of → drive, as being "directed towards the object", in view of a qualitatively determined relationship and not as being "directed towards the experiencing of pleasure", in view of a pure and simple release of accumulated tension (as asserted by S. Freud). They all, therefore, put into perspective the Freudian emphasis on sexuality and the rigid association between drive and erogenous zones. They reformulated the → Oedipus complex in terms of a defence against ambivalence emerging in the phase of transition from the "mother–baby" dyad to the family "triangle". In the same way, they were distrustful of the Freudian concept of "death instinct", considered to be lacking empirical support; even less did they support the typically Kleinian idea that every conflict can be reduced to the tension between libido and death instinct. As a result of this, although in agreement with Klein in considering envy as being an archaic and destructive emotion at the basis of many pathologies, they refused to consider it as being a drive in itself and as the innate expression of the death instinct. They viewed it, rather, as the "product of the disintegration" of the instinctual drives and as a reaction conditioned by the response to these drives. In common with the Kleinians, they also put an emphasis on the pre-Oedipus Complex and on unconscious fantasies as the cause of psychopathology; but they considered the relationship of the Ego with the "internal objects" (that these fantasies depict) as being a defensive deformation, and, so to speak, the shadow of real relationships in the external world, usually generated by the failure of the relationship with the "primary figures": in the mother–baby dyad (Winnicott) and in the first attachment relationships (Bowlby). In fact, what is "internalized", according to the Independents, are not so much the "objects" in which one has invested emotionally, but the "object relations" with significant figures or with aspects of these. This has various consequences: they viewed the splitting of internal objects and the existence of disassociated relationships with individual aspects of the self as leading inevitably to the splitting of the Ego and/or the disassociation of the Self, which would impact negatively the ability of the person to establish healthy relationships. In other words: they viewed internalized object relations act as being a form of intersubject relationship with the external world. Therefore, according to them, the → repetition compulsion (that Freud interpreted as a manifestation of the death instinct) had to be understood as the pathological outcome of conditioned learning from infantile experiences and as an automatic representation of defences erected as a response to some traumatic experience (single traumatic episode or many micro-traumas experienced in relation to primary carers). On a more general note, psychanalysis, conceptualized by Freud as a one-body psychology was reconceptualized as a two-person psychology and as being open to confrontation: on the theoretical front, with empirical psychology and any other behavioural science; on the clinical front, with the patient having a real and complex relationship with the psychoanalyst (that goes beyond simple → transference).

CONCORDANCE OF TECHNIQUE AND CLINICAL STYLE. Even more than theoretical convergence, the British Independents where in agreement on the practical level regarding technique and clinical style. They believed, in fact, that for therapeutic purposes, the nature of the analyst–patient relationship is at least as important as the → interpretations; particularly when one is not dealing with minor conflicts, but with the process of repairing wounded structures at the heart of the psyche. Therefore, when dealing with a "schizoid Ego" (Fairbairn), an "Ego regressed to the womb" (Guntrip), a "basic fault", that is, a "primary defect" (Balint), a → false Self (Winnicott), a "perverted Self" (Khan) or forms of "insecure attachment" (Bowlby) the analyst must not rush to make interpretations, because premature interpretation of the primary defences, in particular those related to destructive attacks against internal objects (typical of Kleinian processes), are systematically misunderstood by the patient and interpreted as being rebukes or, at best, experienced as being the traumatic imposition of categories from the analyst-adult to the patient-infant. This has a negative effect on the relationship and pushes the patient towards adopting conformist simulations/dissimulations that will reinforce the "false Self" and interrupt the regressive process.

For many patients, especially those having a "basic fault" (to be intended as an objective "defect" and not as a subjective "feeling of guilt"), a prolonged and profound regression within a secure relationship appears to be necessary for the analytic process. Only by internalizing the substitute relationship (that is, one that is different to the pathological relationships experienced in the past) is it possible to re-integrate parts of the Self that have been split or disassociated. This "secure relationship", under whose shelter old fears can be revisited and overcome, is called → holding, that is, containment (Winnicott, Bowlby): a term that evokes the image of a baby in the arms of his mother. Analogously, the Kleinian school of thought (W.R. Bion, D. Melzer), influenced by the Independents, viewed the holding as being a fundamental aspect in every relationship → container–contained and, therefore, for the development of the capacity to "mentalize" (→ mentalization). This does not mean that the relationship with the patient has to be naively "selfless", otherwise it can result in the patient experiencing a "malignant regression" that cannot be utilized within the therapeutic context, rather than favouring a "benign regression" (Balint). The Independents are, for this reason, as respectful of neutrality and abstinence as the Orthodox Freudians, although in a different and less distant manner. The Independent analyst seeks to be neither rigid nor self-sacrificing, but presents himself as a "sufficiently good therapist" (Malan) similar to the concept of the → good-enough mother (Winnicott), that promotes growth but also allows for distance. So as to be able to calibrate the quality of the relationship, the importance of the → countertransference is acknowledged, but, in contrast with the Kleinians, they refused to consider it as being only a form of "projective counter-identification" (emotional content "fed into the patient by the analyst"). For the Independents, feelings emerging from the countertransference are also a reflection of the nature of the real relationship taking place within therapy, for which both the patient and the therapist are both responsible. In spite of the emphasis on the nature of the relationship, interpretation (drive, anguish, defence) is also considered by them as being important. Malan insisted on the necessity of re-examining at the very least the principal conflict several times at every level (in the present, in the past, in the transference): no "dynamic psychotherapy" can consider itself as being concluded if this practice has not taken place. In fact, for them, interpretation starts from the holding and support for the capacity for mental representations, but also has the function of consolidating, on the cognitive level, what the patient has acquired on the emotional level; in this way they change the self-representation of the patient in the Ego. Moreover, certain interpretations, (for example of envy and of destructive acts), although necessary, require the analyst to pay special attention to the timing of the interpretation and to its wording. *[L. Symington]*

CONTRIBUTIONS OF INDIVIDUAL "INDEPENDENTS". Amongst the specific contributions of individual authors of this school of thought, one cannot but mention : the "schizoid position" of Fairbairn (as an alternative to the concept of the → "schizoid–paranoid position" put forward by Klein); the concept of the mother as not only being an "object" but also an "environment" (Winnicott) and as the source of every infantile representation of the world (Balint); the so-called failure of the "primary love" that Balint himself viewed as the origin of the basic fault, and the polarities of character to be found in the states of "ocnophilia/philobatism" (need for/ fear of proximity with the love-object) as the alternative outcome of this failure. Additionally, the Winnicottian notion of the "real Self/false Self" and "transitional object"; Khan's analysis of the different forms of perversions, in particular the concept of the fetish as being a false and deformed version of the transitional object; → attachment theory (secure, resistant, avoidant, disorganized) put forward by Bowlby in an area somewhere in-between psychoanalysis and ethology, and developed in his footsteps by M. Main and M.D.S. Ainsworth. *[S. Caruso]*

REFERENCES. Balint M., *Primary love and psycho-analytic technique*, 1953; Id., *The basic fault: Therapeutic aspects of regression*, 1979; Bowlby J., *Attachment and loss. Vol.1: Attachment*, 1969; Id., *Attachment and loss. Vol.2: Separation*, 1972; Id. *Attachment and loss. Vol.3: Sadness and depression*, 1969; Fairbairn W.R.D., *Psychoanalytic studies of the personality*, 1952; Guntrip H., *Personality structure and human interaction*, 1961; Khan M., *The privacy of the self*, 1974; Id., *Alienation in perversions*, 1979; Id., *Hidden selves*, 1983; Kohon G. (ed.), *The British School of Psycho-Analysis: The Independent tradition*, 1986; Malan D.H., *Individual psychotherapy and the science of psychodynamics*, 1979; Rayner E., *The Independent mind in British psychoanalysis*, 1991; Winnicott D.W., *Through paediatrics to psychoanalysis*, 1958.

PSYCHOANALYSIS (LACAN'S)

Jacques Lacan has always declared himself "Freudian", the term he used to name the school he founded (École freudienne de Paris). He has always believed that if post-freudians followed the standard cure model promoted by Freud, they did not follow its spirit: according to Lacan, the direction of the treatment is without standard, but not without principles. And this is the reason of his return to Freud. Unlike post-freudians, Lacan considered that it would not have been sufficient to follow standards in order to name psychoanalytic an experience of the word. His rejection of the standard fixed time of sessions was the ground for his "major excommunication" by the International Psychoanalytic Association. According to Lacan, the principle from which an analysis begins is the taking into account of the formations of the unconscious, and a conducting of the treatment in adherence to the status of the unconscious itself. The fundamental principle is that the only medium of treatment is the word. Nevertheless, not any word, but a word that strictly adheres to what Freud has called the fundamental rule: the patient "must say everything that comes into his head, no matter how unpleasant, irrelevant or senseless" it may be. Lacan emphasizes the reversal between thinking and saying. The analytical treatment is made possible only by following the opposite of what is actually done in life, where one thinks before speaking, while in analysis one must let go and speak, thus having an effect on thinking itself. This reversal favours the patient's acceptance of the symbolic order and its functioning, a *sine qua non* condition for all analytic treatments. The patient will then recognize that his symptom tells a truth that upsets him, a truth that he ignores and about which he wants to know nothing. In Lacan's words, "the symptom is the [→] signifier of a [→] signified that has been repressed from the subject's consciousness". Another fundamental principle: what the patient says must be expressed in the presence of another person who can become the standard-bearer of the unconscious. This is the function of the analyst, a function that requires not only his word but also his presence in flesh and blood. Lacan has strongly insisted that he who believes himself able to fulfil this function must have elaborated his subjective position so far as to have reached a logical end to his personal analysis and must have taken responsibility for the act he makes as an analyst. Hence, here is Lacan's aphorism: "a psychoanalyst authorizes himself only by himself", a famously misunderstood sentence if left out of context, which refers to personal responsibility and that of other analysts (the School), since "only the analyst, not anyone else, authorizes himself". A psychoanalysis starts from the demand of a person who is suffering either in the body or in the mind, a necessary condition, but not a sufficient one. In fact, it is necessary that such a question be not only a simple request for help which other professionals could answer. The demand for analysis differs from the request for help, because it involves the hypothesis made by the patient that the symptom he is suffering, because of its repetition, must have some significance, even if he does not understand its meaning. This is what drives one to speak to an analyst. It is up to the analyst to first verify the patient's hypothesis and make sure that the symptom he complains about be not only of a medical nature. Moreover, even when the symptom is clearly of a psychic nature, it is necessary to make it analyzable. To this aim, it is necessary that the patient recognizes a personal implication in his symptom. Therefore, it is not enough to complain about it or to lay the responsibility on someone else, family members or others, whatever the suffered traumas may be; because the subject does suffer his symptom, but at the same time is pleased with it in such a way that he is not able to get away from it. Lacan calls this pain that grips the subject and that he cannot do without, *jouissance* (enjoyment). At the beginning of a treatment, it is essential to trace the two faces of the symptom: the representation face, where the symptom appears as a subject's metaphor and the enjoyment face, which is the cause of the symptomatic repetition. In order to bring out such a subjective implication, the analyst provides a series of sessions intended to be preliminary to the actual beginning of the cure. These preliminary sessions (Lacan's true innovation) are carried on for as long as necessary. During this preliminary period, the patient rebuilds the cartography of the various moments of the struggle he has undertaken and is still undertaking against that driving force that, although familiar, gives him no rest, but rises above him, dominates and defeats him with regular repetition. By recalling a Hegelien figure, Lacan talks about revealing to the patient, as Freud did with Dora, his position of "beautiful soul". In so doing, the analyst operates a "rectification of the subject's relations with reality (*réel*)" that has the power to put the unconscious at work and to encourage the emergency of → transference. The activation of the unconscious is produced by the encounter between the symptom, as the subject's transferal → signified, and the analyst himself who is the → signifier to which the demand is addressed. The analyst is not the one who knows, but the one who, being invested from his patient's unconscious, operates by running the "subject supposed to know", which is the Lacanian name for unconscious, which appears in the mobilization of removed signifiers, who are always related to the field of libidinal investments, thus having them emerge in unconscious formations (dreams, lapses, faulty acts, wits and so on). This mobilization is synthesized in the Lacanian aphorism "the unconscious is structured as a language". But this aphorism does not say everything. In fact, the unconscious that functions "as" a language – and that produces symptoms that speak, dreams to be interpreted and so on – circumscribes a "real unconscious", which is, for every human being, the left nucleus of jouissance that may reveal itself as a source of invention and creation. In treatment, the "subject supposed to know" is the pivot of the transference, which is the love directed to the "unconscious knowledge". The duty of the analyst answers to the work of the patient, whom Lacan calls the analysand, because he is the one doing the work. In fact, the analyst is not the one who gives meaning to the symptoms, dreams and other unconscious formations, as this would be giving fodder to the unconscious, while the purpose of analysis is to force the unconscious to express its reasons, to allow the analysand to properly decipher those hieroglyphics that are his symptoms and to grasp that nucleus of jouissance that Lacan calls the object a. The object a is not situated in front, but "behind" the desire. It is not the object that the desire tends to, but the object that causes it: to the oral and anal objects, Lacan adds the gaze, the voice and the "nothing". For Lacan, it is the analysand who interprets, with the help of the analyst who encourages and brings out the interpretation by underlining, punctuating and cutting, always guided by that essential function of the treatment that Lacan calls "the analyst's desire". The analyst's desire is the function that guides every analyst, one by one, so that the analytical operation proceeds according to "the ethics of psychoanalysis". Freud thought that analysis was suitable for neurotics (→ neurosis). We now know that the analytical experience is not precluded either to psychotics (→ psychosis) or to perverts. However, the analyst must be able to identify the structure of the patient – neurosis, psychosis, perversion; not to give him a label, but in order to operate in an appropriate way. The analysis could indeed turn out negatively for the psychotic if the psychoanalyst (given a badly calculated manoeuvre) let himself be invested by the function of the "subject supposed to know" on an axis with the function of the Other: evil and persecutor. In this case, there would be a favourable conjuncture that could bring about an outbreak of psychosis. It must be stated that generally the pervert prefers to execute his fantasy in reality, rather than seeing an analyst to elaborate it. Most of the so-called perverts who are driven to analysis are in reality neurotics or psychotics with some traits of perversion that are functional for themselves. How do analyses end? Lacan gave different formulations, which are not in contradiction with each other. The first and the simplest one is that analysis ends when "the analysand thinks he's happy with his life". Concretely, this occurs when his conscious will agrees with his unconscious desire. Other formulations are to be considered, especially those that seek to specify in logical terms the end of the analysis, essential for those who authorize themselves as analysts. A formulation concerns the logic rendering of the subject being "nothing"; another states it in the so-called crossing of the fantasy where the analysand takes the articulated value between the phallic function and the obstructing imaginary object. In a third and final formulation, Lacan emphasizes the metamorphosis that takes place in the symptom itself, which reveals the face of an enjoyment that is now a sign of the subject knowing how to deal with the drive, and that is what Lacan called "*sinthome*", thus using the ancient French and Italian spelling. *[A. Di Ciaccia]*

REFERENCES. Freud S. (1909), *Notes upon a case of obsessional neurosis*, in *The Standard Edition*, X, 1974; Lacan J. (1953), *The function and field of speech and language in psychoanalysis*, in *Écrits*, I, 1974; Id. (1957), *The instance of the letter in the unconscious or reason since Freud*, in *Écrits*, I, 2006; Id. (1958), *The direction of the treatprogressment and the principles of its power*, in *Écrits*, 2006; Id. (1967), *Proposition of 9 October 1967 on the psychoanalyst of the School*, in «Scilicet», 1977, 1–4; Id. (1973), *Television*, in *Television: A challenge to the psychoanalytic establishment*, 1990, 45; Id (1975), *Conférences et entretiens dans des universités nord-américaines*, in «Scilicet», 1976, 6–7; Id. (1959–1960), *The seminar, Book VII, The ethics of psychoanalysis*, 1992; Id. (1960–1961), *Le séminaire. Livre VIII, Le transfert*, 1991; Id. (1962–1963), *Le séminaire, Livre X. L'Angoisse*, 2004; Id. (1964), *Le Sèminaire, Livre XI, Les quatre concepts fondamentaux de la psychanalyse*, 2003; Id. (1975–1976), *Le séminaire. Livre XXIII, Le sinthome*, 2005; Miller J.A., *L'inconscio reale*, in «La psicoanalisi», 2007–2008, 42–44.

PSYCHODRAMA

A brief premise regarding the term "psychodrama": in Italian the word "drama" is associated more with tragedy than it is with comedy, more with problems rather than their solution. On the contrary, in English, the suffix of the word psychodrama, which is "drama", is closer in meaning to that of the ancient Greek from which it is derived ("action"), and means "theatre". For this reason, in Italy today, the old translation of psychodrama has now been replaced with the denomination "psychoplay", a term that is able to better convey the optimistic style of this therapeutic method that is based on play, theatrical action and group encounters. The two terms (psychodrama and psychoplay) can therefore be considered as being interchangeable.

This therapeutic and expressive formula was introduced at the beginning of the nineteenth century by one of the founding fathers of group psychotherapy, Moreno, doctor and sociologist, author of other therapeutic forms such as socioplay, → sociometry, the action-methods and → role playing. Moreno had the courage to propose, at the time and in the city of S. Freud, an → interpersonal model of psychopathology and psychotherapy. His interpersonal approach to the origin and the resolution of conflict (as opposed to the intrapersonal approach of Freud) was so innovative that (with psychodrama *in situ*) it even foresaw the possibility of transferring the → setting from the medical clinic to the real environment and to the real groups in which patients lived. This proposal, which, within a few decades would influence other models of the psyche, started in Vienna. Moreno, a young, unconventional doctor, used to cure his patients free of charge and recounts that he had gone through a "theological syndrome" that, in an era of atheism and agnosticism, led him to embrace the ideal of "I–God", from the work of the philosopher and theologist M. Buber, that gave life to the "Theatre of Spontaneity" (*Das Stegreiftheater*). The new formula combined encounter and representation and contrasts with the rigid conventions of a society that was in deep political and cultural crisis. "My attraction to the idea of God," asserts Moreno,

> started in early childhood. The most important Being in the universe was God and I liked being tied to him. The first session of psychodrama took place when I played the part of God at the age of five years in 1894.

Moreno held his first session of the "Theatre of Spontaneity" in Vienna, in 1922, a year after the stormy first night of *Sei personaggi in cerca d'autore* of Pirandello, in Rome. The Theatre of Spontaneity" is an improvised theatre, without script or actors, that invites the spectators to get on the stage to act out the events of the day. Psychoplay, in Moreno's formulation, is not only a modern invention, with its own theory and technique, but represents the discovery of the archetype of the theatre itself; theatre in its purest state, that is accessible to everyone, not only actors, in a revolution that is both cultural and psychiatric. The model is articulated thanks to the concepts of role, social atom, creative spontaneity, → *tele* (the empathic understanding between two people, at the opposite end of → transference). With hindsight, the meaning of the proposals put forth by Moreno lies in the fact that he revolutionized the meaning of → catharsis, a term referred to by Aristotle in his *Poetics*. In contrast with what happens normally in a theatre, every spectator has, in psychoplay, his own personal catharsis, that ranges from being a spectator to being an actor on the stage where he is able to act out his history, thoughts and feelings. Another historical first by Moreno (that will be confirmed and given technical support through the interactivity of the internet) is the proposal to apply psychoplay to visual recording techniques and even transmission on television. In this way, a "Theatre of Time" is born, that extends the group participation to thousands of people.

At the beginning of the twentieth century, psychoplay, thanks to the interchangeable nature of the roles activated by play and by group dynamics, aimed at transforming every spectator into a playwright, producer and actor in their own life. A similar objective also characterizes sociodrama (or socioplay), that, instead of treating every single patient in the group, works on the problems of all the members of a "real" group, where the members share social, racial, political, economic, cultural problems on a small or vast scale. The analogies and the synchronicity of this revolution with the theatre of Pirandello are striking, most of all with the trilogy of the "theatre within the theatre": *Sei personaggi in cerca d'autore* (1921*), Ciascuno a suo modo* (1924) and *Questa sera si recita a soggetto* (1929). However, Moreno distinguishes psychoplay from the enactment of a scene in a psychological drama such as those of Ibsen, O'Neill or Chekhov. He also distinguishes it from "theatre-therapy", intended as a creative work that is rehearsed and then acted out in a theatre in the form of a show.

From a technical point of view, a classical psychoplay is carried out in different stages: starting from the organization of the space and of the instruments, the introduction of the leader and the members of the group; the warming up that, as a starting ritual, helps the members of a group overcome social barriers; the entering into a dimension that offers the patients space and the possibility of touching, seeing, participating, imagining, travelling in time; the choice of the first protagonist of the session; the description of the roles and the assigning of roles to different members of the group; and finally, the play itself, made up of role reversals, doubling and other therapeutic techniques that continue until the protagonist, with the help of the therapist, has completed his catharsis. The play can therefore vary in length from a few minutes to one or more hours, and requires a considerable investment of attention and energy. The restructuring of the emotional problem being re-enacted takes place in a similar way to S. Ferenczi's "active analysis". This phase leads the patient to experience a greater amount of freedom, awareness and spontaneity, and is carried out with what C.G. Jung would define as an active intelligence of a theatrical nature. During the final phase, the therapist encourages the "mirroring" of the play by the group and invites everyone to share their analogous life experiences with the patient. If necessary, the therapist intercepts and blocks attacks stemming from envy, that are lacking in meaning, moralistic judgements and pseudo-analytic comments from the other members of the group. At the end of the session, some psychodramatists also verbalize their analytic interpretations of the play and of the group dynamics.

What distinguishes Moreno from Freud, from an ideological point of view, is a profound faith in society, which renders possible a therapy characterized by mutual acceptance and by the meeting between human beings that is not made up exclusively of unconscious drives. From the point of view of technique, it is the use of the group, of action and of two types of codes: those of the left hemisphere of the brain and those of the right hemisphere. All this is implemented using a creative and holistic perspective, that the exponents of analytic psychodrama (born in Europe in the 1950s) try, on the other hand, to minimize, with a predominance of the analytic interpretation over the theatrical aspects. From a philosophical point of view, Moreno's approach to psychotherapy appears to be on the same wavelength as that of Jung, in that he is more attracted to symbols of the future than to the signs of the past. If we compare the active analysis of Ferenczi with psychodrama, it is evident that in the setting created by Moreno, the therapist does not interact with the patient alone, but makes him "play" with auxiliary-egos. The two remain within the framework of the public eye. This kind of setting, being in certain ways hypnotic, allows the therapist to obtain quick and profound regressions. But the presence of the group intervention, if well managed, tends to keep the risk of them falling into a collective delirium somewhat at bay. A psychodramatist who is alert has to distinguish between what is real and what is acting, using his clinical competence to interpret the meaning of the spontaneity of the play, in function of the different diagnostic frameworks.

Through the years, Moreno's theory has been increasingly empirically organized and has gained the approval of psychiatry, of universities and of the institutions. The first abstract and prophetic ideas have been supported by techniques of therapeutic interventions that are concrete and measurable. From America, where Moreno emigrated in 1926, this method spread progressively to the rest of the world, arriving in China, India and Japan. In 1932, Moreno finalized the concept of "group psychotherapy" – in relation to a psychotherapy project in the prison of Sing-Sing – and presented it to the congress of the American Association of Psychiatry. He also studied a community of teenage females in a detention centre in collaboration with H.H. Jennings, from a sociometric point of view; that is, he measured the emotional tensions and levels of proximity, distance and reciprocity between the different members of this group. From this experiment, psychodrama and role playing were discovered to be effective, both in the world of communication (for training, prevention, in schools, in the community, in cultural events) as well as in group analysis and in psychotherapy. Today there are tens of thousands of psychologists, psychiatrists and social workers that make use of Moreno's psychoplay and perpetuate the use of his innovative techniques. *[O. Rosati]*

REFERENCES. Moreno J.L., *Psychodrama first volume*, 1946; Id., *Theater of spontaneity*, 1947; Id., *The Autobiography of J.L. Moreno*, 2011; Moreno J.L., Moreno Z.T., *Psychodrama, Vol 1*, 1959; Id., *Psychodrama, Vol 3: Action therapy and principles of practice*, 1969; Rosati O., *Da storia nasce storia*, 1993; Schützenberger A.A., *Psychodrama*, 1979.

PSYCHODYNAMIC DIAGNOSTIC MANUAL → PDM

Psychodynamic paradigm → Please refer to the opening chapter, "The eight paradigms and their respective theoretical-applicative models".

PSYCHODRAMATIST

It is the person leading a → psychodrama, promoter of the action and director of the scenic representation. More often called "director", to express the active role that characterizes his presence, he is the "chief therapist": he starts the session by committing the group to relational activities that are likely to create cognitive and emotional ties between people and to free spontaneity; then, when a protagonist emerges, he starts the scenic representation, stimulating the subject to explore his inner world, with the cooperation of other members of the group (auxiliary-egos). His interpretative function is carried out through his strategy in the selection of scenes to be represented. He is also careful to keep alive the attention of those who are not involved in the action on stage and follow the representation from the audience. *[G. Boria]*

REFERENCES. Boria G., *Psicoterapia psicodrammatica. Sviluppi del modello moreniano nel lavoro terapeutico con gruppi di adulti*, 2005; Boria G., Muzzarelli F., *Incontri sulla scena*, 2009; Moreno J.L., *Psychodrama first volume*, 1946; Moreno J.L., *Who shall survive?*, 1953.

PSYCHOLOGICAL DIAGNOSIS

A diagnostic model of functional type. Opposite to → psychiatric diagnosis, psychological diagnosis conceptualizes the set of variables (personal, environmental, interactive) that influence psychical life and behaviours and contextualizes them inside a theoretical coherent system. It follows that, contrary to psychiatric diagnosis, which is overtly a-theoretical, every psychological diagnosis explicitly refers to theoretical constructs and concepts that derive from clinical research and from psychotherapeutic approaches of reference. In fact, an important characteristic of psychological diagnosis is its orientation towards the operative aspects of diagnosis: building schemes of action that make a diagnosis clinically usable, considering it as a guide for successive phases of psychological (for example of → support and

→ consultancy) and psychotherapeutic intervention. Psychological diagnosis is multidimensional and multi-instrumental. Multidimensionality emerges from the attention paid to all biopsychosocial aspects that influence psychical life (cognitive, emotional, motivational, behaviour patterns), as well as relational (interactional models, communicative dynamics) and social (socio-environmental and cultural variables) aspects. In this perspective, psychological diagnoses can also differ on a theoretical and methodological level in relation to the conceptualization of the problem. This aspect has often been a source of confusion amongst those who rigidly support a diagnostic medical model (→ medical diagnosis), and it has been the main cause of accusations of poor use of scientific methods, which in some cases were directed at psychological functional diagnosis. On the contrary, being a psychological diagnosis, the expression of the continuous progress of techniques and of theoretical and conceptual epistemological frameworks of reference – in other words of operative perspectives –, it represents the operative perspective, which has proved to be the most useful in guiding clinical and psychotherapeutic work with mental disorders. The multi-instrumentality of psychological diagnosis refers mainly to the use of psychometric (→ psychological tests) and of → assessment tools, which integrate the main source of every psychological assessment: the clinical session. The high number of psychometric possibilities of the functional study of behaviour (for instance → projective tests, personality tests, intelligence tests, aptitude tests) changes depending on the goal, which can be clinical, statistical, of research or orientation. In addition, psychological diagnosis is often requested in the forensic field, to investigate one's psychic conditions in juridical, civil and penal trials. *[R.]*

PSYCHOLOGICAL TESTS

Instruments used to acquire information on the psychological state or the psychological functioning of an individual. These tests are standardized in the procedures of administration and in the interpretation of the results, with the aim of obtaining an evaluation that is the most independent possible from the individual variables and from the contest. There are tests that measure intelligence, attitudes, cognitive functions, personality, interests and values. To these we can add the numerous symptomatologic rating scales as well as projective techniques.

Developed with the aim of scientific research, these tests are nowadays used in a wide variety of contexts that vary from the selection of employees of large organizations, to educational and career orientation, from → psychological diagnosis to the evaluation of psychological treatment, from the general evaluation of personality to the study of cognitive functioning in childhood. *[R.]*

PSYCHOLOGICAL THERAPY

Term derived from the Greek language, meaning: "cure", "healing". According to Hippocrates therapeutic instruments include: "the touch", "the remedy", "the word". In the field of psychology, the term psychological therapy is used to refer, on the one hand, to all those → techniques, instruments, acts, modes of communication and of relating, and strategies for → problem-solving that seek to favour change by means of the → interaction between two and/or more individuals within an organized relationship having this aim; on the other hand, it refers to the influence that this process has on the individual affected by the problem. Therefore, therapy excludes the use of drugs, medicine, surgery and invasive psychiatric techniques.

Frequently it is described using the expression "talking therapy", but this definition does not give merit to the multiple possibilities of therapeutic → influence that one can observe within the different → models of therapy. *[R.]*

PSYCHOLOGICAL TYPES

In Jungian theory, the combination of all the characteristics and generalized → attitudes that are recurrent in many individual forms and that are habitually taken up by the conscious and by the → Ego. The problem of typology, according to Jung, was born in the clinical field, where he observed the presence of consistent differences in the personality characteristics present between the people suffering from hysteria and those suffering from early onset dementia. In the former, he observed an intensity of relationship with the object that is above the norm; in the latter, one that is below the norm. According to Jung, → extroversion has a centrifugal movement of the → libido; → introversion a centripetal one. These observations went from the clinical setting to the study of normality and ended with the establishment by Jung of two fundamental attitudes of → personality; the first, extroverted and directed towards the object; the second directed towards the subject. The two attitudes marry with the four → functions of personality: two that are rational (thought and feeling) and two that are irrational (sensation and intuition), which, in turn, can be classified as being introverted or extroverted. From this, eight basic personality types are derived, that, within the conscious/unconscious dialectic present some areas of consciousness that are more differentiated and other, corresponding, unconscious areas that are archaic and undifferentiated in nature. Therefore, for every conscious element there is a corresponding specific hue of the personal → unconscious. The thinking-type will have an inferior function, and vice versa; the feeling-type will have a mode of thinking that is poorly differentiated. The same phenomenon is present in the irrational types. The four functions, when they are differentiated, are specialized attitudes, ways of interpreting reality according to a selective point of view. The thought investigates the logic of things; the feeling their value; the sensation the tangibility of things; and, finally, the intuition their potential. The result of this is a highly complex dynamic of the psyche, an interweaving between differentiated and undifferentiated functions, between extroverted and introverted attitudes, with continuous metamorphoses and conflicts that are created between ways of living and thinking that are not homogenous. This complexity creates complications between individuals with different typologies, but also difficulties at a subjective level, in the relationship with oneself.

Finally, typology for Jung is used to explain the conflict between S. Freud and A. Adler. The former would appear to represent the psychology of extroversion, of sexuality and its vicissitudes; the latter that of introversion, of the superiority complex, of the aiming towards supremacy as a means of overcoming feelings of inferiority. Both perspectives have, therefore, their reasons, but also their limits with respect to the opposite perspective. With Jung's typology, the hermeneutic dimension enters into the discipline of psychology and, far from establishing a closed system of classification, opens it up to the infinite possibilities of the human soul. *[M. Gay]*

REFERENCES. Jung C.G. (1907–1959), *The psychogenesis of mental disease*, in *Collected Works*, III, 1960; Id. (1921), *Psychological types*, in *Collected Works*, VI, 1971.

PSYCHO-NEURO-ENDOCRINO-IMMUNOLOGY

Born from H. Selye's studies on → stress, this discipline was developed, above all, in later researches carried out by Ader, who is considered the real father of psycho-neuro-endocrino-immunology (PNEI). Not only did Selye provide a precise definition of stress, but he also contributed to the description of the complex processes activating on a neurophysiological level in a human body under stress. These studies paved the way to many others that better specified the devastating effects occurring whenever the human body endures an extended period of stress. PNEI also highlights that the three main systems in the human body (nervous system, immune system and endocrine system) do not act separately – as they were believed to do – but interact with each other. But the true innovation is the demonstration that psychological processes, mental attitudes and emotions influence these three main systems. The researches carried out by Ader, Cohen and Felten, confirm the following principles: the immune system works as a sensory organ and a cognitive network; the immune system, the nervous system and the endocrine system are connected to the mind; their molecules can work as neurotransmitters, hormones and cytokines; one's own lifestyle, eating habits and mind play an essential role in maintaining healthy conditions and treating illness. This new perspective on the human body paves the way to a new foundation of health disciplines and a new conception of healthcare in which mental processes are pivotal. *[G. Pagliaro]*

REFERENCES. Ader R., Felten D., Cohen N., *Psychoneuroimmunlogy*, 1981; Biondi M., *Mente Cervello e Sistema immunitario*, 1997; Pagliaro G., Martino E., *La mente non localizzata*, 2010.

PSYCHOPATHOLOGY → PATHOLOGY

PSYCHOPHYSIOLOGY

A scientific discipline that studies the correlation between physiological indices and psychological and behavioural states. The methodology utilized is not invasive and is based on the use of skin sensors that are able to measure the variation of some physiological functions that are linked to psychological functioning, such as respiration and heartbeat, electrical resistance of the skin (psychogalvanic reflex), electromagnetic cerebral functions (electroencephalogram, evoked potential, magnetoencephalography), the activity of the digestive system (electrogastrography), musculo-skeletal activity (electromyography, stereophotogrammetry) and ocular movements (electrooculography, digital visual scanning). A vast body of literature in the field of general and experimental psychology can be found with regard to the correlation between basic psychological processes (for example → memory, → attention, → learning, → perception, → emotion) and psychophysiological responses. In addition, a significant degree of correlation was also found to be present between psychophysiological indices and psychological states related to psychotherapeutic processes. *[R.]*

PSYCHOSIS

A term introduced in 1845 by E. von Feuchtersleben with the meaning of "mental illness" or "madness". Over time this term has been defined in different ways, none of which, however, has obtained a universal consensus. In general, it indicates that the presence of a serious disturbance of the psychological equilibrium of the individual, with the reality testing of the individual being compromised, that is, the capacity to analyze reality according to the beliefs and interpretations of the social environment to which he belongs. Psychosis, as in → neurosis, can be understood from different theoretical points of view and is treated differently according to the school of psychological thought to which one adheres to and the psychotherapeutic model of reference. Psychotic disturbances are characterized by a disturbance in the thought processes of the individual (for example, in the flow of ideas leading to the flight of ideas and in the associative links) and in the content of thoughts (delusional ideation and sensory-perceptual disorders such as auditory, visual, olfactory, tactile and gustative hallucinations). The factors that give rise to this type of disorder have not as yet been identified in a definitive manner but the hypothesis that it results from a combination of biological, genetic, psychological and social factors is widely recognized. *[R.]*

PSYCHOSYNTHESIS

A school of psychology and a psychotherapeutic model created by the Italian psychiatrist R. Assagioli, who was a member of the Freudian Circle in Zürich and learned about psychoanalysis through C.G. Jung. Assagioli formulated psychosynthesis in the 1920s, continuing and developing the psychoanalytic approach, and was a leading pioneer of humanistic-existential and transpersonal psychology. Psychosynthesis is mainly present in these three areas and considers man on an evolutionary path tending to completeness in the direction of the realization of his more profound identity, in a process of progressive synthesis of the personality considered as a play of multiple forces. It is a school of psychology that expresses itself in many fields: therapeutic, self-development, educational and interpersonal and social, but it is in psychotherapy that it finds its richest and more original applications. Psychosynthesis psychotherapy is, in fact, a therapeutic process in which obstacles and delays of the path of development can be faced. The wide vision of the human path is present, in its potentials, along an axis of progression (evolution) and regression (limitations and obstacles). One must remember this axis during illness, which can be an expression either of a difficult process of development or of a distancing from progress and consequent regression, or of a combination of both. At the basis of the theoretical model there is a wide consideration of the unconscious, subdivided into the lower unconscious (personal dimension), the middle unconscious (contents close to the conscious level), the collective unconscious (the archetypical dimension) and the transpersonal unconscious (the essential and creative potentials, feasible in future development). Emphasis is laid, from an existential perspective, not only on the unconscious, but on the conscious and on identity. The first indicates the importance of awareness and of its development in the psychosynthetic process; the second underlines the research and affirmation of subjectivity, the expression of a deep identity called the Self, which it is possible to experience both on an ordinary conscious level (I or personal Self), and on an extraordinary level (the transpersonal Self). It is the Self that represents the goal and also the guide of the psychosynthetic process. Suffering and pathology are expressions of distancing from the Self and from its centre, that remains submerged in the multiple identifications of the whole personality that often are in disagreement. In order to get a clear picture of the psychic complexity and to guide the psychotherapeutic work, psychosynthesis has created several "maps". One of these is that of the seven psychic functions (→ star diagram) that characterize seven basic human typologies. The will is the central function that represents a meaningful contribution by Assagioli to modern psychology, giving a complex and articulate vision of the process of the will, a deep expression of subjectivity and intentionality. It is not by chance that the will is considered in psychosynthesis, together with the conscious, a function of the Self, so that the experience of one leads to the experience of the other and vice versa. In that sense, the will completes awareness, living direction and synthesis to conscious integrations of the material of the unconscious, which acquires value above all in relation to the psychosynthetic process of the person in his existential uniqueness. Another map is that of the subpersonalities, an original psychosynthetic construct that describes psychic reality as a theatrical scenario in which the multiplicity of desires, emotions, qualities, etc. organizes itself in substructures similar to the global personality around a central element, generally a basic need. The work on subpersonalities includes dialectics with the unconscious and the intrapsychic relations between parts. A third map is that of the three levels of the personality – body, emotions, mind – that particularly concerns the expressive ways at the basis of the various typologies that serve to modulate the choice of the best technique in the psychotherapeutic approach. The body is present in each phase of the psychosynthetic process and sometimes is used directly as the place for psychotherapeutic intervention. The maps underline the importance given to the structural organization of the person, and not only to the contents. Pathology, according to psychosynthesis, can develop through the break in dynamic equilibrium between the parts, and can germinate from conflicts that create separation on various levels: intrapersonal (between subpersonalities), interpersonal (in interpersonal relationships) and transpersonal (between the personal and transpersonal dimensions). not only to the contents. The psychosynthetic process is characterized by phases that sometimes take place in temporal succession, sometimes in a different order or with integrations and alternating phases within the same phase of the process itself. The general approach, both as an evaluation and as an initial therapeutic phase, is constituted by a bifocal vision of the person, considered in his conflictual and suffering part, and also in the so-called "healthy parts", that represent resources and potential; each person's unique language is considered in the verbal and nonverbal sphere, and the techniques are adapted to this through various body–mind modalities (words, images, writing, body-expressions). In psychosynthesis, evaluation and existential understanding begin from a conscious situation: values, social-environmental relations, etc. This phase activates the presence of the "observing" I, aware of his own being in the world. That is part of the path of awareness that extends then to the analytical phase, of dialogue with the unconscious. This phase, which reaffirms the psychodynamic roots of psychosynthesis, opens up to the work with the dimensions of the unconscious, dealing with resistances, defences, the transferral relation, through both associative methods and imaginative-symbolic methods, dream-work or work on expressive material: drawing, writing, body language. The interpretation that gives meaning to the unconscious contents follows a subjective perspective, open to the multiple meaning of the unconscious material in which personal aspects may find themselves united with archetypical and transpersonal aspects. Another specific aspect of analysis in psychosynthesis is the alternation and integration between the analytical phase and that of disidentification, transformation and synthesis (fractional analysis). The process of disidentification–self-identification is the creation of inner distance from the various contents in the impartial observation where the subject-observer is aware of self (self-identification) as distinct from the contents (disidentification). This experience, which anyway is gradual and follows a process, may be used to favour the affirmation of subjectivity as the ability of inner mastering, and to contact the multiplicity of the psyche with greater intensity and freedom. Such contact, first with the personal Self and then the transpersonal Self, is part of the reorganization of the personality around a new centre, the basic goal of the ulterior process of transformation-healing. The transformation-synthesis delineates the final and more advanced force of the psychotherapeutic process, even if sometimes synthetic phases are a premise to analytical phases from the start, because situations exist of particular pathological destructuring of the personality. Transformation and synthesis are also spontaneous; in this phase they are consciously directed by a conscious and wilful Self, also with the use of those techniques that psychosynthesis defines "active". The person practices such techniques in the session with the therapist, repeating them alone, collaborating in his own development. If the transformation implies work with a linking of the functions, promoting coordination and change in the passages between emotions, thoughts, images and actions, synthesis represents the most creative aspect of the process in which new realities are formed, that include the preceding constituting parts while transforming them. The transpersonal potentials participate in these constructive aspects; they are not only the goal of the process but the synthetizing means of the personality. This is an example of the relation of integration and synthesis between the personal and the transpersonal dimension. A further example is psychosynthetic psychotherapy addressed to the treatment of transpersonal psychopathology with manifestations of suffering that precede, follow or accompany the process of opening to the transpersonal potentials. Here it is important to work on the recognition of the developmental nature of psychopathology, consolidating and containing the personality in order to integrate certain dimensions. Finally, it must be remembered that it is important, in the psychotherapeutic relation, to consider the aspects of → transference and → countertransference and the position that the therapist has of guiding, as also the human reality of the I–You relation. Regarding the → setting and the techniques, it may be said that the former has a certain degree of conscious flexibility, with a large number of techniques used in a non-eclectic way, but synthetically in a sense of process and in relation with a co-constructed therapeutic plan, by the patient and the therapist together. The following groups of techniques can be noted: analytical techniques of awareness; techniques for mastering, transformation and synthesis; meditative techniques; expressive techniques; → anchoring techniques and relational techniques. This last area represents also the specific application of psychosynthetic psychotherapy to groups, couples and the family. *[M. Rosselli]*

REFERENCES. Alberti A., *Psicosintesi: Una cura per l'anima*, 2008; Assagioli R., *Psychosynthesis: A collection of basic writings* (rev.ed.), 2000; Assagioli R., *The act of will*, 1983; Id., *Psychosynthesis typology*, 2010 (1977); Guggisberg Nocelli P., *La Via della Psicosintesi – Una guida completa con una biografia di Roberto Assagioli*, 2011.

PSYCHOSYNTHESIS PSYCHOTHERAPY → PSYCHOSYNTHESIS

PUER–SENEX

In analytical psychology, it is the archetypal couple of opposites, that appears in the individuation process, with whom the Ego is related. These are two poles of a single dynamic aspect, which is played inside an attraction field striving for the *coniunctio*. In the absence of this reciprocal affiliation, *puer* and *senex* embody a libidic splitting. Both elements can be referred to a bivalent psychological dimension, with a positive and a negative side. The *puer* represents the child in his becoming nature, anticipation of future developments, real openness towards beginning and opportunity of renewal. On the contrary, the *puer aeternus* may indicate one's difficulty in separating from places and figures, showing both a difficulty in living his own current life and the liveliness and impatience of imagination activity, with a continuous and unfulfilled wish to begin. In its positive meaning, the *senex* has the psychological traits of balance, wisdom, generosity, far-sightedness, responsibility; in its negative side, it has the traits of authoritarianism, strict conservatism, lack of imagination, failure in the renewal process and a hardening in the willing of power. The *puer* that "does not meet" the *senex* risks insecurity, the dangerous passion for flight and the refusal of facing paternal depression. So, the *puer* may remain crystallized in a never-ending state of "youthful promise". On the other hand, the *senex* without the *puer* takes the risk of a depressive shadow and a decreased psychic life: a hardening functioning as negative *senex* and sadic father, which alchemists identified with Saturn, "governor of the prison" and extreme judge. The *puer–senex* conflict resolution depends on the mediating function of the anima, which is connected with the unconscious and connects the opposites. Without the anima, the *puer* may commit suicide and the *senex* can meet destructiveness. *[V. Lingiardi]*

REFERENCES. Hillman J., *Puer aeternus*, 1999; Jung C.G. (1940–1941), *The child and core: Two archetypes*, 1981; von Franz M.-L., *The problem of the puer aeternus*, 2000.

PUNCTUATION

Whitin interactional-systemic therapy and communication psychology, the term "punctuation" indicates a modality of definition and classification of a sequence of events or elements. As stated by Watzlawick, Beavin and Jackson, problems of punctuation represent a typical dysfunctional communication pattern: during a long communicative sequence, a verbal exchange can be differently read (that is, punctuated) by the individuals involved in it; therefore, the same behaviour could be interpreted either as cause or effect of a certain action. For example, a man can declare himself withdrawn to protect himself against his wife's complaints, while the woman punctuates this behaviour as the cause of the complaint itself. The same facts are punctuated in very different ways, with dysfunctional effects at a communicative and relational level. *[G. Castelnuovo, G. Pietrabissa, E. Molinari]*

REFERENCES. Watzlawick P., Bavelas J.B., Jackson D.D., *Pragmatics of human communication: A study of interactional patterns, pathologies, and paradoxes*, 1967.

PUNISHMENT

In the behaviourist paradigm the meaning of this term is substantially different from the common meaning attributed to it of an ethical or judicial nature; in these contexts the term refers, in fact, to the penalty or punishment inflicted as a result of breaking a rule; in psychology it refers, instead, to the event following a behaviour that reduces its frequency, intensity or duration. In this way, for example, the prison sentence that is the legal punishment of a crime, is, from a behavioural point of view, ineffective: the criminal, once he has terminated his prison sentence, frequently returns to committing the same crime. From a behavioural perspective, the context in which the concept of punishment is defined is that of the functional analysis of the contingencies that accompany every behaviour: antecedent and consequent, as described by the acronym ABC (antecedent–behaviour–consequence). The punitive value of an event cannot be identified *a priori*, but only in reference to the behaviour B, to which the event is a consequence. If this behaviour persists, what follows is defined as being → reinforcement; if it diminishes, or it is extinguished, punishment. Even for the person who has carried out the behaviour that has been reinforced or punished, the consequences are antithetical: reinforcement increases a person's capabilities, enhancing motivation to try new things, whilst punishment inhibits them and has negative secondary effects, such as for example, anger in the child who has been punished. *[R. Anchisi]*

REFERENCES. Skinner F.B., *Science and human bevavior*, 1953; Id., *Difesa del comportamentismo. Saggi recenti su istruzione e personalità*, 1992.

PURPOSIVE BEHAVIOUR

In neo-behaviourism, a behaviour where a person clearly identifies an object-goal and efficient ways to achieve it. In order for a behaviour to have these features – proactive, or intentional – a simple behavioural, automatic or reflexive response is not sufficient. In fact, the achievement of a goal expresses the intention of a subject, and it assumes a cognition, that is, the expression of the will to reach a goal that does not only aim at the satisfaction of a physical need (like hunger), but also at the pursuit of values and/or rewards. *[G. Lo Savio]*

REFERENCES. Tolman E.C., *Purposive behaviour in animals and men*, I– II, 1932.

Q

QUALITATIVE METHOD → QUANTITATIVE AND QUALITATIVE METHODS

QUANTITATIVE AND QUALITATIVE METHODS

In the literature, the distinction between qualitative and quantitative methods is often used in order to define alternative research paradigms, which refer to wider epistemological antinomies. Among these, the main one compares the reference to an ontological reality (realism) to the idea according to which reality emerges essentially as a social construct (antirealism). The quantitative method stands on the first side of the dichotomy and it is often associated with positivist scientific paradigms. It usually uses highly structured survey-based instruments, experimental and statistical procedures. It aims to identify random relations among empirical variables that are appropriately operationalized and defined. In psychotherapy, the typical example of the application of quantitative methods is the use of psychometric tests to determine a diagnosis or to conduct psychopathological research. Therefore, quantitative methods represent a nomothetic (→ idiographic) approach that aims to explain the phenomena and to generalize the results. This is achieved by following a logic that privileges the context of the justification as opposed to the context of the discovery. Researchers who apply this method are interested in rejecting *a priori* hypotheses since, in the first place, they have to verify the validity of the scientific theory used to represent the studied phenomenon. On the contrary, qualitative methods stand on the epistemological side, which tends to problematize the reference to an external reality (independent from the observer). They are frequently used within interactionist and constructivist paradigms. They privilege observation methods and instruments, which are useful in tracing narratives or other textual material. Their main goal is to reconstruct the individual subjectivity or the complex interaction among individuals. They represent an idiographic approach that is oriented towards the comprehension and the exploration of the meanings through which people generate contextually valid social realities. This cognitive logic, therefore, aims to discover local theories and belief systems, which are culturally mediated and socially organized. In psychotherapy, the most widely used qualitative method is the one based on clinical interviewing (→ therapeutic talk) as an elected instrument of the therapeutic practice. The formal contrast between qualitative and quantitative methods partially leaves space to perspectives that, ignoring the epistemological purism, take on a pragmatic attitude (→ pragmatism) according to which the combined use of the two methods is encouraged because it is more effective than the single approach. Therefore, the quantitative–qualitative distinction can be represented as a *continuum* whose poles consist of, on the one hand, an ontological psychologism, and, on the other hand, radical forms of → constructivism, with the possibility of manifold intermediate shades. *[R.]*

QUATERNITY

In Jungian analytic psychology, this term is intended as the deconstruction of a totality and, together, as the four "minimal" aspects that contribute to constitute it through their interactions, is conceived as a constant of the collective imagination that refers to differentiation and endopsychic integration and, therefore, to the process of → individuation. In particular, the quaternity is considered to be a symbol of the → Self, intended as a totality composed of at least four elements that appear not only in their cultural forms or in religious traditions, but also in dreams, or, in general, in the unconscious productions of the individual. The orientations of the "collective unconscious" of a particular epoch and of the religious representations of transcendence, as in that expressed by the Trinity of the Christian religion, would also tend to eliminate from the totality the "fourth element": for example, evil (as an interactional factor with the "good") or the less differentiated functioning of the psyche, in this way rendering difficult the endopsychic integration that psychotherapy tends to favour. *[E.V. Trapanese, S. Fossi]*

REFERENCES. Jung C.G. (1951), *Answer to Job*, in *Collected Works*, XI, 1973.

QUESTIONNAIRE

List of questions submitted in writing to a select group of individuals, aimed at collecting information on preferences, behaviour, attitudes and opinions. Questionnaires include a number of "tools" such as checklists, rating scales and inventories. The questions include open or multiple-choice answers. The responses are subjected to statistical analysis and can lead to general considerations. The choice of a specific questionnaire in a clinical setting is justified with respect to the type of information that the psychologist wants to obtain: global profile of the person, identification of various problems, the possible quantification or quantification of the extent to which the person possesses a certain trait or psychological state. *[G. Sacco, D. Kakaraki]*

REFERENCES. Ercolani A.P., Perugini M., *La misura in Psicologia. Introduzione ai test psicologici*, 1997; Sanavio E., Sica C., *I test di personalità. Inventari e questionari*, 1999.

R

RACKET

Denomination appertaining to transactional analysis, related to a phenomenon studied at both an intrapsychic and a relational level. In an intrapsychic sense, it describes the presence of ancient emotions, therefore tied to unresolved childhood experiences (→ Ego-state), which can be reactivated in the adult individual; these experiences are felt in place of the person's natural emotions in the present, and are also defined as "parasite emotions". Fear, sadness, anger can show the nature of a racket and need to be distinguished from the homologous emotions tied to the → here-and-now. From a relational point of view, these ancient experiences create particular dynamic relationships, called racketeering, in which their expression provokes, in a manipulative way in the other, the assumption of three dramatic roles used in the theory of psychological → games (Persecutor/Saviour/Victim), without, however, arriving at the role change that is part of the game. *[M. Novellino]*

REFERENCES. Berne E., *«Hello!». . .and then what?*, 1972; Moiso C., Novellino M., *Stati dell'Io*, 1982.

RATIONAL ANALYSIS → DISPUTING

RATIONAL EMOTIVE BEHAVIOURAL THERAPY

Psychotherapeutic theory and practice founded by the American psychologist Ellis at the end of the 1950s. Originally denominated as rational emotive therapy (RET), it can be considered as being the "mother" of all cognitive-behavioural psychotherapies, in that it was primarily due to the influence that the works of Ellis exerted on the principal exponents of behavioural theory that, towards the beginning of the 1970s, led to the emergence of the cognitive-behavioural paradigm; in 1993 Ellis, in fact, decided to modify the name of the model of psychotherapy he had created to that of rational emotive behaviour therapy (REBT), adding the B of Behaviour, with the aim of emphasizing the behavioural aspects of rational emotive therapy. The fundamental assumption of rational emotive behavioural psychotherapy is that our emotional reactions and our behaviour are greatly influenced by our vision of reality, or rather the way we perceive, interpret and evaluate what happens to us. This assumption originates from the teachings of some great oriental masters, such as Lao Tze and Buddha, and the stoic philosophers such Epictetus and Marcus Aurelius, by whom it appears Ellis had been strongly influenced. Rational emotive behavioural psychotherapy also recognizes the influence of physical conditions, past learning experiences and → conditioning mechanisms. Cognitions, emotions and behaviour are considered to be aspects of human experience that are closely interconnected, so much so that, although some emotions can be triggered by external events or biological conditions, their persistance or intensification is, in the majority of cases, influenced by our thinking processes.

THE ABCDE MODEL. The essence of rational emotive behavioural psychotherapy is summarized in the ABCDE model, by means of which both the process that leads to dysfunctional behaviours as well as the process involved in changing them are described. The five letters are a mnemonic system to aid in remembering the five elements of the model, which are: A, the activating event; B, the belief system; C, the emotional and behavioural consequences; D, disputing the irrational beliefs; E, the effects of the transformation. The activating event (A) is the external or internal situation (therefore activating events also include memories and dreams) that people experience. The term belief system (B) refers to the totality of those cognitive processes in the form of thoughts, considerations, interior comments that appear in the mind of the individual regarding the activating event. These convictions can be either rational or irrational. The consequences (C) are those emotional and behavioural reactions that are commonly believed to be caused by the activating event whilst, according to this model, they are heavily influenced by the belief system. The ABC component of this sequence synthesizes the model of emotional reactivity formulated by Ellis. The dispute (D) is the process by means of which one tries to prove the veracity and the logical consistency of the irrational beliefs, with the aim of transforming those ways of thinking that are harmful. The effects (E) of this process of confutation consists of changes at a cognitive, emotional and behavioural level. Within the model of rational emotive behavioural psychotherapy, a thought is considered to be rational if it is flexible, logical, congruent with the external reality and functional, and, therefore, favours the psychophysical wellbeing of the individual and his ability to follow his adaptive goals. On the other hand, with regard to the irrational beliefs, these are characterized by illogicity, assumptions that are not verified, erroneous deductions, absolutist notions, exaggerations and undue generalizations. This model therefore deals with a way of thinking that hinders the ability of the individual to pursue fundamental goals and to achieve a state of wellbeing, leading to negative emotional states that are excessively intense and prolonged. Rational emotive behavioural psychotherapy does not propose a form of thought that is "positive", but a way of thinking that includes a realistic vision of events, without magnifying the negative aspects, but, on the other hand, also by not trying to avoid them. Within this context the rational individual is not to be understood as being a person who is "cold", detached, cerebral and lacking in the ability to be affectionate, but as a person who is able to turn to forms of thinking that are constructive and functional in facing difficulties, so that, although still experiencing unpleasant emotions when faced with adversity, he will still be able to deal with them without feeling overwhelmed by them. Within the rational emotive behavioural model of psychotherapy, the individual's past is considered as being relevant, in that it is in the past that many ways of thinking have been learnt. However, from the moment that discovering the past is usually of little help in changing the present, the therapist, after having gathered the essential information about the life of the patient, will not engage in an "archeological exploration", but will focus his attention on strategies that can help the patient face the difficulties in his present.

THERAPEUTIC TECHNIQUES. Rational emotive behavioural psychotherapy makes use of a variety of therapeutic interventions, that are divided into cognitive techniques, emotional techniques and behavioural techniques. The best-known and most elegant cognitive technique is called → disputing, or rather the challenging and the confutation of the irrational beliefs. With regard to the emotional techniques, the best known is the Rational Emotive imagery, whose aim is that of transforming cognitive → insight into interiorized emotional insight. The behavioural techniques that are most commonly used in rational emotive behavioural psychotherapy are: shame-attacking exercises; risk-taking exercises; stepping out of one's own role; → in vivo desensitization and contingency management (→ reinforcement and → punishment). In the utilization of the various procedures the aim is that of producing a → change that is consistent and enduring in the way of thinking and in the belief system of the patient, rather than simply the elimination of some symptoms. The duration of therapy is relatively short, with an average number of around 15 to 20 sessions, rarely extended for more than a year, unless one is dealing with complex personality disorders. The aim of rational emotive behavioural psychotherapy is that of enabling the individual to be able to learn a method of management of his emotions and behaviour that he can continue to apply to himself in his life even when the therapeutic process has ended.

Rational emotive behaviour psychotherapy shares many objectives with the psychotherapeutic paradigm of the humanistic-existential paradigm (please see the opening chapter, "The eight paradigms and their respective theoretical-applicative models"), although it is essentially anchored in scientific research, and it is therefore in line with the most modern evidence-based approaches (refer to the Appendix, "Empirical research in psychotherapy"). The principal fields of application of rational emotive behavioural psychotherapy are anxiety disorders, depression, couple therapy, anger management, chronic pain, terminal illness, some personality disorders and childhood and adolescent disorders. In recent years the principles and methods of rational emotive behavioural psychotherapy have also been applied in the psychoeducational field, by means of a procedure called rational emotive education, considered as being a means of primary and secondary prevention of psychological disorders in childhood. The professional training of the rational emotive behavioural therapist takes place through a series of intensive training sessions accompanied by an accurate supervision of the videotaped sessions of the trainee therapist. *[M. Di Pietro]*

REFERENCES. Di Pietro M., *L'educazione razionale emotiva*, 1992; Ellis A., *Overcoming destructive beliefs, feelings, and behaviours*, 2001; Ellis A., MacLaren C., *Rational Emotive Behaviour Therapy: A therapist's guide*, 1998.

RATIONAL EMOTIVE THERAPY (RET)

Term used in the period between 1961 and 1993 to indicate what is today known as rational emotive behavioural psychotherapy (REBT). The combination of the terms "rational" and "emotive", in spite of appearing to be antonyms, would indicate the possibility of utilizing modes of thinking that are constructive, logical, functional (rational) with the aim of overcoming emotions that are harmful and counter-productive. *[M. Di Pietro]*

RATIONAL THERAPIST

He who practiced the first form of rational emotive therapy created by Ellis, who, however, afterwards refused to accept the title of "rational therapist" and in various writings emphasized the fact that cognition, emotion, and behaviour are interdependent processes, and that therefore the cognitive dimension cannot be examined separately from the other two dimensions (→ rational emotive behavioural therapy). This aspect has frequently been ignored in cognitivist environments and the position of Ellis has been at times mistakenly assimilated with rationalism, so much so that in the debate between the constructivist position (→ constructivism) and the rationalist position, the psychotherapists that practice rational emotional behaviour psychotherapy have been considered as being rationalist therapists and placed therefore within the rationalist framework. In reality, the second model of psychotherapy developed by Ellis and his associates does not consider reason as being an entity that is superior to human beings; on the contrary, he has a very pragmatic vision of rationality, which is considered by him as being a mode of thought oriented towards favouring the emotional wellbeing of the individual and the overcoming of their personal difficulties. *[M. Di Pietro]*

REFERENCES. Ellis A., *Humanistic psychotherapy: The rational-emotive approach*, 1973.

RATIONALIZATION → DEFENCE MECHANISMS

REACTION FORMATION → DEFENCE MECHANISMS

REALITY PRINCIPLE → PLEASURE PRINCIPLE

REALITY THERAPY

William Glasser, trained in traditional psychiatry, encouraged by his teacher and supervisor, G.L. Harrington, first developed reality therapy in a mental hospital and extended it in a correctional institution in California in the 1950s and 1960s. Other professionals viewed Glasser's ideas as questionable and contentious even though they appeared rooted in the work of Alfred Adler. Both Glasser and Adler believed that behaviour is purposeful and that human beings are social creatures. Glasser added human choice and personal responsibility as explicit components of effective therapy.

REALITY THERAPY: CURRENT STATUS. More recently he derived the theoretical basis from the cybernetic system of brain functioning known as control theory. Because of the emphasis on choice in the practice of reality therapy, Glasser renamed its theoretical basis choice theory. A further development of reality therapy is the current formulation, the WDEP system (Wants, Doing, Self-evaluation and Plan of action), developed by Robert E. Wubbolding. He has made applications to managing, supervizing and → coaching employees as well as to classroom management and organizational development. Choice theory and the practical methodology for implementing it, reality therapy, comprise a mental health system rather than a mental disorder modality. From this point of view, mental health problems are replaced, not merely remediated. Reality therapists focus on healthy behaviours more than on diagnosable and ineffective actions, cognitions or emotions. More specifically, reality therapists help patients improve their interpersonal relationships as a way to address and at least alleviate most presenting problems. Wubbolding has incorporated the Ericksonian principle that there is not a one-to-one correlation between the problem and the solution. Often, the most effective treatment plan *seems* to be disconnected from the problem. Yet, when patients improve their interpersonal relationships, i.e. fulfill their need for belonging in a more satisfactory manner, other issues become less intense: acting out, depression, schizophrenia, attention deficit disorder, conduct disorder and others.

FOUR PRINCIPLES OF CHOICE THEORY. The explanation for the functioning of the human mind, choice theory, provides the foundational principles and theoretical basis for the delivery system formulated as WDEP. All human beings are motivated by five genetically encoded primary → needs: survival or self-preservation; belonging and love; power, achievement and inner control; freedom and independence; fun and enjoyment. These motivators are universal, not limited to any culture. They are general, not specific. Human beings develop specific wants related to each need. As they interact with the world around them they discover need-satisfying experiences and insert them as quality images into their inner world of wants, or quality world. Especially important are images of caring and compassionate people. Satisfying specific wants results in a condition of mental → homeostasis. Lacking fulfilment of wants, human beings generate *total behaviour* composed of actions, cognition, emotions and physiology. While not all behaviours are easily controlled, reality therapists treat them "as if" they are chosen, especially the action component of total behaviour. Behaviour is purposeful. The first goal of behaviour is to impact the external world for the purpose of gaining something from it. The more explicit goal is to achieve a perception of wants and need satisfaction. The second purpose is to communicate with the outside world, i.e. to send a message to the people in one's environment. When information from the outer world is received as perceptions, it is filtered through three lenses: a labeling lens, a relationship lens and a valuing lens. The labeling lens gives a meaning to the information; for instance, a chair receives the label "chair". The relationship lens connects chair and functionality; the chair is designed to support a human being. The valuing lens creates a positive or negative value for the chair; a cherished family heirloom receives a positive value, a broken chair a negative value. As an internal control theory validating the WDEP system of reality therapy, choice theory provides a basis for therapists to perceive clients not as powerless victims but as responsible individuals capable of making choices for satisfying their five internal motivators and their specific wants.

THE WDEP SYSTEM OF REALITY THERAPY. If choice theory, the explanation of human motivation, is the train track, then reality therapy, the delivery system, is the train. Because Glasser founded reality therapy prior to systematizing choice theory, the theory and the practice are often referred to simply as reality therapy. It has been applied to psychotherapy, parenting, supervising employees, family and community relationships, education, criminal justice and more. Common to all applications of reality therapy is the foundation of a warm, safe relationship between the practitioner and the person or group seeking help. Specific characteristics of the therapeutic relationship include appropriate boundaries, informed consent, clear expectations, as well as firmness, fairness and a willingness to listen. This → therapeutic alliance facilitates the successful use of interventions or procedures summarized as the WDEP system. Each letter represents a cluster of possible therapeutic interventions. W: With the guidance of the reality therapist, clients clarify and formulate their specific wants as they relate to their five needs, e.g. what they want from parents, children, job, co-workers, community, hospital, religious institutions, from the therapy itself and from themselves. Because many therapeutic relationships consist in a single session the effective reality therapist asks such questions as: "How would you like your life to be different as a result of our time together today?" Early in the therapeutic relationship the therapist helps patients determine their level of commitment, i.e. how hard they want to work at improving their lives. Level of commitment includes three degrees of intensity: "I don't want to do anything" is often the theme of the patient coerced into therapy. "I'll try. I might" represents a person desiring an outcome but is tentative about his/her willingness to change; "I will" illustrates a willingness to make efficacious choices.

Part of the W of the WDEP system includes an exploration of clients' perceptions, especially their perceived locus of control. Patients feeling oppressed by external forces are often unaware of opportunities for satisfying their wants and needs. The reality therapist helps them identify choices for gaining a sense of inner control or need satisfaction. D: Human beings have the most direct control over actions and secondarily over thoughts or cognition. Therefore, reality therapists help their patients describe both what they are doing and the underlying self-talk accompanying their actions. The key to the effective use of this component is facilitating a discussion of precisely how the patients spend their time as well as identifying such self-talk statements as "I can't" or "I will continue to make the same choices even though they are ineffective". Reality therapists acknowledge feelings but do not encourage continuous discourse about them due to the fact that human beings change emotions by altering actions. E: The cornerstone in the practice of reality therapy is self-evaluation. People change behaviour only when they have judged that their current behaviours have not been effective, i.e. have not resulted in want and need satisfaction. The question, "Is what you're doing helping or hurting you or the people around you?" is the royal road to behavioural change. A second self-evaluation consists in determining the attainability of wants and goals. "Is what you want realistically attainable?" lies at the heart of the efficient use of reality therapy. P: Plan of action. From the point of view of reality therapy effective treatment planning is SAMIC: Simple and uncomplicated; realistically Achievable; Measurable answering the question "when?"; Immediately doable; Controlled by the planner not dependent on others' actions and Committed to, rather than tentative. *[R.E. Wubbolding]*

REFERENCES. Glasser W., *Reality therapy*, 1965; Id., *Choice theory*, 1998; Id., *Defining mental health as a public health issue*, 2005; Kaiser H., *The problem of responsibility in psychotherapy*, in «Psychiatry», 1955, 18; Powers W., *Behaviour: The control of perception*, 1973; Wubbolding R., *Reality therapy for the 21st century*, 2000; Wubbolding R., *Reality therapy*, in J. Frew, M. Spiegler (eds.), *Contemporary psychotherapies for a diverse world*, 2008; Wubbolding R., *Reality therapy: Monograph psychotherapy series*, 2010.

RECOGNITION

In transactional analysis the need for recognition, which Berne identifies as a "hunger", to underline the importance it has for survival, is closely connected with "the quest for special kind of sensation that can only be supplied by another human being"; in particular, recognition is considered to be any sign suggesting recognition of one's existence, of one being seen. Physical stimuli, which are essential for the healthy growth of a child, are also desirable by adults but as time goes by grown-up individuals learn to get them in other forms. A smile (or an insult) can substitute them. However, it is better to receive a negative stimulus rather than no attention at all. According to Berne "a unit of recognition" exists called → stroke, that is "whatever act that implies recognition of the presence of the other". *[A. Ferrara]*

REFERENCES. Berne E., *Games people play*, 1964; *What do you say after you say hello?*, 1972; Stewart I., Joines V.L., *Transactional Analysis*, 1975.

REDECISION

Intrapsychic process of change, central to the transactional analysis approach to psychotherapy. It is excluded from parallel applications, such as those of → counselling. This process is placed in the strategic phase of → deconfusion, and consists of three stages: the → awareness of a childhood scene, called "protocol" (→ script), in which the person has established a → script decision (the latter is meant as a defensive position through which the child tries to give meaning to the suffering that derives from the weight of the → injunctions transmitted by the parental figures); the elaboration of the emotions that the child repressed at the moment in which he made the script decision; → insight about a new possible alternative that the patient can pursue once he overcomes the repressed emotions. In the "redecisional" school (→ transactional analysis) of B. and M. Goulding, the re-decision is searched for through a Gestalt type of work, therefore, cathartic; while in the psychodynamic transactional analysis school of M. Novellino and C. Moiso, it is through interpretive elaboration work of the transfer and countertransfer dynamics. *[M. Novellino]*

REFERENCES. Goulding M., Goulding R.L., *Changing lives through redecision therapy*, 1983; Novellino M., *Seminari clinici. La cassetta degli attrezzi dell'analista transazionale*, 2010.

REDEFINITION

Way of leading patients to review their interpretations and the way they give meaning to events. This technique can be used as a vehicle for change, for example in the case of rationalist therapies, or as a way of consolidating therapeutic changes that have been obtained through the implementation of other therapeutic techniques. Redefinition is different from → reframing precisely because it is oriented towards the attribution of meaning and not towards the perspectives adopted or to be adopted with regard to reality. *[R.]*

▷ In transactional analysis, redefinition is meant by Schiff as the "mechanism people use to maintain their established view of themselves, other people and the world, in order to advance their own → scripts". Redefinition allows us "to defend ourselves against stimuli which are inconsistent with our 'frame of reference'", which is the result of "an overall perceptual, conceptual affective and action set". The frame of reference acts as a filter of reality that allows us to define and integrate it. *[A. Ferrara]*

REFERENCES. Schiff J.L., *Transactional Analysis treatment of psychosis*, 1975.

REDUCTIONISM

Theory according to which scientific disciplines or forms of knowledge are organized in a hierarchical manner, according to their degree of importance. The first and most fundamental science is physics, followed by, in order of decreasing importance, chemistry, biology, psychology and finally sociology. The terms used by a discipline would therefore be translatable without loss of meaning in terms of one of the disciplines that have a higher position in the hierarchy. According to this thesis, therefore, the terms that are frequently used today in psychology are explainable without loss of meaning (→ semantics – meanings) by disciplines such as biology and neurophysiology. In other words, what is relative to the "mental" and "psychic" sphere can be described and explained by the study of more fundamental phenomena, such as the activity inherent to the central nervous system. The reductionist hypotheses therefore negate the theory that systems of reality are composed of many levels, and that many different aspects of truth or meaning can co-exist within the same system; negating the possibility of the emergence of new levels of meaning, freed from the preceding ones, and existing in function of the increase in complexity of the system. Reductionism therefore negates the epistemological autonomy of the various disciplines, reducing them to mere epiphenonemena of physics. The term reductionism is frequently used as a synonym of → reductivism, that has instead a different meaning. *[R.]*

REDUCTIVISM

Theory that considers the complex manifestation of reality as being reconducible to one or a few simple primary principles, that have an explicative power over them. In other words, reductionist thinking seeks to identify those simple elements that, by interacting or aggregating with each other, form a complex phenomenon; it is enough, according to this way of thinking, to study and to understand the functioning of these elements to be able to understand the complex phenomenon from which they are derived.

Frequently this term is used as a synonym of → reductionism, but this use is incorrect, in that between the two terms there is a fundamental difference: reductionism hands over the sceptre of knowledge from a more superficial discipline to a more profound one, whilst in the case of reductivism one goes from a variety of complex events or phenomena to one or a few explicative principles that make up its foundations, always remaining within the same discipline. For example, in classic psychoanalytic theory, the reductivist theory affirms that the various neurotic manifestations are all conducible to a particular vicissitude of the → libido. A reductionist theory would, on the other hand, propose, as S. Freud himself wished, to leave to biology or to neurophysiology the task of explaining in organic and observable terms the central concept of the libido and the ways in which changes in this psychic energy translate into behaviours that are neurotic or normal.

A hypothesis, however can be both reductionist and reductivist at the same time: for example, asserting that any given behaviour is caused by a certain gene is a theory that is both reductivist, because it leads a phenomenon to a primary principle that on its own is able to explain it, but also reductionist, because at the same time it identifies an object of study in psychology – behaviour – as being an object of study of biology – by looking at genes. *[R.]*

REDUNDANCY

As affirmed by Bateson, the content of a message is said to contain redundancy "if, when the sequence is received with some items missing, the receiver is able to guess at the missing items with better than random success". According to Bateson's definition, redundancy provides the means to predict or model particular events, and, thus, it meets the basic need of every human being and every living organism to find stability in, and to adapt to, chaos. Whenever a living system acquires the ability to store information about their achievements, this will use some forms of behaviour more frequently in the course of their adjustment, thus establishing certain rules above others in their action. The formation of rules and laws is a vital need of living organisms; life would not have become possible without them. Once rules and laws are established, they also have a self-solidifying tendency to turn into unshakable truths, as certain psychological experiments, the so called "non-contingency experiments", or the strategic concept of "redundant → attempted solutions" have sufficiently proved. Human beings do not tend to correct their obsolete assumptions that are the products of a once successful past adaptation, but try to develop them further instead. In other words, people have often a tendency to replicate those redundant scripts that were proven functional in the past (or in similar contexts), even when they appear to be dysfunctional (→ functional balance). Whoever experiences a panic attack, for example, with the feeling that their body "lets them down" and, therefore, tries to control their autonomous functions voluntarily, only generates further imbalance and the feeling of a stronger loss of control (→ logic of paradox). Similarly, whoever feels unsure of themselves in certain situations can increase momentarily their sense of security by asking others for help, but they become even more dependent or insecure in the long term. In strategic therapy, once the therapist has reduced the complexity of a problem in the therapeutic process (by means of the → strategic dialogue, for example), and has identified the main redundant and dysfunctional attempted solutions that maintain the specific problem, the redundant perceptive and reactive script of the client (→ perceptive-reactive system) might be unblocked and, thus, the → change can be enabled. *[D. Birkas]*

REFERENCES. Bateson G., *Steps to an ecology of mind*, 1972; Milanese R., Mordazzi P., *Strategic coaching*, 2015.

RE-EVOCATION

In general terms, it can be defined as a recall to the mind of information belonging to the past and previously memorized, or rather stored in the long-term → memory. Objects of recall can be the contents of declarative – or explicit – memory, which is, in turn, divisible into episodic (regarding personal experience) or semantic (regarding general knowledge about the world independently of the situation in which they have been learnt) memory. However, the contents of procedural or implicit memory (regarding the knowledge that we use automatically and unconsciously on how to do something) cannot be the object of recall, in that these are not directly accessible to consciousness.

Recall can be intentional, therefore associated with a voluntary effort made by the individual, or unintentional, and therefore determined by a series of mental associations that are not voluntarily guided by the individual. In experimental research on the functioning of memory, recall is studied through the administration of specific tests (for example, the memorization and the successive recall of a list of syllables, of numbers or of pairs of words). In this case, recall can be free or guided by the help of clues that facilitate the recovery of information. In the absence of trauma or of other pathological conditions, the better the process of memorization (as a result of the depth of elaboration, of the use of mnemonic technique, the vast number of other elements of knowledge that have been memorized, to the emotional meaningfulness of the information to be remembered and so forth), the easier it will be for recall to take place. The lack of ability to recall information, whether this be partial or total, of past experiences or of information determined by a multiplicity of factors, is defined as oblivion. The majority of psychodynamic psychotherapies have centred their methods around the recall of traumatic experiences. However, systematic studies have shown the process of recall to be unreliable, in that it is influenced by the emotional, cognitive and behavioural state of the individual in the present. *[R.]*

REFERENTIAL ACTIVITY

In → multiple code theory, W. Bucci, defines with this term the mental activity aimed at connecting emotions and somatic and sensory perceptions with verbal language. Referential activity is a variable that can be measured (with suitable methods developed by Bucci) to evaluate different levels of emotional intensity and cognitive integration between nonverbal experiences of the patient and the words used to express them. The evaluation of referential activity allows the study of the therapeutic process, as the oscillations of this variable in verbal exchanges between patient and therapist indicate micro-changes, within the sessions, in the patient's ability to use the therapist's interventions to boost their own referential activity. *[A. De Coro]*

REFLECTING TEAM

In the area of conversational therapy, it is the name given to a small group of observers – the team (→ observation) – openly discussing their experiences of a clinical situation while the → client and therapist listen to the team's comments. It is an intervention process developed in systemic family therapy by the Norwegian psychiatrist Tom Andersen in 1985. Several variations of the process have evolved in therapy, training and management. What they hold in common is a basic theme of offering people a unique opportunity to see themselves and their situation through the eyes of others. Typically, the team consists of two to six professionals who sit behind a one-way mirror and observe, as a therapist conducts the main part of an interview. Towards the end of the session, the therapist gives the client an opportunity to hear the team's comments. Team members do not address the client directly (except to introduce themselves); they talk to each other about the conversation they have just witnessed. Comments are offered as resonant experiences, tentative speculations and alternative perspectives; they are not intended to be prescriptive or advice-giving. Priority is given to affirming statements and acknowledgment of the competencies of the client. After 2 to 15 minutes of reflection, the therapist invites the client to respond to the team's comments. Clients (and therapists) are often moved by the reflections, so that therapy can proceed at a new level. *[K. Tomm]*

REFERENCES. Anderson T., Katz A., Lax W., Davidson J., Lussardi D., *The reflecting team: Dialogues and dialogues about the dialogues*, 1991.

REFRAMING

Reframing is a therapeutic technique (also known as restructuring) used in various psychotherapeutic approaches (→ cognitive reframing, → strategic reframing technique) based on the assumption that emotional responses are closely related to how people assess events and give them meaning. This assessment is influenced by the → beliefs they have about themselves (→ self-concept) and others. As a result, changing the way they assess events, seeing them from another point of view, and literally "putting them in a different frame", can completely change their emotional response. In reframing the patient's assessment of reality, the therapist does not reject the assessment itself, but helps the patient to consider it as a hypothesis, and to advance other hypothetical interpretations of the same events. This reframing aims to change the patient's stable bent, which is responsible for making them assess events in the same way, giving them a negative meaning, and consequently feeling negative emotions. *[G. Melli]*

REFRAMING AS A THERAPEUTIC OBJECTIVE

Reframing, besides being a therapeutic technique, can be considered as being the objective of every form of psychotherapy, in that the concept also means a → change in the ways in which a subject perceives and attributes meaning to his or her own reality. The concept of → therapeutic change in any form necessarily includes the attainment of this objective. *[R.]*

REGRESSION → DEFENCE MECHANISMS

REIFICATION

Within the clinical sciences of the psyche – psychotherapy among them – reification is a cognitive distortion that consists in identifying a psychological term with the "thing-in-itself". Reification causes the loss of the conventional, metaphorical, analogical feature of psychological language, which is essentially relational: a certain "construction", such as "personality", "introversion", "conscience" or "psychopathy" is transformed in a factual, existing entity, also due to the effects of the verb "to be" and discourse rhetoric (performative effect). This distortion may lead to a modification of evaluative attribution, for instance by turning the adjectives that categorize and evaluate a behaviour into substantives and, accordingly, into features or predicates of personality (transitive, tautological effect). In this case, the unaware effects of reification result in a confusion between the judgement of a behaviour and the objective properties of the subject, which are, therefore, identified with the traits explaining that behaviour and connoting that specific person.

The same phenomenon may happen on the side of patients/recipients, who, by playing the role of a self-observer and adopting these judgments (diagnoses), take on a psychic reality, a character, a way of being that turns into a → self-fulfilling prophecy. To this self-attributive distortion may also contribute the judgements and diagnoses expressed by others (self-representations).

Reification is present in the clinical sciences of the psyche and reflects the "factual" and regulatory needs of common sense and language (literalism).

An attributive, perceptive and explicative distortion due to the epistemic, positivistic matrix it derives from, but also to the imitation of medical language and thought: a cognitive scheme creating a representation of mental and behavioural processes as if they were real entities or existing objects. *[A. Salvini]*

REINFORCEMENT

In the behavioural paradigm, reinforcement is a stimulus that follows a specific behaviour and increases the probability of its emission. This effect can be obtained through a → reward, in the case of a → positive reinforcement (R+), or through the elimination of an adverse condition, in the case of a → negative reinforcement (R-). In relation to a behaviour, a reinforcement can be primary, if it is directly conditioning, or secondary, if it is indirectly conditioning. The latter facilitates the access to primary reinforcements and it becomes direct only after a generalization and valorization process. Reinforcements linked to physiological needs (food, water, sexuality) are considered primary, while those linked to social (attention, affection, recognition) and symbolic (money, titles, votes) needs are secondary. Experimental schedules can be implemented to represent the functioning of reinforcement in nature. These schedules can be based on the supply of the reinforcement on regular time-frames (fixed interval) or variable time-frames (variable intervals), or based on its supply after a number of fixed and repeatable (fixed ratio) or intermittent (variable ratio) → responses. The latter is the most efficient, as it is unpredictable. *[A. Tamburello, E. De Monte]*

REFERENCES. Hill W.F., *Learning: A survey of psychological interpretations*, 1963; Skinner F.B., *Science and human bevavior*, 1953.

REINFORCEMENT SCHEDULE

In neo-behavioural psychotherapy, a methodology used to enhance learning processes. The success or failure of such learning processes depends on the "planning" of the consequences resulting from the learning itself (→ law of effect); therefore, it is important to know "when and how often" a consequence follows a certain behaviour. There are two main types of reinforcement schedules: continuous (where → reinforcement always follows a correct answer) and intermittent (where reinforcement only follows it occasionally). The latter is divided into four subtypes: fixed ratio (the number of responses leading to the reinforcement is fixed); variable ratio (the number of responses leading to the reinforcement is unpredictable); fixed interval (the first response appearing after a set amount of time is reinforced); variable interval (the first response appearing after a variable amount of time is reinforced). A continuous reinforcement schedule is especially recommended in the initial phases of the consolidation of learning. Once the performance shows some stability, one can gradually move to intermittent schedules to keep the learner attentive and maintaining a good rhythm of study and work. *[V. Poerio]*

REFERENCES. Hilgard E.R., Bower G.H., *Theories of learning*, 1981; Skinner B.F., *The science of learning and the art of teaching*, in «Harvard Educational Review», 1954, 24, 2; Id., *The technology of teaching*, 1968.

RELATIONAL FRAME THEORY

Contextualized theory of language and of human cognition that introduces into the theoretical corpus of the behavioural paradigm (please see the opening chapter, "The eight paradigms and their respective theoretical-applicative models") a new class of operant responses (→ behavioural model of operant conditioning) of a superior order, called the "repertory of relational responses applied arbitrarily". Developed in the middle of the 1980s by Hayes, relational frame theory has given several stimuli both to fundamental research and to applied research, from which other clinical approaches can also benefit, as in the case of acceptance and commitment therapy. Hayes' theoretical work is centred around the concept of a response to a relationship that exists between two or more stimuli that can be non-arbitrary in the case of physical dimensions (for example tall–short, long–short), but that is arbitrary in the case of language, as in the relationship present between an object and its name. Hayes describes different relational frames (contexts, or organizational and relational forms): coordination, opposition, distinction, challenge, hierararchical or deictic. This new approach, empirically founded, can provide a heuristically valid story to the behavioural analysis of complex human behaviour, with particular reference to language and to the cognitive sphere, and is a point of dialogue between behavioural and cognitivist positions. *[G. Presti]*

REFERENCES. Hayes S.C., Barnes Holmes D., Roche B. (eds.), *Relational Frame Theory: A post-Skinnerian account of human language and cognition*, 2001; Törneke N., *Learning RFT: An introduction to relational frame theory and its clinical applications*, 2010.

RELATIONAL PSYCHOANALYSIS

A psychoanalytical school deriving from the concourse of a few post-Freudian traditions (→ object relations, interpersonal psychoanalysis, Self-psychology) and organized around a new paradigm that goes beyond "classical" psychoanalysis based on the → drive model. These developments started in the

United States in the 1980s and led to the establishment of a specific "relational track" in the post-doctoral programme of the New York University in 1988. At the same time in Italy, on a parallel but independent pathway in the late 1970s, a group of psychoanalysts collected around the work of David Rapaport and his followers and, animated by a critical and reformist approach to the classical model, an independent relational psychoanalysis was born with the creation in 1985 of SIPRe (Società italiana di psicoanalisi della relazione), the Italian Society of Relational Psychoanalysis. The work characterizing the reflections of Italian and American psychoanalysts focused on overcoming the limitations and aporias of Freudian metapsychology with the aim of building a theory of the mind capable of going beyond the fruitless opposition of intrapsychic and interactional and of moving inside an "open" view of knowledge, capable of integrating the data deriving from clinical experience with those deriving from research on the psychological development of infants. It is well known, in fact, that after the revolution of 1897, Freudian theory's focus on fantasy led to the disappearance of the object from the scene of psychic development. Freud's quantitative choice in favour of drives funnelled developmental dynamics into the bottleneck of a conflict that takes place only intrapsychically, where the rebound from sexuality to defence and back was a guarantee of the model's "positivity". The intrapsychic and drive models were then merged and any position deviating from this conceptualization was labelled as "naive environmentalism". On the other hand, it is true that the reaction to this theoretical setup was just as dramatic, even if it was often concealed and hidden so that it seemed almost invisible. From this position we can, in fact, explain the theory of deficits that tried to explain adult pathology as deriving from environmental failures. By signalling the relevance of material experience in the child's psychological development, this theory allowed a wider and more complex articulation of interactive exchanges. But the deficit model also dangerously unbalanced the aetiology of distress by "reactively" leaning onto the object, not to mention its consequences at the level of psychoanalytic technique: after a theory of development based on deficits, there followed a reparative therapy that seemed to try to compensate damages by substitution, at least to the extent that the aims of therapy and the therapist's role were oriented to healing, considered as making up for the deficits. Relational approaches derive exactly from the need to overcome the old opposition between intrapsychic fantasies and experiences deriving from the actual other in order to build a bridge between areas traditionally seen as antithetic: intrapsychic/interpersonal, external/internal, dispositional/contextual. The author who worked most at this creative integration was S. Mitchell. His reflections started from the consideration that all these traditions (object relations, interpersonal psychoanalysis, Self-psychology), beyond their undeniable differences, describe human beings and their mental development as deeply rooted in a social context of relations with significant others, the parents first of all. This means that we have here a paradigm that is "other" than drives. But if this is true, we need to change the way we look at a psychic subject: no longer an isolated, separate individual whose wishes are in deep contrast with external reality, but an intersubjective field within which the subject is born and develops psychologically. The concept of "relational matrix" indicates this interactive psychic space that gives rise both to transactional models and to their intrapsychic level. In this conceptualization, an individual is not seen as a passive victim of the so called "environmental failures" but as the active producer of meanings that invest relations and turn them into stable relational configurations. In addition, as they do not have relations as objects, these configurations are also inevitably conflicting. This stress allows Mitchell to highlight his intention of not leaving the area of conflict to classical theory, which had traditionally explained it along the drive–defence axis, but to explain its logic by means of relational configurations. And, in fact, Mitchell calls his theory the "model of relational conflict". Conflict will then concern the psychic dynamics of relations (e.g. the conflict between separation and individuation) or the social network of relations (e.g. one relation against the other) or the dialectics of historical relations/possible relations. In this view, conflict is located between the repetition of historical modes, necessary for the survival of identity, and a new possible space containing diverse and heterogeneous potential. According to this conceptualization, then, psychopathology should be seen as unconscious devotion to inaction and deep loyalty to what is familiar (in Mitchell's metaphor *familia* were the slaves serving patrician families in ancient Rome). This purview obviously entails immediate consequences also at the level of the theory of technique. Moving from a mono-personal conception of the mind to the constructivist approach in epistemology, the immediate consequence is the challenging of the concepts of "neutrality" and "anonymity" that were based on the possibility to provide the observer with an "objective" view of events. Relational psychoanalysis sees the analytical relationship as an exchange between two related subjectivities, both present and mutually affecting data. This means that the analyst's interventions, including interpretations, no longer come from a neutral, offline somewhere. On the contrary, the very concept of interpretation changes: from a one-way explanation coming from a knowing "authority", it becomes a "complex relational event" or a "bipersonal and mutual communication process" that contains cognitive-introspective and affective-experiential aspects. In this complex relational intertwining, interpretations are the outcome of co-construction. This constructivist conceptualization derives from the idea that it is impossible to interpret the unconscious structures and meanings of a given organization and the motives for their existence outside the relational context where they appear and reproduce (it is not possible, in other words, to have direct access to the other's intrapsychic) and the qualitative contents of the analytical relationship cannot be seen only as expressions of the patient's structures and organizational levels, but also as material manifestations of the asymmetric agreement between analyst and patient. For this reason, relational interpretations are addressed to the relationship, i.e. the unconscious meaning underlying the relation, and in this sense, we talk of relational analysis. All this does not mean that we can, or should, cancel the basic asymmetry of the analytical relationship. The mutuality in data production does not imply any symmetry in roles and responsibilities. It only means that, as Aron wrote, an analyst can still stand behind the couch, if he wants, but he can no longer hide behind it. The relational model is not a doctrine and not even a homogenous theoretical corpus, but a systematic effort at starting a resetting based on a critical reconstruction of the models underlying the analyst's therapeutic action, capable of stopping the oscillation of the psychoanalytical pendulum "between the question of guilt and that of responsibility", as Mitchell wrote. This challenge has not been easy and cannot be considered completed. In Italy, for example, the current developments of relational psychoanalytical thinking are more and more oriented, especially in M. Minolli's thinking, towards an epistemology of complexity that finds its most pregnant heuristic image in the metaphor of non-linear dynamic systems. *[S. Zito]*

REFERENCES. Aron L., *A meeting of minds: Mutuality in psychoanalysis*, 1996 (*Menti che si incontrano*, 2004); Benjamin J., *The bonds of love: Psychoanalysis, feminism, and the problem of domination*, 1988 (*Legami d'amore*, 1991); Gill M., *Psychoanalysis in transition: A personal view*, 1994; Minolli M., *Psicoanalisi della relazione*, 2009; Mitchell S. A., *Relational concepts in psychoanalysis: An integration*, 1988.

RELATIONSHIP

A collection of rules that governs the → interaction between individuals and that establishes the meaning that is to be attributed to the message contained in the → communication (as the very same expression acquires different meanings according to the relational context in which it is expressed). Interpersonal relationships can be symmetric or complementary (→ pragmatics of human communication) and are expressed primarily through nonverbal communication. In fact, frequently, relationships are not explicitly negotiated through the use of → language, rather, the more a relationship between individuals is spontaneous and functional, the more it will fade into the background. On the other hand, in situations of conflict it frequently can occur that the reason that triggers this conflict actually consists of a disagreement on who should punctuate (→ punctuation) and define the relationship (and how it should be done); in other words, on who has the right to have "the last word". The relational dimension considered up to now involves the involvement of two or more persons (self–other relationship). However, two other relational dimensions exist: that between the self and the self; and that between the self and the world (intended as a collection of cultural and social norms perceived by the individual as being an unchangeable fact). In the therapeutic field, the relationship together with language and with → therapeutic strategies, constitutes one of the essential aspects in triggering, as well as in sustaining, the process of → change. In some psychotherapeutic models the relationship is considered to be the therapeutic element *par excellence. [R.]*

▷ In Gestalt therapy, a relationship is the development of contacts between a specific "human-animal organism" and a part of its environment (human or non-human). Gestalt therapy studies the → here-and-now of the relationship, defined as the occurring, the being revealed of the experience co-created by organism and environment in contact. The term contact implies the interest in the experience generated by the concreteness of the senses, hence in the aesthetic and procedural values of the relationship. The → contact boundary is the place where the self unfolds and the → phenomenology of the encounter, with the phases of fore-contact, contact, full contact and post-contact, includes backgrounds (past acquisitions) and figures, i.e. current determinations looking to the future (→ figure–ground dynamic). Aggressiveness, being the spontaneous deconstructing force of survival, supports the experience of going towards the other and creative adjustment enables the individual to differentiate her/himself from the social context, but also to be fully and meaningfully part of it. The therapeutic relationship is the being-there-with of therapist and patient; they create an experiential field in which the spontaneous (not anxious) development of the self at the contact boundary is possible and the intentionality inherent in the patient's request for treatment can come to pass. *[M. Spagnuolo Lobb, P.A. Cavaleri]*

REFERENCES. Cavaleri P.A., *Vivere con l'altro. Per una cultura della relazione*, 2007; Spagnuolo Lobb M., *La relazione terapeutica in psicoterapia della Gestalt*, in P. Petrini, A. Zucconi (eds.), *La relazione terapeutica negli approcci psicoterapici*, 2007; Id., *Il setting in psicoterapia della Gestalt. La co-creazione dell'esperienza terapeutica nel qui-e-ora*, in C. Loriedo, F. Acri (eds.), *Il setting nelle psicoterapie*, 2009; Id., *L'incontro terapeutico come co-creazione improvvisata*, in M. Spagnuolo Lobb, N. Amendt-Lyon (eds), *Creative license: The art of Gestalt therapy*, 2003.

RELATIONSHIP QUESTIONS

In family therapy, questions that help the therapist and the → family to establish a meaningful relationship, which needs to be constantly nourished to create a fruitful structural coupling. The therapists "dance with the family" and try to have friendly contact with all the members. They pay attention to both coordinate relationships (for example, the parental couple) and subordinate relationships (for example, parents and children). Through relationship questions, the therapist fraternizes with the family and uses different accommodation techniques, such as: maintenance, tracking, mimesis. Maintenance highlights the → here-and-now of the observed interactions (for example: "Does it always happens that others get distracted when you talk?") and allows the therapist to affect relationships. When therapists perform tracking, they pay attention to communication and behaviour of family members, ask clarification questions and comments of approval and show themselves as an interested interlocutor. With mimesis, therapists adapt to the emotional style of the family, share the same experiences and dynamically wait for the system to be ready to restructure its internal consistency and move towards more functional modalities. *[F. Bruni, P.G. Defilippi]*

REFERENCES. Haley J., *Problem-solving therapy*, 1976; Minuchin S., *Families and family therapy*, 1974; Whitaker C.A., Bumberry W.M., *Dancing with the family*, 1988.

RELATIVE INFLUENCE QUESTIONING

In → narrative therapy, relative influence questioning is used to express a problem by producing new narratives through restructuring redefinitions (for example: "Could you indicate an episode where you did not surrender to the problem?", or: "Do you remember an instance where your relationship could have been overwhelmed by the problem and you have carried its burden instead?"). These questions help unique situations of lived and neglected experiences to emerge and become alternative stories to those dominated by the problem. In this way, they help people to review their individual "narrative", relations and problem. They allow individuals to distance themselves from the problem and be less paralysed, to discover situations that become "unique stories" with new descriptions of themselves, others and relationships. These stories are alternative to the predominant ones saturated by the problem that describe its influence on life and on the relationship with family members. These stories are placed in specific time and space, in an intelligible plot, and propose a reinterpretation of the events and suggest new possibilities. Multiple descriptions of the same event, depending on the point of view from which it is observed, encourage family members to make new distinctions and create new responses. There are two sets of relative influence questions: questions that help the effects of the problem to emerge in order to go beyond a statically rigid vision by introducing flexibility and new viewpoints (kaleidoscope); and questions to identify the influence of people and their relationships on the problem itself, highlighting competences and resources available to deal with adversity (fostering → resilience). *[F. Bruni, P.G. Defilippi]*

REFERENCES. White M., *Narrative means to therapeutic ends*, 1992.

RELATIVISM

Relativism is one of the main problematic issues, as well as one of the most significant epistemological contributions of cultural anthropology to the social sciences. Assuming that all cultures provide systems of values and shared meanings (→ context) that can be fully understood only within their own borders, cultural relativism invites reflection on the scientific status of anthropology itself, marked by a fundamental tension between universal explanation and circumstantial and situational understanding. As can be deduced from this premise, it is possible to specify different forms of relativism at various levels: epistemological relativism, in reference to the impossibility of generalizing cognitive processes; cultural relativism, in reference to the non-comparability between cultural experiences and habits; and psychological relativism, in reference to the unrepeatability of personal experience and to the importance of the study of individual differences. In this sense, it is possible to identify a contrast between two different research approaches to the study of cultural diversities: the first, inspired by the natural and physical sciences, whose explanations are characterized by causal and predictive concepts (nomothetic approach); and an approach to research and therapy influenced by → hermeneutics and humanistic disciplines, where possible interpretations and analysis of meanings and methods are proposed as elective (idiographic approach). At the same time, in the practice of psychotherapy, one can differentiate approaches that rely for their efficacy on the execution of standardized intervention techniques, and others that view the clinical session as the privileged context for the study and the modification of meanings linked to problematic life events. *[R.]*

RELAXATION

A psychophysiological state that is evidenced by the reduction of a state of tension. Relaxation tends to reduce cortical, hypothalamic and sympathetic excitability, decreasing in this way the intensity of emotional states. It can be objectively measured by galvanic skin response, EEG, EMG, respiration rate and heart rate, while at the subjective level it is measured by collecting introspective data about the sensations experienced by people. In 1958, J. Wolpe – exponent of behavioural psychotherapy – used E. Jacobson's progressive relaxation in the technique that he called → systematic desensitization. Other relaxation techniques adopted in other psychotherapeutic areas are H. Benson's relaxation response, → autogenic training, → transcendental meditation, → biofeedback technique etc. *[G. Sacco – D. Kakaraki]*

REFERENCES. Goldwurm G.F., Sacchi D., Scarlato, A., *Le tecniche di rilassamento nella terapia comportamentale. Manuale teorico pratico*, 2003.

RELEARNING → TRANSACTIONAL ANALYSIS

REPARATION ACTS

In strategic family therapy elaborated by Madanes, the expression refers to a → strategic treatment protocol that identifies 16 steps to resolve and repair interactions that have generated a trauma. It is a process that tries to be therapeutic for both the victim and the aggressor, and for every member of the family. The steps to reach the reparation are: account of the offence; opinions about the negative effects of the offence; focus on the spiritual pain of the victim and the aggressor; detection of other similar traumas in other family members; extension of the pain in every family member; expression of sorrow and repentance by the offender; apology by family members who have not given protection; the potential impact of relapse; discussion (only with the victim) about the trauma; identification of a protector for the victim; identification of a reparation gesture; reorientation of the life of the aggressor and the victim; restoration of love for the aggressor; the offender's reintegration in the → family; forgiveness of oneself. *[G. Ganda]*

REFERENCES. Madanes C., *Sex, love and violence*, 1990; Madanes C., *Strategic family therapy*, in A.S. Gurman, D.P. Kniskern (eds.), *Handbook of family therapy*, 1995.

REPETITION COMPULSION

In Freudian psychoanalysis, this expression can have different meanings. It may indicate the active repetition of an experience that was lived passively; or the repetition of actions that are considered corresponding to the necessity of the moment but which actually are the repetition of past experiences or behaviours not necessarily functional to the current situation; or a manner to consider transference (as a true time machine). Clinical perspectives do not always allow us to identify normal conflicting dynamics, the effects of infantile experiences and the realization of a wish. Therefore, these aspects are often neglected to favour the meta-psychological dimension. According to the latter, repetition compulsion is the manifestation of a tendency to return to previous conditions; that is, the tendency of what is living to come back to an inanimate condition from which it originated. This mechanism is connected with death instinct (→ drive) and to instinctual conservatism. This mechanism has been distinguished from the impulse to repeat a previous condition (→ regression). Repetition compulsion re-establishes a previous condition only during an initial phase, but after that it distances itself from it, and the sequence is repeated without changes. Regression would lack the progressive phase of repetition compulsion and entail a unidirectional change and not a negation of change. *[G. Fossi]*

REPLICABILITY

Characteristic of a model of intervention that can be reutilized with different patients that present the same type of problem – whilst at the same time maintaining its characteristic of → efficacy and → efficiency. Replicability is a fundamental property of a therapeutic intervention → protocol, in that, together with the concept of → transferibility, it confirms its intrinsic value, which goes beyond the single situation and the single patient to which it is applied. *[R.]*

Characteristic of a model of intervention that can be reutilized with different patients that present the same type of problem – whilst at the same time maintaining its characteristic of → efficacy and → efficiency. Replicability is a fundamental property of a → therapeutic intervention protocol, in that, together with the concept of → transferability, it confirms its intrinsic value, which goes beyond the single situation and the single patient to which it is applied. *[R.]*

REPRESENTABILITY

In Freudian theory, one of the defence mechanisms of the oneiric work that provides for the transformation of latent oneiric thoughts into manifest oneiric content, in its turn sustained by another mechanism of the transformation of the dream, displacement,

> in the sense that a colourless and abstract expression in the dream-thought, is exchanged with a pictorial and concrete one (because) a thing that is pictorial is, from the point of view of a dream, a thing that is capable of being represented.

Freud specifies that this transformation into "pictorial language" sustains the "interests of condensation and of censure" and allows the regression to visual images, through which the passage through the "concrete terms" of language and the establishment of new connections is able to take place. *[F. Munari]*

REFERENCES. Freud S. (1900–1901), *The interpretation of dreams*, in *The Standard Edition*, IV–V, 1953–1974.

REPRESENTATION

The term comes from the philosophical tradition of modern psychology of Wundt, for whom "significant general representations" bring together a large number of psychic events that exercise a critical control on mental activity. Durkheim speaks of collective representations as the texture of social life; they emerge in the relations of individuals and groups and between the individual and society. Freud utilizes the term to indicate the element of the object that is transcribed in mnemonic systems. In the *Interpretation of Dreams*, he describes how the dream treats "words as things", using them in combinations that lead to "strange and unusual creations"; later, he refers to the acts in the psyche in diverse "transcriptions", with the possibility of being transported from the system of the → unconscious to that of the conscious. Jung, on the contrary, will speak of "images", fantastic representations that do not substitute concrete reality and are distinct, as "internal" images, from sensible reality. An important exception, noted by Moscovici, is that of social representations; these come from his study of the image of psychoanalysis deployed in the French press, and on the consequent perceptions that emerge within that culture. For Moscovici, social representations render the strange familiar, "anchoring" unusual ideas in ordinary categories and everyday contexts, and objectifying the abstract in concrete terms. *[P. Meringolo]*

▷ In psychoanalysis, representation is the permanency of the psychic image in the absence of a corresponding perception. Originally, it aims at neutralizing a lack with the hallucination of a previous satisfaction. Therefore, representation depends on real perception (→ reality principle), while at the same time it reveals the underlying domination of the → pleasure principle. The representation, together with the → affect is inextricably tied to the → drive, in that it permits the psychic expression of otherwise unknowable impulses. The scope of representation and affect are diverse and specifically tied to various psychopathological conditions: representation is repressed, affect displaced, converted. The distinction between representations of "things" and of "words" establishes the difference between the unconscious, based only on the former, and the preconscious and conscious in which both are present. *[G. De Renzis]*

REFERENCES. Durkheim É., *Suicide*, 1897; Freud S. (1900–1901), *The interpretation of dreams*, in *The Standard Edition*, IV–V, 1953–1974; Id. (1914–1916), *Papers on metapsychology and other works*, in *The Standard Edition*, XIV, 1953–1974; Jung C.G. (1921), *Dictionary of analytical psychology*, 1987; Moscovici S., *La psychanalyse, son image et son public*, 1961; Id., *The phenomenon of social representations*, in R.M. Farr, S. Moscovici (eds.), *Social representations*, 1984; Wundt W., *Principles of psysiological psychology*, 1874.

REPRESENTATIONAL SYSTEMS

In neuro-linguistic programming, the first stable form of encoding of the experience linked to the five senses. Neuro-linguistic programming has shown that information coming from the external and internal environment are firstly encoded in the shape of images (the visual system V), sounds (the auditory system A) and sensations (the kinaesthetic system K). The kinaesthetic system involves tactile experience, proprioception, visceral experience (internal organs), vestibular experience (sense of equilibrium) as well as olfactory perception and taste. The representational encoding of experience happens in response to emotional charge, which determines retention of information in medium- and long-term memory. This process is mediated by three processing mechanisms: → deletion (incomplete encoding), → distorsion (formal divergences) and generalization → (flattening differences). Analogical encoding (the similarity principle), which involves representational encoding systems, is followed by digital or linguistic encoding (the all-or-nothing principle), in which the effect of previous mechanisms is stronger. *[S. Boschi]*

REFERENCES. Bandler R., Grinder J., *The structure of magic*, 1975; Id., N*eurolinguistic programming: The study of the structure of subjective experience*, 1979.

REPRESENTATIVENESS

Described by Freud as the psychic aspect of the drive: "as a measure of the demand made upon the mind to work in virtue of its connection with the body". At times, it appears that Freud considered the concept of representativeness as coinciding with the drive itself, "drive representativeness"; at other times he appears to consider it to be the representational expression of the drive, "ideational representativeness". In the first case it is the drive that is designated as being the "psychic representative" of the stimuli that originate from within the body and are received by the psyche; in the second instance, Freud appears to mean a → representation or a group of representations that have been invested at the service of those drives that have a certain amount of psychic energy. *[M. Vigneri]*

REFERENCES. Freud S. (1915), *Instincts and their vicissitudes*, in *The Standard Edition*, XIV, 1953–1974; Id. (1915), *Repression*, in *The Standard Edition*, XIV, 1953–1974.

REPRESSED

In the field of psychoanalysis, the term, used in the first Freudian works, is synonymous with the → unconscious, indicating those contents that escape the consciousness of the individual and that constitute a separate psychic group confined within the unconscious and regulated by the laws of the primary process. In his metapsychological works, Freud identifies in primary repression, built by the ideational representatives of the → drive, a kind of pole of attraction with regard to those elements that will subsequently be repressed. *[N. Dazzi]*

REFERENCES. Freud S. (1914–1916), *Papers on metapsychology and other works*, in *The Standard Edition*, XIV, 1953–1974; Id. (1932–1936), *New introductory lectures on psycho-analysis and other works*, in *The Standard Edition*, XXII, 1953–1974.

REPRESSION → DEFENCE MECHANISMS

RESEARCH

In the field of psychotherapy, the term is used with a double meaning. It can mean the verification and the validation of psychotherapeutic models, of a single therapeutic technique and of the psychotherapeutic paradigms in general through the use of controlled individual or group empirical studies (refer to the Appendix, "Empirical research in psychotherapy"). Or else it can be intended as being synonymous with → heuristics, referring to the exploration of new linguistic and communicative, relational and technical modalities, aimed at the evolution of the efficacy of the therapeutic work as well as at the adaptation of psychotherapy to socio-cultural changes and contexts that influence the expression of psychopathology. In the latter case, in fact, it is well known that forms of psychological suffering are constantly and profoundly modulated by the cultural, social, familial, linguistic and developmental context, and for this reason – in order to be dealt with in an effective manner – the basic instruments of psychotherapy, including → language, the → therapeutic strategies and techniques utilized, are in need of continuous adaptation and refinement. *[R.]*

RESILIENCE

Resilience is the ability to pick oneself up after a → crisis, more flexible, more aware and more balanced than before. It is the instinct to overcome suffering without succumbing, and to learn from what happened. Resilience is a process of cognitive, emotional, behavioural and spiritual reframing of one's representation of → pain that leads to overcoming losses, grief and traumas with the desire to rebuild, although lacking energy. This reframing helps to differentiate weakness from vulnerability and to reinforce a person's character. Resilience elicits physical, mental, relational and moral strength, awareness of being alive, and gratefulness for any additional time in which new horizons can unfold, even those which before the crisis seemed non-existent. During the critical period, resilience leads to the reinforcement of emotional detachment to what is happening, protects against excessive pain and nourishes hope that things will change. After the event, resilience brings awareness that the worst belongs to the past and stimulates the deep understanding of the wounds. This rapid transformational process of the meaning distracts from negative thoughts and feelings, recovers willpower and passion for the possible, and rediscovers the value of living. Resilience invites us to look to the future, conscious of what can and should be done, to work together with the destiny that has given us another chance. In order to boost resilience in patients it is useful to raise awareness that the past is past and that, starting in the present moment, they are directed to the future. *[C. Casula]*

REFERENCES. Casula C., *La forza della vulnerabilità*, 2011; Short D., Casula C., *Speranza e resilienza*, 2004; Walsh F., *La resilienza familiare*, 1998.

RESISTANCE

In Freudian theory, "anything in the actions and in the discourse of the analysand that can be an obstacle to the therapeutic work". The concept of resistance has played a fundamental role in the birth, and the development, of psychoanalytic technique. Already in his *Studies on Hysteria* Freud attributed the difficulties of the therapeutic work to the activation of a "resistance" that would manifest itself by making the images recalled by the patient confused and full of lacunae. Although presenting itself as an obstacle that risks impeding the progress of the therapeutic work, resistance also allows the recognition of pathogenic memories as they emerge. The painful character of these memories led Freud to hypothesize that the resistance evidenced by the patient to the re-emergence of these memories was due to the reactivation of defences, of repression, and that it was therefore a manifestation of the same force that, in pushing memories away from the conscious "had co-operated in the genesis of the hysterical symptom". The difficulty with which these memories re-emerged, and the reluctance with which the patient would communicate them, had now become clues that were able to guide the therapist towards the discovery of repressed memories; therefore therapy could be conceptualized as being the psychological work necessary in order to "overcome in the patient a psychic force which opposed the pathogenic idea from becoming conscious". In this way, having given up hypnosis and hypnotic suggestion and having turned to the → free associations technique, his therapeutic work ended up revolving around the recognition of resistance. Progressively, starting from the 1920s, Freud placed increasing emphasis on the defensive aspect of resistance and brought back the analysis of resistance to the analysis of the defences of the Ego (→ mechanisms of defence). *[N. Dazzi]*

REFERENCES. Breuer, J., Freud, S., (1893–1895), *Studies on hysteria*, in *The Standard Edition*, II, 1953–1974.

RESISTANCE TO CHANGE

A natural tendency of all human systems (individual, couple or family) to resist change to the existing conditions, maintaining a homeostatic equilibrium (→ homeostasis), even when this is clearly dysfunctional (→ functional balance). The resistance to change, being an inescapable characteristic of living organisms, represents one of the central themes of all psychotherapeutic orientations, even if it is conceptualized and managed differently according to the different models of therapy. The term appears, therefore, with different connotations throughout the history of psychotherapy, from S. Freud and his followers up to the Palo Alto School and M.H. Erickson, to quote some of the greatest scholars of this theme.

Two principal orientations in tackling resistance to change can be identified, to which different corresponding modalities in the structure of the logic of the therapeutic intervention and in the choice of the type of communication utilized by the therapist exist. On the one hand, there are those models that tackle resistance as something that needs to be eliminated in a direct manner, through its interpretation (psychodynamic approach) or rationalization and understanding (cognitive and behavioural approaches).

Although exhibiting significant theoretical and methodological differences, these models utilize an ordinary → logic of intervention as well as utilising modes of communication that are of a rational-explicative nature. On the other hand, there are approaches in which resistance is circumvented or utilized in the direction of → change (systemic and strategic approaches), thanks to the utilization of non-ordinary logic and modes of → communication that are suggestive and injunctive. According to this point of view, the fact that a system is not alerted in a direct manner regarding its possible change leads to the reduction to a minimum of its resistance, and therefore one can achieve the desired change in a manner that is decisively more rapid and with less difficulty. *[R.]*

RESPONDENT CONDITIONING → CLASSICAL CONDITIONING

RESPONSE

In the behaviourist paradigm this refers to a → behaviour that is induced by a particular → stimulus or in some way associated with it. For example, the perception of an earthquake taking place (S) can evoke feelings of fear and escape (R). Experience can favour new S–R associations that were not meaningful before the event (for example, the oscillation of a ceiling lamp will recall the same fear and escape response). *[M. d'Ambrosio]*

REFERENCES. LeDoux J., *The emotional brain*, 1998; Le Ny J.-F., *Le conditionnement*, 1961.

RESPONSE FREQUENCY

In the model of operant conditioning, it is one of the parameters characterizing a learned behaviour (→ behavioural model of operant conditioning). It describes the number of times that such behaviour has been emitted by a subject (in a minute, an hour, a day, etc.). If the → frequency is related to a behaviour learned by classical or Pavlovian conditioning (→ behavioural model of classical conditioning), the term "elicitation frequency" needs to be used. *[F. Fois]*

RESPONSE PREVENTION

In cognitive behavioural psychotherapy, it is the patient's exposure to a feared thought, image or event, while ensuring that the subject withstands the impulse to perform rituals and/or reassuring avoidances.

Exposure is a therapeutic behavioural technique consisting in facing feared situations, objects or thoughts that generally are avoided by the person, both in a gradual way (→ graded exposure) and in → flooding.

Both exposure and response prevention lead to a more functional management of anxiety, with a consequent increase of one's personal sense of self-efficacy. *[B. Rainieri]*

REFERENCES. Dèttore D., *Obsessive-compulsive disorder and thinking illusions*, in «Psicoterapia Cognitiva e Comportamentale», 2011, 17(3); Sanavio E., *I comportamenti ossessivi e la loro terapia*, 1978; Id., *Psicoterapia cognitiva e comportamentale*, 1991.

RESPONSIBILITY

In the field of law, but also in that of philosophy, the concept of responsibility is of significant importance, with regard to the fulfilment of an obligation, or the effects of an action. In psychology, different schools of thought talk about responsibility as being a subjective and internal attitude, even if it has different shades of meaning, according to the fundamental premises underlying the meaning. S. Freud describes the passage from being an irresponsible child to that of becoming a responsible parent as "maturation", and this takes place through a healthy → identification with the father. Some of his followers have moved from the idea of identification with authority to the capacity of being answerable for one's actions and their consequences: responsibility means, therefore, the capacity to manage a contractual relationship.

The meaning attributed to this term is, however, different in those psychotherapies that make out of the assumption of responsibility for oneself a fundamental objective of change. This is the position taken by Gestalt psychotherapy, whose representatives assert that one can talk about responsibility every time that there is contact with facts or events, relationships, feelings, ways of being, behaviours. Being responsible means being able to provide an answer to the awareness of one's internal states, to the awareness of the way in which we determine their existence and their meaning. Responsibility is, in fact, part of the process of self-regulation of the organism. In view of this theoretical position, responsibility is therefore configured as the "capacity to respond", which means being able to choose a behaviour, with the aim of managing one's own sensations and emotions, as well as managing those events to which an individual is exposed. *[R.]*

RESPONSIVENESS TO MINIMAL CUES → ERICKSONIAN HYPNOTHERAPY

RESTRUCTURING → REFRAMING

RETROACTIVE ANNULMENT → DEFENCE MECHANISMS

RETROFLECTION

In Gestalt psychotherapy, the function of the self that is defined by Perls as being "originally directed from the individual towards the world, that instead changes direction and is directed backwards, towards the person from which it originated". A healthy exercise of retroflection allows the individual to contain impulses in order to delay their expression to a time and situation that will allow for a more effective satisfaction of these needs. A chronic attitude towards retroflection involves a habitual retention of one's needs, with the consequent behaviours of self-inhibition that are likely to be an obstacle towards a healthier osmosis between the needs of the individual and the possibility of contact with the resources of the environment. *[R. Zerbetto, R. Versaci]*

REFERENCES. Perls F., Hefferline R.F., Goodman P., *Gestalt therapy: Excitement and growth in the human personality*, 1951; Zerbetto R., *Gestalt: la terapia della consapevolezza*, 1998.

RÊVERIE

In the psychoanalytic theory of Bion, rêverie is defined as one of the factions of the "alpha function" of the mother that corresponds to a "mental state that is open to receiving all 'objects' originating from the loved object; that state, therefore that is able to take in the → projective identifications of the child". Bion in fact postulates the existence in the personality of a → function, that he calls precisely the alpha function, which operates on the sensorial and emotional impressions, transforming them into elements that can be utilized for thoughts, dreams, memory and in order to establish the distinction between conscious and unconscious. If the alpha function is blocked or inverted, the contact with internal or external reality will produce only indigestible elements (beta elements), that cannot be reutilized or assimilated but only evacuated into the surrounding field (into the soma or into the environment) through projective identification. The structuring of the alpha function depends highly on the mother–child relationship in the earliest phases of life. If the relationship is sufficiently good, the newborn projects onto the mother sensory stimuli that he is not yet able to metabolize, in order for the mother to receive them, process them and return them in a form that is utilizable. Reintrojecting the transformed elements, the child introjects also their transformative function. The term reverie is utilized by extension in clinical practice, where it indicates the mental attitude of the psychoanalyst towards the therapeutic work, intended as the capacity for non-linear and oneiric thinking, which allows for the reception and containment of the emotions emerging from the patient. *[C. Neri, L. Selvaggi]*

REFERENCES. Bion W.R., *Learning from experience*, 1962; Id., *A theory of thinking*, 1962.

REVERSAL → DEFENCE MECHANISMS

REVERSAL OF PERSPECTIVE

A Bionian concept, according to which a series of facts can be viewed from one or two different perspectives, just as certain ambiguous figures. For example, there is a famous figure that can be seen as a vase or as two faces (→ figure–ground dynamic). This can happen sometimes creatively and at other times to interrupt the therapeutic progress. For example, an interpretation that, if accepted in the way the analyst intended, would give rise to disturbance, is accepted as a mere definition and therefore it is of no concern to the patient. *[J. Symington]*

REFERENCES. Bion W.R., *Elements of psychoanalysis* 1963.

REVERSING THE FAMILY HIERARCHY

In strategic family therapy, a technique developed by Madanes to counter incongruous hierarchies (→ hierarchy). Children try both to change and to protect parents with their symptoms; a disturbed child appears as both dependent on parents and superior to them, obtaining the "victory of the defeated". During the intervention strategy, the therapist manipulates and redistributes power by promoting communication sequences in order to form a proper hierarchy, while opposing at the same time the sequences that disqualify it. The therapist tries to ensure that parents have a superior position to children. Parents are enabled to express expectations and rules for children, as well as the consequences of transgression. *[G. Ganda]*

REFERENCES. Madanes C., *The prevention of rehospitalization of adolescents and young adults*, in «Family Process», 1980, 19; Id., *Strategic family therapy*, 1991.

REWARD

Gratification, also known as reward, that an individual receives after having exhibited operant behaviour, within the context of a learning process by → operant conditioning. A more adequate term in this context is that of → positive reinforcement. *[F. Fois]*

RIGIDITY

In the field of strategic family psychotherapy, the psychological difficulty of including points of view that are different from one's own; a defensive attitude that closes off any possible doubts regarding one's convictions; poor levels of permeability within the family "boundary", lack of ability to alternate between complementary (→ complementarity) and symmetrical (→ symmetry) positions, being emotionally closed-off in such a way as to interrupt the temporal and spatial cycle of the family, leading to a state of suspension that stops the individual at a precise point of his life, most commonly in the phase in which a → trauma occurs, a critical event, a loss; a mechanical repetition of identical relational modalities, even when the contest changes. *[M. Menafro]*

REFERENCES. Cancrini L., La Rosa C., *Il vaso di Pandora. Manuale di psichiatria e psicopatologia*, 1991; Chianura P., Schepisi L., Dellarosa A.C., Menafro M., Peruzzi P. (eds.), *Le relazioni e la cura*, 2008; Menafro M., *La psicoterapia infantile sistemica: l'uso relazionale della fiaba inedita*, in P. Gritti, E.L. Di Caprio (eds.), *Le nuove prospettive della psicoterapia sistemico-relazionale*, 2006.

RITE

A procedure that is consolidated or even coded. The power of the rite has been recognized in its ability to help make a society more stable and cohesive, protecting individuals within an interaction, and safeguarding the image one has of oneself. In a neurotic disorder the rite becomes an instrument that protects the individual from that which he is afraid of. Its structure can be an action, physical or mental, carried out and repeated according to a precise scheme that originates from an internal pressure that is experienced as being uncontrollable, which pushes the individual to enact certain behaviours in spite of the fact that he is aware of their lack of real or practical usefulness.

To the primary → anguish, from which the individual attempts to protect himself by means of the rite, a second is added relative to the omission or the doubt of not having carried out the rite in an adequate-enough manner. The therapeutic power of the rite is recognized in its capacity to help to endure and overcome difficulties, to mediate and overcome conflicts or as a therapeutic technique that activates a process of healing; it is used, with a greater or lesser degree of awareness, to promote → change in psychotherapy, whether this consists of the structure of the → setting or the regularity of the scheduling of the sessions, the payment or whether it originates from specific therapeutic manoeuvres. Particular attention has been given to the rite in the form of an → ordeal by those who acknowledge its presence in all types of therapy and who have developed it as a technique aimed at removing the power of the symptom by provoking a level of discomfort that is equal to that caused by the symptom itself. In the more evolved strategic approaches (→ brief strategic therapy Nardone's model) a series of → counter-ritual techniques have been developed for the treatment of obsessive-compulsive patients. *[R.]*

▷ In the enactment of rites, attention is prevalently focused on the experience of the sacred, on representations of nature, the world of humans and events that are considered to be worthy of being included in the collective memory. By means of ceremonies and sacred cults, or by means of the telling of a story and other events, the mythical and religious beliefs actualized by the rite are used to reinforce the emotional states of the individual that have been induced by the symbols. The amplifications that in psychotherapy allow the the psychic events of the patient (for example, a dream) to be put alongside a particular ritual is possible, according to Jung, precisely because, in the rite, universal needs, symbolically expressed are manifested: for example, the symbolism of the Catholic mass. One of Jung's criticisms of modernity is based on the idea of an obsolescence of the (transformative) psychological value of the rite. From this, the focus on the conscious narrative of the patient and on the unconscious material offered to the psychotherapist developed. According to Jung, this unconscious material aspires to become conscious in that it is an expression of an innate tendency of the processes of the psyche. This interpretative-curative line of thinking is referred to by all those who see in the rite a universal need of the human psyche, in contrast to those who believe that the rite is a culturally coded expression that does not conform to the idea of the psyche as being objective and ahistorical. In this second point of view, the rite would be one of the forms of the perception of reality (internal and external) that can be utilized in order to access the collective dimensions, to which the psyche of an individual inevitably makes reference. *[E.V. Trapanese, S. Fossi]*

REFERENCES. Jung C.G. (1912), *Transformation symbolism in the mass*, in *Collected Works*, XI, 1969.

RITE OF PASSAGE

A ceremony that in various Scandinavian cultures marks the transition between various life stages or the progression of class and of specialization, in addition to establishing differences within social → groups. Australian narrative psychotherapy gives a certain amount of emphasis to rites of passage, so much so that at the end of therapy with children and adolescents a "diploma" is awarded that is visible to friends and relatives (because, in order for a new narrative to have an effect on the identity of a person, the presence of others with whom it can be shared is necessary); this marks the passage from being a "patient" to becoming an "expert", able to put his own experience at the service of other children who have a similar problem. *[M. Giuliani]*

REFERENCES. Van Gennep A., *The rites of passage*, 1960; White M., Epston D., *Narrative means to therapeutic ends*, 1990.

ROLE-PLAYING

According to Moreno, father of → psychodrama, it is the key instrument to perform an improvised representation of a patient's life in a group. The "play" begins after the narration of the patient, when the therapist asks the patient-protagonist to assign roles in their story to other patients who work as actors or "auxiliary Egos." The game proceeds with various techniques, like role reversal, the double, the mirror, the soliloquy. According to Moreno and A.A. Schützenberger, the techniques of active intervention are more than 300. The patients gradually play adult roles and states of mind and free themselves from the conditionings exerted by the family and by all the alienating contexts. They move towards the "catharsis of integration", where the psychodrama culminates. The role-playing continues with the final sharing of experiences in the group, which aims not so much at analysis, but rather at creating empathy and existential encounter. Moreno claims that role-playing precedes the emergence of the Self: the roles do not emerge from the Self but rather the Self can emerge from the roles played in life and in therapy. The theory of psychodrama considers role-playing from various viewpoints: training, distribution, assumption, creation, definition, dynamics, dominance, measurement, perception, stability and, above all, pathology. Pathogens role-plays, such as parentification, take place in families where the functions of the real role of a child overlap with the alienating pressure of a father's or mother's idealistic role assigned unconsciously to the child. For example, the old custom of giving a baby the name of an ancestor can make a child the unaware and involuntary interpreter of an intergenerational family ghost. The alienating pressure of such a role affects children's lives and is likely to affect their freedom. From a therapeutic perspective, thanks to Moreno, the role-playing technique has become part of many forms of psychotherapy: from Gestalt therapy, to → Ericksonian hypnotherapy and systemic therapy. This is also used in → family constellations where role-playing becomes dangerous due to the authoritarian interference of the leader, who chooses, assigns and interprets, in their own way, all the roles of the participants. *[O. Rosati]*

REFERENCES. Moreno J.L., *Psychodrama first volume*, 1946; Moreno J.L., Moreno Z.T., *Psychodrama, Vol 1*, 1959.

ROLE REVERSAL

It is the most typical technique of → psychodrama, which makes a person (a member of the group, a protagonist) assume, for a time, the role of another person. This "other" is usually a significant real person, but it can also be the personification of an object, an idea, a fantasy, a part of oneself. The reversal makes the images of others concrete and perceptible, giving shape to the perceptions of the subject. As it requires a decentralization from oneself, role reversal leads to reflection on personal experiences and to understanding – in the other's shoes – new elements that will then be integrated into the context of one's own individual perceptions: the other becomes less mysterious, more differentiated, and the protagonist has a better acknowledgement of his/her own individuality. *[G. Boria]*

REFERENCES. Boria G., *Psicoterapia psicodrammatica. Sviluppi del modello moreniano nel lavoro terapeutico con gruppi di adulti*, 2005; Boria G., Muzzarelli F., *Incontri sulla scena*, 2009; Moreno J.L., *Psychodrama first volume*, 1946; Id., *Who shall survive?*, 1953.

S

SANDPLAY THERAPY

Analytical therapy defined during the 1950s by D.M. Kalff, student of C.G. Jung. Used initially with children and adolescents, it rapidly found effective application also with adults. The theoretical and clinical basis is Jungian psychoanalysis, in particular several cornerstones of Jungian thought such as: the → individuation process, creativity, → fantasy, imagination, → symbols. It is also necessary to mention the contributions of M. Lowenfeld, M. Klein and D.W. Winnicott to the scientific corpus and the practical therapy of sandplay. The very nature of sandplay requires the rules of analytical → setting. The space of the patient–analyst relationship is constituted by a room; here the patient has two trays available (76 × 54 × 7 cm) with a blue inner bottom, symbolizing water (sea, rivers, lakes), each containing either dry or humid sand and, along walls, shelves full of miniature reproductions of human figures (current and past civilians and soldiers), animals (pets, birds, fish, wild animals, dinosaurs, dragons), trees, flowers, buildings and household furniture and decorations, means of transportation, boats, pieces of wood, stones, shells, modelling clay. By placing such objects in the sand, the patient creates a three-dimensional representation. The symbolic value of each individual object, the relationship established amongst the various objects, the type of contact of the patient with the sand and the state of the sand itself (dry, humid, manipulated), all contribute to the emergence of the psychic state of the patient. An unconscious problem is staged and internal conflicts are made visible. Subsequently, the sandplay image needs to be connected to the context of the analytical room: objects used; sequence and timing of their disposition; emotions expressed or not; words pronounced before, after or during the creation of the sandplay image; signs of transference movements; countertransference resonance of the analyst. The contact of the patient's hands with the materials, the plasticity of the sand, the utility of objects, the evocative power of sandplay images, all reveal the possibility of psychic transformation. Psychic transformation, however, only becomes possible when the therapist accepts, contains and interprets the sandplay image produced by the patient (miniature objects used, method and timing of choice of the objects, manipulation or not of the sand) as a symbolic element (union of internal and external aspects) of the entire psycho-analytical process. The training of sandplay therapist is an additional specialization beyond the basic Jungian psychoanalytical training: it also requires a specific analytical training based on the assisted analysis of the therapist's own sandplays. *[M. Garzonio]*

REFERENCES. Garzonio M., *Theatre of earth, water and hands*, in M.I. Wuehl (ed.), *In the room of the Jungian analyst*, 2002; Kalff D.M., *Sandplay and its therapeutic impact on the psyche*, 1966.

SATORI

In Gestalt psychotherapy, as in the zen tradition, satori is a state of privileged consciousness characterized by a singular experience of the presence of → awareness, integrity, acceptance and widening of the state of consciousness. This state can be momentary or more enduring and is similar to the state of illumination – nirvana or *samadhi* in the respective Buddhist and Hindu traditions – with which one can associate, generally, a state that is more enduring. A self-limiting condition of the structure of the Ego appears to be able to tune into a dimension of wider belonging in which the individual feels that he is "part of the whole" and as being part of a plan that gives him a meaning that is more vast than his singularity. The experience of → insight represents, in particular in the psychoanalytic tradition, a moment of profound understanding regarding contents that had previously been perceived as being confusing or obscure. In the Gestalt tradition, Perls used the expression "aha" experience to refer to an experience of awareness that does not limit itself to the phenomenon of intellectual understanding, but that also includes an emotional and holistic dimension of the individual. Quoting Perls:

> One of the most spontaneous and surprising experiences of satori happened to me around twelve years ago on a Miami beach . . . Like a stroke of lightening the world became overwhelming in its existence, tri-dimensional, full of colour and life, like clarity "without" life, but with a full sense of satisfaction of: "This is real". This was a complete awakening, the returning to my senses, and my senses that were returning to me, and my senses made sense.

[R. Zerbetto, D. Santabbondio]

REFERENCES. Daishi Y., *Il canto dell'immediato satori*, 1994; Perls F., *Here and now*, 1969; Zerbetto R., *Gestalt: la terapia della consapevolezza*, 1998.

SCALE TECHNIQUE

A technique arising from the → brief solution-focused therapy developed by Shazer and Berg. It consists of asking the patient: "If today you had to evaluate your situation on a scale of zero to ten, where zero represents how things were in your first session and ten being when the therapy will have been concluded successfully, what number would you give to describe your present situation?" De Shazer defines "zero" as being the moment in which the client has asked for help and not when their situation was at its worst point, so that the point of reference will not be a period of time that may have been very long ago, which therefore would not allow the therapist to underline the resources that the patient has employed in order to improve his situation. If, to this question, the client answers: "I feel that I am at zero", the therapist can ask: "Therefore, what have you done so far to prevent things from becoming worse?" or "How come things did not become worse?", always from the point of view of orienting the therapeutic investigation towards the 'positive. This technique is introduced when the therapist has managed to develop an adequate description of the → miracle question, in such a way that the scale technique will promote the attainment of every single therapeutic objective. In this way, the psychotherapist is able to highlight what has already improved and what the client has done to achieve this improvement. Additionally, the scale will enable the therapist to translate the "miracle" from the point of arrival (a score of ten) into a series of steps, creating in this way a process in which every step has corresponding thoughts, emotions, behaviours and interactions that are associated with the different areas of the life and of the reality of the client. *[G. Nardone]*

REFERENCES. De Shazer S., Dolan Y., Korman H., Trepper T., McCollum E., Berg I.K., *More than miracles: the state of the art of Solution Focused Brief Therapy*, 2007.

SCIENTIFIC METHOD IN PSYCHOLOGY AND PSYCHOTHERAPY

The study of healthy and pathological phenomena (in the etymological sense of "states that create suffering") can be considered scientific when it follows the criteria of rationality, empiricism, quantification, operationalization, theorizing and epistemological awareness. In summary, these principles can be so described: the phenomenon is investigated in its functioning through the data coming from the experience (empiricism, rationality); observations are catalogued and made accessible and repeatable by others (quantification, operationalization); the collection of observed phenomena is used to build a pattern of relations and an explanatory model (theorization); researchers are aware of the principles/assumptions that lead both their observation and their theorizing (epistemological awareness). There are several possible ways to apply these principles to the study of psychology and psychotherapy. The different scientific practices can vary depending on the phenomena being studied and on the instrumental limitations of the investigation. There are three main methods used in psychology and psychotherapy. The experimental method: controlled variables are manipulated by the researcher in order to prove the truth/falsity of a hypothesis. A variable can be "dependent" (measurement of the effects), "independent" (directly manipulable by the researcher in order to study its effects on the dependent variables) or "constant" (not directly manipulable by the researcher). This is the main method used in psychology to study mental processes such as → memory, → perception, → learning, thinking, reasoning, emotions, etc. In these cases, the researcher creates an experimental situation characterized by the presence of independent variables and constants, and he/she studies the changes on behaviour and psyche (dependent variables). The application of the pure experimental method to psychotherapy is difficult due to the complexity and number of variables involved, compared to more limited phenomena, such as those related to mental processes. Nevertheless, testing the clinical efficacy of different psychotherapeutic intervention models in relation to the various types of psychopathological problems is now an established practice. Another method is empirical observation: the systematic observation of a process or phenomenon where the variables involved are measured and isolated to understand how they work. The observational method is adopted when a direct manipulation of the variables is impossible (or impractical), but also when, as for example in the preliminary stages of a study, the variables to be controlled later need to be identified. In psychology, the observational method involves many areas of application, from social psychology studies to those on child behaviour. The observational method implies an ecological context, that is, a natural environment where, very often, observer and observed systems affect each other. Finally, the clinical method is the scientific method of choice used in clinical practice and psychotherapy. It is the study of changes determined by therapeutic interaction on the behaviour and the psychology of the individual. Taking a scientific attitude towards the study of reality should never be confused with the concept of infallibility or → truth. In fact, a key assumption of the scientific approach is the idea that scientific development is a process of constant correction, falsification and paradigm changes, according to new observations and/or theories. *[R.]*

SCREEN MEMORY

Expression coined by Freud who, in a brief space of time, defines it in three different ways in succession, each complementary to and at the same time different from the other. The first definition deals with the "earliest memories relative to infancy" that have a peculiar characteristic: "their official content is made up of banal and indifferent impressions, that have not made a significant emotional impact upon the child when experienced". The second definition represents a correction of the first and designates memories, or better, "fantasies related to infancy", in which the "the mnestic image does not reproduce the episode [faithfully] but rather another psychic element, tied to the one that has been rejected by means of close association"; the apparent insignificance of the content that arises from censorship and displacement. Finally, the last definition referred to "memories" that in reality will turn out to be "reconstructions". *[L. Sarno]*

REFERENCES. Freud S. (1899), *Screen memories*, in *The Standard Edition*, III, 1953–1974.

SCRIPT

In Berne's transactional analysis, a particular neo-psychoanalytic conception of → transference neurosis. It consists of the intrapsychic and relational manifestation of the → protocol, understood as that infantile organization of defensive reactions through which the child reacts to parental messages that inhibit his natural development (→ injunction). The child defends himself, by auto-limiting his cognitive and emotional potential, in order to maintain a → homeostasis with the relational environment. Berne describes different types of script, from the "banal" one, in which the individual auto-limits himself, arriving at a life constructed by programmes aimed at avoiding situations and relationships perceived as risky, to the "destructive" one, in which the individual unconsciously goes towards a tragic end: he can commit homicide or suicide, remain dramatically alone or take refuge in madness. Berne describes how the script expresses itself in group dynamics through the so-called "group image", or rather the unconscious image of one's family group, which is projected onto groups with which the individual enters in relationship in his adult life: work, therapy group, etc. In transactional analysis, the therapist bases his intervention on the analysis of the modality through which the patient "repeats" his script within the therapeutic relationship. The script is meant by Berne also as a process of organization of the identity of the individual, and in this sense of "cultural scripts" need to be understood as the whole of the environmental influences that transmit, through the family, values and expectations about the "normality" of the individual. A special contribution to the study of the male script is made by Novellino, through the analysis of three syndromes: "Pinocchio", "the Masked Man", "Don Giovanni". In these syndromes, Novellino describes three typical psychopathological frameworks, in which the man, compulsively following infantile situations that have impeded a healthy development of his male identity, constructs three different defence mechanisms that lead him to take refuge in the pathological use of lies (Pinocchio syndrome), to repress feelings of weakness and fragility (the Masked Man syndrome), to obsessively pursue the seduction of women (Don Giovanni syndrome). *[M. Novellino]*

REFERENCES. Berne E., *"Hello!" . . . and then what?*, 1972; Novellino M., *Psicoanalisi transazionale*, 2004; Id., *Viaggiando con Frodo: alcuni adolescenti diventano uomini, alcuni uomini rimangono adolescenti*, 2007.

SCRIPT DECISION

In transactional analysis, psychological position that the child fixates on, in different moments in his psychological development, when he has to face and to defend himself from the excessive weight of → injunctions that are transmitted by parents. This position becomes unconscious and determines successive behavioural styles in adult life, in transactional analysis called → script. If, for example, the child finds himself having to suffer from an intense and repeated behaviour of abandonment in his first two years of life (death of a parent, his own hospitalization or that of one of his parents, serious neglect of his basic needs), he will perceive it as an injunction to "not exist" and, to defend himself from the emotional violence that derives from it, could take a position of the type: "I will never lean against anyone, I will think only about myself": this decision will lead him to a script of solitude and of avoidance of intimate emotional situations or, clinically speaking, to a depressive condition. In the theoretical and methodological framework of transactional analysis, it is considered a basic assumption that what has been "decided" can be "re-decided": psychotherapy has the task of helping to realize this change, at both an intrapsychic and a relational level. *[M. Novellino]*

REFERENCES. Berne E., *«Hello!» . . . and then what?*, 1972; Moiso C., Novellino M., *Stati dell'Io*, 1982.

SCRIPT MATRIX

In transactional analysis, diagnostic instrument developed by C. Steiner, at the time Berne's "protégé", which pragmatically sums up the main "messages of the → script" from both the maternal and the paternal sources. The author investigated its nature during his studies on the script of alcoholics, in which he underlines the following messages: messages of → counter-script ("Be a man!", from both the father and the mother); injunction ("Do not be a man", from the mother); programme ("This is how to be a man", from the father). This matrix, which subsequently evolved, essentially maintaining the original pattern, highlights how, in the construction of the script, the child is faced with verbal messages that lead to behavioural models that, in reality, contradict those more profound nonverbal ones given by previous injunctions; to find a mediation between these two levels, which are in profound contradiction, the child takes a → "script decision", which in the case of the alcoholic, will be to become a drinker (often like the father), to act the "role" of a man and to avoid feeling the great pain of not really being able to be one. *[M. Novellino]*

REFERENCES. Berne E., *«Hello!» . . . and then what?*, 1972; Moiso C., Novellino M., *Stati dell'Io*, 1982.

SEARCH-FOR-EXCEPTIONS TECHNIQUE

Within the model of → brief solution-focused therapy, technique that is based on the premise that not all problems occur all the time, everywhere and anywhere; rather, there are always "exceptions" to their occurrence, which, once identified, can be replicated and utilized with a view to finding a solution. An exception is something that takes place instead of the problem, and can frequently present itself without the voluntary intention of the patient, or even without him being aware of it. During the therapeutic session, the patient is invited to search in his past for possible "exceptions" to the presenting problem that, even if small, can be utilized in order to produce small progressive changes, leading to a definitive resolution of the problem itself. The key to this manoeuvre lies in the fact that the therapist acts as if the person has "already resolved this problem, even if for a very brief period of time or in a particular situation. But, for some reason, the aforementioned solution that the individual or the family has tried, and that has been successful, was not maintained or has been forgotten. For this reason, the therapists working within this approach spend a large part of the session attentively investigating all the possible exceptions that have taken place, and when found, will greatly emphasize them, in the attempt at guiding the person towards replicating them.

The research for exceptions is also widely used in the Nardone model of → brief strategic therapy, in two ways. In the first, the therapist prescribes to the patient to pay attention, in the interval of time between one session and another, to the spontaneous occurrence of small but significant exceptions to the problem; in this way a → self-fulfilling prophecy is created that is potentially able to produce a first unblocking of the problematic situation of the patient. In the second, the therapist guides the person during the session to go through his past history to look for possible exceptions to his redundant script (→ attempted solution), or rather for any episode in his life in which he dealt with the same problematic situation in a way that was different to his usual way of dealing with his problem and that has led him to obtain positive results. The exception may have been chosen freely, it may have been imposed on him (dictated by internal or external situations) or spontaneously expressed by the person, so that the person may have realized only later what had actually taken place.

The principle objective of this investigation is that of evaluating if it is possible to take advantage of the resources that the person has already employed in the past in the direction of change, even if these situations have happened only a few times or even only once. If significant exceptions do exist, the therapist can guide the person towards understanding what type of process to induce in order to reapply what has worked and, in this way, create effective solutions. Basing itself on the resources and on the capacities that the person has already employed in the past, the amplification of the exceptions represents the path of least → resistance to change for the patient, and therefore should be given priority every time it is in any way possible to implement it. Because it is extremely productive, the search for the exception is used both in the clinical field as well as in the organizational field (→ coaching). *[G. Nardone]*

REFERENCES. De Shazer S., Dolan Y., Korman H., Trepper T., McCollum E., Berg I.K., *More than miracles: The state of the art of solution-focused brief therapy*, 2007; Milanese R., Mordazzi P., *Strategic coaching*, 2015; Nardone G., *Problem solving strategico da tasca*, 2010.

SECONDARY GAIN

In strategic family therapy, it is the gain obtained by the maintenance of psychological or medical → symptoms. This theoretical construct was introduced, for the first time, by Freud, together with the construct of primary gain. According to the author, symptom formation always promotes a gain for the individual. The term "primary gain" describes the partial drive discharge (→ drive) of unconscious desires, while avoiding → anguish or → sense of guilt; the "secondary gain" concerns any advantage obtained as a result of having a symptom. In addition to negative or painful aspects, a symptomatic expression (physical or mental) can entail potential benefits such as social, economic advantages or draw attention. For example, a physical disease may involve, in addition to physical discomfort, a chance to avoid unwanted responsibilities or unpleasant situations. While the psychodynamic theory considers primary gain more important than the secondary one, potential benefits of a symptom must be taken into consideration in the treatment, as they represent a significant obstacle for the process of → change. Today, the concept of secondary gain has increased in importance in the field of medicine and health care; it emerged from the boundaries of psychodynamic theories and emphasized interpersonal and social aspects. *[E. Molinari, F. Pagnini, G. Pietrabissa, G. Castelnuovo]*

REFERENCES. Freud S. (1915–1916), *Introductory lectures on psycho-analysis (parts I and II)* in *The Standard Edition*, XV, 1953–1974.

SECURE BASE

Secure base behaviour was described by Ainsworth to define a child's inclination to use the caregiver as a safe harbour in case of need and from which to leave again to explore the environment after having been reassured. In secure attachment (→ attachment theory), the phenomenon of secure base indicates the presence of a dynamic balance between attachment and exploration. Instead, this aspect is missing in insecure attachments: in the "avoiding" model, there is an inability to turn to the parent in case of need, in response to an excessive exploration; in the "ambivalent" model, the lack of reassurance provided by the parent inhibits the exploratory potential of the child. *[A.M. Speranza]*

REFERENCES. Ainsworth M.D.S., Blehar M.C., Waters E., Wall S., *Patterns of attachment: A psychological study of the Strange Situation*, 1978; Bowlby J., *A secure base: Clinical applications of Attachment Theory*, 1988.

SEDUCTION

Act of attracting another person to oneself for sentimental, sexual, relational purposes, or to obtain other intangible benefits (for example, power and control) or material benefits (for example, goods). The ability to fascinate others is a personal quality that goes far beyond the mere aesthetic component, as it is, rather, related to the psychic characteristics and the → personality of individuals. In terms of communication, seduction uses nonverbal → language made of voluntary and involuntary signals, gestures, implicit messages, which can arouse strong and durable emotions in the interlocutor. The concept of seduction was first used in psychotherapy by Freud in his first theory on the etiology of psychoneurosis. Within the therapeutic → setting, seduction can be used consciously by the therapist as a communication tool to persuade and influence the patient, leading him to behaviours that are functional to his → wellbeing. From the patient's perspective, however, it takes on the characteristic of an attitude, generally unaware, put in place to control the processes of → influencing and → change that are experienced as threatening or frightening. *[R.]*

▷ In psychoanalysis, the concept of seduction was introduced by Freud in 1893, to explain neurotic symptoms, and it was interpreted as a "childhood sexual trauma" suffered because of an adult. This sexual event is traumatic because it is unexpected; it generates a sudden increase of drive excitement and, finally, being incomprehensible, given the psycho-affective immaturity of the child, it cannot be integrated but only dissociated, and constitutes "the first time of the trauma". It remains silent until another event of a sexual nature, "the second time of the trauma", associatively linked to the previous one, revokes and mobilizes defences such as repression and neurotic symptoms: Freud uses the term *Nachtraglichkeit* to indicate the deferred action of a trauma, which on the one hand, is the basis of neurotic symptoms, and on the other, is the starting point for a possible therapeutic re-signification. In the letter to Fliess of September 21, 1897, Freud renounced the seduction theory, noting that, for many hysterical patients, the childhood sexual trauma was, in actual fact, just a fantasy of seduction. For Freud, it was a very relative renunciation, since he never stopped believing that hysteria was a traumatic neurosis; moreover, by enhancing the fantasies of seduction, he opened psychoanalysis to the wider horizons of infantile sexuality and of the → Oedipus complex. *[E. Mangini]*

REFERENCES. Freud S. (1887–1904), *Letters to Wilhelm Fliess*, 1961; Id. (1851), *Project for a scientific psychology*, in *The Standard Edition*, II, 1976–1980.

SELF

In the context of analytical psychology, it is the central → archetype and the goal of the individuation process; in Jungian thought, the Self represents, at the same time and paradoxically, both the psychic wholeness and the "overarching" core of the personality. "The Self is not only the center but also the whole circumference, which embraces both consciousness and unconsciousness." The achievement of this goal has to do with the transcendence of the opposites, *complexio oppositorum*, "where opposites are united", "play of light and shadows". The Self, promoter or "organizing principle" of the personality, acts with the aim of the individuation process; by doing it, the Ego works for the Self and "dwarfs the → Ego in scope and intensity". The archetype symbols of the Self include "figure of the superordinate personality" (the king, the prophet, the saviour), "geometrical structures containing elements of the circle and quaternity" (→ mandala), to which Jung ascribes therapeutic properties for psychic fragmentation. Emphasizing the distinction between concept and experience, intellectual vision and subjective phenomenology of the Self, Jung argues that "the Self is no mere concept or logical postulate; it is a psychic reality" and so it "can only be expressed by means of symbols": it does not permit scientific evidence and has a numinous nature. Jung's work on the self is at the centre of his investigations on the religious function of the mind. The idea that the mystical experience is the result of a shift from the Ego (centre of consciousness) to the Self (the centre of conscious and unconscious) offers an explanation of the inexplicable and ineffable quality of this experience. *[L. Lingiardi, M. Luci]*

REFERENCES. Jung C.G. (1928), *The relations between the ego and the unconscious*, in *Collected Works*, VII, 1967; Id. (1944), *Psychology and alchemy*, in *Collected Works*, XII,1968; Id. (1942–1948), *A psychological approach to the dogma of the Trinity*, in *Collected Works*, XI, 1970; Id. (1947–1954), *On the essence of Psyche*, in *Collected Works*, VIII, 1969.

SELF-ACTUALIZATION

It is the actualization of the growth potential, the development and use of talents and abilities inherent to every human being. The concept, essential for therapies adopting the existential humanistic paradigm, was developed by Maslow (→ need; → existential-humanistic paradigm) and placed at the top of the "pyramid of needs" described by him. Rogers outlined the concept of tendency towards actualization, to illustrate the tendency of every person to develop their skills, if these are not obstructed by emotional blocks or by an altered self-concept. The central theme of Goldstein's theory on personality is self-actualization or self-realization. With this the author intends to attribute human motivations to people's drive to develop their own innate potential, which must necessarily act according to and in harmony with the social and cultural context of individuals.

In psychodynamics, C.G. Jung has formulated the concept of → individuation, which similarly illustrates one's ability to implement their particular individual qualities, distinguishing themselves from the conforming drives of collective consciousness. From an → empowerment perspective, self-realization is expressed in increasing opportunities for a person to make a choice. Empowered people have a greater sense of self-efficacy, feel a sense of control over events and exhibit a greater sense of confidence in a positive outcome of their actions. These characteristics ensure individuals achieve their potential and expectations more easily. Together with the presence of significant social relations, → wellbeing, vitality and congruency with oneself were considered essential for psychological growth. The degree of gratification of basic needs and self-realization seems positively correlated with the degree of psychological health of the individual; wellbeing would be the result of the realization of those needs that lead to the development of human nature and to the realization of one's own potential. Therefore, self-realization is a goal common to all forms of therapy. *[R.]*

▷ In client-centred therapy, the term self-actualization indicates the inherent motivational dynamism that presides over the process of personality development and growth. It was originally introduced by Goldstein and developed later in the field of humanistic psychology (by A. Angyal, C. Bühler, K. Horney and E. Fromm in particular) and it was recently resumed by system theory (→ system) through the concept of → autopoiesis in Maslow's hierarchy of needs. Self-realization is considered the highest level of motivation that characterizes a healthy and mature individual, positively involved in developing and expressing their full potential. In Rogers's work, self-realization indicates the regulative aim of the therapeutic process, as it represents a constitutive trait of a "fully functioning person", congruent with their organismic experience and dynamically open to change. Self-realization is linked to the fundamental postulate of "actualizing tendency", according to which every living organism has an innate and essentially positive driving force that directs them spontaneously and constructively towards self-preservation, growth, expansion and self-enrichment, and against which the therapeutic intervention exerts a "non-directive" function of liberation and facilitation. *[D. Bruzzone]*

REFERENCES. Bruzzone D., *Carl Rogers*, 2007; Goldstein K., *The organism*, 1939; Maslow A.H., Maslow A.H., *Motivation and personality*, 1954; Maturana H.R., Varela F.J., *Autopoiesis and cognition*, 1980; Rogers C.R., *Client-centered therapy*, 1951; Rogers C.R., Kinget M., *Psychotherapy and human relations*, 1962.

SELF-ANALYSIS

A process whereby a person psychoanalyses themselves. Freud's self-analysis has been the founding act of psychoanalysis: the Oedipus complex, child sexuality and the meaning of dreams have been "discovered" through it. However, the limits of the self-analytic process are obvious: since the defences and resistances are unconscious procedures, it is impossible for the person to recognize them in herself without help. Moreover, as a solitary process, self-analysis does not allow the development of the dynamics of → transference and → countertransference. After all, Freud conducted his self-analysis in the context of an epistolary dialogue with his friend, W. Fliess, who became for the occasion analyst *ante litteram*. Every psychoanalyst, after their analysis and training, is inevitably engaged in a process (more or less successful) of constant self-analysis, which can be of great help, both in clinical activity and in private life. *[F. Gazzillo]*

REFERENCES. Anzieu D., *Freud's self-analysis*, 1978; Freud S. (1887–1904), *Letters to Wilhelm Fliess*, 1961.

SELF-CONCEPT

In the context of cognitive-behavioural therapy, a process by which people construct a feeling of continuity and uniqueness that allows them to cope with endless changes in life while maintaining stability in the sense of → personal identity. The feeling of continuity allows an individual to cope with and integrate discontinuities or emotional discrepancies; the feeling of uniqueness allows them to cope with and integrate otherness. The construction process of the Self is, according to James, an incessant circularity of the two "ingredients" of the self in every moment. Guidano writes:

> the *Self* is multimodal and multilevel. It is multimodal because knowledge is not just cognitive, but also emotional, sensory, perceptual, kinaesthetic and procedural. It is multilevel because the emergence of language and its articulation causes, for us, the experience to take place simultaneously and continuously on a double level: the immediate experience and the conscious image we have of ourselves.

In accordance with the cognitive-constructivist model, the self-concept represents the core of man. Man self-organizes (→ self-organization) with autopoietic ability (→ autopoiesis), and actively constructs his own personal meaning within attachment relationships (→ attachment theory), and therefore their identity, which develops throughout life. *[M. Dodet]*

REFERENCES. Guidano V.F., *La complessità del sé*, 1987; James W., *The principles of psychology*, 1890; Maturana H., Varela F., *Autopoiesis and cognition*, 1980; Neisser U., *The perceived Self*, 1993.

SELF-CORRECTIVENESS

Ability of a strategy to self-correct during its execution based on the effects produced by the intervention itself. A model of therapy is self-correcting when it can correct the course of the intervention phase by phase, depending on the responses given by the patient to the therapist's instructions. If the provided indication does not produce the effect desired and anticipated by the therapist, this can adapt their intervention on the basis of → feedback obtained from their mistake. The concept of self-correctiveness is closely related to that of → predictability, that is, the faculty of the therapist to anticipate all the possible effects of their intervention. Self-correctiveness and predictability, for a long time ignored in the context of psychotherapy, have become central constructs in the most recent evolutions of the strategic paradigm, thanks to the constant work of action-research and construction of treatment protocols handled by G. Nardone and his collaborators. The self-correctivity of a therapy model, allowing the re-adaptation of the intervention session by session, is a guarantee of greater speed and efficiency of the intervention itself. *[R.]*

SELF-DISTANCING

In logotherapy, the ability to observe oneself from the outside with awareness and, consequently, the freedom to assume new attitudes towards our own existential condition or events that influence us. The term is part of Frankl's anthropological vision; its therapeutic application translates into distancing from fears and anxiety-inducing ideas and knowing how to "understand the comical side of things". The technique of → paradoxical intention devised by Frankl consists in bringing out the humorous aspects, turning fear into desire. *[A. Bartoletti]*

REFERENCES. Fizzotti E. (ed.), *Il senso come terapia. Fondamenti teorico-clinici della logoterapia di Viktor E. Frankl*, 2007; Frankl V.E., *Man's search for meaning: An introduction to logotherapy*, 1946.

SELF-ESTEEM

Evaluation or consideration that an individual has of themselves. This construct is considered essential for a person's psychological balance as it involves directly cognitive, emotional, motivational and behavioural aspects. Moreover, it is connected to the feeling of psychological → wellbeing. W. James defined self-esteem as the relationship between the perceived self (corresponding to the qualities and skills that a person believes he possesses) and the ideal self (which represents how a person would like to be). In this case, self-esteem becomes a crucial aspect of a person's psychological balance, so that the vast majority of those who require a psychotherapeutic intervention has a relatively low level of self-esteem. Other types of patients declare (provocatively or due to self-deception) high levels of self-esteem which, however, are strongly in contrast with their personal efficacy. Given its importance, self-esteem is an anamnestic (→ anamnesis) and a diagnostic (→ diagnosis) assessment criterion and it is also used to evaluate the therapeutic process, as the ultimate goal of any psychotherapy is to achieve a good level of personal self-esteem. *[R.]*

SELF-EVALUATION SCALE TECHNIQUE

Technique of the → brief strategic therapy Nardone model, inspired from the → scale technique developed by S. de Shazer and I.K. Berg (→ brief solution-focused therapy). The technique of the self-evaluation scale is employed in order to evaluate the degree of change achieved by the patient and to gradually push him towards the total resolution of his problem. The technique consists of the following question: "If we had to evaluate your current situation on a scale of 0 to 10, giving your situation when you had your first session as being 0 and 10 representing the total resolution of the problem that brought you here, what score would you give yourself?" This evaluation is carried out when the problematic situation has started to be resolved in a relevant manner and the patient has started to engage in behaviours that are different to those that were typical of his old redundant repertoire of behaviours (→ attempted solutions). The technique of the self-evaluation scale helps the therapist and the patient have a "numeric" and shared measurement of the therapeutic change from the point of view of the person who is actually experiencing the problem. This is useful not only to highlight the change that has taken place but also as an incentive towards the implementation of further changes. Departing from this technique, Nardone has developed a successive therapeutic prescription that, employing the logic of the → self-fulfilling prophecy, guides the patient to go beyond their current situation in order to arrive at the final objective. For example, if the person evaluates himself as having a score of 6, the therapist can prescribe the following:

> From now until the next time we meet I would like you to, every day, during the course of the day, observe what is happening, looking for an indicator that will enable you to say that you have progressed from a 6 to a 7 on our scale. Towards seven o'clock I would like you to make this sort of self-evaluation: if something has happened in a spontaneous manner that would enable you to assert that you have moved a step, good, you will not have to do anything and you will be able to postpone asking yourself this question to the following day. If one evening you evaluate that, nothing has happened spontaneously, you will have the rest of the evening to do something in a voluntary manner that will enable you to move to a score of 7, but make sure it is not more than 7.

Based on this → illusion of alternatives technique, this → prescription becomes an indirect injunction, as a result of which change will be inevitable because, whether it takes place spontaneously or in a voluntary manner, it will have to, in any case, take place. The technique of the self-evaluation scale is very useful during the phase of consolidation of therapy, in the third stage of psychotherapy (→ strategic therapy phases). *[G. Nardone]*

REFERENCES. Nardone G., Balbi E., *The logic of therapeutic change*, 2015.

SELF-FULFILLING PROPHECY

This term refers to a prophecy or assumption that, as a result of the fact that it has been formulated, makes the predicted event come true; in this way, it confirms its own veracity. Watzlawick analyzed in a detailed manner the phenomena associated with this kind of non-ordinary → logic, which completely overturns the logic of linear causality (→ causalism) and asserts that it is the cause, located in the past, that will produce an event in the present. In the case of the self-fulfilling prophecy, on the contrary, it is an event anticipated in the future that produces events in the present, in this way causing the predicted event to come true. Numerous studies have been conducted on this phenomenon. Rosenthal studied the surprising effects that the expectations of teachers have on the intelligence quotient of their students and their academic performance. Szaz and Rosenhan have researched and documented the way in which diagnostic psychiatric "labels", once made, can transform themselves into "diagnoses that are self-fulfilling" in the eyes of the patient, of his family and the specialists themselves (→ anti-psychiatry). Finally, it is also important to refer to the numerous studies regarding the renowned → "placebo effect", a fascinating phenomenon that highlights the enormous power that a prophecy that is self-fulfilling can have not only psychologically, but also at a physiological level, causing changes at an immunological level and in other bodily systems. It is precisely because it is able to literally produce a reality without which it would not have taken place, that the logic of the self-fulfilling prophecy has important implications for certain types of psychotherapeutic models such as the brief strategic therapy model of G. Nardone. Thanks to the utilization of this phenomenon, both within the therapeutic communication and in the formulation of particular therapeutic → prescriptions, the psychotherapist guides the patient towards changing his reality, transforming his personal dysfunctional prophecies (→ functional balance), frequently the cause of the persistence of psychological and relational problems, into functional prophecies. For an example of a therapeutic technique that utilizes this logic one can refer to the → "as if" technique. *[T. Garcia-Rivera, R. Milanese]*

REFERENCES. Rosenhal, D. L., *On being sane in insane places*, in «Science», 1973, 179 (4070); Rosenthal R., Jacobson L., *Pygmalion in the classroom*, 1968; Szasz T.S., *The myth of mental illness: Foundations of a theory of personal conduct*, 1962; Watzlawick P., *The invented reality*, 1981.

SELF-MONITORING

In cognitive-behaviour therapy, self-monitoring is the first phase of → self-regulation, aiming at measuring the self-regulatory skills (→ self-regulation capability) of the client. It is widely used to obtain information on behaviours, emotions and cognitive representations in life contexts. According to the goal, standardized forms are filled in by the client, where the designed variable is recorded: emotional state or information related to the target behaviour, e.g. eating habits in the case of obesity, number of weekly cigarettes in the case of smoking, daily activities in the case of depression. Standardized forms for the self-monitoring of emotional episodes, reporting the main variables (behaviour, body sensations, internal dialogue and images) are particularly useful to study feelings from an internal perspective for clinical, training and research purposes. *[S. Borgo]*

REFERENCES. Borgo S., *Il vissuto emozionale: un nuovo metodo di studio*, in «Idee in psicoterapia», 2008, I; Karoly P., Kanfer F.H., *Self-management and behaviour change: From theory to practice*, 1982.

SELF-OBJECT

In the field of Self psychology, the experiencing of what is external to the object as being an integral part of the subjective experience of a human being. This "other" is fundamentally another individual, but can also be an activity, an artistic expression, an ideology, etc. This "other" becomes indispensable to the maintenance of the equilibrium and the wellbeing of the individual. This relationship with the other is experienced as being an integral part of the individual's identity. According to H. Kohut, the experience of the Self-object is considered as being a normal part of psychological development and a source of internal cohesion and wellbeing during the span of a lifetime. In the course of their development, all human beings experience a constant need for Self-objects: these exhibit a process of transformation from being archaic Self-objects to infantile, adolescent and finally adult Self-objects over the course of human development. *[G. Nebbiosi, S. Federici]*

SELF-OBJECT TRANSFERENCE

In the field of Self psychology, the concept of → transference underwent a profound change with respect to that of classic psychoanalysis. If, on the one hand, transference is recognized in its more orthodox meaning (projection onto the therapist of the parental figures or of parts of them), on the other hand, value is given to the way in which the therapist experiences the patient as a self-object, that is, as another that is indispensable to the maintenance of the equilibrium and personal wellbeing. Self-object transferences have three configurations: the idealizing self-object transference: "You are perfect and I am part of you"; the mirroring self-object transference: "I am perfect and you are part of me"; and the twinship self-object transference: "We are both the same and in this sameness lies our perfection".

The good management by the therapist of self-object transferences is considered as being crucial for the good progress of therapy. *[G. Nebbiosi, S. Federici]*

SELF-ORGANIZATION

In post-rationalist psychology, it is the tendency to organize subjective experience and interaction with the environment using modalities consistent with the knowledge structures already available. When significant changes in environmental conditions occur, a system capable of self-organization can maintain a state of equilibrium by developing increasingly complex forms of internal organization. The concept of self-organization and the processes that characterize it follow partially from Piaget's concepts of assimilation and accommodation. In the post-rationalist cognitive psychotherapy proposed by V. F. Guidano, self-organization allows individuals to protect and perpetuate their sense of identity (→ personal identity); alternations to this process are considered as an element of vulnerability to psychopathology. *[R.B. Ardito, M. Adenzato]*

REFERENCES. Guidano V.F., *Complexity of the Self*, 1987, and *The Self in process*, 1991; Piaget J., *Genetic epistemology*, 1971.

SELF-ORGANIZING SYSTEMS

Any physical, biological, social system whose functioning depends on its internal organization and not on environmental perturbations. A self-organizing system possesses an internal organization that cannot be modified by the environment, unless the system itself is destroyed in its entirety. The environment can only activate the behaviour of the system, but is not able in any way to establish the ways in which it can change, its direction or its development. *[D. Liccione]*

REFERENCES. Ashby W.R., *Principles of the self-organizing dynamic system*, in «Journal of General Psychology», 1947, 37.

SELF PSYCHOLOGY

The theory of development and of psychotherapeutic technique developed by Kohut, who revisited the classical psychoanalytic model that attributes a fundamental importance to the narcissistic development (→ narcissism) and to the integration and consolidation of the → Self. The difficulties encountered with patients with narcissistic personality disorders, who present with symptoms related to low self-esteem, poor sense of self and problems in establishing relationships with others, led Kohut to experiment with and to integrate different models of therapeutic techniques. This led him to underline the importance of → empathy (also known as vicarious introspection) as the principal instrument of observation of psychological phenomena. Empathy is, from Kohut's point of view, a type of listening that allows a person to immerse himself profoundly into the internal life of another person, and it is through empathy that the mother is able to recognize the psychological state of the child in any given moment; it is also through empathy that the mother is able to modulate her reactions, which can be adapted to a greater or lesser degree to the needs that the child is expressing.

Kohut's observation and analysis of patients with narcissistic personality disorders led him to hypothesize and then to assert, in his formulation of a model of psychological functioning, that this type of pathology originates from narcissistic deprivation that resides in the structure of the self and, in particular, in the difficulties present in the original empathetic relationship with the mother or with the primary carer of the child. According to Kohut, the infant is born as a joyful being that comes into this world with the need to be taken care of and affirmed in the various expressions of his being. These include those related to aggressiveness, which is, according to Kohut, aimed at self-assertion. It is the experience of the mother, intended as → Self-object, that will determine the way in which his narcissism will develop, in other words the love that will develop towards himself, as well the establishment of a Self that, from being rudimental at birth (lacking in reflexive awareness), will develop into a structured psyche, the nuclear Self. The term Self-object refers to the subjective aspect of the function of a relationship. The needs expressed by the infant from birth are those of finding in the mother a mirroring reaction that is adequate and an objective for his self-idealization. A mother who consistently fails to respond in an adequate manner to the needs of the child (as a result of, according to Kohut, the presence of pathology in her own Self) will result in the repeated failure of the Self-object, causing the development of a narcissistic personality disorder. In the exchange between the mother and the Self of the infant the so-called optimal frustrations play a fundamental role, as they produce the "transmuting internalizations", a process that gradually consolidates and structures a Self that is mature, able to nourish a healthy narcissistic love, that is able to envision ideals and work towards achieving them, that is able to channel its aggressiveness towards the affirmation of the self and the attainment of one's goals. Patients with narcissistic personality disorders have, instead, remained stuck to archaic configurations of the Self that are grandiose and/or archaic objects that are overestimated and invested with narcissistic libido.

Nevertheless, according to Kohut, patients with narcissistic personality disorder are different from psychotic patients and patients with borderline personality disorder, in that they have, however, achieved a cohesive "Self", in the sense of a mental structure that has both functions that have been traditionally attributed by classical psychoanalysis to the → Id, → Ego and → Superego, as well as having characteristics of an active agent with its own qualities and own relationships with Self-objects, although these are still archaic.

This cohesiveness of the Self allows patients with narcissistic disorder to establish with the psychoanalyst a narcissistic transference (→ Self-object transference), that will reactivate the archaic structure of the Self without the danger of regression and fragmentation. By means of the Self-object transference, the patient will be able to re-live in the analytic relationship the early developmental phases of the infant: the phase of grandiosity (grandiose Self) and those of idealization. In this way, an idealizing transference (emerging from the patient's need to find in the therapist the idealized imago: in this sense the function of the Self-object becomes that of allowing the patient to attribute to the therapist unlimited capabilities and power, with the aim of saving something of the missed narcissistic experience); a mirroring transference (as a result of the reactivation of the grandiose Self: in this case the function of the Self-object is that of allowing the patient to see in the therapist an image of himself with the aim of finding confirmation of his own existence and vitality); and, finally, a twinship or an alter-ego transference (with the aim of meeting the patient's need to find similarities with the other: in this sense the function of the Self-object is that of allowing the patient to share with the therapist his abilities and competence). In therapy, as in the development of the infant, the optimal frustrations (failures of the therapist that are non-traumatic and therefore ones that the patient is able to tolerate) are necessary for transitory reactions of retreat to take place that will enable him to re-dimension the expectations of the grandiose Self and modulate it, in order to make them more realistic. Through the empathic resonance of the therapist (which in Kohutian therapy constitutes the cardinal method of understanding the patient and of understanding the countertransference of the therapist), the patient will feel accepted and understood by the therapist. The working through of the Self-object transferences by means of interpretation (which constitute the more advanced stages of this same empathy, in the sense that they are not intellectual constructions, but explanations offered with the warmth that is created also as a result of the desire of the analyst to "tune into" the feelings of the patient), together with the genetic reconstructions, will unblock, in the Self of the patient, the potential for development that had become stuck.

The goal of the therapeutic process, therefore, is to carry out a sort of restoration of the Self, that has deficiencies on the narcissistic level caused by prolonged inadequate reactions of the mother and of the environment surrounding the infant at the time of his birth. It is important to emphasize how, for Kohut, the need for Self-objects, with their relative functions, is also present in adulthood: this affirmation implies that a revision of the drive theory as formulated by S. Freud is required. Kohut affirmed that:

> Narcissism, or the love for oneself, the investment of the Self in itself and for itself, has its own mode of development, its own specific developmental stages. Narcissism has its own epigenetic sequence, that is no different to the love towards objects.

In this new formulation, the libido follows two areas of development: one referring to the object libido, which leads to the development of a mature love for objects; the other, a narcissistic libido, which leads to a mature love for the Self. In the process undertaken by the narcissistic libido, Self-objects are not loved, in and for themselves; rather they are experienced as parts of the Self or are used in order to preserve the love for the Self for narcissistic purposes. Through the course of his life, therefore, the individual will love objects (object-love) and will need objects that will provide him with love and attention and that will guarantee the persistence of the narcissistic love. In other words, the individual will acquire, over time – and if necessary through analysis – an independence that will never be separate from the Self-objects and that will endow him with a mature capacity to utilize them.

Kohut also revized the concept of the → Oedipus Complex, in light of his observations of narcissistic personality disorders and his formulations on the psychology of the Self. "Drive theory and its developments explain the guilty Man but do not explain the tragic Man". If, in fact, the Freudian model looks at the consequences of the non-resolution of the Oedipus Complex as an incapacity of the psyche to resolve conflicts, the Kohutian model asserts that it is the structure of the Self that determines the way in which the infant will experience the Oedipus Complex. If the child has a strong sense of Self, in the oedipal phase he will experiment with feelings of affirmation of the Self, sexual desires and feelings of possession towards the parent of the opposite sex, and feelings of self-confidence and competition towards the parent of the same sex. Once again, the empathic reactions of the parents, to a greater or lesser degree, will determine the outcome of this developmental phase: parents that respond to the new accomplishments of the child with joy and pride will help him to experience the oedipal phase as being one in which the libidinal and aggressive tensions are vital for his sense of Self and for the relationships he is able to establish with Self-objects. On the contrary, a conflict that is experienced as being too intense, and the appearance in this phase of an excessive degree of anxiety, aggression and anguish, are expressions of a failure in the relationship with the Self and the Self-objects, as a result of which a strong sense of Self fails to be established. According to Kohut, the consolidation of the Superego is connected to the end of the oedipal phase, but the author emphasizes an origin and a meaning that is narcissistic, deriving its formation from the transfer of the idealized image of the Self (in its original configuration) onto an external figure that is idealized, transformed into an internal system of idealized values. For Kohut, at the centre of human experience, there is always, tragic, as in the case of Ulysses, the search for the Self, an endeavour that is very different from the conflict associated with oedipal guilt. *[P. Cruciani, N.Delicato]*

REFERENCES. Kohut H.T., *The restoration of the self*, 1977; Id., *The Kohut seminars*, 1987.

SELF-REFERENCE

A term borrowed from logic, designating both the reference to itself of a statement and the capability of systems to regulate and self-organize themselves (→ system, → self-regulation capability). The second meaning has gained importance in psychology thanks to Maturana and Varela's studies. In psychotherapy, the term has acquired a negative value, indicating a statement that justifies its validity by referring to itself. In fact, when applied to psychological theories and psychotherapy, self-reference is the process of validating a theory using the concepts of the theory itself, thus giving rise to a recursive and self-confirming mechanism. Asserting that a person is suffering from panic attacks because he/she is anxious or that a person is depressed because scarcely motivated, are examples of self-referential thought. Another expression of self-reference applied to therapeutic theories is so-called "confirmation bias", which consists in the involuntary selection of information and/or distortion of observations to confirm a therapist's reference theory or some diagnostic hypothesis. In regard to this, it is important to remember that modern scientific epistemology, to which most of the psychotherapeutic models refer, emphasizes the concept of "refutationism" proposed by the philosopher K. Popper, who claimed that the scientific nature of a theory or a psychological assertion lies in the possibility of it being subjected to falsification. *[R.]*

REFERENCES. Maturana H., Varela F., *The tree of knowledge*, 1987.

SELF-REFLECTION CAPABILITY

It belongs to the broader generative property of mind that, in accordance with social cognitive theory, is seen as able to reflect on its own thought processes and therefore to regulate itself. From this perspective, individuals do not simply react passively to environmental pressures, but act in advance with, and with awareness of, the aim of actively transforming the environment. *[F. Celi]*

REFERENCES. Bandura A., *Self efficacy: The exercise of control*, 1997; Caprara G.V., *Bandura*, 1997.

SELF-REGULATION

In the context of Gestalt therapy, a fundamental psychological process by which the organism adjusts to the environment spontaneously and creatively, so that acting becomes consistent with feeling. The importance of self-regulation is stressed by many authors, particularly Perls. In Gestalt therapy, every incomplete situation and every unsatisfied desire do not become a → figure following a predetermined decision, but happen quite spontaneously. The → contact between organism and environment, the experience of the "field" (→ field theory), takes place and is organized always on the basis of the "spontaneous conscience" of the predominant need. The intentionality of the organism, the choice of priorities and the planning of the appropriate action are all moments that are necessary to lead to the unblocking of the uncompleted situation. Fixing attention, or an excess of intentionality, are, on the other hand, the basis of a "neurotic self-regulation". *[M. Spagnuolo Lobb, P.A. Cavaleri]*

REFERENCES. Cavaleri P.A., *Dal campo al confine di contatto. Contributo per una riconsiderazione del confine di contatto in psicoterapia della Gestalt*, in M. Spagnuolo Lobb (ed.), *Psicoterapia della Gestalt. Ermeneutica e clinica*, 2001; Id., *La profondità della superficie. Percorsi introduttivi alla psicoterapia della Gestalt*, 2003; Perls F., Hefferline R.F, Goodman P., *Gestalt therapy: Excitement and growth in the human personality*, 1951.

SELF-REGULATION CAPABILITY

In cognitive behavioural therapy, self-regulation capability allows a person to direct their behaviour towards objectives set by the person themselves, to make predictions about the likelihood of achieving these objectives and to assess their actual achievement. Along with → self-reflection capability, → symbolization and → vicarious learning, self-regulation can explain conscious and planned human behaviours. In psychotherapy, it can be used to overcome the idea that responses are automatically triggered under the pressure of internal or environmental stimuli. In this way, a patient can be helped (for example, a hyperactive child) to realize that they can self-regulate their behaviour. *[F. Celi]*

REFERENCES. Bandura A., *Social learning theory*, 1977; Id., *Self efficacy: The exercise of control*, 1997; Harris K.R., Danoff F.B., Saddler, B., Frizzelle R., Graham S., *Self-monitoring of attention versus self-monitoring of academic performance: Effects among students with ADHD in the general education classroom*, 2005.

SELF-RELATIONS PSYCHOTHERAPY

Self-relations psychotherapy has been developed by Stephen Gilligan over the last three decades, inspired by Milton Erickson, Gregory Bateson, Buddhism, Aikido and other sources. In contrast to other approaches, self-relations does not see symptom disturbances as inherently negative experiences that must be fought with "flight, flight, or freeze." Based on Milton Erickson's → utilization principle, self-relation therapy instead takes the more positive view that a → "symptom" signifies that some major identity change is trying to "awaken" into a person's life. Such transformational attempts occur at various points in each life, especially around major life events and experiences – for example, a family birth, death, or marriage; a job or residence change; an illness or trauma, etc. Whether such intensive experiences are positive or negative depends on the human relational connections with them. Thus, a symptom represents a core life experience that has been related to in a negative way – by self or others. Hence, self-relations psychotherapy seeks to identify and implement the positive human connections with an experience that will transform it from a negative symptom to a positive resource. This basic idea means that there is no inherent meaning, value or form to a core experience. For example, a young patient underwent therapy due to "chronic anxiety" issues, which had emerged since childhood, when he witnessed some psychotic symptoms of his father. The anxiety presented by the above client is sensed in its more primary form as the feeling of fear. This is not inherently bad; its meaning and consequent unfolding depends on how it is held and regarded. For the client, there was no human presence to witness it, positively connect with it, and allow it to be a helpful learning. Instead, its isolation from human connection led it into its frozen form as negative "anxiety" that subsequently was to be avoided. The therapeutic approach of self-relational psychotherapy looks to create a positive context—in the body, the mind and the social context—that will allow the core experience to be connected to in a more positive way. Thus, in our example, the therapist made sure the client felt relatively relaxed and in good connection with the therapist. Then she suggested that he imagine a situation in which the tension had occurred, and to gently attune to what this tension felt like. Here the therapist made sure she felt a welcoming attitude towards whatever the client would experience. The client described the feeling as an uncomfortable pressure in his chest. When the therapist now calmly asked him whether he felt connected to this feeling, the client said he did. The therapist gently suggested that the energy in the chest was a positive presence that could be welcomed, that it was a gift and not a problem, and guided the client in terms of how to similarly connect with the energy. In this way, the client began to develop a positive connection with the energy, and it subsequently unfolded as a helpful feeling, rather than as symptomatic anxiety.

THREE MINDS AND THREE LEVELS OF MIND. To work positively with a person's experience, self-relational psychotherapy emphasizes three different minds – Somatic, Cognitive and Field – each of which can operate at three different levels – Primitive, Ego and Generative. The somatic mind is the intelligence within the body; it operates "beneath and before" the thinking of the verbal cognitive mind. The somatic mind is basically the mammalian consciousness – embodied, without self-awareness, but with tremendous energy, relational attunement and feeling. It is the first (but not only) "unconscious mind", connected to ancestral histories and tremendous resources. We can see it operate in its pure form in animals and young children. The cognitive mind is the second mind, the Ego-intellect "in the head". It is based on verbal rules, social maps, beliefs, plans and meanings. It represents and seeks to maintain identity (of a person, a family, a culture, etc.) Operating on its own, it can easily become rigid and context-insensitive, locked in its maps and fixed understandings; yet connected with the other minds, it is the basis for an exceptionally generative consciousness. The third mind is the field mind. A field is the contextual space within which human beings operate. Examples include family, history (memory "field"), culture, workplace, physical environment and emotional environments. These contexts significantly shape and influence human experience and behaviour in many ways. Self-relational psychotherapy posits that they have an "intelligence" independent from somatic or cognitive knowing. As noted, these minds can operate at three different levels. The primitive level is the lowest; it has awareness but no self-awareness, so it responds spontaneously and instinctually. Consequently, it is unstructured and non-linear, able to move freely through multiple associations and meanings. Again, this can be negative or positive, depending on the human presence connected with it. This human presence also operates at the second level of Ego consciousness. Here we have awareness of awareness, but typically at the price of dissociation from the primitive realm. Ego consciousness is accomplished via muscular tension that separates the observer from the observation, thereby creating a disembodied intellect, where the body, nature and others are experienced as "otherness". That is, most Ego awareness is achieved by muscularly suppressing primitive consciousness, resulting in a managerial type of consciousness interested in control, analysis and conceptual order. This limited self-awareness is a tremendous evolutionary leap from the first level of the primitive, because of the possibility of operating with verbal-symbolic → language in its many forms – intention, plans, symbolic representation, linear time, simulations, etc. However, when it is disconnected from the primitive – e.g. the body, nature, feelings – it can mistake its maps for reality itself, with many pathologies resulting, most notably the attempt to unilaterally dominate and subjugate "otherness" (violence) or a feeling of loss of enjoyment, energy or direct connection to life (alienation and apathy). The third level is the generative, where self-awareness includes both the part(s) and whole at the same time. A key definition of "generative" is the capacity to create something that has never existed before; contrasted to the gross, muscle-based consciousness of the Ego-level, generative consciousness is based on subtle awareness. Examples are experiences of wellbeing (e.g. gardening, meditation, cooking, walking in nature, connecting to a loved one), mastery (the experience of flow, being in the "zone", feeling centred), and love. In such experiences, a person is connected to both an individual self and something greater (what self-relational psychotherapy calls the field) at the same time. The primitive and Ego levels integrate into a higher consciousness capable of transformation, healing, subtle awareness, the capacity to hold multiple truths, and integrative thinking. While this level is often thought to be available under exceptional positive conditions where there is no threat or → stress, self-relational psychotherapy specifically addresses how to help clients achieve this level to face their difficult challenges, as it is only at this level that transformation and healing occur.

A BRIEF THEORY OF SYMPTOMS AND TRANSFORMATIONS. The three levels of consciousness allow us to realize a general theory of how and when problems develop, and how they either remain problems or are transformed into solutions.

The development of a social identity (or → "Ego-state") is the movement from the primitive to Ego consciousness. For example, a child starting with mostly primitive consciousness learns the verbal rules, social skills, reality maps and cultural traditions to create a stable Ego-sense of self and the world. A person developing other social roles (for example, as a teacher, athlete, businessperson, parent) goes through similar Ego development. Of course, each person develops many different Ego states – for example, one client had identities as a son, a father, a Jew, an American, a man, a depressed person and a highly educated person. Such Ego states are necessary to navigate the world. Of course, we can get lost in any one of them, mistaking our Ego state for our deepest consciousness.

All Ego-states are impermanent, and each identity will go through "death and rebirth" cycles across their lifetime. That is, a person must periodically release back into their primitive consciousness, one way or another, either for rest/renewal or transformation/healing of their Ego identity. The destabilizing of Ego identity can happen in many ways. One is normal life changes (e.g. a family birth or death, starting or completing school, starting or ending a job, puberty, leaving home, getting or losing a job, marriage or divorce, etc.). A second is negative experiences (e.g. trauma, significant illness or injury, job loss), which can shatter a person's identity at many levels. A third is voluntary initiation of altered states (for example, by intoxication, meditation, dancing, venturing into totally novel environments or challenges). In each of these contexts, the normal "box of identity" is dissolved, and consciousness moves from the Ego-identity level back to the primitive. What happens next determines whether a problem or solution develops.

The Ego response to the primitive consciousness determines its value, form and subsequent unfolding. If a person, or those in his community (e.g., family, society), takes a negative relationship to it – for example, fear, rejection, dissociation – it becomes a negative experience. As long as this "fight, flight or freeze" connection to the primitive consciousness continues, it will remain negative, perhaps even growing in symptomatic intensity. However, if a positive relationship is taken, the primitive experience will become a solution.

THE MOVEMENT TO GENERATIVE CONSCIOUSNESS. To transform a negative state to a positive one requires a generative level of consciousness. This, then, is a core practical focus of self-relations psychotherapy. The generative level of the somatic mind is aligned and centred; it carries high levels of relaxation, absorption, fluidity (flexibility) and openness. The generative level of the cognitive mind is oriented around the Ericksonian relational principle of accepting and positively utilizing whatever is there. It involves practices of resonant intention, acceptance, complementarity, generating multiple representations of an experience and integrating parts into a whole. The generative level of the field mind involves opening beyond the focal content (e.g. the problem) to a larger field of awareness that includes resources. The therapist thus attunes to helping the client to do this, thereby creating a positive context in which an experience might be transformed to its highest level. *[S.G. Gilligan, S. Kessler]*

REFERENCES. Gilligan S.G., *The courage to love: Principles and practices of self-relations psychotherapy*, 1997.

SELF-REPRESENTATION

Sub-system of the concept of the Self (theoretical hypothesis formulated by a person that contributes to the definition of the idea of the Self) that represents the part that is operational, interpersonal, situational, empirically produced, projected onto the assumption of roles and attributions regarding one's identity. Self-representations, as an explanation of a process of self-knowledge, are built within a system of → relationships (→ interpersonal, → symbolic and socio-cultural) into which the person is inserted and which are made accessible on the basis of the emotional states present at that moment and in that situation; these influence the meaning attributed to events, the judgements formed, the selective social comparisons, the interpretations of one's own role; they also act on the subjective motivation to undertake particular actions, on the organization of psychological difficulties, on the willingness or lack thereof to change. The tendency of individuals to self-confirm their self-representations through → feedback given by others, implies the search for other interactive situations of "negotiated symmetry", functional to the maintenance of the desired Self, and the consequent tendency to select information that is confirmatory. This process is defined by some authors as being "self-deception" (→ logic of self-deception). *[R.]*

SELF-SCHEMA

Concept introduced by Markus in 1977 to describe the cognitive representations that an individual has of himself. The self-schema are cognitive structures that perform the duplicate functions of the organization of the relevant information one has about oneself and that of modulating the acquisition of new knowledge regarding oneself and one's own psychological characteristics. Since the mid-1980s, self-schema have been considered as being → Self-representations (→ Self-concept) not only of a cognitive nature, but also of an affective-emotional nature, from which the concept of an emotional-cognitive representation of the self develops. The concept of self-schema emerges within the context of a structuralist and rational conception of the human mind. Already in Kantian philosophy the human mind is provided with an *a priori* collection of schema without which it would be impossible to understand experience and create a mental representation of oneself, of others and of the world. The concept of → mental scheme, from which the concept of self-schema is derived, has been widely used by F. Bartlett (in the study of human memory), from theorists of Gestalt psychology (in order to explain some characteristics of perception), by J. Piaget (in the study of developmental epistemology), and by U. Neisser (in the field of the cognitive psychology of personality). *[D. Liccione]*

REFERENCES. Markus H.R., *Self-schemata and processing information about the self*, in «Journal of Personality and Social Psychology», 1977, 35.

SELF-SYSTEM

Within the framework of Sullivan's interpersonal theory, self-system defines the organization of experiences in order to protect the Self, keep the "not-me" out of awareness and avoid the development of anxiety. In protecting the individual from anxiety, such "dynamism" plays both a defensive and a selective role in that it selects which experiences may be incorporated into the Self. In this way, it organizes the formation of personality and maintains those portions referring to → "good-me" inside consciousness. To this end, the system applies a set of "security operations" – apathy, selective inattention, dissociation – in order to avoid anxiety and focus on other mental material. If the self-system fails, security operations collapse. Depending on how much anxiety has entered the Self, an individual may develop a personality based on a range of critical issues from low self-esteem and complete lack of confidence to psychosis. In Sullivan's view, whilst self-system should be regarded as an operational system, the Self should be viewed as the container of anxiety-free representations. *[A. Cresti, S. Brizzi]*

REFERENCES. Greenberg J.R., Mitchell S.A., *Object relations in psychoanalytic theory*, 1983; Sullivan H.S., *The Interpersonal theory of psychiatry*, 1953.

SELF-THERAPY

In rational-emotive behavioural therapy, it is the ability of a person to activate, encourage and provide for himself everything that can be therapeutic, healing and balancing. Self-therapy activates the psychological resources that people use to maintain mental health and also develops the abilities to cope with stress. Most mental disorders, in fact, affect people whose skills in dealing with personal and relational problems are not well-established. Traditionally, the term "therapy" is reserved for the dual relationship that involves a therapist and a patient, who searches in this therapy, often in a passive way, for a solution to his psychological pain. Self-therapy actively involves the person in the resolution of personal or psychological problems or at least in the attempt to resolve them by activating resources of awareness and psychological mastery. The subject can be a spontaneous or naive self-therapist, who uses the self-narration of subjective experience in an intuitive way, or "methodical conscious", when he draws from subjective experience the methodology, or rather, a "technology of the self" that will be transmitted together with the evidence of the care pathway performed. Another point of view about self-treatment can be learned from Ellis. Human beings are active developers of their own reality, and assume a central role in their suffering but also a role as promoters of wellbeing. The patient is responsible for his change and the therapist is the "research supervisor," who actively monitors and directs the patient towards change. Among the various forms of self-therapy, there are also groups for self-help and self-medication. Self-help groups are composed of people who share the same problem (for example alcoholism). The objective is, while discussing together about a shared problem, to provide emotional support and improve the psychological abilities of the participants to be aware of the problem and also to find personal resources to deal with it. People who make up the group are all at the same level, and this makes them co-responsible for the mutual support provided: they are both users and providers of the psychological aid. Self-help groups contribute to the release of passivity created by the sense of impotence and lack of self-confidence, which often governs these people. Group activities are usually self-financed and self-managed, and conducted in an informal and spontaneous way; they are an additional resource to psychotherapeutic treatment to support people with mental health problems. The introduction of a professional facilitator (helper) has been part of the evolution of self-help groups. The main focus is on the quantity and quality of the relationship between the facilitator and the self-help group: some studies have shown that this collaboration, if properly conducted, contributes positively to the achievement of the objective of the group. The facilitator should have an active but non-directive attitude, he should help changing processes to emerge without controlling or directing them, and he should help group members to make these processes explicit, in order to promote autonomy and independence. Some studies about the performance of self-help groups have highlighted that, without the facilitator, the cases of early conclusion increase; the presence of the helper is useful to allow optimal progress and conclusion of the work of each component of the group; instead, in cases where the presence of the helper is prolonged, the effect would be rather counterproductive. Another form of self-therapy, as has been said, is the one known as "self-medication", through which is meant both the activity of a subject who takes drugs – prescribed or not – without consulting the doctor, to treat minor pathological conditions (e.g. a cold) but also the act of taking alcohol or drugs in order to alleviate one's psychological pain; the first form of self-medication is useful, provided that it does not expose the person to harmful side effects of the drug that he does not know about; the intake of substances such as drugs or alcohol is an inappropriate attempt at self-care, which results in a further burden being placed on top of the initial psychological suffering. In this regard, Khantzian argues that the use of psychoactive substances by some schizophrenic patients is aimed at reducing feelings of suffering and pain related to negative emotions, anxiety and depression, but can cause isolation and social withdrawal. Moreover, in these psychotic patients, the use of these substances worsens the progress of the disease and affects adversely the acceptance of the pharmacological treatment that is necessary to cure them. *[M. Procacci, C. Petracca]*

REFERENCES. Ellis A., *How to stubbornly refuse to make yourself miserable about anything – yes, anything*, 1990; Foucault M., *Technologies of the Self*, in *Technologies of the Self: a seminar with Michael Foucault*, 1988; Francescato D., Leone L., Traversi M., *Oltre la Terapia*, 1993; Ghezzani N., *Autoterapia: guarire la propria psiche con strumenti personali*, 2005; Khantzian E.J., *The self-medication hypothesis of substance use disorders: a reconsideration and recent applications*, in «Harvard Rev Psychiatry», 1997, XLIV, 4(5); Maton K., Leventhal G.S., Madara E.J., Julien M., *Factors affecting the birth and death of mutual-help groups: The role of national affiliation, professional involvement, and member focal problem*, in «American Journal of Community Psycology», 1989, XVII, 5; Semerari A., *I processi cognitivi della relazione terapeutica*, 1991; Silverman P.R., *Mutual help groups: Organization and development*, 1980.

SELF-TRANSCENDENCE

In logotherapy, a fundamental dynamic of personality that, according to Frankl's → dimensional ontology, belongs to the spiritual (noetic) dimension of human beings and expresses their intentionality. In franklian logotherapy and existential analysis, self-transcendence represents "the essence of existence" and constitutes an original motivational principle that is independent from the hierarchy of needs (Maslow) of the psycho-physical organism. According to Frankl, → self-actualization is a "collateral effect" of self-transcendence. Human beings, driven by the → will to meaning, are originally oriented towards something or someone beyond themselves (a goal to reach or a person to love); every narcissistic withdrawal (search for pleasure, power or happiness) is fundamentally neurotic.

The therapeutic technique of → dereflection aims at promoting self-transcendence in cases of excessive self-observation or hyperintention (i.e. sexual neurosis). Self-transcendence displays the capacity of the spiritual person to distance himself from the psychophysical organism and to face external conditionings by taking decisions; it represents the basis of spiritual strength and psychological → resilience. *[D. Bruzzone]*

REFERENCES. Bruzzone D., *Autotrascendenza e formazione*, 2001; Id., *Viktor Frankl*, 2012; Frankl V.E., *The doctor and the soul*, 1946; Id., *Pschotherapy and existentialism*, 1967.

SEMANTICS

Field of linguistics that studies the meaning of linguistic signs, that is, of words, of expressions, of phrases and of text. It is a discipline that analyzes how linguistic signs acquire the property of transmitting meaning: the scope is that of associating the meaning of signs (that is, the object that they indicate) with the process of assigning meaning. The study of semantics lies in the field of philosophy of language (the study of the phenomena that guide the process of assigning language) or of linguistics (study of the system of signs belonging to a language, the way in which they are manifested or the way they interact in the linguistic system). Frequently, both disciplines deal with the semantic analysis; as a result of this it becomes difficult to assign a procedure to one rather than to another. Descriptive semantics examines what signs mean in the different languages: for example, they deal with identifying what constitutes a verb or a verbal phrase or a noun and a nominal phrase. This analysis is used by anthropologists in order to study how the signs expressed in a language are correlated to the perception of the world of which they speak. Theoretical semantics, on the other hand, is the research into a general theory of meaning in language.

In psychology, indications for the description of mental processes of understanding and for research into how meaning is acquired are derived from semantics; in etiology, semantics deal with the ways in which other species communicate and the study of the content of the communications of various animals. Within the field of psychotherapy, semantics, as in → hermeneutics, is the instrument for the interpretation of the meanings attributed to reality, as well as a linguistic vehicle for therapeutic → communication, focused on the meanings and on the linguistic codes that produce such meanings. *[R.]*

SENEX → PUER–SENEX

SENSATION

Emotional and visceral experience associated with sensory experience. In psychotherapy, the term is used primarily to refer to feelings, affection, an emotional connotation connected to → perception, and in particular deriving from our somatic proprioception. This definition was primarily proposed and adopted by C.G. Jung. In this sense, sensation can be defined as the perception of one's own → emotions. This meaning is different to that normally used in general psychology and the neurosciences, where the term "sensation" refers to the process of sensorial transduction that is preliminary to perceptive integration and principally associated with the information derived from the sensory organs. Sensations play a fundamental role in the therapeutic relationship. These are, in fact, both a source of evaluation, understanding and diagnosis for the therapist, and a useful parameter of evaluation of the feeling of → wellbeing attained by the patient as a result of the work carried out in therapy. In addition, being close to the intuitive aspects of perception, sensations orient the therapeutic intervention at a par with rational evaluations and make possible all those processes of therapeutic → problem-solving on a heuristic basis. Some attempts have been made to classify the basic sensations that, if, in part, can be superimposed onto some of the primary emotions (pain, joy, sadness, disgust, anger, surprise, fear), are separate in that they represent an emotional experience that takes place at an even more "basal" level. *[R.]*

SENSE → WILL TO MEANING

SENSE OF GUILT

An expression indicating the unpleasant feeling of having committed harm or having transgressed a socially shared rule. From an evolutionary perspective, the purpose of such a feeling is to induce pro-social behaviours in individuals, such as remedying a mistake or compensating the other person for the suffering inflicted. In psychoanalysis, it may be conscious or → unconscious and it is the result of a → conflict between → Superego and driving needs. This conflict can take various neurotic forms: it can be expressed through obsessive rituals, through which the Ego tries to keep forbidden desires under control or it can turn into strong self-accusation, as in melancholic depressions. There is an unconscious sense of guilt behind many self- or hetero-destructive behaviours, as well as behind many of the failures in one's own life. In Gestalt therapy, guilt is like a "projected resentment": who feels guilty has previously projected (attributed) his/her own resentment onto another person, which, as a projection, is perceived as coming from the environment and induces the feeling of having done something evil.

Therapy consists in discovering and expressing the reason behind one's resentment, and in expressing, explicitly, desires and requests to another person. In the context of existential therapy, a sense of guilt is seen as an indispensable human condition; therefore, the goal of therapy is not to eliminate it, but to understand the message and harmonize it within one's own existence. Other interpretations (also belonging to that model) consider the sense of guilt as feeling indebted towards their own missed chances in life; such a sentiment would often be obscured by boredom, → anxiety, depression or → anguish. In psychopathology, a lack of sense of guilt in an individual who commits reprehensible actions (murders, violent acts, crimes) is called psychopathy. *[R.]*

SEPARATION

Freudian theme revisited by Lacan from a structural perspective. The individual that is split, divided, is represented by Lacan with a $, to indicate the separation of the speaking being from the signified of his own speech. He is not to be viewed as the consequence of a pathogenic accident, but he constitutes the regular structure of the Lacanian individual, being the result of the signifying chain. The theory of subjective causality identifies in alienation/separation the two fundamental operations that, at the same time, separate and generate the individual to himself. The first, highlights the inclusion in the discourse of the Other, the second the movement of separation of the signifying chain obtained through an object that has a different nature from that of the signifier. *[S. Guido]*

REFERENCES. Lacan J. (1964), *The four fundamental concepts of psychoanalysis*, in *The seminars of Jacques Lacan XI*, 1977; Id. (1964), *Posizione dell'inconscio*, in *Scritti*, 1974.

SETTING

English term used to describe the temporal-spatial area in which the psychotherapeutic encounter takes place. It is the context that defines and delimits the relationship between psychotherapist and patient, whether this be an individual (individual setting) or a group (group setting). The concept of the time at which the session takes place, the fee of the therapist and the modes of payment, the frequency of the encounters, whether it is possible to meet outside of the agreed schedule and the particular nature of the relationship between the therapist and the patient (for example the physical distance, the possibility of bodywork, the presence of an armchair, sofas, desk) are all included in the concept of the setting of therapy. All therapeutic models agree on the necessity of having a setting that is clear and well-defined for the proper conduction of therapy. However the variability of the setting between one therapeutic model and the other is very wide: some therapists prefer to ask the patient to lie on a sofa, others ask them to sit on a chair; some prefer to sit in front of the patient, others place the patient behind them; there are even some therapists that invite the patient to lie on a cushion or mattress to induce in him a greater degree of relaxation and to predispose him to a better externalization of his feelings. The frequency of the sessions can vary from four to five times a week to once every two weeks or a month. The term setting is also used in psychological → research and designates the context and the rules that have to be followed in order to ensure that an experiment or the administration of a test be considered as scientific. In this case, the setting defines the time and the way in which it is administrated, or an experiment conducted, the type of communication and the relationship between the experimenter and the subject/subjects, the neutrality of the procedures and of the evaluation of the subjects. *[R.]*

SEXUAL IMPOTENCE

In the past, a term used in sexology to indicate an erectile dysfunction and the consequent impossibility of performing a sexual act effectively. Sexual impotence is called primary when it appears from the beginning of sexual activity, and secondary when it occurs during a sexual act. The most common causes of erectile dysfunction are of psychogenic nature (performance anxiety, conflict between partners, guilt, excessive emotionality, etc.), but they can also be organic or iatrogenic (for example, as a result of a surgery or use of psychotropic drugs). *[R.]*

SEXUALITY

According to Freud, human sexuality is not just a reproductive function – rather it is, above all, an expression of sensual pleasure that runs parallel to biological functions and human activities. According to Freud, sexuality becomes activated already in early childhood; therefore, the somatic areas presiding over eating, defecating and urination have been defined as "erogenous zones". In this perspective the → "pleasure principle" – the search for pleasure – overlaps and often conflicts with the "reality principle" – that is to say, the instinct for safeguarding the survival of the individual and the species. Sexuality is central in Freud's psychoanalytic thought and he considered it responsible for the onset of → neurosis. Early on, Freud believed neuroses to be the effect of sexual traumas sustained in childhood (theory of precocious seduction). Later on, he replaced this theory with that of the persistence – in the guise of fantasies – of mnestic traces of sexual traumas dating as far back as human prehistory. Subsequently Freud clarified that, in childhood, sexuality emerges "leaning on" the vital bodily functions (theory of analysis) therefore arousal sets on as "collateral effect of internal processes as soon as the intensity of these [. . .] has [. . .] overcome certain quantitative limits". It is understood that the sexuality with which psychoanalysis occupies itself, is that pertaining to childhood – individual childhood as well as the infancy of humankind. This possesses a traumatic valency and – according to clinical psychology that defines sexual perversions as the paradigm of a subconscious → fixation of pre-genital sexuality of which a neurosis represents the negative side – is defined as psychosexuality. The first representation of a psychic conflict (first topography) is between the → Ego, as a self-preserving need and sexuality enslaved to the pleasure principle. Later on, when the presence of a libidinous component was recognized in the Ego, the conflict came to be described as being between an object-libido (directed outwards toward objects and an "Ego-libido" (inward-directed → libido, or narcissism). Subsequently Freud conjectured that the conflict arose between an anti-vital need (death → drive) and a vital need (life drive). Therefore, sexuality became associated with drives towards life; yet Freud's reflection on masochism demonstrated that the death drive operates at the core of it, and if extroverted, it determines its opposite – sadism. The close relation between sexuality and destructivity stressed by clinical psychology opened the question as to whether destructivity becomes eroticized under the cover of sexuality, or whether it must be supposed that an intrinsically non–self-preserving aspect might be present at the core of the sexual drive. It becomes therefore necessary to distinguish between a sexuality linked to the purpose of the self-preservation of the individual and the species, and an unbridled sexuality – submissive only to the pleasure principle and in conflict with self-preservation. *[F. Conrotto]*

▷ For Jung sexuality, not reducible to the Freudian construct of the drive, represents a fundamental experience of progressive psychification–self-reflection of a pre-psychic instinct-motivation assimilated to an "already existing psychic complexity", within the dynamic of reunification of opposites characteristic of the → individuation process. In it, sexuality founds and expresses the relationships with the world of objects, already implicated in the original psychic complexity of the individual.

Through sensuality-sexuality, the individual creates and discriminates the world in terms of objects, producing the possibility to access a real dimension of sense and intimacy that reassembles the primitive relationship, first unconscious-undifferentiated, in a relationship between a subject and an object that is both intimate and separate, corporeal and imaginary, as well as reciprocally internal and external one to the other. The transpersonal-relational nature of sexuality is evidenced by its presence in the relationships with the world of objects in general, as in artistic productions or in religious inspiration, as well as in all the relationships between self and objects as evidence, for example, in the vicissitudes of → transference or in psychopathology. *[S. Carta]*

REFERENCES. Breuer J., Freud S. (1893–1895), *Studies on hysteria*, in *The Standard Edition*, II, 1953–1974; Id. (1887–1904), *Letters to Wilhelm Fliess*, 1961; Id. (1901–1905), *A Case of Hysteria, Three Essays on Sexuality and Other Works*, in *The Standard Edition*, VII, 1953–1974; Id. *On narcissism: An introduction*, 1914; Id. (1920), *Beyond the pleasure principle*, in *The Standard Edition*, XIV, 1953–1974; Id. (1924), *The economic problem of masochism*, in *The Standard Edition*, XIX, 1953–1974; Green A., *The chains of Eros*, 1997; Jung C.G. (1935), *Principles of practical psychotherapy*, in *Collected Works*, XVI, 1966; Laplanche J., Leclaire S., *The unconscious and the Id: A volume of Laplanche's problématiques*, 1999; Id., *Elementi per una metapsicologia*, 1991.

SHADOW

In analytic psychology, this term refers to the dark side of the individual, to all aspects of himself that he would like not to have and that are considered to be negative, but also all that does not reside in the conscious because it is incompatible with the way the individual would like to see himself. Jung considered the Shadow as being an indelible part of our personality, with which we have to find a way of coexisting. According to Jung, everyone has a shadow as part of his psyche, otherwise we would not be human. According to him, the shadow is expressed through projection, the dark part of ourselves that has been repressed is projected onto others, (*he* is negative, not I). At other times, positive or valued aspects of the self are repressed, that, if brought to awareness, would lead to an enrichment of one's personality. If it remains in the unconscious, the Shadow acquires a life of its own and a strong emotional charge; it escapes the control of the Ego and constitutes a nucleus that is completely split from the rest of the psyche; for this reason, in psychoanalytic therapy, the problems related to the Shadow are the first to be dealt with. The Shadow is a moral problem that tests the entire personality, because it inevitably leads to the issue of personal responsibility with regard to evil. Becoming aware of our Shadow leads to a transformation of our psyche, where one is able to meet with the "other" residing within us, leading to a greater awareness of the negative aspects of ourselves as well as allowing the Ego to regain control. The acceptance of the Shadow as an integral part of our personality is necessary in order to activate the process of → individuation. Jung also refers to a collective Shadow, that represents the evil that is carried out collectively, of which we are not conscious. An example could be represented by Nazi ideology that considered the destruction of others as being "good and lawful", (→ persona). *[A. Benvenuti]*

REFERENCES. Jung C.G. (1921), *Psychological types*, in *Collected Works*, VI, 1971; Id. (1951), Jung C.G., *Aion: Researches into the phenomenology of the self*, in *Collected Works*, IX/II.

SHAPING

In the field of cognitive-behavioural psychotherapy, procedure – also known as modelling – that allows for the acquisition of a desired behaviour that does not form part of the repertory of the individual through the → reinforcement of progressive approximations, always closer to the desired final behavioural response. During the therapeutic intervention, behaviours that are similar, even if only slightly, to the desired behaviour are reinforced, and when these have been acquired, the therapist moves on to behaviours that are even more similar to the objective, extinguishing the previous ones. In the construction of a shaping programme, it is important to specify the end behaviour that one wants to attain in order to be able to programme, even if in a flexible manner, the successive approximations by means of which the behaviour will be modelled. *[P. Orifiammi]*

REFERENCES. Martin G., Pear J., *Behaviour modification: What it is and how to do it*, 2007.

SHORT-TERM PSYCHODYNAMIC PSYCHOTHERAPY

Short-term pychodynamic psychotherapy is expected to be as short as possible and as long as is needed. Research shows four to six sessions as average but the contract is flexible according to need.

The focus and time-frame are mutually agreed by client and therapist. The focus is circumscribed but may also be renegotiated. It is the strategic focus that is important and this will be where the emotion is. Sessions may be spaced, which allows more time for homework and adaptation to individual needs. This model has the expectation that problems stem from the past and it draws on the psychodynamic tradition and also on the newer therapies. Experienced therapists of this model fuse together an awareness of → transference and → resistance to change with aspects of Gestalt, transactional analysis, cognitive-behavioural therapy, art, fantasy and other therapeutic tools. These are used flexibly to help the client. The aim is to be alongside the client, facilitating their search for freedom and to teach the client to become their own therapist. Teaching can circumvent resistance and highlight transference issues and help the client to understand psychological processes. This aids → motivation. Motivation for change and understanding is essential for therapy. The problem presented is the starting point from which difficulties rooted in the past can be accessed, unraveled and the emotions revisited and dealt with appropriately. This is to enable the client to deal with the present and future, free of the unfinished business of the past. The first session is crucial in speeding up the process; in this session it is important to touch the client's pain and to begin the work of therapy.

The approach demands activity and involvement of both client and therapist. The therapist's expectation of change in a brief period is necessary and inspires hope. The approach is intense, incisive, focused and flexible in every aspect. It requires skill, experience and great sensitivity to be at all times in tune with the client. It is in the energy created by this activity and involvement of both client and therapist that the mysterious essence of therapy happens. *[P. Rawson]*

REFERENCES. Rawson P., *A handbook of short-term psychodynamic psychotherapy*, 2005.

SHOULD

Auxiliary verb in English that conveys the meaning of a rigid "duty" or "obligation". Rational-emotional behavioural therapy considers this term as being one of the principal expressions of those absolute expectations (→ must-urbation) that are the origin of the great majority of emotional difficulties. This happens when in the habitual ways of thinking "shoulding" prevails; for example, "He absolutely should not have done this to me", or "I absolutely must obtain this". In particular, "shoulding" towards oneself ("I have to behave well and be approved by all the persons that are important to me, otherwise I am a total failure and this would be terrible"); towards others, ("Others should treat me well and behave in the way that I think they should behave, otherwise they are pigs, scoundrels and deserve to pay for it"); regarding life conditions, ("Things that happen to me have to be the way I expect and everything should be easy and pleasant, otherwise life is unbearable"). The therapist that works within the model of rational emotive behaviour therapy does not have the dogmatic belief that the shoulding behaviour has to always lead to emotional problems, but believes that people who maintain an attitude that is more realistic and more flexible have a greater chance of avoiding the development of dysfunctional emotions when facing difficult situations. The rational alternative to these absolute expectations are thoughts that indicate preferences, desires and aspirations. *[M. Di Pietro]*

REFERENCES. Dryden W., Neenan M., *The rational emotive behavioural approach to therapeutic change*, 2004; Ellis A., *Overcoming destructive beliefs, feelings, and behaviours*, 2001.

SHOULDISM

In Gestalt therapy, it is the attitude that considers duty a priority over an organism's need, that is, the tendency, regarding behavioural choices, to refer to considerations concerning one's sense of duty rather than the organism's real current needs. Instead, these needs are central to the Gestalt approach. Human beings are considered as an organism dealing with survival, with all the problems that this entails in relation to their habitat, which is not only their natural one, but also to the specific human context to which they belong. The needs of the context are often different and opposed to those of the organism. Consequently, a person needs to adapt to them by renouncing those needs pushing from the inside, which are more authentic but potentially dangerous for the social order. In this way, a person can develop an "outward" personality, which allows the subject to socially survive without undue difficulties but it alienates them from their authentic experiences and turns them into someone who is at the service of social order. This situation has a very high cost in terms of "meaning of life" and becomes, in many cases, the cause of various symptoms. From a Gestalt perspective, shouldism is one of the main sources of mental disorders. The therapy consists of both helping people to reconnect with their profound needs, that is, with the organism's needs, and developing behavioural styles that allow them to fully express their needs and satisfy these needs as much as possible. The psychological work is oriented towards the direction of creating a more complex behavioural language that can better connect the intrapsychic level with the outside world. *[P. Quattrini]*

REFERENCES. Kierkegaard S., *Fear and trembling*, 1843; Id., *Either/Or*, 1843; Montefoschi S., *Il senso della psicoanalisi. Da Freud a Jung e oltre*, in *Opere*, I, 2001; Naranjo C., *Techniques of Gestalt therapy*, 1973; Perls F., *Ego, hunger, and aggression*, 1969.

SIGNIFICATION

Within the field of narrative therapy, definition that implies the non-existence of "facts" in themselves, in that it is the meaning that we attribute to them that will make them psychologically meaningful. The individual and human systems (→ system) are engaged in an incessant negotiation of meanings and attributions of meaning to reality and to the relationships in which they are involved: in this way, psychotherapy becomes an endeavour aimed at discovering the meaning of events and of → symptoms. *[M. Giuliani]*

REFERENCES. Anderson H., Goolishian H., *Human systems as linguistic systems: Preliminary and evolving ideas about the implications for clinical theory*, in «Family process», 1988, 27(4).

SIGNIFIED

The signified is, for Lacan, an elusive content in that it is constituted as an effect of the signifying chain. Lacan dissolves the bond between signified and signifier of the linguistic "sign" of F. de Saussure through the accent placed on the importance of the bar and in this way establishes a double net of relationships between elements that do not cover themselves. The Lacanian individual emerges from this process internally divided as a result of the language and of the action of the signifier: this is translated, in linguistic-structural terms, into the Freudian concept of repression. From here, the hypothesis is that the signified can never be accepted as an object, but that it slides under the bar as the result of a concatenation of the signifiers. In this way the "illusion that the signifier responds to the function of representing the signified" can be dismantled and the repressed object (signified) has to make use of the formations of the unconscious (condensation/metaphor and displacement/metonymy) to return to the "spoken" in the code of an enunciation and in the symptom. *[F. Quesito]*

REFERENCES. Lacan J. (1953), *The function and field of speech and language in psychoanalysis*, in *Écrits: A Selection*, 1977; Id., *Il seminario, Libro XVII, Il rovescio della psicoanalisi*, 2001.

SIGNIFIER

That which represents, as written by Lacan, "a subject for another signifier". Subverting the concept of "sign" belonging to the structuralist linguistics of F. de Saussure (that predicted the unity of the sense of signified and signifier) Lacan gives importance to the bar inserted between the S and the s of the algorithm (S/s), as a factor of separation. The bar indicates the impossibility of the relationship between signifier (S) and signified (s), because the correspondence between the word and object is excluded by the existence of language. The sense of the spoken language is constituted only in the articulation between signifiers, and signification emerges as the effect of the chain of signifiers. The bar in the algorithm that separates the symbolic aspect of the signifier from the imaginary aspect of the signified is the same as that which Lacan describes as being the descriptive element of the divided subject. Lacan in this way confirms the total division between language as a pre-existing system and the subject of the act of speaking as the result of the separation between signifier and signified, in that the articulation constitutes that part of the discourse of the subject that remains innately separate from repression. *[F. Quesito]*

REFERENCES. Lacan J., *The function and field of speech and language in psychoanalysis*, in *Écrits: A selection*, 1977; Id., *The seminar of Jacques Lacan: The other side of psychoanalysis*, XVII, 2007.

SKINNER-BOX

Cage created by B.F. Skinner for the study of operant conditioning (→ behavioural model of operant conditioning). This permits the animal on which the experiment is being carried out to perform actions (for example, pressing a lever) in order to receive a → reinforcement (for example, food) or in order to avoid → punishment (for example, an electric shock). The release of the reinforcer can be regulated by the experimenter based on the number of → responses of the animal and on the interval of time that passes between the occurrence of one reinforcer and another. *[A. Couyoumdjian]*

SMALL DISORDER WHICH PRESERVES ORDER

In the → brief strategic therapy Nardone's model, this term refers to a type of → strategic reframing technique formulated by G. Nardone and used for the treatment of particular cases of obsessive-compulsive disorder (OCD). Clinical-empirical research carried out by the Centro di Terapia Strategica in Arezzo has demonstrated that there is a large percentage of cases of OCD present with compulsions that do not follow a predetermined sequence of actions when carrying out the rituals. These compulsions consist of actions and thoughts that are "preventative" in nature, that is, aimed at protecting and maintaining a form of order considered by the individual as being the "perfect" order. An example of this would be the attempt to maintain one's house as a "temple of cleanliness", defending it from any possible form of "contamination", for example, by preventing anyone from entering the house or obliging them to carry out extensive rituals of cleanliness. Or else it could be a preventative ritual aimed at defending one's loved ones from bad luck or aimed at achieving total control over life, with the idea that this will allow them to avoid making mistakes, etc. The individual can, for example, continue to correct the positioning of certain objects around the house until they are considered to be "in perfect order", in order to prevent something terrible happening to themselves or to their loved ones. In all these cases, in which the compulsions do not have a specific sequence, it is rather difficult and limiting to prescribe the use of → counter-rituals with a predetermined sequence (for example those typically used in treating reparatory compulsions). The strategic psychotherapist, therefore, has to first of all intervene on the beliefs underlying these behaviours (→ logic of belief) and on the rigid and idealized perceptions of the patient, in order to guide him in a gradual manner towards change. By means of the use of → strategic dialogue, the therapist starts to introduce doubt into the patient's idea of total perfection (for example the idea of perfect cleanliness, purity, order, total control, etc.). The patient is guided, through the use of a series of questions with the illusion of an alternative (→ illusion of alternatives technique) and the use of successive restructuring paraphrasing, to question his rigid perceptions. In this way, the therapist starts to prepare the patient to accept the idea that, in order to get rid of his fears and his obsessions, he needs to avoid protecting himself from disorder, in that it is precisely this that makes him so vulnerable and distressed. He is led to understand that his goal should not be that of looking for and desiring total perfection, which is an impossible task in this imperfect world, but rather that of immunizing himself from disorder. By means of the use of strategic dialogue, that pits "fear against fear", the patient realizes that the only way of escape from this trap is to immunize himself in order to become stronger.

At this point the prescription becomes an inevitable request, a joint discovery. Even the most resistant of patients usually accepts the prescription of a "small daily dose of a little disorder in order to maintain the order". In this way, the role of the therapist becomes that of guiding the patient in this process of immunization, inviting him to voluntarily introduce a small disorder or risk in his rigid order. This will lead him to undergo a second-order change (→ first- and second-order change), in that the therapeutic prescription works upon the reaction (preventative compulsion) and on the perception (obsession) of the patient. *[C.Portelli]*

REFERENCES. Nardone G., Balbi E., *The logic of therapeutic change*, 2015; Nardone G., Portelli C., *Knowing through changing*, 2005.

SOCIAL ADAPTATION

The process by which the individual comes to a balanced relationship with the social context in which he lives, anticipating and assuming the regulatory and cultural point of view as a guide for his actions. The criteria that pre-order the definition and evaluation of social adaptation are not fixed and universal because they refer to a set of rules and vary depending on the historical moment and the specific socio-cultural context. According to many authors, it is a sign of good overall functioning of the person and a sign of mental health. Often psychotherapy steps into areas where there is a form of social maladjustment (expressed as the distance between the social reality, which is objectively defined and institutionalized, and the subjective reality of the person who carries a deviant behaviour), with the aim of readjusting the individual to the violated normality and bringing them back to a socially "appropriate" behaviour. *[R.]*

SOCIAL COGNITIVE THEORY

Theory of → personality according to which man, rather than being subjected to → drives or → scripts that are predetermined and not controllable, possesses the capacity (also called agency; → human agency) of predicting, anticipating, deciding and changing events. Social cognitive theory has fundamental implications for the practice of psychotherapy because, departing from its assumptions, it highlights the possibility of instilling in the patient a process of → cognitive reframing that places him at the centre of his process of → change. *[F. Celi]*

REFERENCES. Bandura A., *Social learning theory*, 1977; Galeazzi A., Meazzini P. (eds.), *Mente e comportamento. Trattato italiano di psicoterapia cognitivo-comportamentale*, 2004; Goslin D.A. (ed.), *Handbook of socialization theory and research*, 1969.

SOCIAL FEELING

Social feeling is a fundamental instance in individual psychology, and is viewed as a feeling of belonging as well as a feeling of community spirit and cooperation. It expresses the intersubjective and relational nature of the human mind: the innate potentiality of biological and intrapsychic structures for aggregation and a force that unites the individual with others and the environment so he or she can connect and communicate. It rebalances the self-assertive drives of striving for power and allows units of ideo-affective meaning to function synchronously. Innate and environmental potentialities harmonize the needs of social feeling with the perspectives of the → creative Self. In psychotherapy, transformative communication is a function of the creative interaction of the social feeling of the patient and therapist. *[A. Bianconi, E. Cairo]*

REFERENCES. Adler A., *The practice and theory of individual psychology*, 1920; Rovera G.G., *La psicologia individuale*, in G.B. Cassano, P. Pancheri (eds.), *Trattato italiano di psichiatria*, 1999

SOCIAL IMITATION

Within the behavioural paradigm, social imitation – or modelling – is the process of → learning a behaviour by observing what other people do. It can happen unintentionally and unconsciously. People tend to especially imitate behaviours of others identified as models, which are reinforced by their environment (the reinforcement of a model's behaviour, making it more easily imitable, is called "vicarious" reinforcement). A good model has similar characteristics to those of the observer (e.g. age, sex, etc.), and it is perceived by him/her as authoritative, competent and experienced. *[G. Melli]*

REFERENCES. Bandura A., *Social learning theory*, 1977.

SOCIAL INFLUENCE

As human beings belong to a social species, they are inevitably subject to processes of mutual influence that manifest themselves in relationships at all levels (→ interpersonal, group, community) and in various fields concerning contact and → communication (family, school, amicability, organizations, mass media). Thus, social influence is a global and pervasive phenomenon, which results from a real or imagined presence of other individuals in a person's life. This phenomenon is closely connected with the process of creation of implicit and explicit judgments that "others" may or might formulate on the behaviour and opinions of the subject, who is therefore often influenced both consciously and unconsciously. Due to its global and pervasive character, social influence can be interpreted as a process tending towards pure conformity (majority influence) and more generally to the conservative tendency of social systems (tradition). In this sense, social influence carries a negative meaning, as it seems to contradict every idea and human aspiration towards freedom and personal autonomy. Social influence can also express itself as innovation and conflict in theoretical models that have demonstrated the ability of active minorities to change deeply the positions of majority groups. Therefore, when integrating two models, social influence can be understood as an expression of conservative and innovative tendencies in local cultural contexts. It defines and delimits – but it does not eliminate – the expressive possibilities of individual freedom, which is also historically determined. → Persuasion and → suggestion are terms associated with social influence but they are not overlapping in meaning. They are considered specific forms of communication aiming at producing changes in judgement and → behaviour. They can be attributed to rational arguments or to emotional → manipulation. *[S. Smiraglia]*

REFERENCES. Mucchi Faina A., *L'influenza sociale*, 1996; Smiraglia S., *Le vie della persuasione sono infinite*, 2009.

SOCIAL REWARDS

According to the behavioural paradigm, the term → reward refers to an event that increases the frequency of a behaviour. The social reward consists of praise, signs of approval or attention, originating primarily from significant others (relatives, teachers, friends), that can reinforce a certain type of behavioural → response. *[G. Palmieri]*

REFERENCES. Kendall P.C., Braswell L., *Cognitive-behavioural therapy for impulsive children*, 1985.

SOCIAL RITE

Collective ceremony that takes place on occasions that involve crucial changes in the cycle of life, in different cultures and traditions; the most important social rites take place at birth, in the passage to the age of adolescence and that of adulthood, at marriage and at death. As V. Turner highlights, every rite has three crucial stages: the separation, that is the abandonment of the previous state; the exclusion, that is the period of transition in which the individual no longer possesses the characteristics of the preceding state, but neither has he acquired those of the successive state; the aggregation, that is, the re-admission into society in a new state. The social rites, with their potential psychological involvement, are responsible for the subjective and emotional reality of each one of us; we find them in this way, also in the rigorous → setting of the room of the psychologist as in the rituals of cure present in psychiatric hospitals. A complex system of symbolization is at work, similar to that present in works of art, in myth and in poetry, that can be made explicit only by means of a careful analysis of the situations in which such symbols are expressed. The symbolic character and its therapeutic potential also demonstrate how rites accompany the psychological development of the individual and the collectivity, and the multiplicity of rites that are part of the construction of the → identity of man. Rites form part of the most diverse realities of everyday life and are present in the archaic rites as well as in post-industrial civilizations. The rite belongs to man and is there for man and always plays a role in psychotherapeutic processes. *[R.]*

SOCIETY

In Fromm's vocabulary (humanistic paradigm; please see the opening chapter, "The eight paradigms and their respective theoretical-applicative models"), the term refers both to the concrete organizational configuration of a group of individuals, and to their respective ideological and psychological structures. A society, in fact, besides promoting a determined amount of material production and establishing precise relationships and procedures in a community of men, tends to stabilize itself from a psychological point of view. Through an operation of "filtering", it allows the awareness of contents that are functional to its continuation, promoting different types of social characters in the groups of which it is composed. In this way, Fromm writes, 'the energy of the individuals is channelled in such a way as to make them productive forces indispensable to the functioning of society". *[L. Corti, E. Benelli]*

REFERENCES. Fromm E., *Escape from freedom*, 1941; Fromm E., Suzuki D., De Martino R., *Zen buddhism and psychoanalysis*, 1960.

SOCIOMETRY

In → psychodrama, the term designates a set of techniques and tools that allow the quality of affective relationships within a group to be represented using mathematical tools and graphs (pen-and-pencil sociometry) or the same psychodramatic representation (action sociometry). The first type of sociometry leads to the construction of sociograms, i.e. of diagrams in which the forces of attraction and rejection and the situations of indifference, present at a certain time in a group, appear quantified. Action sociometry allows the structure of the social relations in a group to be represented using psychodramatic techniques. The latter – instead of paper, pencil, graphic symbols, numbers, segments – uses the psychodramatic space of the stage and the members of the group as a means of detection and representation. Attraction and rejection are indicated by placing each person in a spatial relationship of closeness or distance referring to those towards whom we want to make evident the quality of the relationship; a more specific definition of this quality is further expressed by the posture (rigid, flexible, squatting, from behind, etc.), the mimicry (smile, disgust, kindness, ridicule, etc.) and by the tone and content of a verbal message. *[G. Boria]*

REFERENCES. Boria G., *Psicoterapia psicodrammatica. Sviluppi del modello moreniano nel lavoro terapeutico con gruppi di adulti*, 2005; Boria G., Muzzarelli F., *Incontri sulla scena*, 2009; Moreno J.L., *Psychodrama first volume*, 1946; Moreno J.L., *Who shall survive?*, 1953.

SOLILOQUY

In psychodrama, means by which the individual freely expresses what goes on in his mind, in a way that makes others perceive this as something that is not addressed to any person other than the individual himself. In this solitary talking (monologue), thoughts emerge and are articulated without following the rules of logic or the needs of completion of a story; rather they are regulated in their concatenation by the variable and unpredictable flow of emotions. The therapist can be induced to ask for a soliloquy when he considers it fruitful that a subject expresses the emotions felt in himself in a certain → here-and-now; or when, at the launch of a scene, it is useful for the → protagonist to synthetically express antecedent facts; or, again, when the protagonist, in a situation of dialogue, says things that – even if justified by the context – do not seem to coincide with what he really lives in that moment: in this case the director of psychodrama encourages the subject to stop and to express, thanks to the dialogue between himself, his real feelings (similar to the theatrical "apart", when the actor says something that looks as if it is in brackets, as if thinking aloud). *[G. Boria]*

REFERENCES. Boria G., *Psicoterapia psicodrammatica.* Sviluppi del modello moreniano nel lavoro terapeutico con gruppi di adulti, 2005; Boria G., Muzzarelli F., *Incontri sulla scena*, 2009; Moreno J.L., *Psychodrama first volume*, 1946; Moreno J.L., *Who shall survive?*, 1953.

SPLITTING → DEFENCE MECHANISMS

SPONTANEITY

According to Berne, the ideal aim of a process of change through transactional analysis is the reaching of autonomy, which is "achieved when one liberates or regains three abilities: [→] awareness, spontaneity and [→] intimacy". "Spontaneity means option [. . .] it means liberation from the compulsion to play games and have only the feelings one was taught to have". Stewart and Joines, taking from Berne, put spontaneity in relation with the → Ego-states and underline that one can react with spontaneity starting from any one of these: Parent, Adult or Child. "For example one can react as a Parent proposing, again, the emotions and behaviour [acquired] from parents or parental figures". James and Jongeward reckon that to be spontaneous means "to be free to make your own personal choices" accepting "responsibility" and being free means leaving a pre-determined lifestyle and "exploring new ways to think, to feel and to re-act", with the presence of the Adult. Spontaneity enables the expressions of natural emotions, stimulates curious exploration, intuition and creativity. It keeps alive the contact with the naturalness of the free Child, a function of the Ego-state that can be reawoken or made more active in favour of authenticity in the response, congruent with what happens in actual reality and not conditioned by limiting messages that come from the past. *[A. Ferrara]*

REFERENCES. Berne E., *Games people play*, 1964; James M., Jongeward D., *Born to win*, 1971; Stewart I., Joines V., *Transactional Analysis*,1975

STAR DIAGRAM

In psychosynthesis, the star diagram depicts the physiology of the psyche as it was defined by Assagioli.

The circle in the middle represents the field of consciousness of the → "egg diagram". In the middle there is the conscious Self or "I" (8) and all around, the will energy (7); then, the six points of the star represent the different functions of the psyche. The seven functions are: sensation (1), emotion (2), desire, impulse (3), imagination (4), thought (5), intuition (6).

The will function, for its peculiar role and its connection with the I and with the other functions, is represented in a different way. It is rather a "meta-function", that is, a function holding power to act over others, making those active and co-ordinating to an aim. A function, that is, a way of functioning of the psyche, must not be confused with its various elements: there is, for example, the thinking function and there are specific thoughts. *[D. De Paolis]*

REFERENCES. Assagioli R., *The act of will: A guide to self-actualization and self-realization*, 1973.

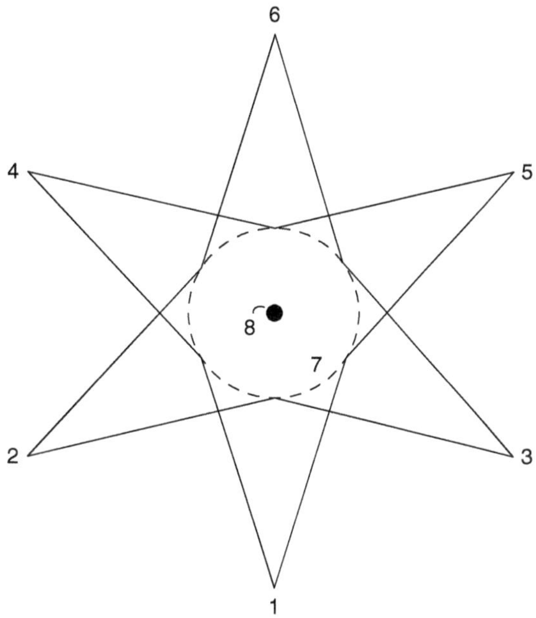

Figure 2 Star diagram.

STEREOTYPE

In 1922, in a book that would become a classic of communication studies, Lippmann used, for the first time, the term stereotype, arguing that, in most cases, we do not define something after seeing it, but before, complying with what our culture has already defined for us, and we tend to perceive it in the form that has been "stereotyped" for us. Stereotypes, socially shared generalizations about objects, ideas, individuals or groups, are "legitimating beliefs", that make plausible the status quo, turning "what is" into "what should be" and making undoubtedly true a psychological, social and economic event. They are also used as working hypotheses to be confirmed with further information, underestimating dissonant statements and also influencing the memory of the past: more likely, for example, we recall the positive information related to our own group and the negative ones related to the external group. And finally, stereotypes can become → self-fulfilling prophecies, because those who undergo them may react, with the socially expected behaviour, and, in doing so, paradoxically reinforce them. We talk about "stereotype threat", in fact, about the evaluation of the underachievement of some pupils, which may exacerbate their marginal situation, preventing a different view of themselves and therefore a more suitable behaviour. *[P. Meringolo]*

REFERENCES. Brown R., *Social psychology: The second edition*, 1986; Howard J.W., Rothbart M., *Social categorization and memory for in-group and out-group behaviour*, in «Journal of Personality and Social Psychology», 1980, 38; Lippmann W., *Public opinion*, 1922.

STIMULUS–RESPONSE RELATIONSHIP

Within the behavioural paradigm, a stimulus (S) is defined as any environmental variation that is able to provoke a response in the nervous system of an organism, whether this activity consists of a primary reflex → response or whether it is a reaction that is expressed in one or more behaviours. The variation in the environment can always be defined in physical-chemical terms, but in psychology one is not only interested in the physical-chemical dimension that has the ability to provoke a specific response (R).

A stimulus can more correctly be defined as a "stimulus situation" or "stimulus event". Stimulus and response are interdependent (if a response exists there must be something that it is responding to and a stimulus exists because there is a response to it) and have to be conceptualized and studied as reciprocal events in a field where every change in one also provokes a change in the other. The psychological event is a function of a stimulus and a response, but also of the history of the individual, the environment in which stimulus and response take place and the means by which the organism and the environment come into contact with each other. The functional properties of the stimulus and of the response are determined by the interaction between the organism and the stimulus-object. The stimulus function represents the description of a specific action of one part of the environment on a specific individual and can depend both on the natural characteristics of the stimulus and the history of interactions of every organism. Many functional stimuli have been experimentally studied and grouped into classes of functions: an eliciting function (produces R); a discriminative function (orients R); a reinforcing function (reinforces R); and a penalising function (weakens R) *[P. Moderato]*

REFERENCES. Moderato P., *Interazioni umane*, 2010.

STORIES

Narrative psychotherapy assumes that interpersonal relationships mould events and happenings into stories. In turn, stories shape the construction of meanings and the emotional responses to new events, and convey a sense of predictability of the environment. Stories integrate characters, contexts, individual motives with the observer's perspective. Stories account for events in a more or less coherent, aesthetically convincing and emotionally viable way. Within a clinical/therapeutic context, the inherent intersubjectivity of the construction of stories allows the drafting of new, more coherent, aesthetically convincing and emotionally viable accounts. Psychologists can adopt different techniques to promote alternative stories when working with clients, that is, including in the setting different → generations, highlighting narrative discrepancies, proposing different → punctuations, and integrating dissociated emotional states. *[V. Cigoli, F. Aschieri]*

REFERENCES. Byng-Hall J., *Rewriting family scripts*, 1995; White M., *Maps of narrative practice*, 2007.

STRANGE SITUATION

Ideated by Ainsworth within the field of → attachment theory, the Strange Situation is a standardized method of observation, lasting for about 20 minutes, created in order to evaluate the equilibrium between the attachment system and the exploration system and to illustrate the individual differences in the attachment models of infants. It is also utilized to evaluate the attachment model in babies between 12 and 20 months. This procedure permits the observation of the capacity of the child to use the parent as a "secure base" to explore his environment and as a refuge to return to in order to receive comfort and security when he is frightened or distressed, for example, when facing a new situation, a new person or brief separations. The attention of the observation is focused mainly on the interactive style adopted during the reunion with the parent. The procedure consists of seven episodes, each lasting for around three minutes, within which separations and reunions with the parent take place. *[A.M. Speranza]*

REFERENCES. Ainsworth M.D.S., Blehar M.C., Waters E., Wall S., *Patterns of attachment: A psychological study of the Strange Situation*, 1978.

STRATAGEM

In the art of war, a clever expedient employed in order to defeat an enemy who is stronger, frequently by using his own strength against him (as in some martial arts). In the art of rhetoric, it is the trick of persuasion that is an alternative to cogent argumentation. The extensive use of the "therapeutic stratagem" in the solution of human difficulties is owed to M.H. Erickson, but the development of the theory behind the use of the stratagem in therapy is owed to radical constructivism (→ constructivism) and to the Nardone Model of Strategic Therapy, where the stratagem (also known as a "behavioural trick") is an instrument aimed at building "planned casual events", at restructuring (→ strategic reframing technique) and at persuasive reasoning to provide the patient with → corrective emotional experiences that are able to substitute his dysfunctional mental constructions with others that are more functional (→ functional balance). The stratagem can be considered as the application of non-ordinary → logic to therapy, and presupposes the use of non-conventional modes of definition and resolution of problems. *[M. Rampin]*

REFERENCES. Nardone G., *Cavalcare la propria tigre*, 2003; Nardone G., Balbi E., *The logic of therapeutic change*, 2015.

STRATEGIC DIALOGUE

In the context of → brief strategic psychotherapy Nardone's model, a therapeutic technique used to conduct the first session, aimed at directing the subject, trapped in pathogenic perceptions and pathological reactions, towards new ways of feeling and reacting in respect to their problem. Developed from the work of Nardone, strategic dialogue represents the quintessence of the strategic approach to psychotherapy, as it uses targeted and strict persuasive and suggestive communication techniques to induce the person to change their own personal disposition towards reality. Strategic dialogue encompasses five specific communicative manoeuvres: questions with an illusion of alternatives; restructuring paraphrases; evoking sensations; recap to redefine; prescription as a joint discovery. The "questions with an illusion of alternatives" are questions with two possible answers, to induce the interlocutor to focus on the goal of change. The alternatives offered through the questions highlight possible perceptions of the problem and possible ways to solve it. Therefore, the interlocutor, with their response, must "decide" which of them fits their case. In this way, during the phase of investigation itself, patients spontaneously venture into territories that are different than those they already know. Their perception of the problem begins to change, since the strategic questions show them the problem from new perspectives, or because they highlight potential critical points. This communicative manoeuvre refers to the → illusion of alternatives technique adopted by M.H. Erickson to break down the resistance of the patient to follow the prescriptions. However, in the strategic dialogue, this is not used to prescribe actions but to induce responses. The interlocutors, persuaded by their own responses, transform autonomously their own way of perceiving things and consequently their way of reacting to them. Therefore, they will change their vision and their → attempted solutions. In this way, a dialogue using well-constructed "questions with an illusion of alternatives" acts often as → corrective emotional experience. The strategic questions with an illusion of alternatives move from more general questions first and then, in a spiral process, to more specific questions based on the responses concerning the details of the situation. This means that both the sequence and the questions do not follow a rigid plan, but they fit the logic of the interlocutor. The specific questions and the response alternatives are based on this logic and on the consequent assumptions. These must lead to undermining the subject's perceptions and then to reorientate them towards more functional directions:

> the process is a sort of "interactive dance" where questions create answers and answers allow the construction of successive strategic questions. This continues until the interlocutor declares that he changed his position following the new assumed perceptions yielded by the discoveries acquired through the dialogue.

Any sequence of two or three questions with an illusion of alternatives is followed by a "restructuring paraphrase", the second of the five strategic dialogue manoeuvres. The therapist uses the answers to formulate a definition of the problem that verifies their correct understanding. No "interpretation" is proposed to the interlocutor. Instead, he is asked a diagnostics "check" of how the problem functions ("otherwise please correct me . . ."). In this way, the subject has the feeling of being considered and respected rather than forced or disqualified, as the expert, to whom they applied, asks for confirmation rather than proposing judgements. "This creates a climate of collaboration between the two, bypassing any resistance and misunderstanding, and this is already a therapeutic component of the dialogue". The person feels not only accepted but put in the position of being an active part of the process of knowledge. In addition, the confirmation of the correct diagnosis by the interlocutor acts as a mechanism of self-persuasion. On the contrary, if they do not agree with the "paraphrase", this indicates that the therapist is off track and needs to adjust. Therefore, strategic paraphrasing can induce change in the interlocutor or in the investigation. The act of paraphrasing the answers to strategic questions that have highlighted failed attempts to handle the problem, directs the interlocutor's attention in this vicious circle. This concrete experience triggers the need of the person to change their attitude. By proceeding in this spiral funnel made of questions, answers, paraphrases and confirmations, gradually the interlocutor's attention moves from the problem to the mechanisms that maintain it and to what needs to be done to solve it. The third of the five steps is to "evoke sensations", that is, to induce change through what the interlocutor "feels" during the strategic dialogue. For this purpose, an evocative language is used:

> it makes no difference if one makes use of aphorisms or metaphors, anecdotes or concrete examples, a quote or a poetic narrative, an argument or a counter-argument, as long as it evokes a sensation that triggers an emotional effect that leads to the persuasive scope.

Evoking sensations should not be a mere literary exercise, but a lever to produce the desired reaction: the strategically evoked sensations should arouse "aversive" emotions towards the attitude that needs to be interrupted and "exciting" emotions towards the reaction that needs to be incremented. In addition, the formulation should be tailored in the communicative style and personal characteristics of the subject persuaded, so that the rhetoric structure selected corresponds to their usual representation systems. Essentially, the persuasive strategist should be able to select the most appropriate rhetorical expedient for the person and the situation to be changed, introduce it in the most efficient verbal and nonverbal manner and use it at the most suitable moments throughout the dialogue. Once the investigative-discovery phase is completed and new perspectives are induced, one should proceed with a conclusive recap. This fourth manoeuvre is called "recap to redefine", that is, retracing the crucial points of the entire strategic dialogue and connecting the discoveries made around the problem to what maintains it and what would have the power to solve it. However, the solution is not declared directly, but proposed as a logical consequence of the acquired knowledge:

> proposing to the patient a conclusive frame ensures that this will soundly anchor him and become the mnemonic representation of something already fulfilled, and not something that still needs to be acquired. The operative consequences that will follow will be perceived as an effect of known fact and not of a threatening unknown reality.

Through this manoeuvre, a sensation of reassuring knowledge regarding the problem and the perception of it is created, as well as what is necessary to arrive at its solution. The subject's positive expectations and their sense of control are incremented by recapping what has been said during the dialogue to redefine the terms of the problem and by recapping what has been already done to try to solve it and what still needs to be done. Also, it is important to consider the importance of the suggestive effects of the hypnotic redundancy that characterizes the whole process. The phase "recap to redefine" helps to reinforce and increment all the previously induced effects and makes them converge on change. The last phase of the strategic dialogue is "prescription as a joint discovery". At the end of the session, when all the previous phases of the strategic dialogue have been implemented, the interlocutor needs to agree on what should be done to ensure that the changes of perspective, made during the session, become operative actions in the real life of the person who asked for help. This is the phase of the therapeutic indications where what has been discovered, agreed upon and redefined during the dialogue, needs to be translated into tasks (things to do or to think): "this is the phase of the strategic dialogue that is essentially the same therapeutic style as the brief strategic therapy we were conducting ten years ago". However, there is a difference in how it is performed: there is no "separation" between investigation phase and the therapeutic injunctions; the whole sequence of dialogue flows smoothly and the interlocutor is ready to accept the indications as a natural effect of the dialogue conducted together. In this way, the communicative exchange becomes a therapeutic tool, as it acts simultaneously on the four fundamental levels of the psyche: perception, emotion, behaviour, cognition. The strategic dialogue changes the traditional approach to the first session that is commonly used for investigation and diagnosis: it becomes the concrete beginning of the therapy. Also, the role of the therapist changes. The therapist does not play the role of the expert who listens or explains, but acts to make the patient an active part of the discovery path. In doing this, the patient increases their sense of control by eliminating any resistance and orienting their perception towards alternative directions. Moreover, thanks to what happened during the dialogue, the patient is ready to accept the therapeutic indications that end the session. *[S. De Antoniis]*

REFERENCES. Nardone G., Salvini A., *The strategic dialogue*, 2007.

STRATEGIC DIRECTIVE PSYCHOTHERAPY

Mode of intervention developed in the 1960s by Haley and other collaborators of the → Mental Research Institute (MRI) of Palo Alto. It places the therapist in an active role with regard to the patient in such a way as to utilize, even in an implicit fashion, interpersonal influence and an evocative style of communication in order to achieve change. According to Haley, the therapist has to take the initiative of everything that takes place within the therapeutic context, developing a type of intervention that is focused on the problem.

This type of intervention is different in its theoretical presuppositions, in its aims and in the therapeutic style to the "non-directive" style of therapy derived from the work of Rogers (→ client-centred therapy). According to Rogers, in fact, the individual has an innate tendency towards self-fulfilment and the role of the therapist is that of stimulating the emergence of these innate capacities; this is why the sessions takes place in a less structured manner. For Haley, on the contrary, the individual lives constricted by structures and relationships of a hierarchical nature, and when he arrives in therapy he finds himself in such a state of confusion and suffering that he is not able to use his potentialities (other than in a dysfunctional manner). Therefore the principal task of the therapist, according to Haley, consists of assuming the responsibility of conducting in the first person the "game" (described by P. Watzlawick as "taking control of the ship") in order to guide the patient in the process of → change. This kind of therapy is based on phases that are more structured than they are free, where the client is asked to follow precise instructions, because, according to Erickson, the patient has to receive the order to do something and this something has to be linked to his problem. *[F. Petruccelli]*

REFERENCES. Erickson M.H., *Collected works of Milton H. Erickson*, E.L. Rossi (ed.) 2008–2015; Haley J., *Uncommon therapy*, 1973; Id. (ed.), *Conversations with Milton Erickson*, 1985.

STRATEGIC FAMILY THERAPY

Strategic family therapy is a development that stems from the strategic therapy of Milton Erickson. It includes diverse approaches but all of them have certain characteristics in common. A primary feature is that the responsibility is on the therapist to plan a → therapeutic strategy for solving clients' problems. The therapist sets clear goals that always include solving the presenting problem. The emphasis is on designing a strategy for each specific problem. Since the therapy focuses on the social context of human dilemmas, the therapist's task is to design an intervention in the client's social situation. A problem is defined as a type of behaviour (→ pattern) that is part of a sequence of acts between several people. The approach emphasizes a distinction between identifying a problem presented in therapy, and creating a problem by applying a → nosography or by characterizing an individual or a family in a certain way. Psychiatric and psychological diagnostic criteria (→ psychiatric diagnosis; → psychological diagnosis) are seldom used, and the first task of the therapist is to define a presenting problem in such a way that it can be solved. The approach is sensitive to and includes a social network wider than the → family, particularly involving professionals who have power over the person with the presenting problem. When an adolescent is hospitalized, the social unit for the therapist is not only the young person and his family but also the professionals with power over medication, hospitalization and discharge. Similarly, when someone is on probation, the power of the probation officer and the court is such that they must be included in the therapist's plans. Therapists are expected to influence teachers and school personnel, who can determine the way a child is identified and labeled. Sometimes it is necessary to make the dissension among professionals the focus of therapy. The strategic approach emphasizes the analogical language in the way it conceptualizes a problem. It is assumed that a symptom, analogically or metaphorically, expresses a problem and is also a solution, although usually an unsatisfactory one, for the people involved. The focus of therapy is often on changing analogies and metaphors. The goals of therapy are primarily to prevent the repetition of unfortunate sequences of interaction and to introduce more alternatives and complexity. The therapy is planned in steps, or stages, to achieve the goals. Every problem is defined as involving at least two and usually three people. The therapist first decides who is involved in the presenting problem and in what way. Next, the therapist decides on an intervention that will shift the family organization so that the presenting problem is no longer necessary. Usually change is planned in stages, so that a change in one situation or one set of relationships will lead to another change in another relationship and then to yet another until the whole situation changes. Interventions are planned to involve family members with one another or to disengage various family members from one another. Often the therapist first creates a new problem and solves it in such a way that the change will lead to the solution of the problem originally presented by the family. There is a concern with → hierarchy in this approach. Parents are expected to be in charge of their children, and cross-generational coalitions, such as one parent siding with a child against the other parent, are blocked. There is also a cautious concern about where the therapist is in the hierarchy, so that he or she does not inadvertently form coalitions with members low in the hierarchy against those who are higher. Interventions usually take the form of directives about something that the family members are to do, both inside and outside of the interview. These directives are designed to change the ways in which people relate to each other and to the therapist. Directives are also used to gather information by observing the way people respond to the instructions. The approach assumes that all therapy is directive and that a therapist cannot avoid being directive, since even the issues she or he chooses to comment on and his or her tone of voice are directive. In this therapy, directives are deliberately planned, and they are the main therapeutic technique. Directives may be straightforward or paradoxical, simple and involving one or two people, or complex and involving the whole family. Sometimes the therapist gives directives in metaphorical ways, without making explicit what she or he wants to happen. Since in strategic family therapy a specific therapeutic plan is designed for each problem, there are no contraindications in terms of patient selection and suitability. The approach has been used with the whole age range and all socioeconomic classes, with presenting problems of various kinds, such as psychosis, brain damage, marital problems, loneliness, fears, delinquency and psychosomatic symptoms. In each case, the therapist designs a strategy; if, after a short period of time, the strategy is not successful, a new strategy is formulated. This is not an approach where the therapist continues to do more of the same when he or she is failing. The approach allows the therapist to borrow in turn from all other models of therapy any techniques that could be useful in solving a presenting problem. As part of my contribution to strategic family therapy, I have developed a treatment method that has proven successful both in halting violence and preventing its recurrence. The most important aspect of this method is its focus on the spiritual → pain of both the victim and victimizer. Certain kinds of physical harm perpetrated by one human being on another cause emotional damage and harm the soul and inner essence of the victim and victimizer, shattering the integration of their minds, bodies and spirits. To heal the minds of victims and victimizers, we must also heal their spirits, and the only way to do this is to heal their relationships. The method consists of 15 steps that lead the perpetrator to take full responsibility, in front of the whole family, for his or her actions; to understand the spiritual pain involved; to express sorrow and repentance; and to make reparation to the victim. Another one of my contributions to the approach has been the concept of levels of emotional and spiritual development. There are five dimensions in terms of how people relate to one another and there are specific challenges associated to each dimension. *The Need to Dominate and Control.* The first dimension is the need to control the environment and our own life. This is the lowest level of spiritual development where people are mostly concerned with dominating and exerting power over others. Power is used for personal advantage and people are mainly motivated by the wish to satisfy selfish needs. Relationships are mostly exploitative. The individual's goal is to dominate for his or her own benefit. The main emotion is fear. The therapist needs to help the person to transition away from issues of fear, control and selfish desires and towards the wish to be loved.

The Need To Be Loved. The second dimension is the need to be loved. The person is mainly focused on being cared for, nurtured and loved. This level is emotionally and spiritually higher than the first, but the person is still selfishly focused on themselves. The main emotion is desire. The wish to be loved can bring out the best qualities in people, but it can also result in irrationality, selfishness and harm.

Rivalry and violence can be based on the desire to be specially favoured. When people are stuck at this level, their needs never seem to be fulfilled and there is always frustration and discomfort. The therapist needs to lead the person away from the wish to be loved and to the desire to give love and protect others. *The Need to Love and Protect Others.* At the third dimension, the need that predominates is the wish to give love and protection to others. The wish to love and protect can bring out our highest qualities of compassion, devotion, generosity and kindness. It may also elicit intrusiveness, possessiveness, domination and violence. When people get stuck at this level, the main emotion is despair. The person can become desperate from the frustration of not being able to give sufficient love and protection to his or her loved ones. The therapist needs to lead the person away from excessive desire to give love and protection and towards the need to repent and to forgive. *The Need To Repent and To Forgive.* In the fourth dimension the main issues are to be able to repent for what the person has done wrong and to forgive those that have done wrong to us. Everyone makes mistakes and, wittingly or unwittingly, hurts others. And everyone, in the course of their life, has been hurt by others. What is important is to be able to repent for the wrong that one has done and to forgive those who have harmed us. This is a high spiritual level but, when people are stuck here, there can be grief, isolation and the main emotion can be shame. The therapist needs to move the person to be able to change the focus to one where the main issue is how to contribute. *The Need to Contribute Beyond Oneself.* In the fifth dimension the main issue is to go beyond repentance and forgiveness, to set all that aside and to focus on contributing to others, to a mission, to the world. This is the highest spiritual level. It's not a trade. The therapist needs to move the person to contribute but not in order to get something. When a person is able to focus on contribution, time disappears and even one's self disappears. This is truly a state of flow and happiness. The need to contribute, however, can become excessive and the person loses track of their other needs. If this is the case and the person is focused on contributing at the cost of their health or perhaps the wellbeing of their children, the therapist needs to move the person back to the first dimension and to the need to dominate and control their own life and their own environment. The five levels are a continuum and the therapist needs to identify where the person is in these dimensions and help them to move to the next level. During the course of a person's life the dimensions are like a spiral and what is desirable is not to get stuck at any one level. *[C. Madanes]*

REFERENCES. Haley J., *Strategies of psychotherapy*, 1963; Haley J., *Advanced techniques of hypnosis and therapy: The selected papers of Milton H. Erickson*, 1967; Haley J., *Problem-solving therapy: New strategies for effective family therapy*, 1976; Herr J. and Weakland J., *Counselling elders and their families*, 1979; Madanes C., *Strategic family therapy*, 1981; Madanes C., *Behind the one-way mirror: Advances in the practice of strategic therapy*, 1984; Madanes C., *Sex, love and violence: Strategies for transformation*, 1990; Madanes C., *The secret meaning of money*, 1994; Madanes C., *The violence of men*, 1995; Madanes C., *The Therapist as humanist, social activist and systemic thinker . . . and other selected papers*, 2006; Madanes C., *Relationship breakthrough*, 2009; Montalvo B., *Aspects of live supervision*, in «Family Process», 1973, 12; Montalvo B., Haley J., *In defense of child therapy*, in «Family Process», 1973, 12; Palazzoli M.S. *et al.*, *Paradox and counterparadox*, 1978; Watzlawick P., Weakland J., Fisch R., *Change: Principles of problem formation and problem resolution*, 1974.

STRATEGIC REFRAMING TECHNIQUE

This therapeutic technique can be considered the most powerful communication strategy of → brief strategic therapy Nardone's model. Reframing is based on the constructivist assumption (→ constructivism) according to which there is not a unique true reality, but several ones that change, thanks to the point of view taken by the observer. "Reframing" means relabeling the images and the sense of reality of the patient, as if he has become, temporarily, a totally different person. Through this technique the therapist brings out several points of view about the situation and the idea of the problem explained by the patient. The therapist tries to guide the patient in a reconceptualization of his observation perspective of reality.

Through hypothetical doubts, rational explanations, → metaphors or an evocative language, the psychotherapist brings the patient to change his own → perceptive-reactive system. The therapist, by implementing a reframing, does not change what the patient reports to him, but only the meaning referred to by that content. Without denying the patient's ideas, the therapist brings him to perceive reality in a different way. Thanks to this technique, it is possible to change

> the background or the conceptual and/or emotional viewpoint in relation to which a situation is experienced and to place it in another frame which fits the facts of the same concrete situation equally well or even better, and thereby change its entire meaning.
>
> (Watzlawick, Weakland, Fisch)

Reframing can be carried out by using various communication methods: hypothetical doubts and/or surprising and provoking manoeuvers that force the patient to change his perceptive-reactive perspective. The therapist uses storytelling or metaphors including aphorisms, mottos or → particular prescriptions, that transmit specific messages and alternative points of view. The aim of this process is to encourage a behavioural, cognitive and an affective-emotional change to establish a new functional adaptation through the adoption of new meanings and values. In other words, as Watzlawick suggests, the therapist facilitates a change of the "second-order reality", which is constructed by "the attributed meanings, significance, or value that people give things" (→ first-order reality and second-order reality). It could be argued that reframing can be considered not only a therapeutic technique, but the ultimate purpose of any kind of therapeutic intervention (→ reframing as therapeutic purpose). *[A. Barsotti, G. Desideri, F. Di Nucci]*

REFERENCES. Nardone G., *Suggestione → Ristrutturazione = cambiamento*, 1991; Nardone G., Watzlawick P., *The art of change*, 1993; Watzlawick P., Weakland J.H., Fisch R., *Change: Principles of problem formation and problem resolution*, 1974.

STRATEGIC THERAPY PHASES

During the course of a strategic treatment, it refers to distinct periods that share common goals and techniques. The specific treatment model utilized by the therapist theoretically determines how many phases of therapy are defined and on which tasks the therapist will focus during each phase.

The → brief strategic therapy Nardone's model defines four phases of therapy: start of the game; unblocking the pathology; reorganization of the rules of the game and consolidation of treatment; end of the game. The addition of the consolidation phase has the advantage of preventing relapses and yielded more successful long-term outcomes than traditional strategic therapy (→ brief therapy MRI's model). The start of the game entails defining the problem, identifying the type of resistances (→ resistance to change), investigating → attempted solutions and initial therapeutic interventions. Unblocking the pathology entails redefining the first stage for the patient and changing the rigid → perceptive-reactive system, stimulating more changes and blocking the return of previous attempted solutions. Reorganization of the rules and consolidation entails measuring the changes that have occurred thus far in therapy, facilitating the acquisition of a new, more flexible perceptive-reactive system, and furthering progressive change until the goals of treatment have been met. The end of the game entails helping the patient (re)gain complete personal autonomy, focusing on the patient's strengths in overcoming the problem, closing the interventions, and following up (→ follow up) with the patient. *[C. Hybarger]*

REFERENCES. Nardone G., Portelli C., *Knowing through changing*, 2005; Nardone G., Watzlawick P., *Brief strategic therapy*, 2005.

STRATEGIC TREATMENT PROTOCOL

In → brief strategic therapy Nardone's Model, a clinical intervention model, specific to a determined type of disorder, composed of specific → strategies and techniques, organized in a progressive sequence of therapeutic stages (→ strategic therapy phases) with specific objectives to be attained. The formulation of treatment protocols represents the passage from general theory on the formation and on the resolution of problems, developed by the → Mental Research Institute (MRI) of Palo Alto (→ brief therapy MRI's model) to specific formulations relative to the functioning of the specific psychological disorders and their resolution in brief periods of time. Intervention protocols are in fact made up from a planned sequence of therapeutic procedures that are adaptable and self-correctible (→ self-correctiveness) based on the evolution of the intervention itself in such a way so that the therapeutic action presents in a systematic and rigorous manner at a structural level, but is also flexible and elastic in terms of direct application. Their development in the Centro di Terapia Strategica in Arezzo by Prof. Nardone and his team, started from their study of a particular type of disorder (obsessive-phobic disorders) and through empirical experimentation in a systematic and rigorous fashion on which interventions were producing effects and which were the redundant → attempted solutions that were being interrupted. This first → intervention-research was followed by others on other types of disorders, such as eating disorders, sexual disorders, depressive disorders and post-traumatic stress disorders. During the development of a treatment protocol, once the less-effective techniques are removed, those that have proven to be more effective in producing change are selected and new protocols are developed *ex novo*.

In the moment in which a solution "fits" the problem and produces effective results, one tries to adapt it and use it in an increasing number of cases. Only the techniques that continue to produce changes, when replicated on problems of the same type, are considered to be empirically effective. With this method, bit by bit one tries to select the techniques that are most adapted to the particular type of disorder, inserting them into a pre-established sequence, and hypothesizing possible variations, in such a way as to optimize to the maximum the → efficacy and the → efficiency of the intervention, literally "fitting" it to the problem. Gradually, through refining and adding to various manoeuvres, a first, ordered sequence of possible manoeuvres and counter-manoeuvres is identified. This strategy represents the treatment protocol of the particular disorder being studied. To be considered valid, a strategic treatment protocol has to present specific characteristics: a degree of effectiveness that is greater than 70 per cent, average effectiveness of fewer than 20 sessions, → replicability, → transferability, → predictability and the ability to correct itself. This last characteristic is a guarantee of the safeguarding of the individuality of the individual and ensures that the protocols are able to predict all possible variations. On the basis of the individual responses of the patient to the therapeutic prescriptions, in fact, the therapist always chooses the most profitable mode of action from a variety of possibilities: it is always the way in which the patient reacts that will guide the choice between the various possible options of successive manouvres. A second principle of complete self-correction completes and amplifies the first: the ability of the therapist to change strategy when that which is being applied is not working. A treatment protocol represents, therefore, a model of → problem solving that is built *ad hoc* for redundant → patterns at the level of the structure of the problem, that, however, needs to be adapted to the uniqueness of every single person and context. By virtue of its predictive power, that is, its ability to anticipate the possible evolutions of the therapeutic interaction, the protocol in this way allows for a constant and continuous self-correction of the model of intervention on the basis of the effects that are detected phase by phase. *[F. Cagnoni, R. Milanese]*

REFERENCES. Cagnoni F., Milanese R., *Cambiare il passato*, 2009; Muriana E., Pettenò L., Verbitz T., *I volti della depressione*, 2006; Nardone G., *Brief strategic solution-oriented therapy of phobic and obsessive disorders*, 1996; Id., *La dieta paradossale*, 2007; Nardone G., Rampin M., *La mente contro la natura*, 2005; Nardone G., Verbitz T., Milanese R., *Prison of food*, 2005; Nardone G., Watzlawick P., *The art of change*, 1993; Watzlawick P., Weakland J.H., Fisch R., *Change: Principles of problem formation and problem resolution*, 1974.

STRESS

More properly defined as General Adaptation Syndrome (GAS), this term was introduced by the biologist H. Selye in 1936 to define the systemic effects on the organism of defence responses induced by somatic, sensory, psychic and social stimuli, both acute and chronic. These stimuli may exceed a person's habitual adaptive and physiological resources and activate responses of "alarm", "resistance" and "defence". If prolonged, these responses may provoke a situation of breakdown resulting in psychosomatic pathologies in different organic systems (the cardiovascular system or the immune system, for instance) or emotive response disturbances (such as anxiety and depression). Situations that are perceived as threatening, especially if recurring, can cause the hyperactivation of neuro-vegetative and endocrine responses generating an organic pathology such as, for example, a hypertensive cardiomiopathy. Although the biological response to the "general adaptation syndrome" is aspecific and, consequently, independent of the nature of the stressor, the psychological response is specific, since it is a function of the meaning attributed to a stressing event. The relevance of the subjective interpretation of events has resulted in researchers attributing increasing importance to the personal, social and cultural meanings ascribed to stressors, and, consequently, to relational, situational and personal variables. For the sake of prevention and therapy, great importance is attributed to de-conditioning (→ autogenic training) and relaxation practices such as → biofeedback or different types of meditation techniques (→ meditation). Psychotherapy is often used to modify people's conditions and modalities of reaction, or to act upon → attempted solutions (such as avoidance, escape into illness or the surrender of a sense of self-efficacy), to change relational behaviour styles, or to modify adrenergic psychosomatic hyperactivation or the escape into depressive symptoms. *[A. Salvini]*

STROKE

In transactional analysis, a stroke is defined by Berne as an "unit of recognition" that meets the need to exist through being "seen", an adult form that replaces physical contact. Strokes can be verbal ("I like you") and nonverbal (for example, a smile); there are also negative strokes ("stupid"). Strokes satisfy the natural need of stimuli: it has been demonstrated that rats treated with electric shocks, despite the pain, grow better than others left without any stimulus. The most satisfying strokes are the unconditional ones, referring to what a person is, not to what they do. When people give meaning to the strokes received based on their reference system (that is, their own way of defining the world) and change their meaning and value, this action is called "stroke filter". According to transactional analysis, it is important to learn how to ask for strokes: it is not true that, if requested, they are worthless. In order that a stroke exchange can be genuine and effective, this should be managed by the Adult → Ego-state. McKenna uses a specific diagram to evaluate and balance how much a person gives, takes, asks or refuses to give in terms of strokes. It is important to stroke oneself, and recognize and communicate to others one's own positive results. *[A. Ferrara]*

REFERENCES. Berne E., *«Hello!» . . . and then what?*, 1972; McKenna J., *Stroking profile*, in «*TAJ*», 1974, 4, 4; Steiner C., *The stroke economy*, in «TAJ», 1971, 1; Stewart J., Joines V., *TA today: A new introduction to transactional analysis*, 1987.

STRUCTURAL HYPOTHESIS → TOPOGRAPHICAL MODEL OF THE MIND

STRUCTURALISM

Structuralism constitutes a general orientation of philosophical, sociological and psychological thought (and not only) that, in contrast principally with functionalism, highlights the research of a basic order (structure) that lies at the heart of the different processes involved in the different behavioural expressions of the individual and of society. "Structural" and "structure" are terms that therefore refer to all that makes up the behaviour of the individual and society. According to F. de Saussure, linguistic structuralism deals with the research into the fundamental organizational rules of the *langue*–language that is both necessary and sufficient, beyond the local diachronic and synchronic varieties of the *langue*–language, to explain the human ability of expression and communication. In short, structuralism researches what keeps a structure stable, guaranteeing the evolutionary continuity and explaining its variations without detracting from the value of the same explicative principles. In this way, in sociology, structuralism – referring significantly to the Marxian interpretation – explains the behaviour of individuals and of the masses with reference not so much to the representations and convictions, although these may be present in the local culture (intended as a superstructure), but to the general laws of economy and to the specific conditions with which the relationships of production take place.

In synthesis, according to structuralist theory, it is the social structure that explains social behaviour. In psychology, the affirmation of the structural paradigm is, above all, the work of J. Piaget. His structural interpretations can be better understood with reference to the distinction between maturation and learning (→ development stages (Jean Piaget's)). The child cannot learn if the biological and developmental premises (maturation) are not consolidated, as these make possible the manifestation of the ability and functional and cognitive competences of the child. Even the different models of psychotherapy can be subdivided between those that are structuralist and those that are functionalist in nature. *[S. Smiraglia]*

STRUCTURE

According to E. Berne the concept of structure is closely connected with that of Ego-states, which are "the primary object of transactional analysis". The → Ego-states are Parent, Adult and Child, a consistent set of thoughts, emotions and behaviour that forms the "content" of personality, the structure, in fact, from which manifest behaviour emerges, giving life to functions. The structural model is based on "memories and strategies stored in our memory". The Ego-states "are not useful ideas [. . .] they refer to phenomena" based on actual reality. The Child Ego-state is a reflection of childhood, whilst that of the Parent is the incorporation of the models transmitted from the parental figures. One is in the Adult state when the way of being and behaving responds with flexibility and congruence to the experiences that one is living in the present. *[A. Ferrara]*

REFERENCES. Berne E., *Transactional Analysis in psychotherapy*, 1961; Id., *What do you say after you say hello?*, 1972; Stewart I., Joines V., *Transactional Analysis*, 1975.

SUBJECT

In psychology and in psychotherapy, the individual understood as he who acts or who knows (in contrast with an → object, he who is on the receiving end of an act), and who possesses initiative and autonomy of action. More generally speaking, the individual who is at the centre of psychological research, of psychotherapy, of an experiment, is also denominated as being a subject. In Freudian psychoanalysis, the subject loses, at least partially, the idea of autonomy and freedom of action, in that this theory views him as being "subjected to" → desires that escape awareness and that influence free choice and responsibility. On the contrary, humanistic psychology has attempted to recuperate the notion of the subject understood as being an active and free individual, inserted into a complex system of relationships with the world, and perceived from a holistic point of view (→ holism), with a particular personal history, needs, hopes and individual motivations. The different models of psychotherapy, which possess very different languages, all converge on the idea that the individual is capable of change, if helped in the correct manner, through the acquisition of awareness, of new behavioural models, and enriched through emotional experiences and new styles of relationships with themselves, with others and with the world. *[R.]*

SUBLIMATION→ DEFENCE MECHANISMS

SUGGESTION

Communicative process that induces an individual to accept in an acritical manner that which is suggested to him; it can also include the induction of behavioural responses. Frequently, the suggestive effect is obtained by means of allusions, presuppositions, implications or other linguistic and communicative forms that elicit responses in an indirect manner, that is, by circumventing the logical-critical capacities of the recipient. The effects of suggestion can also be referred to oneself (self-suggestion); this can induce a state of bodily relaxation or induce an analgesic effect on oneself. Also well-known is the phenomenon of mass suggestion, as in the "crowd effect" of G. Le Bon, or the "Lucifer effect" studied by P. Zimbardo. A considerable part of the research in this area has concentrated on identifying the structure of messages that can induce a hypnotic effect; other researchers have focused on the variables of the personality of the individual that is receiving these messages, developing the concept of "suggestibility" to indicate the degree to which an individual is prone to being influenced.

In the context of psychotherapy one can observe very different perspectives regarding this construct. Some approaches would like to totally eliminate the presence of suggestive phenomenon, giving priority to logical-rational demonstrations as being a form of communication that is most suited towards inducing a change in the beliefs or convictions of the patient; others, deriving from a tradition of hypnosis and strategic approaches, instead make deliberate use of indirect communication with the aim of circumventing → resistance to change; yet others minimize the value of suggestion in the therapeutic process, although within their therapeutic → techniques one can actually detect a significant presence of the use of hypnotic suggestion. *[R.]*

SUPERCONSCIOUS

In psychosynthesis, it is the most evolved level of the unconscious, the source of intuitions, creative inspiration, ethical imperatives, impulses towards altruistic actions, states of ecstasy and illumination. Various techniques of psychosynthesis, – amongst which one can find → meditation, internal dialogue, visualization, the ideal model – can facilitate the access to the superconscious. However, frequently, a separation from the superconscious is achieved by resorting to the → defence mechanisms described by psychoanalysis. There are various factors that can induce the use of defence mechanisms: the fear of the unknown; as an escape from responsibility; unease towards that which is perceived as not being compatible with the structure of one's personality; the fear of the intensity and the power of the transpersonal world; the fear of psychological disintegration. Usually, the influx of energy and the contents of the superconscious are experienced as being a positive and gratifying experience – that which Maslow describes as being the "peak experience", and therefore highly significant within the context of psychotherapy. In the case of a psychological organization that is weaker, however, inflation, disorientation, hyperstimulation can take place. In general, however, the experiencing of the superconscious is felt as being regenerative, illuminating and, at times, as providing resolution. *[P. Ferrucci]*

REFERENCES. Assagioli R., *Psychosynthesis, a manual of principles and techniques*, 1965; Maslow A., *Toward a psychology of being*, 1962.

SUPEREGO

This term belongs to the lexicon of Freud's second topography (→ topographical model of the mind). It was introduced in *The Id and the Ego* in 1922. In this work, both the → Ego and the Superego are formations that, genetically speaking, derive from the → Id and are differentiations of the Id. However, elements that fall under the scope of the Superego's activities were already present in the first topography. Indeed, the Superego is an agency that exercises what, in the first topography, was referred to as ethical conscience, self-preservation and the Ego ideal. The new development in the second topography was to bring these activities together in the psyche with distinct and autonomous characteristics compared to the other two agencies (the Ego and the Id). The statement that the Superego evolves out of the Ego is not sufficient to fully explain how it is generated. It is necessary to introduce the activity of the triangular oedipal relationship (→ Oedipus complex), triggering a twofold identification with the father and with the mother that is expressed through the fundamental prohibition that, in the ultimate analysis, explains the genesis of the Superego from the Id, that is to say, out of the field of instinctual cathexes. In effect, the outcome of these two identifications in the sexual phase of the oedipal complex consists of the formation or alteration within the Ego of an agency that stands in opposition to the Ego, and which is known as the Superego. In this sense, the Superego is a remnant of the Ego's earliest object choices (cathexes) and therefore, like the Ego, part of it is unconscious. The Superego refers essentially to the Ego, towards which it takes a dual stance. On the one hand, it admonishes: "It is thus (like the father) that you must be", while on the other it admonishes: "You are not permitted to be thus (like your father)"; in other words, "You cannot enjoy all of his prerogatives". The two faces of the

Superego may be explained by the fact that, in the oedipal complex, the father positions himself at the same time as an ideal and as the agent of → castration, that is to say, as the barrier to incestuous sexual fulfilment. Through the intervention of repression (→ defence mechanisms), the infant Ego strengthens itself by erecting the very same barrier within itself. In consequence, the Superego is destined to retain the father's features; the stronger the repression of oedipal impulses, the more strictly the Superego will exercise its rule over the Ego. During the course of psychotherapeutic treatment, the analyst often occupies the Superego's position, as it is from this position that mutative interpretations may occur. *[P. Valerio, M. Bottone, R. Vitelli]*

REFERENCES. Freud S., *On narcissism: An introduction*, 1914; Id. (1922), *The Ego and the Id*, in *The Standard Edition*, XIX, 1953–1974.

SUPERIOR QUALITIES DEVELOPMENT

In psychosynthesis, superior qualities are psychic qualities that are potentially real or that are already partially actualized, such as love, joy, beauty, health, peace, energy, patience and many others. They have a vital existence and importance and they cannot be explained as simply being → defence mechanisms or derivations of other levels of the unconscious. Superior qualities can become an essential point of reference in psychotherapy and the subject of → meditation and visualization. They can be cultivated and developed, giving them attention and value. In this way they become an alternative focal point to the pre-existing neurotic nucleus. In this way they gradually substitute the pre-existing disorder, becoming a source of new emotions and new ways of thinking; they give life to the whole personality. *[P. Ferrucci]*

REFERENCES. Ferrucci P., *La forza della gentilezza*, 2005.

SUPPORT

Activity related to the emotional, cognitive and existential aid that characterizes every type of psychological and psychotherapeutic intervention, aimed at the prevention of suffering, at the promotion of wellbeing and at the rehabilitative and enabling intervention in the psychological field. Support can be directed towards a person, a group and a community. The clinical interview, the → communication and the → relationship represent the main channels through which the helping and supportive relationship is expressed; through the utilization of methods and instruments of knowledge that refer to clinical psychology and psychotherapy (for example, → empathy, understanding, analytical ability, critical analysis, principles of health psychology, psychopathology, etc.), the psychologist is able to establish a relationship that has the ability to activate the resources of the individual (or a group) aimed at helping the individual or group overcome, improve or manage better the presenting problem. Therapeutic support touches upon all the areas of functioning of the individual, (perception, emotion, cognition, relational capacity), without necessarily constituting a psychotherapeutic intervention. In fact, the increase in and improvement of the individual's personal abilities, and the development of autonomy, represent the principal objectives of a supportive intervention. As a result of the fact that it constitutes a fundamental element of the psychological and/or psychotherapeutic helping relationship, the supportive intervention is legally recognized as being a prerogative of the profession of the psychologist. This term is also used with a specific meaning in the field of Gestalt psychotherapy. *[R.]*

SUPPRESSION → DEFENCE MECHANISMS

SURPLUS ENJOYMENT

In the field of Lacanian psychoanalysis, this term is defined in conjunction with the notions of "phallic jouissance" and "Other jouissance". For Lacan, these terms outline the three characteristic stages of enjoyment. The phallic jouissance is the energy dissipated with a partial discharge (such as sexual pleasure derived from the masculine organ, in an essentially solitary sense), and for "phallic functioning" he refers to any part of the body that renders possible, or impossible, the access to external pleasures. The jouissance corresponds to pleasure withheld, which the phallus prevents from going out; the word "plus" or "surplus" indicates that the part of the energy that is not discharged is a surplus that constantly increases internal tension; this remains anchored to the erogenous zones from where it stimulates a permanent state of erogeny and from which develops the push of desire. Finally, Other jouissance, a state that is fundamentally hypothetical, corresponds to the ideal situation of absolute pleasure of the female narcissistic desire of love. *[F. Quesito]*

REFERENCES. Lacan J. (1972–1973), *The seminar of Jacques Lacan: Encore*, XX, 1975.

SYMBIOSIS

In the field of transactional analysis, according to Schiff, "symbiosis occurs when two individuals behave as if they formed one person". It is a natural phenomenon from conception until children gain a certain autonomy, but it becomes pathological when it is the result of passiveness or of an unresolved dependence. Schiff describes it in terms of → Ego-states. Basically, in a relationship one individual puts in their own Ego-states Parent and Adult, whilst the other puts in the Child. According to Berne, symbiosis does not permit autonomy; that, in the transactional analysis model, is based on having the capacity to be spontaneous, aware and intimate. The experiences of symbiosis at a mature age sustain the life → script and represent attempts to fulfil needs that have not been satisfied during childhood. In symbiosis of second order, the natural roles are inverted: for example, a child takes the role of a parent towards their own real parent. Symbiosis manifests itself through passive behaviour: doing nothing, over-adaptation, agitation, incapacitation, or rather a paralyzing refusal to think or take responsibility and, finally, violence. *[A. Ferrara]*

REFERENCES. Berne E., *Games people play*, 1964; Schiff J.L., *Transactional Analysis treatment of psychosis*, 1975.

SYMBOL

According to Freud, a symbol is an indirect representation based on analogic connections that can vary widely in nature. In his reflections, however, it assumes specific and binding demarcations; the most significant of them is the unconscious quality of what is symbolized. Connected to the discovery of the → unconscious, the symbols studied by Freud are produced as an effect of repression (→ defence mechanisms) and operate in the subsequent conflict between the tendency to repress and the repressed psychic content. For these reasons, symbols can be found in dreams and in psychopathological symptoms. Even if they are part of the constellation of experiences of every single individual, they find their universal foundation in the shared general interests of human beings, as well as in the basic modes of functioning of the psyche. For this reason, symbols meant in this way, can be also found in → myths, in → folklore, in literature, in religions; this also explains the frequency of the "typical dreams", which are independent of the particular characteristics of the dreamer and of the associative material. As a result of the unconscious connotation of symbols, in the Freudian conception, the relationship between the symbolized and the symbolizer always moves in a centrifugal direction, from the inside of the psychic organization towards the external world. When one keeps in mind that symbolic content comes from a universal matrix and is organized according to modes of psychic functioning that are equally universal, one can understand the innate inequality between the relative availability of symbolizers and the restricted number of the symbolized, which are reducible to the body with its elementary needs and the associated physiological functions, sexuality, generativity, life and death. *[G. De Renzis]*

▷ Jung strongly affirms the distinction between sign and symbol, and this fact highlights the difference in his point of view from that of Freud.

> A conception that defines the symbolic expression as being the best possible, and therefore as the formulation that is most clear and characteristic that one can enunciate at present, of something that is relatively unknown, is symbolic [. . .]. An expression that is proposed for something well known still remains a mere sign and will never constitute a symbol.

The symbol embodies an excess of meaning, which refers to an "ulterior" meaning that is not predictable and not necessarily finite. Something is no longer "either this or that", but this and that and even something else. Following the rules of formal logic, this excessiveness is equivalent to uncertainty, in virtue of the fact that the Jungian symbol can never be decoded in a definitive manner:

> A word or an image is symbolic when it implies something that is beyond its obvious and immediate meaning. It possesses a wider aspect, "unconscious", that is never defined with precision or completely explained [. . .]. When the mind explores the symbol it is brought into contact with the ideas that are beyond rational capacities.

If the symbol exhausts its meaning and becomes a "dead symbol", it loses that predictive function that the "live" symbol possesses, which, by indicating what we do not know, opens the door to becoming. The transcendental function of the symbol can restart the blocked psychic dynamic present in neurotic conflicts. From this, the importance of the symbolic attitude in therapy is derived. *[A. Benvenuti]*

REFERENCES. Freud S. (1900–1901), *The interpretation of dreams*, in *The Standard Edition*, IV–V, 1953–1974; Jones E., *The theory of symbolism*, 1916; Jung C.G. (1921), *Psychological types*, in *Collected Works*, VI, 1971; Id., *Man and his symbols*, 1964.

SYMBOLIC

Relative to the meaning of things, images, ideas, gestures, the content of which refers to something that goes beyond their purely exterior form, but that maintains its analogous relationship with it. The symbolic quality is that which allows the establishment of relationships between concepts that cannot be reduced to formal and abstract rules of logic, or that can render intelligible to the human being what would otherwise escape his simple formal reasoning.

In psychoanalysis, dreams, lapsus, → symptoms, are "symbolic" in that they are a manifest expression of a latent content that lies at an unconscious level. For S. Freud, the activity of the unconscious operates through the "symbolic thought" that makes it possible to carry out operations of displacement, condensation and substitution (→ defence mechanisms of), in that the energy of the psyche flows from one representation to another according to the → pleasure principle. From a different point of view, Piaget (→ development stages (J. Piaget's)) talks about the "symbolic thought", with reference to the capacity of the child, from the age of 18 months onwards, to build representations that will allow him to mentally configure objects that are not present in the immediate environment; in parallel, "symbolic play" will develop, characterized by the capacity of the child to "pretend", or rather to utilize elements of reality to represent things that are present in his fantasy (for example, the child that puts a bottle near his ear pretending that it is a telephone).

In all cases, one can define as being symbolic any human expression, or process in which a "representation" is used in order to connect concepts and meanings. The → symbolic interactionism in W. James and E. Goffman deals with the development of models for the study and utilization of symbolic interactions between human beings. This approach represents the foundation of some of the modern forms of psychotherapy. *[R.]*

SYMBOLIC-EXPERIENTIAL FAMILY THERAPY (WHITAKER'S)

Whitaker's symbolic-experiential approach is the evolution of the earlier formulation of an "experiential non-rational psychotherapy", a → model developed by Whitaker in collaboration with Malone. In those years, psychotherapy was being recognized as an autonomous discipline and psychotherapists were required to clarify the nature, the fundaments and the roots of their enterprise in order to legitimize the discipline and its validity. Symbolic-experiential therapy is an approach based on experience, which, throughout the therapeutic process, is oriented towards the expression and integration of the patient's – be it an individual, a couple or a → family – feelings and experiences. Whitaker assigns a particular value to the expression of the patient's and the therapist's subjective, implicit and explicit, feelings, fantasies and thoughts; the therapy is the space for the expression of the drive and imaginative world. In his definition of the therapeutic process, Whitaker emphasizes the → here-and-now, the present. In the symbolic-experiential therapy the → interpretation, the → insight, the analytical methods for the exploration of the patient's past, are seen as collusive modes that are used in order to avoid anxiety, to reduce the emotional "temperature" of the therapeutic encounter, to protect himself from the possibility that something significant happens, to obstruct the therapeutic process, and thus to limit both the patient's and the therapist's growth and emotional integration in the present; as Whitaker underlines,

> the present is time's most delicate part, the one that is usually avoided, [. . .] sharing the same memory is a performance, it is not an experience. Sharing memories is not a way of communicating our inner self, but only a strategy to avoid to be what we are, while at the same time talking about who and when we used to be, about things we already know.

THE THERAPIST'S ROLE. "The dynamics of psychotherapy lies in the person of the therapist": this is what Betz and Whitehorn used to say. By locating the therapeutic relationship and its interpersonal dynamic at the centre of the therapeutic process, Whitaker is undoubtedly the family therapist who has focused on the therapist's person the most. As Loriedo has underlined in his introduction to *Midnight Musings of a Family Therapist*, Whitaker's position is close to that of some psychoanalysts who worked on schizophrenia, such as H.F. Searle and H. Racker. The first has emphasized the importance of the therapist's willingness to go through his own insanity and embrace the patient's sickness. The latter underlined the need of co-transfer within the general economy of a therapeutic relationship. Therapy is grounded on persons and relations, not on technical interventions and theoretical abstractions; theories and techniques "come to life only when are filtered through the therapist's person". Whitaker underlines vigorously that the therapist must not assume the patient's responsibilities and has to avoid helping and supporting the patient. When the therapist takes the place of the patient, trying to help him find a way out of his problems, the therapist "prevents the pearl taking form"; it weaken the patient's resources, his abilities, his power; in so-doing, the therapist makes the patient inept, powerless and dependent. On the contrary, if the therapist endures the anxiety, the conflict, the tension of the real encounter, if he tolerates the increase of emotional temperature, if he does not take refuge in a hidden repertory of techniques and theories, he can assume his own responsibilities, and avoid making his self-confidence depend on the patient's approval; only in this way will it, perhaps, be possible to offer authentic support and help to patients in their attempt to become real persons:

> as a matter of fact, the all business of helping them is frightening. It is humiliating, because it is like saying that our way of living is better than theirs [. . .] I'm mindful of any patients' attempt to delegate the responsibility for their life. It is their game, not mine. My responsibility lies in making them accept their own responsibility for the life they live.

If the therapist accepts the responsibility for his own feelings and allows himself to be a real person, he gives the patient the permission and the right to be equally real, thus to be fearless of his own fantasies, his own unacceptable feelings such as jealousy, rage, envy, etc. If the therapist allows himself to be hostile, annoyed, depressed or weak, the patient is given the possibility to accept himself, his own way of being.

THE STRUCTURE OF THE THERAPEUTIC PROCESS. The different stages of Whitaker's therapy can be schematized into three phases: the initial, the central and the final one. The evaluation is a fundamental part of this therapeutic approach; it begins with the first phone call and continues in the first live meeting. There are two elements that guide the evaluation: on the one hand, the therapist's attempt to access the family and to create a relationship based on → empathy aimed at identifying the elements of distress that can drive the patient to change; and, on the other hand, what in Whitaker's terms can be defined the "stimulation of the labour pains". The latter of these two elements has different forms and can be conducted in multiple ways, such as "the battle for structure" and the "battle for initiative". The battle for structure is basically the process that defines the rules of the therapy → setting and its beginning is marked by the therapist's request to make the whole family participate in the therapy. In order to strengthen his credibility towards the family, the therapist must win this battle. By playing the role of the "symbolic parent" or "adoptive-temporary parent", the therapist makes clear that he belongs to a different generation – that is, he assumes a hierarchically different responsibility in the relationship – and that the therapy occupies "a different level than that of the family's everyday life". The therapy is not an *inter pares* dialogue; a meta-position has to be created in order to generate a common space, an "us-position", that can include the therapist without simultaneously making the therapy get enmeshed in the internal dynamics of the family. This is the actual meaning of the battle for structure, which has often been misunderstood and interpreted as a technique of power. Once the structure of the therapy is set, the initial phase can continue through the battle for initiative, that is, the definition of the "self position" within the family. In this phase, the family must take the initiative and has to define the direction that the therapy has to take; "the ball is in their hands and even if I'm their coach, I can't take the ball and throw it into their life and into their efforts to make that life better". According to Whitaker, in the initial phase of the therapy it is important that the therapist keeps, in relation to the family, the position of a foreigner or a guest; at this point of the relationship, too much benevolence or fake cordiality would, in fact, risk leaving a legacy of mistrust and suspicion to the rest of the therapy. Furthermore, for Whitaker, co-therapy is the ideal methodology to apply: "the presence of another therapist makes each therapist free to act as a real person, and not as a mere symbol". A co-therapy is not just the sum of two therapists; it is instead an articulate structure in which the relationship between the two therapists becomes in itself a constitutive part of the therapy, to the point that Whitaker names it "the third therapist". It is then particularly important for the therapists to become able to offer, through the example of their reciprocal interaction, alternative models of relationship. The correct achievement of the battle for structure and the battle for initiative generates the → therapeutic alliance; to keep this alliance alive, rather than to consider the family as a simple sum of autonomous parts, the therapist has to look at it as a multifaceted organism in which multiple interconnections take place: "out of my experience, I know that the family members feel my interest in them as a unity". The therapist needs to be sure to be able to move in and out of the emotions of the family, without being included or expulsed by the family members. Once the rules for the therapeutic relationship and the initial level of reciprocal involvement between the family and the therapist are set, the central phase of the psychotherapy begins. It focuses on how to deepen the therapeutic meaning of the relationship and on how to achieve the → change. Whitaker invites therapists to be aware of two frequent risks that characterize this phase: the danger of being absorbed by the family (like a parent that becomes a whole with their sons) and the danger of becoming the opposite, that is, a distant and indifferent figure (like a parent who is never free to be childish and play with their sons). Once these risks have been avoided, the therapist has to get closer to the family in order to activate the sense of self-protection of the family. To be efficient, the therapy needs the relationship to be profoundly significant, both for the family and for the therapist; thus, all sorts of emotions belonging to the therapeutic relationship have to be stimulated; for example by demonstrating how inadequate traditional models of relationship are compared to the relationship between the therapist and the family, or by using sudden strategies of emotional provocation and modification. It is equally important to establish a relationship that goes beyond symptomatic behaviours. For instance, the therapist can expose his own fantasies in order to get around the tendency of the family to create a relationship only focused on the → designed patient's symptoms. The therapist suggests his own fantasies without interpreting them, so as to push the patient and the family to acknowledge the existence of a number of factors beyond the symptoms and to accept engaging in a personal relationship with the therapist. The final phase and the separation begin when the change becomes visible and begins to consolidate, when it is possible to see the first signals of a renewed autonomy of the family from the therapist and the predominance of a certain degree of flexibility. The roles within the family are no longer rigid and stereotypic, subgroups become mobile, triangulations become elastic enough to be painless; at this point, the flexibility of the family makes the therapist feel at ease and gives it the possibility of moving comfortably: "therapists, like the parents of an adolescent that is about to become an adult, feel marginalized". At this point, if the therapist does not feel more involved than is useful, and if he does not need to defend himself from the difficulties of the therapy, a delicate balance can emerge and the final phase becomes a natural development. The separation begins when the family starts to reject the therapist's values and models in order to create its own, when it starts to see the therapist as a person rather than a role, when family members become "their own therapists", the only ones responsible for their lives. Often, this is a difficult moment for the therapist, who can find in the co-therapist the needed support to overcome his bond with the family and face the "empty nest". Later, the family itself will support the therapist: to speak about one's own difficulties and emotions connected to the separation between the family and the therapist can be very useful in these situations.

> I feel a sense of loss, similar to the one parents feel when their sons leave to go to college. However, I bless them and they are free to come back whenever they want. But they never leave empty-handed; the impact of the therapeutic experience that we had together is now woven into the weft of their life.

[C. Loriedo, M. Jedlowski]

REFERENCES. Betz B., Whitehorn J.C., *Effective psychotherapy with the schizophrenic patient*, 1975; Whitaker C.A., *Il gioco e l'assurdo. La terapia esperienziale della famiglia*, 1984; Id., *Midnight musings of a family therapist*, 1989; Whitaker C.A., Bumberry W., *Dancing with the family. A symbolic-experiential approach*, 1988; Whitaker C.A., Malone T.P., *The roots of psychotherapy*, 1953.

SYMBOLIC INTERACTIONISM

A theory introduced in the United States in the early twentieth century in continuity with the pragmatist philosophy of W. James and Ch. S. Pierce. This theory was systematized in the 1930s and then expanded in the 1960s and it can be summarized in three assumptions. The first is the focus on the subjective sphere, that is, on the meanings given by individuals to the world in which they live. The second is the interest in the negotiating character of social life, that is, in the social and symbolic interaction processes by which individuals construct these meanings. Social interaction emphasizes the role of cooperative exchanges among individuals belonging to a common social group. This kind of group is understood as a set of collectively regulated relationships, which transform subjective experiences in organized activities. Instead, symbolic interaction emphasizes the processes which, through and beyond → language, become manifest in shared meanings (norms, values, institutions). Symbolic interaction underlies mutual expectations of behaviour, which represent the "social role" and the ability to summon up others' point of view – to assume the role and therefore orient one's own actions – through which the "mind" emerges . → Identity is constructed by the dialogue between the organization of other people's internalized attitudes, which represents the socialized aspect of behaviour (Me), and the response of the individual to such attitudes (I). The perennial exchange between these two elements generates the Self. Finally, the third assumption of symbolic interactionism is the active role of individuals in both the interpretive process through which they construct reality and in the process responsible for the emergence of the Self. In psychotherapy, some approaches refer directly to symbolic interactionism as theoretical foundation. *[R.]*

SYMBOLIZATION

According to → social cognitive theory, the capacity to internally represent one's own experiences through the use of → symbols, mainly verbal but also iconic, and to attribute a meaning to them. It represents the overcoming of trial-and-error learning, where a person has to make a mistake and suffer the negative consequences in order to learn to not make the same mistake again. The ability to symbolize allows us to test possible solutions through mental operations before acting. As in many other aspects of social cognitive theory, symbolization also highlights the active role that man has in changing his life and the environment around him. *[F. Celi]*

REFERENCES. Bandura A., *Social learning theory*, 1977; Id., *Self-efficacy in changing societies*, 1995.

SYMMETRY → COMPLEMENTARITY

SYMPTOM

State of malaise or a change in a person, related to particular physical reactions, emotions, thoughts, behaviours and relationships. In psychotherapy, the seriousness of the symptom depends on the measure to which it conditions and limits the potential of a person, and his level of autonomy and adaptation to the surrounding environment. The symptom experienced by the person can be "Ego-dystonic", and therefore incompatible with the perception that the individual has of himself and of his own → wellbeing, or else "Ego-syntonic", in other words in concordance with these perceptions. When the symptom is "Ego-syntonic", the person tends to refuse treatment, in that he is not aware of having a disorder (for example, people affected by psychotic disorders or personality disorders), or else, although he is aware of this, still believes that the symptom meets his needs in other aspects that for him are more important, (for example, the anorexic patient or the bully).

For the approaches of the psychodynamic paradigm, the symptom represents the superficial expression of a deep emotional conflict that one needs to uncover. For those who work within a behavioural paradigm, it is the same as the pathology to be cured, whilst for those that work from a systemic-relational paradigm, it is the manifestation of the disequilibrium in the family relationship. This is an example of how the different perspectives in psychotherapy have formulated different definitions of the construct of the symptom and of the strategies for its treatment. *[R.]*

SYMPTOM PRESCRIPTION

In brief strategic therapies MRI and Nardone's model, it refers to the classic paradoxical intervention (→ logic of paradox) that commands a person to continue a problematic behaviour, thought or emotion in order to bring the problem to its own resolution. The power of this interventions lies in its ability to decrease resistance (→ resistance to change) and create an opportunity for the individual to establish a different balance. By telling an individual to continue something considered problematic, a → double bind is established. This will take individuals to a change, both when they follow the directive and when they decide to avoid following it. This intervention is often prescribed when, after an accurate analysis of the problem, resolving it by adopting more conventional means is considered to be difficult. For example, if a child is misbehaving, then the child is told to continue the behaviour and even encouraged to perform it better. When facing this prescription, a child has two alternatives: deciding to comply with the directive or stopping the behaviour entirely. If the child obeys, and therefore he/she continues to misbehave, their "misbehaving" becomes an act of obedience and not of rebellion. If the child rebels and disobeys the directive, then the misbehaviour stops. In both cases, the rebellion is nullified by virtue of the fact that it was prescribed. The symptom prescription is one of the most significant examples of the use of the → "be spontaneous" paradox in psychotherapy. It represents the logical mechanism on which many of the prescriptions of the → brief strategic therapy Nardone's model are based, as for example the → worst fantasy technique and the → hypochondriac check-up technique. *[E. C. Frank]*

REFERENCES. Nardone G., Watzlawick P., *The art of change*, 1993; Watzlawick P., *The language of change*, 1978; Watzlawick P., Weakland J.H., Fisch R, *Change. Principles of problem formation and problem resolution*, 1974.

SYNCHRONICITY

According to Jung, the taking place of events that present a correlation between physical events and psychological states or conditions that, in some cases, are not considered as being a simple coincidence. The concept of synchronicity expresses the correlation between internal states (psychological) and external events (physical) on the three levels of time, space and meaning. The conception of the → libido according to Jungian theory (free and lacking in a fixed reference) allows in fact the establishment of points of connection between the two phenomena, bringing into question the unlimited and unconditional application of the principle of causality as being the only valid criterion of knowledge. Jung's intention was to give importance and visibility to a range of phenomenon that are frequently neglected in that they are considered as "irrational" and at the same time to credit forms of acquisition of knowledge that are different to those of science, based on the principle of finality, aside from that of causality. Synchronicity can be defined as the expression of a "meaningful coincidence", the expression of an event that cannot be explained within a causal relationship and is therefore removed from the chain of scientific knowledge and defined as being irrational. The result obtained by Jung by means of the application of the concept of synchronicity is not the denial or discrediting of scientific knowledge, but of its limitation with respect to a range of phenomena that are usually excluded from the process of scientific knowledge. In the clinical field emphasis is placed on the possibility of an order of knowledge that is different to the rationalist one and, therefore, on the possibility of comprehension of psychopathological phenomenon that are otherwise inaccessible, in that they are considered as "irrational". *[A. Iapoce]*

REFERENCES. Jung C.G. (1951), *Synchronicity: An acausal connecting principle*, in *Collected Works*, VIII, 1982–1993; Id. (1951), *On synchronicity*, in *Collected Works*, VIII, 1982–1993.

SYNDROME

In the biomedical field, a grouping of signs, of unknown origin, that present themselves in association and are connected to one another through physiopathological connections; their → aetiology is therefore unknown (this being substantially different with respect to the definition of disease, which is characterized instead by the empirical knowledge of the organic factors that are its cause). Referring to signs and physiopathological connections, this concept, as, moreover, is the practice in the medical field in general, implicates the necessity of an empirical referent (specifically, the human body) and of diagnostic techniques that are reliable and valid with respect to it. In psychology, in particular the DSM (→ diagnostic manuals), employing a medical model, the term is adopted to describe all the so-called mental disorders, in that they are behaviours that are dysfunctional with respect to the environment in which they are acted out; they are not attributable, however, to causes that are empirically identifiable and connected in a deterministic manner to the effect. Additionally, the criteria according to which such behaviours, defined as being symptomatic, are recognized as being co-morbid are not based on physiopathological connections, but by virtue of their frequent co-presence (a stochastic criterion).

Therefore, if in the medical model the word syndrome is defined according to the theoretical-epistemological presuppositions of the disciplines that medicine draws upon as an operational procedure, in psychology it takes on a different meaning in the face of the incompatibility of these assumptions with respect to an object of knowledge that is not empirically identifiable. *[R.]*

SYNTHETIC PHASE

In psychosynthesis, analysis is only the first part of therapy and should be followed by a synthetic phase, consisting in overcoming conflict and tears and in facilitating the cohesion of the various psychic components into a harmonious whole. The goal is the inclusion of each element, even if apparently different or discordant. The whole is greater than the sum of its parts: the synthesis produces a new reality. In this way, a sense that didn't exist before emerges, as when letters combine to form a word, or words to form a discourse. There is a real qualitative leap. The synthetic phase often happens spontaneously around a unifying centre: a new interest, a project, an ideal, which can become the organizing principle of the psyche. *[P. Ferrucci]*

REFERENCES. Assagioli R., *Psychosynthesis: A manual of principles and techniques*, 1965.

SYSTEM

In the systemic-relational field, theoretical construct that includes numerous other concepts such as, amongst others, complexity, organization, order and dynamic equilibrium. A system can be thought of as a totality of elements whose interdependence confers on the totality itself properties for which the whole is greater than the sum of its individual parts. For this reason, the system evidences its own particular characteristics that are defined as emerging. The → systems theory, developed in particular by L. von. Bertalanffy in the 1950s, constitutes an area of interdisciplinary research that ranges from physics to biology, from ecology to → cybernetics and psychotherapy. Examples of systems can be identified in a complex organism such as the human body, rather than in the environment of the Amazon forest, or even a → family within which difficulties are manifested that require psychotherapeutic intervention. Therefore, in family therapy the attention of the therapist is directed not so much, and not only, towards the person that is the bearer of the pathology as much as it is directed towards the relationships between the members of the family that constitute the pathological humus that finds expression in the → designated patient. Systems can participate – acting as sub-systems – in systems that are even more complex and reflect internally the effects deriving from such an inclusion; in this sense, systems are conceived as being open, in other words as being permeable and dynamically sensitive to the variations in the overall equilibrium. For example, a family system can reveal difficulties that in turn derive from the social and cultural context to which they belong, understood as being a macro-system. *[S. Smiraglia]*

Systemic–relational paradigm → Please refer to the opening chapter, "The eight paradigms and their respective theoretical-applicative models".

SYSTEMATIC DESENSITIZATION

It is one of the most well-known and effective techniques of behavioural psychotherapy; it was proposed by Wolpe for the treatment of simple phobias. It targets the → extinction of conditioned anxiety through the process of → counter-conditioning, that is, purposely creating an association between anxiety-related stimuli and a relaxation → response. The patient is first trained in deep muscle relaxation; then, he/she is asked to develop a hierarchy of anxiety-related stimuli (15 to 20 items); finally, he/she is asked to relax himself/herself, and is exposed to the lowest item on the hierarchy (→ graded exposure), over and over again. When the exposure is no longer a cause of anxiety, maintaining a relaxed condition, the therapist moves to the next step, and repeats the process until the entire hierarchy has been completed. The patient is usually exposed through imagination (→ imaginal exposure), but sometimes also in vivo (→ in-vivo exposure). *[G. Melli]*

REFERENCES. Jacobson E., *Progressive relaxation*, 1938; Wolpe J., *Psychotherapy by reciprocal inhibition*, 1958.

SYSTEMS THEORY

A system is an organized composition of elements. Systems theory, together with → cybernetics, deals with the structural functions and rules of all systems, independently of their material composition. In a way that is parallel to cybernetic theory, systems theory asserts that every system has three characteristics. The totality: the members of a system are in a reciprocal relationship between themselves, in such a way that a change in the behaviour of one of its members causes a change in the behaviour of the other members; from this one can conclude that a system can only be understood if it is considered in a global manner, as a totality of interdependent elements; observing the individual parts or the individual members is not enough (non-sommativity) in order to understand it, in that their organized connection gives the system an "emergent quality" (→ field theory). Equifinality: in "open" systems (in interaction, therefore, with other systems, whereas a "closed" system is a system that does not interact with the external environment), the parameters and the processes internal to the system constitute the explanation of the effects on the system itself; according to this principle, the functioning of an open system is explained by the interaction between its components and not by the initial conditions that would have generated it. The retroaction (→ feedback): the behaviour of a member of the system is at the same time cause and effect of the behaviour of the other members.

Systems theory has been used in order to develop theoretical models of psychotherapeutic work with families (→ family therapy). In a manner that is opposite to theories of intrapsychic → determinism, this theoretical perspective does not consider the behaviour of the individual as being the effect of processes that are purely interior, in that the behaviour of the members of the family-system have to be understood by analyzing the processes of communication that take place between the components of the same system. *[R.]*

SYZYGY

In the Jungian model, dynamic between elements of the psyche of opposing signs. The psyche has a polar structure (→ psychic polarities), that is, it is made up of, and animated by, the conflict between opposing elements (representations, feelings, etc.). The analytic process consists of the work, carried out by the → Ego, of recognizing the unconscious elements, opposite to one's own, without renouncing the latter, and therefore oneself: the Ego therefore finds itself in a state of suspension ("crucifixion") that tends to aim towards achieving psychic wholeness (that is, towards the extension of awareness), at the expense of perfection (absence of contradiction). The agnostic syzygy (union between a god and a goddess) expresses the fact that masculine elements are always accompanied by their corresponding female elements: in general, an opposite is never separated from the other, its antithesis. It therefore symbolizes a tendency towards wholeness, a wholeness in becoming, since the opposites in the psyche will never arrive at a total synthesis, but will remain in a state of tension that is the essence of the dynamism of the psyche. Between the gods of the syzygy there is a union, but not unity: in this way the psyche is always on the road to totality, but the mythical fusion is never achieved. The totality therefore has a position or a value that is superior to the syzygy: this is the two halves of the whole, the tension between opposites from which unity descends. Between many couples of opposites, a particular aspect is that of the "double", where the Ego opposes itself, but that between masculine and feminine is one of the most important in analytic practice and in relationships. *[G.M. Vadala, A. Benvenuti]*

REFERENCES. Jung C.G. (1936), *Archetypes and the collective unconscious*, in *Collected Works*, IX (part I), 1969.

T

TABOO

The word taboo has entered nowadays into our common language, but it originally comes from the Polynesian term *tapù* which indicated "what is sacred, prohibited, separate, or impure". A "forbidden" object can be considered as a taboo, as well as an "untouchable" person, an "unapproachable" place or an act viewed as literally "unthinkable". In the field of psychology, Wundt (1912) was the first to observe that taboos are the oldest legislative code of humankind; however, the restrictions derived from them are different from those derived from our religious or moral codes, since taboos are not justified by the authority of any god or a legal system but are self-evident and appear "obvious" to all of those who share a specific culture. On the relevance of taboos in the history of psychoanalysis, please refer to Freud for incest (→ incest taboo) and one's ambivalence towards it, and to Ferenczi and Suttie with regard to "tenderness". About the broader significance of the term taboo, refer to the many studies that have dealt for many years with "the secret" in psychosis and in the transgenerational transmission of family history. *[F. Borgogno, G. Cassullo, A. Bella]*

REFERENCES. Ferenczi S. (1932), *Confusion of tongues between adults and the child*, in Id., *Final contribution to the problems and methods of psychoanalysis*, 1955; Freud S. (1913–1914), *Totem and taboo: Some points of agreement between the mental lives of savages and neurotics*, in *The Standard Edition*, Volume XIII; Suttie I.D., *The origins of love and hate*, 1935, 1988; Wundt W., *Elemente der Völkerpsychologie*, 1912.

TALE

According to the Jungian school, tales (like dreams and visions) are the purest expression of the psychic processes of the collective unconscious: that is, they reflect, in its simplest form, the basic models of the psyche: → archetypes. Every tale can be considered a relatively closed system, focusing on only one basic psychological meaning, common to all mankind, which is expressed through a series of symbolic images and events. The plot of a tale starts generally from a situation of difficulty and hindrance. This must be overcome by facing obstacles, dangers and the constant risk of failure to arrive at a solution that represents a changed existential condition. The → hero is the archetypal figure able to operate re-establishing a new emotional balance. *[F. Avon, A. Benvenuti]*

TECHNIQUE

Psychological instrument of therapeutic intervention, formalized, repeatable and transferable; in its application it has proved to be effective in the production of → change and/or the resolution or management of different forms of psychological suffering. The concept of psychotherapeutic technique includes both the application of a → problem-solving procedure, as well as a style of communication and interaction (verbal and nonverbal attitude, para-linguistic communication, the construction of a particular emotional atmosphere). There are many possible classifications of the techniques used in the field of psychotherapy: in the psychotherapies that have a constructivist matrix, therapeutic techniques are usually subdivided into direct and indirect interventions. The former refers to all those manoeuvres in which there is coherence between the therapeutic action and the objective to be achieved, for example, the case in which the patient is asked to adopt a specific behaviour that is explicitly aimed at the elimination of a → symptom. In the case of indirect techniques there can be a strong dissonance between the objectives of change and the therapeutic requests. This happens, for example, when the therapist concentrates on producing change on a secondary aspect of the problem (or of minor → resistance) of the patient, producing, in this way, in reality, a change in the principal problem. Typical examples of these are the techniques in which the attention of the patient is shifted onto tasks related to the "study" of the symptom, or those based on the → ordeal and on paradoxical → prescriptions.

There is a debate between authors of different models of therapy on whether or not it is correct to use the concept of technique in the context of the relationship between psychotherapist and patient. According to exponents of Rogerian psychotherapy and according to many Jungians, one cannot talk about technique in psychotherapy, in that they view therapy as being be entirely based on the relationship between therapist and patient, which is always unique and unrepeatable. In contrast, authors that are closer to the cognitivist, systemic, strategic and Gestalt models argue that the application of techniques is very important or even fundamental in order to induce a change in the patient. It appears, however, to be an established fact that every model of psychotherapy consists of a structure around a technique or a collection of techniques that are more or less formalized, that are then taught in the course of the training of the therapist; this is what happened, for example, in the psychoanalytic model, which has maintained the teaching of the free association technique over time, still today considered as being a fundamental technique of this kind of therapy. Frequently, technique is configured as a direct expression of the personality of the author that has created it and as a creative solution suitable for achieving therapeutic results: S. Freud ideated the technique of free association in order to overcome the resistance of patients towards remembering unpleasant events; F. Perls created the technique of the → hot seat in order to be able to achieve → awareness in a more rapid manner; C.G. Jung created the technique of → active imagination to aid in the understanding of dreams; A. Lowen devised a series of methods of working with the body; M.H. Erickson developed an effective and creative expedient to induce a trance (→ Ericksonian hypnotherapy) in the patient. *[R.]*

TELE

In psychodrama, the most simple unit of feeling that is transmitted from one individual to another. The *tele* is the expression of the natural tendency of the human being to put himself in an emotional relationship with other beings; the quality of the emotion that passes through an invisible bridge (*tele* means "from a distance") gives to such a bond the characteristics of attraction (positive *tele*) and rejection (negative *tele*), with a variation that can go from the maximum of attraction to diminishing to indifference (absence of *tele*). The term *tele* includes that which is usually described as reciprocal → empathy, emotional communication that is two-way, emotional warmth, etc.

From a genetic point of view the *tele* appears before → transference: the *tele* constitutes, in fact, a primary mode of functioning (not learnt, already able to take place at the moment of birth), whilst transference is a secondary mode of functioning (learnt, follows the experience). *[G. Boria]*

REFERENCES. Boria G., *Psicoterapia psicodrammatica. Sviluppi del modello moreniano nel lavoro terapeutico con gruppi di adulti*, 2005; Moreno J.L., *Psychodrama volume 1*, 1946; Moreno J.L., Moreno Z.T., *Psychodrama volume 3: Action therapy and principles of practice*, 1969.

TELEOLOGY

Methodological perspective – important in analytic psychology – that interprets psychic processes according to their aims and goals, in contrast to the reductionist method that interprets them according to principles of causality. According to the teleological method, the product of the unconscious is instead interpreted as a symbolic expression that represents, in anticipation, an element of a future psychological development. Every neurosis is, in this sense, also an attempt towards self-healing, the research for a new equilibrium that has been more or less successful. Next to the past, to the causes, to infantile fixations, the future enters in full force as a project, as a research for security, of power with regards to the environment, of self-affirmation, according to the theory of A. Adler (→ individual psychology), as well as the search for new equilibria, according to the principle of the tendency of the Self towards the achievement of wholeness. In this sense, neurosis is always current, being the becoming of time both past and future always present in the research for new solutions and new synthesis. *[M. Gay]*

REFERENCES. Jung C.G. (1921), *Psychological types*, in *Collected Works*, VI, 1971; Id. (1912–1928), *Two essays on analytical psychology*, in *Collected Works*, VII, 1967.

TÉMENOS

In analytic psychology, term (from the ancient Greek language meaning "a delimited area of land consecrated to divinity") that indicates an image used to designate a space, both internal and external, in which all the parts of the → personality that have been split are re-united; a sacred interior boundary that is the origin and the goal of the soul and contains the unity of the conscious and unconscious life. The connotation of sanctity alludes to the delicateness and to the complexity of the analytic task: the centre of the personality is protected, in order to avoid it being attracted to and influenced by the external world. Inversely, the world of daily life is to be separated from the more intimate personality that could invade the individual and/or his environment with destructive acts. Within the sacred fence, an area of the personality that is considered as being taboo (→ taboo), it becomes possible to meet the unconscious through the objectification of its images. The *témenos* protects and does not disperse the plurality of the unconscious images, neither internally nor externally: internally the distractions of the world that are interiorized will not have a disintegrative effect on the psyche; in the relationship with the external world it will not produce destructive effects. The image of the *témenos* indicates, therefore, the necessity of an analytic → setting that includes the definition of both the intrasubjective and intersubjective boundaries, within which it is possible to carry out the analytic process. *[G.M. Vadalà, A. Benvenuti]*

REFERENCES. Jung C.G. (1929–1957), *Commentary on "The secret of the golden flower"*, in *Collected Works*, XIII, 1967; Id. (1935), *On the theory and practice of analytical psychology*, in *Collected Works*, 1977.

TENSION

Element of which the dynamics of the psyche is constituted, in continuation with the antonymic dynamic of the psyche as described by Jung. The tension between → opposites has been a state inherent to the human nature, in that it represents not only the antagonism of the → drives, but also of the intellectual tendencies or of the different aspects of the personality. The normal existence of contrasting tendencies, even the simple ambivalence between wanting and not wanting, choosing between desires that are antagonistic towards each other, that is, between different values, creates tension that frequently can be worked through in a natural manner and resolved. In → neurosis instead, according to Jung, two tendencies act one against the other in direct opposition and, of the two, at least one is unconscious.

For this reason, Jung considered neurosis as being the expression of a tension between opposites that is much more intense than normally takes place in everyday life, that can lead to a relative dissociation between the → Ego and the → unconscious, due to the inability to accept parts of the unconscious that have been rejected (for example, the → shadow) as being part of the Self. A block can, therefore, be created in the ability of vital processes to function. This intense conflict also indicates a desire to re-establish the tie that has been severed. According to Jung, therapy tends, therefore, to render this conflict conscious, restoring to the patient the ability to master ambivalent attitudes that interfere with the development of the conscious, as happens, for example, in the passage from one developmental phase to another more mature one. *[A. Benvenuti]*

REFERENCES. Jung C.G. (1912), *New paths in psychology*, in *Collected Works*, VII, 1967; Id. (1918), *On psychic energy*, in *Collected Works*, VIII, 1969.

TESTING BY THE PATIENT

According to → control-mastery theory, the patient implements a series of tests aimed at the psychotherapist, that have the principal objective of finding a direct disconfirmation of their own → pathogenic beliefs that have been acquired in childhood. In the context of the therapeutic work, the patient tests his pathological beliefs with the aim of disconfirming them by means of the help of the therapist: this can be achieved both by means of nonverbal behaviour, but also through verbal expression. The patient tends to project his tests in such a way as to gather disconfirmation of his beliefs with the minimum risk possible. This can take place through the passive-into-active tests as well as through → transference.

By means of the passive-into-active tests, the patient re-enacts with the therapist the same traumatizing behaviours that one of his parents had adopted towards him, hoping unconsciously that the therapist will deal with it in a manner that is different from that of his mother or his father, so as to be able to learn from it. This concept can be also partly assimilated with the concept of → identification with the aggressor, but in a positive way. The clinical phenomena relevant to this theory correspond, to a greater degree, to the notions of → projective identification and projective counter-identification, but taken from the perspective of a "competent patient" (as opposed to the "resistant" patient) who is trying to feel better and to get rid of his disorder. Subsequently, the patient will try to adopt the modes of response that he has observed in the therapist in his daily life.

In the second case, that is, through the transference test, the patient can test his pathological beliefs in a more direct manner, behaving towards the therapist in the same way that he behaved as a child, hoping unconsciously that he will not obtain the same response from the therapist as he had obtained from his parents. If this hope materializes, the patient can start to disconfirm the belief that it was him that created in the parents the reactions that were traumatizing to him. In this way, a kind of → emotionally corrective experience takes place. The therapist, through his reactions to the test, can put the patient in the condition of feeling safe, so that he is able to face the fears that his pathological beliefs are predicting will be present and to work towards their disconfirmation. The therapist therefore should not be neutral, but must be the patient's ally, and should actively engage in the attempt at discrediting the pathological beliefs of the patient and to help him to pursue his goals. The patient is perceived as being active and competent, rather than being intent towards resisting the therapy. *[M. Casonato, S. Sagliaschi]*

REFERENCES. Weiss J., *How psychotherapy works: Process and technique*, 1993; Weiss J., Sampson H., *The role of pathogenic beliefs in psychic reality*, 1997; Weiss J., Sampson H., Mount Zion Psychotherapy Research Group, *The psychoanalytic process: Theory, clinical observation, and empirical research*, 1986.

THANATOS

Term used by psychoanalysis to designate the death → drive. Freud considers the repetition compulsion that characterizes different situations and clinical facts (such as the manifestations of sadism and masochism, the compulsion to repeat painful or unpleasant situations that is manifested in the play of children, " fate neurosis" and in → transference), to be an expression of a → repetition compulsion, of a principle of functioning preliminary to the → pleasure principle, older than the latter, that aims to restore the state of equilibrium of the organism. The degree of strength of the drive in the manifestations of the compulsion to repeat, and their "demonic strength", reveal a universal aspect of the drive, which can be defined as a "push, inherent in the living organism, towards reverting back to the preceding state [. . .] an expression of the conservative nature of the living being". Developing the hypothesis that "all the drives tend to attempt to restore the precedent state of affairs", Freud reformulates, in an exquisitely dualist interpretation, his drive theory by identifying a fundamental contraposition between → Eros and Thanatos, and therefore between the living drive and the death drive. *[N. Dazzi]*

REFERENCES. Freud S. (1920), *Beyond the pleasure principle*, in *The Standard Edition*, XIV, 1953–1974.

THERAPEUTIC ALLIANCE

An interpersonal interactive process created between patient and therapist, that can establish a relationship of trust and cooperation with the purpose of achieving agreed objectives. The central element of every therapeutic process is the strong link established between patient and therapist. In order for this alliance to be effective, it must be characterized by an active collaboration. Since the first meetings, therapist and patient define, together, the goals to be achieved and the times and manner of the therapy. Therefore, the contractual aspect marks an explicit bilateral commitment for a well-defined course of action and it represents a very delicate moment, where the foundations of the therapeutic process are laid. Through → communication, the therapist tries to create harmony with patients, to make them feel at ease so that they can trust and rely on the therapist and contribute to taking an active role in the process of change with their inner resources and motivation. No good therapeutic technique can succeed if it is not conveyed by a strong therapeutic alliance. This explains why it has been studied by all therapeutic schools. Starting from psychoanalytic theories, it was then an object of empirical research for the construction of assessment tools. In recent decades, research concerning the → efficacy of therapy has been focusing on studying patient–therapist relational dynamics. The entire scientific literature agrees that the quality of the therapeutic alliance affects the process and the outcome of therapy. *[R.]*

THERAPEUTIC CONTRACT

An agreement between therapist and patient on objectives and methods of work, which specifies methods used, fees and terms of payment of the therapist, ethical responsibilities of the therapist and the rights/duties of the patient as well as objectives and duration of the path taken. The agreement is usually expressed in the first session, and can vary according to the theoretical orientation of the therapist. Within the different therapeutic approaches, the therapeutic contract can be explicitly formalized and negotiated with the patient or, conversely, considered implicit. *[R.]*

THERAPEUTIC DOUBLE BIND

A communication between therapist and patient based on paradox (→ logic of paradox) and set to invariably produce a change about the symptom. The structure of this interaction mirrors that of the pathogen double bind formulated by G. Bateson and his group to explain "schizophrenia as a specific communication model" (→ double-bind theory). Therapeutic double bind implies an intense relationship, the one between therapist and patient, which the latter considers of great importance in terms of psychological survival, and an injunction, ordered by the therapist. The injunction is structured to reinforce the behaviour that the patient perceives as wrong and therefore expects to be corrected and to imply that this reinforcement is a vehicle of change; it therefore creates a paradox by telling patients to remain as they are or to try increasing what they would like to eliminate. The therapeutic situation must prevent patients withdrawing into themselves or dissolving the paradox by making comments. An example of therapeutic double bind is the paradoxical technique of → symptom prescription: the therapist redefines the symptom by connoting it positively, and therefore they ask the patient to act it rather than suppress it. In this way, the symptom is put in check: if the patient performs the therapist's injunction, they will prove to have the power to manipulate/modify the symptom (which is the purpose of therapy). Instead, to oppose the prescription they need to avoid the symptomatic behaviour (which is, again, the purpose of the strategy). *[R.]*

THERAPEUTIC OPERATIONS

Techniques presented by Berne as central and characterizing the methodology of transactional analysis. They are described in a logical sequence of eight interconnecting interventions, while remaining in that circular methodology for which the therapist has to manage the real events of the therapeutic relationship, knowing when it is the right moment to return to previous phases of the therapeutic work; in other words, transferring the principles of the methodology to a specific "therapeutic plan" (→ transactional analysis). The use of the principles of the experimental method applied to psychotherapy provides useful parameters to manage the so-called circular methodology. The first six therapeutic operations are: questioning, specification, comparison, explanation, illustration and confirmation. These first six are developed within the strategic phases of → therapeutic alliance and → decontamination; in other words, they characterize the therapeutic work aimed first at the definition of a → therapeutic contract, then at the reinforcement of the → Adult Ego-state. The last two operations are: interpretation and crystallization. These two characterize the strategic phase of → deconfusion, or that part of the therapeutic work aimed at a → redecision with respect to the patient's → script. Berne referred the eight operations to group psychotherapy with transactional analysis, but today they are applied to individual psychotherapy, above all in the approach with a psychodynamic orientation called the transactional psychoanalysis of Novellino: in the latter, in particular, the centrality of interpretation is recovered, an operation that is not used in the other two approaches that are widespread today, that is, the "re-decisional therapy" of B. and M. Goulding and the "integrative psychotherapy" of R.G. Erskine. *[M. Novellino]*

REFERENCES. Berne E., *Principles of group therapy*, 1966; Novellino M., *Seminari clinici. La cassetta degli attrezzi dell'analista transazionale*, 2010.

THERAPEUTIC RELATIONSHIP → ENCOUNTER

THERAPEUTIC RITUALS

Within the approach of the → Milan School of Family Therapy, "a series of actions, usually combined with formulae or verbal expressions, that all the members of the family are required to carry out". The therapeutic ritual is a → prescription by means of which the therapist introduces new rules of interaction without actualy verbalizing them, so that the members of the → family are not able to comment on them or attempt to disqualify them. A well-known case is that of the Casanti family, where the prescription – highly structured in its detail and in its timing – required them to meet every other day so that all members of the family could express their feelings towards the family, during a fifteen-minute period and without being interrupted. Besides legitimizing expression and discouraging reticence, this ritual prevented the formation of hidden coalitions between the members of the family. *[M. Giuliani]*

REFERENCES. Selvini Palazzoli M., Boscolo L., Cecchin G., Prata G., *Paradox and counter paradox*, 1978.

THERAPEUTIC STRATEGY

Logic of solutions applied to psychotherapy and aimed at specific or general objectives related to → change. In the first instance, the strategy is aimed at interrupting the vicious circle of a specific pathology (cessation/diminution of the disorder), whilst in the second, it is oriented at producing an unspecified change (increase of the feeling of → wellbeing). The strategy can be located at a level of abstraction that is different with respect to the single → stratagem. Frequently utilized as a synonym, the strategy represents the programming and the implementation of a finalized and predetermined plan of action, and includes all the steps necessary to achieve this aim: the analysis of the problem, definition of the objectives to be achieved, application of the solutions, achievement and evaluation of the results. However, the stratagem represents a single expedient or intervention used to overcome an individual problematic situation. Metaphorically, the strategy allows the winning of the war, whilst the stratagem allows us to win the battle. The use of strategies in psychotherapy has reached its maximum theoretical-practical systematization in the interactional-strategic paradigm, but it is also common in other forms of therapy, from the cognitive approaches to the psychoanalytic ones. It is, in fact, virtually impossible to think of a form of professional psychotherapy that does not employ therapeutic strategies that guide the actions of the therapist. The choice of the strategies to be adopted varies in relation to the → epistemology of reference of the therapist: the theoretical presuppositions and the working hypotheses play a role in guiding the productive thought of the therapist, and therefore in finding and implementing solutions. *[R.]*

THERAPEUTIC TALK

An essential instrument of verbal psychotherapies to construct the therapeutic relationship and to induce change, where it is postulated that the therapeutic process is realized mainly through the verbal exchange between therapist and patient. The quality of the relationship, which is established during the progress of the verbal interaction, has the power to modify the patient's perceptual, emotional, cognitive and behavioural states. Therapeutic talk is an essential tool of therapeutic intervention, so that each different psychotherapeutic approach recommends specific forms of it and contemplates an adequate preparation during a psychotherapist's training (→ strategic dialogue). *[R.]*

THIRD-GENERATION BEHAVIOURAL THERAPY

A natural evolution of cognitive-behavioural therapy that today has accumulated more evidence of efficacy. The focus of treatment extends beyond the solution of specific problems, to encompass personality disorders and existential problems. Focusing on the importance of context and functions of psychological phenomena, and not just of their form, the third-generation behavioural therapies emphasize contextual and experiential change strategies. Special importance is given to the therapist–patient relationship as a means of change. The experience (behavioural, cognitive and emotional) within the session becomes the main instrument of change. Examples of third generation behavioural interventions include S. Hayes's acceptance and commitment therapy (ACT), Lineham's dialectical behaviour therapy (DBT), R. Kohlenberg's functional analytic psychotherapy (FAP), mindfulness-based cognitive therapy (MBCT) and metacognitive approaches like that of A. Wells. [*P. Moderato, G. Miselli*]

REFERENCES. Harris R., *The happiness trap: Stop struggling, start living*, 2007; Hayes S.C., *Get out of your mind and into your life: The new acceptance and commitment therapy*, 2005; Moderato P., Presti G., Miselli G., *La terapia cognitivo-comportamentale entra nel terzo millennio*, in S. Di Nuovo, G. Falgares (eds.), *Per una psicologia psicologica*, 2008.

THREE-GENERATION MODEL OF PSYCHOTHERAPY

Particular mode of definition and of observation of family relationships (→ family) in their evolution over time. In the relational-systemic approach, starting from the pioneering studies of Bowen and di Framo, great value has been given to the process of differentiation of the self from the individual's family of origin. In other words, in the dynamic equilibrium between belonging and separation, each individual in the course of his personal history should be able to emancipate himself from his family of origin, overcoming his personal need for dependence. Williamson, researcher in the wake of the aforementioned authors, talks about the attainment of individual autonomy once the condition of "intergenerational intimidation" is overcome, a personal autonomy that is not attained at the end of adolescence, but that is "conquered" around the age of around 35 to 40 years of age. This means that the mere "leaving home" of the young adult is not by itself sufficient to acquire that "I position" (well described by Bowen), or rather the capacity of comparing oneself in an adult–adult relationship when dealing with one's parents. In this sense, Andolfi coined the expression "chronic son" in order to describe an adult son who feels obliged to depend emotionally (at times, also financially) on his parents. This is frequently encountered after a painful and unbalanced conjugal separation, when one of the partners ends up "re-entering" the welcoming home of the parents, retaking the role of the son, rather than being able to find within himself the capacity to deal with the loss and take up an autonomous path in his life.

Numerous authors in the field of systemic theories have talked about the triangle as a unit of measurement to observe family relationships in their development: Bowen, Framo, Whitaker, Walsh, Haley, Hoffman, Minuchin, Scabini, Andolfi, to mention the most important; and on the level of research the most recent studies of Fivaz on the "primary triangle". Once the triad is acquired as a unit of study of human relationships, of the relational → patterns of the family group, and even more of the psychopathological emergencies of a member of the family, the observations of reality obtained will be profoundly different from those obtained by who instead uses the dyad as a lens for observation. The modes of clinical intervention and of conducting research will also be influenced by these different presuppositions (one need only consider, for example, the → attachment theroy based on the observations of the mother–child interaction). The term "relational triangles" can therefore be used to mean all the elementary structures of all relationships, including those in which apparently only two people are involved. Even in this case is it possible to see how, for each of the two subjects involved, a figure of reference that acts as a "third" exists in the relationship, even if it belongs to another space, another time or, more frequently, to another generational level.

Those relational triangles in which the persons involved are located on three different generational levels (for example, grandfather, parent, grandchild) are described as being trigenerational; by "trigenerational family" one intends an extended family map, which can be disposed along a vertical plane, crossed by at least three horizontal planes. On each level one can find all those that belong to the same generational level, so that, from top to bottom we can find, respectively, the generation of grandparents, that of the children and that of the grandchildren. These are united in various ways by the relational triangles, spatially identified by a kind of set of "familial co-ordinates" that indicates the persons involved and the level to which they belong. The understanding of the individual and of his developmental processes appears, therefore, to be favoured by the construction of an observational scheme that allows us to "see", according to Andolfi and Angelo, "the current behaviours of a person as relational metaphors, or rather as indirect signals of needs and emotional involvement of the past that find the space and time to manifest themselves concretely in the current relationships". Therefore a piece of information, whether it is verbal or analogic, on "how the relationship between father and son is expressed today" (identified as the second and third generation) has an implicit and complementary aspect that also exerts an influence on how the "parent perceives today the past relationship between himself and his own father", moving in this way the emotional content of the information to a superior level, or rather between the second and the first generation. The complexity increases if everything is also connected to those more abstract images and ideals of "being a father and a son" that each has incorporated to a greater or a lesser degree of intensity within one's own familial and cultural context, and these take on the value of an actual behavioural code.

In this sense the study of "family myths" and their evolution in the development of relationships becomes very useful. The → myth becomes, in this way, a grid of interpretation of reality in which elements of reality and of fantasy co-exist, partly "inherited" from the family of origin and partly constructed by the actual families. Specific events of the life of the family or of the individual, in particular in the critical phases of existence (births, deaths, chronic illnesses, economic failure, accidents, etc.), can elicit strong emotional responses and significant familial tensions that will make each family member take on and maintain over time, different roles and functions according to the position of each individual within that particular "mythic constellation". The myth can be built and can evolve through almost three generations and becomes in this way a matrix of knowledge, representing an element of union and a factor of cohesion for those who believe in this truth. It is equally true that adhering to familial myths uncritically and considering the elements of which they are made up in a static and prescribed way can be very limiting and can trap new generations in repetitive and predictable behaviour.

According to Montagano and Pazzagli, the continuity of the lineage of a family across time, the tie with the ancestors and the descendants, can be represented by the image of the tree, which symbolizes the tie with the past (the roots) and with the future (the shoots), and the unity of the trunk with the multiple branches that originate from it. The "genogram" is, in this sense, the graphic representation of the genealogical tree and a way to help the individual describe the historical development of his family; it can be defined as being a diagram of the extended family relationships, which include at least three generations. The relational psychologist or psychotherapist can turn to the genogram with their clients in order to have a graphical and visual representation of the familial environment, loaded with affective meanings. The genogram includes, apart from the names and ages of all the members of the family, the specific dates of significant events (births, deaths, marriages, separations, etc.,) work activities, university degrees, behavioural models and other relevant information. This exercise, however, does not represent a mere gathering of information, but tends to bring into focus the emotional history of individuals, giving particular attention to the description of family myths and their intergenerational transmission, allowing the person that describes it to view himself within the wider framework of his family.

The genogram brings to light elements that have been repressed or that have remained in the shadows; it helps the individual to re-experience his past and to promote the emerging of a series of memories, feelings, rancour, in the context of the relationships with the family of origin, leading to the discovery and the redefinition of the most significant events in the life of the individual as well as the way in which they connect with each other. The voyage into the history of the family allows the individual to re-interpret it in a critical manner; it uncovers emotional blocks, secrets, myths and alliances: all significant elements that, together with the recovery of a historical memory, give the individual the opportunity work towards a better life project.

In addition to the genogram, which can be utilized both in therapy and in psychotherapeutic training, another modality exists for it use, this time analogic and nonverbal, in order to observe "in vivo" one's family relationships. This is the "family structure", introduced into the field of systemic-relational psychotherapy by Satir; this consists of the "construction" of a visual and spatial representation of the family relationships by one or more members of a family during a session; by means of arranging the members of the family in space, the attitude of their postures and their physiognomy, the play with the closeness and distance between the family members, the direction of their gaze, the "family drama" is given life with all its range of emotions. By means of the sculpture of the family relationships, the need for language and the limits imposed by rational logic can be bypassed, allowing the exploration of the deepest emotions, more intense and more unconscious, amplifying in this way the interpretation of reality. In this way the "mythical images" of the family may emerge, together with the ghosts that accompany them, the stereotypes of gender and the prejudices towards one member of the family or the other, and the emptiness and fullness of the emotional relationships of that group.

In conclusion, one can assert that the trigenerational model is an interpretational tool that is essential in order to explore the process of development and the life cycle of the family, as the research into those problematic areas, once identified, allow the therapist, but more significantly, all the members of the family, to better utilize the resources and competences of each individual. Therefore the illness, the psychological or relational disorder of a person, together with the suffering that comes from it, are not only sources of malaise for the entire family but become "bridges of knowledge", vital occasions to recover a sense of "us" and to rediscover the value of solidarity and reciprocal support. *[M. Andolfi]*

REFERENCES. Andolfi M., *Manuale di psicologia relazionale. La dimensione familiare*, 2003; Andolfi M., Angelo C., *Tempo e mito nella psicoterapia familiare*, 1988; Bowen M., *Family therapy in clinical practice*, 1978; Fivaz-Depeursige E., Corboz-Warnery A., *The primary triangle*, 1999; Framo J.L., *Family-of-origin therapy: An intergenerational approach*, 1992; Haley J. (ed.), *Changing families: A family therapy reader*, 1971; Hoffman L., *Foundations of family therapy: A conceptual framework for systems*, 1981; Minuchin S., *Families and family therapy*, 1974; Montagano S., Pazzagli A., *Il genogramma. Teatro di alchimie familiari*, 1989; Satir V., *Conjoint family therapy*, 1967; Scabini E., *L'organizzazione famiglia tra crisi e sviluppo*, 1985; Walsh F. (ed.), *Normal family processes*, 1982; Whitaker C.A., *Midnight musings of a family therapist*, 1989; Williamson D.S., *Personal authority via termination of the intergenerational hierarchical boundary: A "new" stage in the family life cycle*, in «Journal of Marital and Family Therapy», 1981, 7(4).

T-MAZE

An experimental investigation technique, typical of the behaviourist paradigm, that was in use during the 1930s and 1940s. It was used to investigate how → learning (of guinea pigs) was influenced by previous experience in terms of → reinforcement and/or cognitive maps. This technique was later abandoned. *[P. Moderato]*

TOLERANCE

This word can have different meanings. It can indicate: the capacity to accept limits or to tolerate → frustration; poor tolerance of frustration has been indicated as the cause of multiple neurotic disorders. In the interpersonal field, it indicates the process of acknowledgement and acceptance of the limits imposed by the cohabitation of individuals in the same social environment. Finally, it can designate the diminution in or loss of response to medicine following prolonged use; the concept is frequently used to refer to drug addiction, where it refers to the necessity of the individual to take increasingly large doses of psychoactive drugs with the aim of obtaining the desired effect. *[R.]*

TOPDOG VS UNDERDOG

In Gestalt therapy, a metaphor used to describe one's own inner conflict. Perls conceived inner conflicts as characterized by two "antagonists" that apparently have different power, but in reality, only have different positions. He represented them as a dog barking from an upper position to a dog in a lower position, which seems to lose the sense of confrontation, but actually, because of the passive resistance, the situation is immobilized. By using this metaphor, Perls highlighted that a conflict is never solved with the prevalence of the more "righteous" part, because the other part has always the means to put a spoke in the first one's wheels. A negotiation between the two parts is always necessary. These parts need to find, if not a dialectical overcoming, at least a compromise, to avoid the risk of the person losing energy and capabilities (in this perspective, embracing a sense of duty, as an autonomous value regardless of the context, looks like a failed attempt from the outset to solve an internal conflict by simply suppressing one of the two parts; for example, a scientist who follows their work routine, leaving aside insights that would make the research more complicated, would then have to deal with the dissatisfaction generated by these actions). The metaphor has been lost in contemporary Gestalt therapy, which typically uses the simplest notion of "polarity", coined by the Polster spouses to indicate intrapsychic elements in opposition, without necessarily identifying them specifically. This facilitates people's internal dialogue and it has taken the technique of therapeutic intervention to such sophisticated levels that it makes it appear natural, without artificial stratagems. Regardless of its technical use, the metaphor is still useful to understand the futility of some inner conflicts, and advises the therapist that if the frame of reference does not change, the internal balance of the person will hardly change. *[P. Quattrini]*

REFERENCES. Perls F., *The Gestalt approach and eye witness to therapy*, 1973; Polster E., Polster M., *Gestalt therapy integrated: Contours of theory and practice*, 1973.

TOPOGRAPHICAL MODEL OF THE MIND

In accordance with the etymology of the term (topical, or rather, "relative to a place"), this expression refers to two different descriptions of the functioning of the psyche proposed by Freud in the field of psychoanalytic theory: the first topography, as outlined in the *The Interpretation of Dreams*, introduces the distinction between psychological processes of an → unconscious and of a conscious nature; the second topography was developed in *The Ego and the Id*, in order to better define the specific functions of the three systems → Ego, →Id and →Superego and their location with respect to the different levels of consciousness.

FIRST TOPOGRAPHY: Consists of the topographic representation of the psychic processes: conscious-preconscious-unconscious. Just as only a very small part of the total mass of an iceberg is visible above water, with most of it being submerged under water, so the human psyche consists not just of the conscious manifestations that reveal themselves in logical thought and through verbal language. A second part, equivalent to the level at which the iceberg is floating in the water, to do with thoughts and memories that float between the conscious and the unconscious, is generally identifiable with what is forgotten but can be recalled intentionally through attention and memory. The largest part, which, in the case of the iceberg, sinks into the marine abyss, represents the unconscious level, which, precluded from subjective investigation, interprets the biological components and their expression through drives (→ drive) as well as being the seat of those psychic components that are the objects of repression (→ defence mechanisms).

SECOND TOPOGRAPHY: The theory of the "psychic provinces", the first topography, is superimposed on by that of the psychic processes indicated as being the Ego, Id and Superego, also known as the "structural hypothesis". The psyche is viewed as being a complex unity, made up of three poles that are in relationship with each other but have different functions: the Id (the original drive pole), the Ego (the part of personality that is rational and conscious) and the Superego (the moral conscience). With the second topography, the mode of functioning of the Id, Ego and Superego in relationship with the places described by the first topography is clarified. The Id is the impersonal and chaotic expression of the vital biological forces and is totally unconscious. The Ego is the functional space that is determined through the differentiation of the Id and that responds to the needs of satisfaction of the drives that takes into account environmental and cultural limits: it presents therefore an unconscious and a conscious component. The Superego develops through the interiorization of the values and the moral norms of the parents and of the social environment; it controls and modifies the instincts in order to make them acceptable on the basis of moral values that have been internalized. As in the Ego, the Superego also presents with an unconscious component and a conscious component. *[S. Smiraglia]*

REFERENCES. Freud S. (1900–1901), *The interpretation of dreams*, in *The Standard Edition*, IV–V, 1953–1974; Id. (1922), *The Ego and the Id*, in *The Standard Edition*, XIX, 1953–1974.

TOTE

In cognitive behavioural therapy, a model of analysis of finalized behaviour that extends the model stimulus–response (→ stimulus–response relationship) to the base of learning theory, including those elements of cognitive processing that relate to a cybernetic concept (→ cybernetics) of → feedback. The acronym TOTE describes the four phases of goal-oriented behaviour: Test, Operate, Test, Exit. The *Test* phase matches the sensorial representation of an objective or "desired state" (for instance, the right volume of TV) with perception of the "current state" (for instance, a much-too-high volume). *Operate* phase (for instance, push the volume key to lower the volume) begins if *test* shows a discrepancy between the two previous states (desired and current), till the discrepancy has been eliminated. Finally, *Exit* marks the end of TOTE and of related behaviour. Mostly in cognitive behavioural therapy, TOTE can be used as a model for realizing "well-formulated" objectives, which are then subject to appropriate feedback (verification). Among the most important criteria of well-formulated objectives are realism (an objective should be obtainable), positivity (in a formal grammatical sense, not in terms of content – for instance, "to have healthy lungs" rather than "to quit smoking"), sensory (in terms of a result that can be seen, heard, and touched with one's hands). As far as feedback is concerned, it is necessary to define precise models that include a definition of contents to be verified: who does it, in which way and within what time scale. *[S. Boschi]*

REFERENCES. Miller G.A., Galanter E., Pribram K.M., *Plans and the structure of behaviour*, 1960.

TRAIT

The notion of "trait", intended as a behavioural mode that is stable over time and in different contexts, can be traced back to the philosophy and to the medicine of Ancient Greece. Pythagoras, Hippocrates, Plato, Aristotle, later on Galeno up to I. Kant, up to the founder of psychology, W. Wundt, have emphasized the seductive nature of the typological description of individuals. Trait psychology received a propulsive energy at the beginning of the twentieth century thanks to the progressive increase in the knowledge of statistics, and to the new possibilities of measurement of the characteristics of human behaviour. In fact, thanks to factor analysis, Cattell was able to identify, starting from the classifications that had been developed by other authors, two main types of traits – those that are superficial and those that are source traits – and three modes of expression: ability traits, temperament traits and dynamic traits. In the more modern panorama of the cognitivist paradigm, the trait, intended as a characteristic that is gifted with stability over time and that is independent of external situations, is assimilated with the conceptual definition of cognitive style and of structure. By style, the enduring and internally coherent individual differences in cognitive organization and function is intended. The term refers both to the individual differences in the general principles of cognitive organization, and to the various subjective tendencies that do not refer to the general human cognitive function. It reflects differences in personality and the genetic and experiential differences in cognitive abilities and cognitive function. Every individual has a specific capacity to represent himself and the world through a style that is typical of himself, equipped with a significant degree of internal stability, the rules and elements of which are made up by organizing thought and filtering information in such a way as to ensure that everything falls within a unitary structure of reality. *[F. Vincelli]*

REFERENCES. Cattell R.B., *The description of personality. Foundations of trait measurement*, in «Psychological Review»1943, 50; Dobson K.S., *Handbook of cognitive-behavioural therapies*, 1988.

TRANCE → HYPNOSIS

TRANSACTION

Basic unit of human communication consisting in an exchange, between two individuals, of "motivational bricks" provided by → strokes. The term refers to the main event described by E. Berne's transactional analysis. This exchange involves two or more → Ego-states of the sender and the receiver, with different consequent types of transactions (complementary, crossed, ulterior). Each type of transaction calls for its own rule of communication, which describes the possible "destiny" of that particular communication. A fourth rule of communication, tied to the phenomenon of interpersonal and therapeutic intuition in particular, is described by Novellino. The ulterior transactions, given by a double level of communication – the first social or explicit and aware; the second psychological and unaware – lead to particular interactive patterns called psychological → games; these reactivate unresolved childhood experiences, which lead to a reinforcement of the individual's → script. Specific transactions are those of → transference and → countertransference, and their analysis was developed by the Roman Psychodynamic School and in the → setting of individual psychotherapy by the transactional psychoanalysis movement. In the latter area, further studies of the specific nature of these transactions led to the relational psychoanalysis of unconscious communication. *[M. Novellino]*

REFERENCES. Novellino M., *Psicoanalisi transazionale*, 2004; Id., *Seminari clinici. La cassetta degli attrezzi dell'analista transazionale*, 2010.

TRANSACTIONAL ANALYSIS

Neo-psychoanalytic psychotherapy movement, that is tied to an evolution of the original Freudian model, founded in the 1950s by the Canadian psychiatrist and psychoanalyst Eric Berne. He was a student first of P. Federn and then of E. Erikson. He studied the phenomena of intuition and of group dynamics, arriving at a theoretical and methodological model centred on the analysis of the relational functions of the Ego and on the attainment of the intrapsychic and social autonomy of the individual. His model quickly became widespread, first in America and then in the rest of the world, generating great interest, both by professionals and by lay people, thanks to the simplicity of the technical language that Berne used to distance himself from certain, sometimes inadvertent, obscurities of the language of psychoanalysis. In this he followed the path of pioneers like W. Reich and F. Perls, who also distanced themselves from orthodox psychoanalysis, placing themselves in the larger philosophical environment of humanistic psychology (see the humanistic-existential paradigm in the opening chapter, "The eight paradigms and their respective theoretical-applicational models").

This affiliation, however, contributed to creating a distorted image of transactional analysis as being a "brief" psychotherapy, aimed at treatments of symptomatic behavioural disturbances, an image moreover aided by the enormous success of popular books, like *I'm OK, You're OK* by T. Harris. The epistemological reality of Berne's work is that of a deep psychotherapy, re-evaluated and re-centred, above all thanks to the epistemological and clinical contributions of the so-called "Roman School" of psychodynamic transactional analysis, founded in the 1980s by M. Novellino and C. Moiso, aimed, with particular attention, at the treatment of borderline and narcissistic personality disturbances; the latter referring to the specific clinical situation that derives from infantile omnipotence, typical in the second year of life, which can remain in the adult, with a consequent excess of love of oneself.

METAPSYCHOLOGY. Berne built his psychological theory on a distinctly interpersonal framework, basing his studies of the phenomena of intuition in groups on the research of the neurosurgeon W. Penfield on the coexisting states of consciousness and on the cybernetics of communication of N. Wiener and A. Korzybski. An innovative and pioneering model emerged in which the intrapsychic and the relational were two sides of the same coin: a mind conceived as bi-personal, which surpassed the monadic conception of the Freudian psychic apparatus and anticipated many of the current developments of → relational psychoanalysis. The intrapsychic aspect of the personality is based on two cornestones; the first is the theory of the → Ego-states, understood as systems organized at a cognitive/emotional/behavioural level; Berne describes the *exteropsychic* Ego-state (called → Parent), derived from the introjection of significant parental models; the *archaeopsychic* Ego-state (called → Child), a fixation of infantile experiences, decisive for successive development; the *neopsychic* Ego-state (called → Adult), a dynamic organizer of the psychic competence of contact with the here-and-now. The second cornerstone on which the intrapsychic aspect of the personality is based is the theory of the psychological → script, a conceptual derivation of the Freudian → transference neurosis (a compulsive repeating in the adult life of emotional drama that is unresolved in childhood, like abandonment, escape, etc.), which Berne develops in a relational sense: this consists of the whole of the scenarios of the adult life of an individual unconsciously based on unelaborated infantile experiences of the first models of relational attachment. The relational aspect of the personality is based on another two fundamental chapters, complementary to the first two: the first chapter is that of the theory of transactional analysis, in the strict sense of the term, which studies the rules of communication among the Ego-states of two or more subjects; the → transaction studies the activity (trans-action) that can develop between one or two Ego-states of the individuals and the different outcomes that the communication can foresee; the motivational base of the transaction is given by the natural need that people have to exchange stimuli (defined as hunger for strokes). Among the different types of transactions that Berne describes, the transactions of transfer and countertransfer are to be underlined, which constitute the principle dynamic, both of the disturbances of daily communication and of the relational events that are central to the therapist–patient relationship. Finally, the last fundamental chapter is that of the theory of psychological → games (in the acceptance of transactional analysis), which greatly contributed to transactional analysis becoming widespread. The psychological game consists in a neurotic dynamic, as peculiar as it is frequent: two or more persons communicate on two levels, the first explicit and predominantly verbal (called the *social* level), the second implicit and unaware (called the *psychological* level) and the success of the two parallel communications leads the players to a payoff given by negative confirmations about themselves and about the others and by emotions already experienced during unelaborated childhood events (parasite emotions or → rackets). The co-active repetition of games unconsciously leads to a reinforcement of the thesis foreseen by the psychological script. In sum, the Bernian metapsychology conceives the development of the personality through the contemporaneous taking place of three intrapsychic structures organized according to systems tied to introjected parental models (Parents) and to the correlated infantile reactions (Child), which become Ego-syntonic and Ego-dystonic (or homogeneous or not homogeneous) with the evolution of the structures adapted to the environment based on the perception and the elaboration of the here-and-now (Adult); the remaining Ego-dystonic conflict between the parental models and the infantile reactions leads to the development of a psychological script, which in its turn will express itself relationally with particular communication transference (psychological games). The analysis of these relational modalities can lead both to the understanding of the intrapsychic dynamics and to their therapeutic elaboration.

THE PHILOSOPHY OF THE CLINIC. With transactional analysis, Berne builds a model of psychotherapy that is sensitive to the humanistic orientation, which, in the1960s, characterized the different movements emerging from a vast debate, critical both of the unreliability of orthodox psychoanalysis in terms of efficacy, and of the behaviourist approach considered excessively "medicalized". The psychotherapist had to be neither the neutral and distant analyst nor the directive and detached scientist, but had to present himself as an involved and participating actor in the human reality of the patient. The transactional analyst begins from the positive potential innate in each human being (state of → OK-ness), to be able to profitably guide his patient on a voyage to the roots of his troubles, seen as a consequence of a psychological script and of games carried out to maintain it. The therapeutic relationship is based on two cardinal points, first psychological and then methodological: 1) contractibility, based on a relationship of direct collaboration towards realistic and shared, as well as verifiable, aims; 2) re-decisionality, interpreted as a possibility of changing the infantile position at the base of problems presented in therapy. Among the different metaphors, which Berne was fond of, used to illustrate his vision of the role of the therapist, the "fishing licence" is fundamental to understand the essential nature of his philosophy: the task of the therapist faced with the existential "hunger" of the patient is not to provide "the fish" to satisfy his hunger, but to lead him to get a licence to be able to fish independently.

THE CLINICAL METHODOLOGY. Transactional analysis was born from neo-psychoanalytic roots, given the training of its founder, who, moreover, intended to overcome some of the limits of the Freudian orthodox approach. At his death in 1971, its psychodynamic character was, for a variety of reasons, largely abandoned, in favour of a cognitive-behaviourist line, recently proposed again. In any case, in the 1980s, the Roman School of psychodynamic transactional analysis re-evaluated, also at an international level, the original psychodynamic approach. The work on the Ego-states and on the transference of Moiso, and that of Novellino on unconscious communication and on interpretation, have marked the passage towards a transactional analysis centred on the analysis of the transference and countertransference dynamics in a therapeutic → setting, both of groups and individuals (→ transactional psychoanalysis). The Roman School calls for a careful theoretical distinction between the methodology, understood as the application of the Bernean theory to the therapeutic setting of consequential strategic phases, carried out by specific operative tactics, and the therapeutic plan, resulting from the application of the principles of the methodology in each specific clinical situation, which is assessed by considerations tied both to the diagnosis and to the therapeutic contract. The methodology is organized according to four strategic phases. The first is *alliance*, during which the therapist establishes a dynamic collaboration, both at a conscious level (contract) and at an unconscious one (positive transfer). The second is *decontamination*, aimed at rendering the patient's Adult aware of the ancient influences that condition his problems, both the introjective ones (contamination from the Parent to the Adult) and the regressive ones (contamination from the Child to the Adult); at the end of this phase, the patient is able to acquire social control over his relational behaviour. The third phase, central from the psychodynamic point of view, is *deconfusion*, which follows the emotional elaboration and the resolution of the ancient roots that are at the base of the clinical problem. Finally, there is the *re-learning*, conclusive stage, in which the therapist helps the patient both to verify the stability of the change realized and to elaborate the analytic detachment.

TRANSACTIONAL ANALYSIS SCHOOLS. In the 1950s and 60s, three main branches of clinical application of the Bernean methodology were recognized: the "classical" school of Berne's closest collaborators, who predominantly followed a cognitive-behaviourist interpretation; the "redecisional" school, founded by the couple B. and M. Goulding, who integrated the theory of transactional analysis with the Gestalt psychotherapy technique by Perls, proposing a cathartic approach; the "re-parenting" school of the J. Schiffs, who applied transactional analysis to residential treatments of psychotic patients. Currently, two main lines are identified as confrontational among the transactional analysts: the relational psychoanalytic branch, adhered to, apart from by the Roman School, by the British group of H. Hargaden and C. Sills (relational transactional analysis), and the branch of "integrative" psychotherapy of R. Erskine, a further evolution of the redecisional approach. As has already been said, some people propound a transactional analysis of cognitive orientation; at the moment, however, it lacks an effective methodological character.

TRANSACTIONAL PSYCHOANALYSIS. Transactional psychoanalysis, developed by Novellino as a pillar of psychodynamic transactional analysis, consists of the application of the methodological principles of transactional analysis, understood in a psychodynamic sense, to the individual setting of psychotherapy. Its cardinal points are: the conception of the psychic apparatus as bi-personal, in line with the developments in psychoanalysis proposed by S. Mitchell (relational psychoanalysis); the focus on the dynamics of transfer and counter-transfer; the recovery of the centrality of the Bernian operation of interpretation; the accurate analysis of unconscious communication. The latter refers to transference in therapeutic communication by the patient of unconscious experiences that "mark" the here-and-now of the relationship. From this point of view, the use of the analytic couch was re-proposed, in suitable clinical situations, already described by Berne in the technique of regressive analysis.

APPLICATIONS OF TRANSACTIONAL ANALYSIS. Born as psychotherapy, transactional analysis today develops the operative possibilities innate in its method, even in adjacent fields: Clinical counselling, pedagological counselling and organizational counselling. The training of transactional analysts, in the different fields, is regulated by criteria illustrated by associations, both international (ITAA: International Transactional Analysis Association; EATA: European Association for Transactional Analysis) and national. *[M. Novellino]*

REFERENCES. Berne E., *Transactional analysis in psychotherapy*, 1961; Id., *Principles of group therapy*, 1966; Novellino M., *Psicoanalisi transazionale*, 2004; Id., *Seminari clinici: la cassetta degli attrezzi dell'analista transazionale*, 2010.

TRANSEXUAL PARENTHOOD

The term refers to the experience of parenthood, to the beliefs and feelings linked to the assumption of the parental role by transsexual people. "Parenthood" refers to the universe of meanings that a man and a woman actively generate when they become father or mother, while the prefix "trans" alludes to the parent's gender identity change. Transsexual parenthood involves the self-representation as parent, and the related role assumptions (according to one's own gender identity) impersonated before the person goes through the surgical sex conversion, and the new set of self-images allowed by the surgery. After the transition, the son/daughter will start to interact with a parent whose sex is opposite to the previously impersonated parental role. A second condition of transsexual parenthood occurs in the event that a person becomes a father/mother after the conclusion of the transition; in that case, the operated person will impersonate the parental role in accordance with the assumed gender identity. *[E. Bordin]*

REFERENCES. Faccio E., Bordin E., Cipolletta S., *Transsexual parenthood and new role assumptions*, in «Culture, health & sexuality», 2013, 15(9); Ruspini E., Inghilleri M., *Transessualità e Scienze Sociali*, 2008.

TRANSFERABILITY

The degree to which a model of intervention can be learnt and applied by different therapists in different contexts whilst maintaining the prerogatives of → efficacy and → efficiency. Transferability is a fundamental property of a therapeutic treatment protocol (→ strategic treatment protocol), in that it evidences its value independently from the characteristics of the individual therapist. *[R.]*

TRANSFERENCE

In the Freudian conceptualization, transference – initially considered as being one of the principal obstacles to psychoanalytic treatment – starting from 1912, was considered as being "the essential instrument of the analytic treatment". The term "transference" indicates as much the emotional attitude (positive or negative) of the patient with regard to their psychoanalyst as it does the process through which the patient reactivates, with regard to the figure of the psychoanalyst, emotions, thoughts and behaviours originally directed at people that were in the patient's life before therapy, and, in particular, towards parental figures. In transference, therefore, the patient transfers onto the analyst powerful past experiences and feelings already experimented in precocious relationships with significant figures. Unaware of these connections, the patient re-experiences his own feelings as being pertinent to the present and not as being derived from past situations. Within the different "modern" perspectives – that underline to a varying degree the contribution of the analyst to the relationship with the patient, or rather of all the intersubjective events that take place between two persons – transference is instead defined in reference to past relational configurations, continuously recreated as much in "real" life as they are in the therapeutic relationship, with which the analysand constructs and assimilates his own experience of the analytic relationship. Transference is therefore considered both as the way in which the individual uses the unconscious principles of organization in order to understand what surrounds him, but also as a re-experimentation of the past as it is remembered in the present and not for how it actually happened. *(N. Dazzi)*

▷ For Jung, the analytic situation is a "kind of "dialectic process", a dialogue between two persons". According to Jung, the person is a "psychic system that, when it acts on another person, enters into an interaction with another psychic system". This interaction is regulated by the general psychological dynamic that renders possible the accessibility to and the understanding of the world of objects as a result of the spontaneous circuit of projection–working-through–recovery of psychological contents/schemes that are unconsciously/implicitly solicited. The analytical situation implies the relationship between the "psychic totality" of analyst and patient, or rather between the respective conscious and unconscious systems in which the → countertransference is no longer intended as a reaction or unidirectional response to the transference of the patient, but the countertransference of the analyst, intended as an intersubjective contribution to the circular relationship with the patient, is considered as being the fundamental vehicle and container of the cure (for a Freudian prospective, refer to Heimann, 1950). This is configured as a co-cure that cannot be propitiated by any technical manipulation.

One can therefore summarize the analytic relationship as a relationship, between the conscious of the analyst and that of the patient, that can generate: a → therapeutic alliance; a relationship between the unconscious of the patient and that of the analyst, intended as a regressive reproduction of an undifferentiated state of mystical participation, almost regularly of a sexual nature; a relationship that crosses between the unconscious of the patient and the conscious of the analyst. It is only in the last two cases that we can describe the complex dynamics as being ones of transference. These can be of a personal-complexual nature in which the object represents the → *imago* belonging to the infantile past, or of a collective-archetypal nature; in other words, the activation of an *imago* related to psychological states that have not as yet been experienced and that do not belong to the period of infancy. *[S. Carta]*

REFERENCES. Carta S., *Jung: Tracce dagli Altri*, in «Rivista di Psicologia Analitica», 2007, 22; Heimann P., *On the countertransference*, in «The International Journal of Psychoanalysis», 1950, 31; Jung C.G. (1935), *Principles of practical psychotherapy*, in *Collected Works*, XVI, 1966; Id. (1946), Jung C.G., *The psychology of the transference*, 1957, in *Collected Works*, XVI.

TRANSFERENCE NEUROSIS

Notion derived from the same concept as that of → transference. It refers both to a category of pathological disorders, but also to a phenomenon that arises during the course of psychoanalytic therapy. In *Remembering, Repeating and Working Through*, Freud defines "transference neurosis" as being the consequence of the establishment of transference in the analytic relationship. The conflict that constitutes the original nucleus of the neurosis of the analysand, which is related to his relationship with the most important persons in his past; it is transferred onto the relationship with the therapist, in such a way as to bring it into the present and relive it through the dynamics of the analytic relationship. According to this conceptualization, the neurosis of the patient is gradually substituted by a new "artificial pathology" that can be worked on directly in the course of psychoanalytic therapy, of which it has become a fundamental component. The transference neurosis is therefore a sort of intermediary between pathology and real life. As Freud pointed out in *Beyond the Pleasure Principle*, on the one hand,

> one needs to allow the patient to relive a certain part of his past life and on the other hand ensure that he maintains a certain amount of detachment that will allow him to realize that what to him appears to be reality, is in reality only the reflection of a past that has been forgotten.

As a consequence of the resolution of this new pathological phenomenon obtained through analysis and interpretation the resolution of the original problem also takes place. From a nosographic point of view, Freud observes that it is possible to "undertake the clinical distinction between transference neurosis and narcissistic disorder" and proposes a distinction be made between the different mental organizations that allow the transfer of an important libidinal investment onto the figure of the therapist and those in which this process is hindered by a stable amount of libido bound at a narcissistic level, who therefore, is not able to form new significant relationships with external objects. The impossibility of creating a transference relationship characterizes, therefore, those neuroses that are described as "narcissistic neuroses", pathologies that are more serious and basically not accessible to psychoanalytic therapy, whilst neuroses that allow the transference onto the figure of the therapist, such as hysteria and obsessive neuroses are described as "transference neurosis". The connection between the structure of the personality, and the nature of the relationship with the therapist is in this way confirmed, as is the amenability towards treatment of the patient, that is, the possibility of carrying out the psychoanalytic therapy in an effective manner. *[P. Cruciani]*

REFERENCES. Freud S. (1914), *Remembering, repeating and working through*, in *The Standard Edition*, XII, 1953–1974; Id. (1920), *Beyond the pleasure principle*, in *The Standard Edition*, XIV, 1953–1974; Id. (1923–1925), *The Ego and the Id and other works*, in *The Standard Edition*, XVIII, 1953–1974.

TRANSPARENTHOOD → TRANSEXUAL PARENTHOOD

TRANSTHEORETICAL PSYCHOTHERAPY

The transtheoretical model of behavioural change was developed by Prochaska and Di Clemente to overcome the differences among traditional models of psychotherapy. According to these authors: to improve the process of → change in human behaviour, a particular theory of human beings is not necessary. Instead, the therapy needs to focus on change processes themselves and on their environmental and social variables. Transtheoretical psychotherapy is empirically founded and it is different from evidence-based psychotherapy (see the Appendix, "Empirical research in psychotherapy"), because it does not refer to any existing theory whose → efficacy must be verified or from which the most suitable → techniques to treat a case are adopted.

CHANGE PROCESSES. Systematic studies of change led Prochaska and Di Clemente to promote and induce behavioural change through ten processes. They are listed in hierarchical order as follows: 1) *Self-awareness*. Self-observation in the environmental → context in which a change is required is the basic process for changing, without which a person can remain prisoner of perceptive-regulative frames of mind, leading them to react always in the same way (→ attempted solutions); 2) *Catharsis*. Catharsis leads to acceptance of emotions. It is used as a → defence mechanism against → anxiety and fear of changing; 3) *Self-review*. Change implies not only the modification of a single behaviour, but changing the → script of one's own life according to new goals and values; 4) *Review of environmental context*. Change implies also modifying the contingencies that influence one's behaviour; 5) *Self-liberation*. → Awareness to be free in choosing is another step in the process of change; 6) *Autonomy from the social context*. It implies understanding how one's own thinking is affected by the social context, which can generate inflexible attitudes toward change; 7) *Deconditioning, counterconditioning*. Not only thoughts and prejudices but also automatisms, induced by respondent or operant conditioning, make behaviour dysfunctional. Therapy aims to solve those automatic habits; 8) *Stimulus control*. For the same reason it is also necessary to control environmental stimuli (→ environment) that elicit conditioned responses; 9) *Reinforcement control*. Stimulus control is effective if the consequences of the elicited behaviour are under control, i.e. under a discriminative → reinforcement; 10) *Helping relations*. The development of social skills leads the subject to be socially supported in his changing process.

CHANGE STAGES. Change progresses through five stages: 1) Pre-contemplation. In the first stage subjects do not consider changing and therapy aims to induce them to pre-contemplate that possibility; 2) Contemplation. Subjects are aware of their problems and therapy helps them to examine the advantages of changing; 3) Preparation. Subjects want to change and therapy helps them to define an effective project to carry on the change and to overcome the difficulties; 4) Action. People engage in changing their problematic behaviour and therapy supports them; 5) Maintenance. Subjects succeed in changing. Now the therapy helps them to go on and prevent relapse. Transtheoretical psychotherapy starts by identifying the stage where the subject is, and continues with a flexible approach based on practical evaluations: considering, for example, which aspect of problematic behaviour requires an urgent or priority intervention, to avoid dangerous situations or severe damage for the client, or to reach results more rapidly, so as to motivate the client to pursue more difficult changes.

EPISTEMOLOGICAL FRAME OF TRANSTHEORETICAL PSYCHOTHERAPY. Four basic assumptions characterize transtheoretical psychotherapy. In fact, the processes and the variables of change must: 1) be expressed in operational terms; 2) have been empirically tested; 3) apply to both the therapeutic and natural context; 4) apply to all kinds of human behaviour.

Transtheoretical psychotherapy provides a basic model of change that can be applied to a wide variety of problematic behaviours. A number of longitudinal randomized trials demonstrated its efficacy and efficacy to promote change. *[R. Anchisi]*

REFERENCES. Prochaska J.O., Di Clemente C.C., *Transtheoretical therapy: Toward a more integrative model of change*, in «Psychotherapy: Theory, Research and Practice», 1982, 19; Id., *The transtheoretical approach*, in J.C. Norcross, M.R. Goldfried (ed.), *Handbook of psychotherapy integration*, 1992; Prochaska J.O., Norcross J.C., *Systems of psychotherapy: A transtheoretical analysis*, 1994.

TRANSUBSTANTIATION

The Eucharistic rite of the transformation of the bread and of the wine into the body and the blood of Christ has been given two fundamental interpretations, which Jung contrasts with each other in his work *Psychological Types*. Here he deals with the realist interpretation of P. Radberto and with the abstract interpretation of G. Scoto Eriugena, both philosophers of the Middle Ages, one a French Benedictine abbot, the other an Irish monarch.

The realistic interpretation is more materialistic, more tied to feeling, to the value of the ritualistic encounter, and corresponds, according to Jung, to an extroverted attitude (→ extroversion). The second interpretation is instead associated with an introverted attitude (→ introversion) in that, in perceiving in the Eucharist a rite of memory, it is tied to the *logos* and the subjective, psychological and spiritual value of the presence of the faithful at the conducting of the rite.

Later, in his study on the symbolism of the Catholic mass, Jung contrasts transubstantiation both with the vison of Zosimo of Panopoli and with the process of → individuation, and reflects on how this transformation of something material into something spiritual, beyond the cultural stratifications of the Eucharistic rite, originates from the more archaic structures of the psyche, and on the way in which they present themselves, even to the present day, in the transformative processes of the contemporary individual, visible in the images of his dreams and of his imagination. *[M. Gay]*

REFERENCES. Jung C.G. (1921), *Psychological types*, in *Collected Works*, VI, 1971; Id. (1938–1940), *Psychology and religion: West and East*, in *Collected Works*, XI, 1958; Id. (1942), *Transformation symbolism in the mass*, in *Collected Works*, XI, 1969.

TRAUMA

In the first Freudian theoretical formulation, a trauma is the source of energy that produces, at birth, the activation of the central nervous system, that had previously constituted a closed system that was self-sufficient and self-gratifying (principle of the nirvana or neurotic inertia). The nervous system possesses a barrier against stimuli, but during the traumatic event this is shattered, creating a state of accumulation of energy that is expressed in suffering and in functional disorders. The only possibility of therapeutic intervention, in the first Freudian theoretical formulation, consists of the outward discharge of excess energy → discharge.

REAL TRAUMA. According to J. Breuer, friend and colleague of Freud, the traumatic event takes place during a particular psychological state, denominated as the "hypnoid state" (light state of self-induced hypnosis). Through the induction of a hypnotic trance in patients that develop hysteria following a traumatic event, it is possible to recover the memory of the trauma and to obtain healing. At the start of the collaboration between Freud and Breuer this principle was observed to be present by both. Subsequently, Freud would distance himself from Breuer's theories, as he believed that trauma was sexual in nature. He formulated the hypothesis that its incestuous nature did not allow the memory to remain at the level of the conscious; it is therefore repressed (→ repression), as it is experienced as being Ego-dystonic. The traumatic event that takes place during infancy, according to Freud, causes the subsequent development of pathological symptoms in adulthood. After puberty, when sexual energy has matured, a fortuitous event of minor importance may be enough to trigger the development of the disorder.

IMAGINED TRAUMA. As a result of the ever-increasing experience in listening to the accounts of his hysterical patients, Freud developed, over time, a different conception, and started to believe that a real traumatic event had probably never taken place, and that the memories and reconstructions of his patients could be attributable to projections of their sexual fantasies. At first he tried to save his initial theory, asserting that in the unconscious no distinction was made between reality and fantasy, but he soon came to believe that sexuality is already present in infancy and that these biological drives are able to build incestuous fantasies. If, on the one hand, such a theoretical revolution had built the foundations for the construction of the fundamental concepts of Freudian psychoanalysis (→ drive,→ Ego, → Id, → Superego), on the other hand, it had set in motion the necessity, for the purposes of healing, to discover relevant psychological material in increasingly precocious phases of development (pre-oedipal). Additionally, with the aim of rendering conscious that which is unconscious, the interpretation of the analyst takes the place of memories of events. The theory of real trauma was subsequently picked up and given importance by one of the most influential of Freud's students, S. Ferenczi, who asserted its actual verifiability. *[G. Fossi]*

REFERENCES. Freud S. (1894), *The neuro-psychoses of defence*, in *The Standard Edition*, III, 1953–1974; Id. (1909), *Five lectures on psycho-analysis*, in *The Standard Edition*, XI, 1953–1974; Id. (1915), *Thoughts for the times on war and death*, in *The Standard Edition*, XIV, 1953–1974; Id. (1932), *New introductory lectures on psycho-analysis*, in *The Standard Edition*, XXII, 1953–1974.

TREATMENT → THERAPY

TRIADIC QUESTIONS

A technique developed by the Milan school (→ Milan school of family therapy). For example, in a family session, a mother can be asked to describe the relationship with her daughter. Alternatively, the same question can be asked in triadic form, that is, asking the father how he views the relationship between the two women, and then asking them what they think of the description they have just listened to. These questions produce information, not so much in terms of facts and predicates, but rather of descriptions of relationships and differences between these descriptions. In this way, every → family member becomes an observer of other people's descriptions. Pearce describes the

Milan school's triadic questioning as an example of cosmopolitan communication, as it encourages scepticism towards single-perspective "truth". *[M. Giuliani]*

REFERENCES. Pearce B., *Communication and the human condition*, 1989.

TRIANGULATION

In the field of tri-generational psychotherapy, a concept finalized by Bowen to designate the involvement of a third person in a relationship between two people that is unstable, characterized by poor tolerance of anxiety and subjected to internal and external disturbing emotional forces. Once the anxiety diminishes, the triangle is dispersed, otherwise two of the three members will turn to the external world to "triangulate" another person. Frequently, in family therapy, it is the triangulation of the son or daughter: the involvement of a third in the feelings and in the problems of the parental couple; the poorer this relationship, the more intense this involvement becomes. The process of "de-triangulation" consists of leading one of the parents (Bowen frequently worked with only one member of the couple, when he felt there was a risk of triangulation at the expense of the therapist) to develop a sense of self that was separate from that of the relationship with the son/daughter. *[M. Giuliani]*

REFERENCES. Bowen M., *Family therapy in clinical practice*, 1978.

TRIUMPH

A term used in individual psychology that in an intrasubjective sense indicates experiences of satisfaction or self-celebration in which self-esteem is increased by real or supposed awareness of results that have been achieved. In psychopathology it indicates an excessive exacerbation of the feeling of superiority of one's self, which is defensively perceived as the best and victorious in relation to reality and to others. If supported by aggressive drives and by an inflated striving for power, the compensatory need to perceive oneself as the triumphant party can induce a lifestyle that is abusive and manipulative with regard to others, to the point where the individual carries out harmful acts (malignant narcissism). In psychotherapy, evaluating the dynamic sense of the patient's experiences of triumph is an essential part of formulating a comprehensive diagnosis. *[A. Bianconi, C. Gasparini]*

REFERENCES. Adler A., *Menschenkenntnis*, 1927; Id. *What life should mean to you*, 1931.

TRUE SELF → FALSE SELF

TRUST

In general, a state of certainty due to the conviction of being trustworthy to ourself, others and the world around us, which occurs also in the context of total or partial lack of information, where it is impossible or difficult to have access to valid proof to confirm our prediction of being trustworthy. The subject of the prediction is our perception of the intentions and/or competence of the agents responsible for the expected results. To trust something or someone always underlines a risk, that the subject assumes through a process with variable degrees of consciousness. Trust can be expressed through a threshold measure localized on a statistical distribution that goes from absolute distrust to blind trust with, in the middle, a measure of uncertainty. That capacity positively influences our behaviour, eliminating eventual anxiety and uneasiness that could lead to a closure or avoidance attitude. Regarding theory of games, as well as in every interdependent relationship, to trust means to feel that, given the chance, it is improbable that the person behaves in a way that goes against us. Trust is an influencing factor in decision-making inasmuch as each subject is free to avoid a risky cooperative relationship, going for the most valuable option for everyone. In the field of psychotherapy, the patient's trust of the therapist is a crucial factor in order to induce therapeutic → efficacy, as well as trust in oneself and one's own abilities, which represent a shared goal in all forms of psychotherapy. *[R.]*

TRUTH

Generally speaking, the correspondence between a statement and reality. Plato in *Cratilo* affirms: "true is the speech that describes things as they are, false is that one that describes them as they aren't". In psychotherapy the concept is to be considered in referring to specific theoretical postulates of different models. In psychoanalysis the reaching of truth, thought to be the purpose of the therapy itself, has been intended as: 1) the record of a bad or traumatic event happened in the past; 2) the discovery and acceptance of a drive, push or a desire that the person feels as unbearable or dangerous; 3) the reconstitution of a sense of authenticity (real Self). Achievement of truth in psychoanalysis is also having conscience and overcoming the → defence mechanisms that work to maintain Ego-dystonic contents in the unconscious: these processes, apart from being responsible for symptomatology, obstruct the object perception of the analyst by the patient (→ transference). Therapies that imitate the phenomenological-existential tradition find truth in the evidence with which phenomenal data appear in the element itself. These data are about → awareness arising from corporal sensations, life experiences, necessities and → responsibility in choices with which the person creates their own existence. This discovery, apart from being, itself, at least partially therapeutic, would allow the person to elaborate past traumas, accept Ego-dystonic desires, make themself responsible for their own life experiences and emotive necessities and individuate and live the personal project of spiritual realization. Classical cognitivism, which starts from completely different premises, has, however, kept the idea that the human psyche can come to a correct and true knowledge of the world around it. This approach has concentrated especially on the elaboration processes of information, affirming that neurosis was the consequence of the reiteration of expectations, considerations and false, inadequate, distorted logical inferences compared to a logically and factually correct valuation of reality. Coherently with this postulate, cognitive therapy tries to give preference to the development of realistic thinking processes, and the restoration of ideas and rational convictions that correspond to reality. Constructivist orientations, which deny that truth can be considered objective or independent in relation to the subject, are opposite to these models; what is called truth, or fact, is nothing more than the result of a perception, elaboration and active building of an interior or environmental reality by the individual. About this Von Foerster, one of the fathers of modern → constructivism, says, in support, that

> reality is just the construction of who believe to have discovered and analysed it. What is hypothetically found out is an invention, the inventor of which doesn't know one's own inventing and considers reality as something that exists independently from itself.
>
> (Watzlawick)

Models that accept this epistemic postulate are the cognitive-constructivist orientations, strategic psychotherapy, hypnosis and a part of systemic-relational orientations. In constructivist psychotherapy, the overtaking of the concept of truth is translated into constructs of "operative conscience", "pragmatism" and "efficiency". The constructivist therapist works with the purpose of helping the patient adapt himself to situations that might reveal themselves as difficult, building more functional reality and perceptions and developing strategies of → problem solving, on one side, structured for reaching concrete purposes, but, on the other, so flexible that they can adapt to the constant evolving of situations. *[V. Luzi]*

REFERENCES. Von Foerster H., *Truth is the invention of a liar: Conversations for sceptics*, 1998; Watzlawick P., *Invented reality: Contributions to constructivism*, 1981.

TUNING TECHNIQUE

Technique of → hypnosis without trance, introduced by G. Nardone in the field of → brief strategic therapy – Nardone's model. This consists of adopting the relational and communicative position that is most suitable to induce the interlocutor to modify his own perceptive-emotional position, reducing to a minimum his → resistance to change. There are many techniques deriving from the strategic model that highlight the importance for the therapist of knowing how to adopt the language, attitudes and communication styles of the patient: M.H. Erickson talked about "learning to use the language of the client"; in the field of → neuro-linguistic programming, great importance is given to the pacing technique; S. de Shazer preferred instead to talk about "joining". All these techniques, even if they have different nuances, emphasize the importance of following closely the language of the client as well as his logic, in such a way as to create an impression of similarity.

The technique of tuning, on the other hand, suggests that, in order to get closer to the other person in an effective way (to create syntonization), it is often necessary to assume different positions and to use different styles of language that are complementary with respect to those of the interlocutor. According to this point of view, therefore, the therapist needs to use language and attitudes that are in harmony with those of the patient, rather than identical or similar, adopting a position that is complementary to the → change that he would like to introduce. Faced with a very talkative patient, for example, the therapist will select short but impactful statements, rather than statements that are long and verbose, in such a way as to avoid establishing a useless symmetry in the relationship. At the same time, faced with a depressed patient, the therapist has to absolutely avoid going along with the position of the patient; rather, he should introduce a form of communication, for example language, that is evocative, that is able to restructure (→ strategic reframing technique) the perception of reality of the patient from the first session. *[R. Milanese]*

REFERENCES. Milanese R., Milanese S., *Il tocco, il rimedio, la parola*, 2017; Nardone G., Loriedo C., Zeig J.K., Watzlawick P., *Ipnosi e terapie ipnotiche*, 2006.

U

UNCONDITIONED REFLEX → UNCONDITIONED RESPONSE

UNCONDITIONED RESPONSE

Also known as an unconditioned reflex, this refers to a → stimulus–response relationship that depends on the phylogenetic characteristics of the individual. Therefore, it deals with a relationship that does not develop and that is not modifiable by experience. For example, if you show some meat to a dog that has been deprived of food, the meat (→ unconditioned stimulus) elicits salivary secretion, in other words, an unconditioned response. Another example relates to the blinking elicited by the presence of a puff of air in the eyes. The unconditioned response has to be distinguished from other stimulus–response associations that are similar in their level of automaticity and awareness, but that are learnt (for example, braking suddenly when seeing a pedestrian). In its common usage this term can be used to indicate the physical component of the stimulus–response relationship (in other words, the unconditioned response). *[A. Couyoumdjian]*

UNCONDITIONED STIMULUS

In the field of behavioural psychology this term refers to the sensorial component of an → unconditioned response. It therefore refers to a sensory stimulus that is able to elicit an unconditioned response on the bases of a phylogenetically determined association. Examples of unconditioned stimuli are food placed in the mouth that induces salivation and the puff of air in the eyes that induces blinking. *[A. Couyoumdjian]*

UNCONSCIOUS

The distinction between conscious and unconscious systems can be traced back to the first Freudian topography (→ topographical model of the mind). It represents the turning point of the rationalization effort made by psychoanalysis to interpret behaviours that seem to escape the control of human will and intentions. In particular, the metaphor of the iceberg highlights that what emerges from man's psychic life is minimal compared to the entire amount of unconscious mental processes. Moreover, it indicates that individuals are much less aware of the reasons behind their behaviour than they think. Therefore, the unconscious is interpreted by psychoanalysis as a meaningful universe, rather than a realm of chaos and irrationality, starting from which, S. Freud stated the possibility of producing rational → interpretations of individuals' healthy and pathological behaviour by integrating the understanding of the biological component of human nature (instincts and → drives) with its social component (moral, world and cultural determinations). Descriptively, the term unconscious applies to all the psychic contents that are not included in the field of conscience. This outlines a mental space or psychic system – the unconscious – that is made of elements that are repressed (→ repression) from consciousness since they are in conflict with some powerful biosocial factors regulating human conduct that are related to the laws and norms of psychosexual development (→ libidinal development stages). According to Freud, the unconscious is not only a place where thoughts, → desires (primarily infantile) → and feelings (the "psychic" objects) are collected, but also a specific functional element of mental processes. *[S. Smiraglia]*

REFERENCES. Ellenberger H.F., *The discovery of the unconscious: The history and evolution of dynamic psychiatry*, 1970.

UNCONSCIOUS FANTASY

In the context of Freudian psychoanalysis, it is an imaginative activity, mostly visual, produced outside consciousness or processed consciously and then repressed. The phantasmatic unconscious activity originates from biological processes and undergoes a symbolic elaboration. An unconscious fantasy is the psychic correlate, the representative content of → drives. It depicts the fulfilment of unconscious wishes in a more or less deformed way due to defensive processes. Unconscious fantasies originate from a child's basic needs in relation to the mother; later, they are organized in scenarios that represent the subject in relation to others. Freud noticed that the outside world represents the place where primary internal objects must be found again. Unconscious fantasies represent an implicit meaning of what is latent in drives, affections and sensations. They show how libidinal drive and → destructiveness can be represented in archaic mental processes. Starting from Freud, the psychoanalytic theory tries to explain the stability, efficacy and the relatively organized nature of phantasmatic life underlying thoughts, feelings and motivations. Isaacs elaborated the notion of unconscious fantasy in a systematic way as it had emerged in the early works of M. Klein on children in 1921. Unconscious fantasy characterizes unconscious contents that can become conscious or not: it tends to combine internal drives with the outside world. This occurs both in mentally healthy and ill individuals. *[G. Perfetto, A. Voltolin]*

REFERENCES. Freud S. (1919), *A child being beaten*, in *The Standard Edition*, XVII, 1953–1974; Isaacs S., *The nature and function of fantasy*, in «International Journal of Psycho-Analysis», 29, 1948; Laplanche J., Pontalis J.B., *Originary phantasm, phantasms of origins, origins of the phantasm*, 1964.

UNDERWORLD

By using a Freudian metaphor, Jung often compares unconscious contents to the products of an "underground" world and the process of assimilation of the unconscious to a Dantesque journey that involves a descent into the underworld and the subsequent ascent to the surface. For example, he identified the image of his own concept of → anima in the classical myth of Demeter and Kore. This is intended as a function of the unconscious psyche aiming at integration with the consciousness. This function is partly related to the underworld (which includes the concept of evil and darkness) and partly considered a protective guide towards spiritual creativity when experiencing the wholeness of the Self. Similar is the alchemic metaphor used by Jung to describe the process of integration between consciousness and the unconscious as an immersion in a purifying bath or as a death that leads to rebirth. *[A. De Coro]*

REFERENCES. Jung C.G. (1941), *The psychological aspect of the Kore*, in *Collected Works*, IX/I, 1969.

UNIFYING CENTRE

According to psychosynthesis, a psychological entity able to harmonize and co-ordinate the various components of the personality around its centre. This centre can be "outside" the person, for example, when a man or a woman identifies themselves with their professional role or parenting functions; or, on the other hand, "inside" the person, as in the case of a dominant inclination, a creative task or a dominating tendency. Nevertheless, the real unifying centre must coincide with our real Self, in its different levels of manifestation and consciousness: personal or transpersonal self. All the other unifying centres are temporary, even if some of these efficacious results can last throughout one's life. The concept "unifying centre" is closely connected to "synthesis", because every synthesis is created from the action of a different and higher factor. And we must regard every synthesis as "partial synthesis", or rather temporary: otherwise our growth could stop but, on the contrary, life, with its continuous reshuffling of the cards, asks us, on the one hand, to integrate new parts, on the other hand, to replace elements that do not exist anymore. This process is one of continuous reorganization. *[D. De Paolis]*

REFERENCES. Assagioli R., *Psychosynthesis: A manual of principles and techniques*, 1965; Assagioli R., *Psicosintesi: per l' armonia della vita*, 1966.

UNUSUAL REMARK

According to narrative therapy, an unusual remark in the patient's account points to a discrepancy, revealing a possible alternative vision of the dominant reality; it comes from a subordinate, dimly lit but socially shared, sphere of reality, called the sociological underworld. It presents the therapist with an approachable way of modifying the rigid and symptomatic perception of the story (→ stories) upheld by patients and by their social contexts. Therapists can also use unusual remarks (→ astonishment) alien to patients' views and opinions for therapeutic goals, by adopting persuasive techniques described by classical rhetoric and, nowadays, employed in business and advertising (i.e. amplifying to the point of absurdity patients' own statements, stressing content and emotional tone). *[G. Manfrida, E. Giachi]*

REFERENCES. Berger P.L., Luckmann T., *The social construction of reality*, 1966; Manfrida G.M., *La narrazione psicoterapeutica. Invenzione, persuasione e tecniche retoriche in terapia relazionale*, 1998; Manfrida G.M., *Plausible, convincing and appealing. characteristics and development of therapeutic stories in a shared reality approach*, in «Journal of Systemic Therapies», 2011, 30.

UTILIZATION

Central principle of Ericksonian psychotherapy, defined as the readiness of the therapist to respond strategically to all aspects of the patient or the environment. Utilization can be considered as the trance of the therapist – the condition in which the hypnotherapist assumes an externally focused trance – in comparison to the trance of the patient that is, instead, directed internally. This externally focused trance is characterized by a state of readiness to respond and to seize the moment by capturing and using whatever happens. In fact, if the therapist wants to promote a state of readiness to respond in the patient, he first must be willing to show the same kind of responsiveness. With this in mind, the therapist can use something coming from the environment (such as the pressure of the back of the chair), something coming from the patient (such as an idiosyncratic language), the sequence of the problem or the symptomatic behaviour itself. Even the therapist's family or the therapist's handicaps can be used, as M.H. Erickson demonstrated repeatedly in numerous therapies. Whatever exists in the environment, in the patient, in their history, in their problem, in the therapist's office, can be used.

Utilization indicates that the therapist is an active participant in the process of co-creation of → change occurring in the patient and, as a central construct of the Ericksonian model, it can be used both in → hypnosis and in psychotherapy. Four key principles of utilization can be identified. First principle: the therapist's induction comes first. Second: whatever the patient brings can be used; everything that exists in the therapeutic situation can be used. Third: any technique adopted by the patient to be a patient can be exploited by the therapist. Fourth: whatever answers are obtained by the therapist, he or she must develop them.

The construct of utilization appeared at the beginning of the experimental work of Erickson and has been developed and extended by a large number of important thinkers who followed in his footsteps, such as J. Haley, M. Yapko, S. Gilligan and B. O'Hanlon, just to name a few. All Erickson's followers have turned to the principle of utilization and they incorporated it into their own theories and methods. In fact, it can be said that utilization is, for Ericksonian psychotherapy, what analysis is for dynamic approaches or conditioning for behavioural psychotherapy. *[J.K. Zeig]*

REFERENCES. Zeig J.K. (ed), *The evolution of psychotherapy: The second conference*, 1992; Zeig J.K., Lankton S.R. (eds.), *Developing Ericksonian therapy: State of the art*, 1988

UTOPIA

A term used in individual psychology in an intrasubjective sense to indicate the individual's striving for the ideal Self and to go beyond the limits; in the experiential sense it refers to striving for a gratifying and fulfilling relationship with the world and with others. Striving for perfection substantiates the conscious and unconscious tissue of Self, activates defensive structures, configures some lines of the life project, and modulates lifestyle. A utopian ideal implanted in the power of → creative Self can represent an encouraging and transformative force; in a pathological sense, it can induce melancholic experiences of inferiority and impotence. The ideal of utopia is linked to social feeling, i.e. the individual's ability to relate in a genuinely cooperative way. In the psychotherapeutic relationship, the utopia of perfect healing can help to support a constructive resolution, but it must never deviate into unattainable directions, which would consequently be discouraging. *[A. Bianconi, C. Gasparini]*

REFERENCES. Adler A., *The neurotic character*, 1912, in *The collected clinical works of Alfred Adler*, I, 2002; Adler A., *The practice and theory of individual psychology*, 1920.

V

VERISIMILITUDE

Resemblance to the truth. They can be defined as verisimilar all those statements that do not contain logical contradictions, that do not conflict with the technical knowledge of human societies and that do not deny the possibilities of human behaviour or, more generally, the known natural laws. According to K. Popper, verisimilitude is the highest aspiration of a scientific theory, which can never be considered definitively true. In fact, according to the criterion of falsifiability, a theory can be considered as scientific only when there is a theoretical condition where it can be proved to be false, that is, when it can be refuted. It follows that a theory can be, at the most, verisimilar, that is, approaching asymptotically an unattainable truth. In other words, a theory is verisimilar because it gets closer than other theories to the → truth. A scientist who wants to reach a thorough understanding of phenomena needs to create more and more refined experiments, which may increase the "truth content" of the theories underlying them, making them closer to the truth. *[R.]*

VERTEX

In Bion's thought, the term describes a "viewpoint" or "perspective" starting from which an experience can be psychologically represented. Just as a three-dimensional object can be better understood by being seen from many different directions, so there are many different points of view by which aspects of the psychoanalytic object can be revealed, such as from the perspective of money, medicine, religion or education. *[J. Symington]*

REFERENCES. Bion W.R., *Transformations*, 1965; Bion W.R., *Attention and interpretation*, 1970.

VICARIOUS LEARNING

A typical form of → modelling. According to the views of the first behaviourists, influenced by the epistemological perspective against introspection, learning would take place through associated stimuli (→ classical conditioning) or by the consolidation of reinforced responses (→ operant conditioning). Through vicarious learning, internal elements start to be introduced and individuals are recognized as having an active role in their learning process, which occurs through the imitation of a model. In a therapeutic context, it is important to remember that vicarious learning is more effective if the model is perceived as authoritative or close to the patient. In the latest developments of the → social cognitive theory, the relationship between the subject's active role in vicarious learning, self-efficacy and perceived → human agency has been highlighted. *[F. Celi]*

REFERENCES. Bandura A., *Social learning theory*, 1977; Id., *Toward an agentic theory of the self*, in H. Marsh, R.G. Craven, D.M. McInerney (eds.), *International advances in self research*, III, 2008; Miller N.E., Dollard J., *Social learning and imitation*, 1941.

VOMITING

A term used in → brief strategic therapy – Nardone's model, that was first introduced in the book *Prison of Food*, to indicate a form of eating disorder, distinct from anorexia and bulimia nervosa. It is based on the → intervention-research conducted by the Centro di Terapia Strategica in Arezzo in the 1990s. The "vomiting syndrome" represents a technological specialization of the other two disorders and it is based on the compulsive need to eat and vomit for pleasure, rather than vomiting after binging to avoid putting on weight. The pleasurable sequence of eating and vomiting makes this typical compulsion uncontrollable. This compulsion becomes a true model of pleasure-seeking behaviour that people are no longer able to renounce. Vomiting can therefore be considered a sort of perversion or pleasure-based compulsion rather than a true eating disorder. This is why the disorder presents a considerable → resistance to change and requires an ad hoc treatment protocol (→ strategic treatment protocol), different from those used for anorexia and bulimia (→ postponing pleasurable compulsions). *[R. Milanese]*

REFERENCES. Nardone G., *Al di là dell"amore e dell'odio per il cibo*, 2003; Nardone G., Verbitz T., Milanese R., *Prison of food*, 2005; Nardone G., Selekman M.D., *Uscire dalla trappola*, 2011.

W

WELLBEING

An overall sensation of satisfaction with regard to one's own life, in relation to the gratification of psychological, emotional, social, spiritual and physical → needs and → desires. An individual's wellbeing resides both in the biological dimension of the organism and in the quality of the relationship that the person has with themselves, other people and the world. Among the important factors that generate wellbeing, is the expression of one's own potential and talents and the ability to address and solve problems within one's own life. The modern biopsychosocial vision has allowed the the traditional biomedical view to be overturned; this view defined health and wellbeing in terms of absence of organic diseases, and the body was considered as a machine and malaise as a failure or a malfunction caused by an external pathogenic agent. Nowadays, body and mind are considered integrated dimensions of the individual and wellbeing is seen as a point of balance between all the factors involved. In the modern perspective, also supported by the positions of WHO (World Health Organization), the idea of wellbeing has been increasingly focused on the presence of behaviours that continuously improve one's personal level of satisfaction: wellbeing is thus comparable to a dynamic process that looks for a functional adaptation to the environment, and therefore it maintains a nature of subjectivity, contextual relativity and historical variability *[R.]*

WELLBEING PSYCHOTHERAPY

Traditionally psychotherapy has been dedicated to the understanding and treatment of psychopathological manifestations, with a focus on trauma, syndromes, disorders and deficiencies. This understanding and treatment considers mental health as a mere absence of the symptoms just described. In relatively recent times, as Seligman, Rashid and Parks noted, the focus has gradually shifted towards the positive aspects of life, such as happiness, psychological wellbeing and personal resources. In the past, there were researchers who considered qualities such as self-interest and personal maturity to be the optimal level of psychological functioning; it is only towards the end of the twentieth century that there was real action directed towards the promotion of happiness, such as those proposed by Fordyce; through the emergence of positive psychology other publications have been written such as *Positive Psychotherapy* by Seligman and collaborators, and *Well-being Therapy* by The Fava Group.

THE FIRST CONTRIBUTIONS ON HAPPINESS PSYCHOTHERAPY BY MICHAEL FORDYCE. In the late 1970s, Fordyce reflected on the meaning of "personal happiness" and, in accordance with the prevailing literature, he agreed that a pervasive and continuous feeling of emotional wellbeing can serve as a comprehensive indicator of life satisfaction. Although the research had already provided an ample and consistent framework about the personality and environmental attributes that characterized the people who had reached a high level of happiness, Fordyce noted that, at the time, there was no experimental work about the possibility of permanently increasing the feeling of happiness and wellbeing of individuals. He directed his attention towards college students, with the intention of promoting their happiness and wellbeing through a series of psycho-educational interventions based on accurate information and specific exercises. Fordyce conducted a number of studies aimed at the acquisition and application of information on expressions of human happiness. In one of his studies, the participants of the first group, stimulated by reading his text "Human Happiness: the

Findings of Psychological Research", were able to identify and implement the conduct and habits of the people who were happier. The participants of the second group were encouraged to complete nine activities on a daily basis, deemed by Fordyce to be particularly effective in promoting psychological wellbeing. In a second phase of the survey, students received detailed instructions on the tasks to be performed daily to achieve 14 objectives, such as attitudes and behaviours considered key to achieving a state of greater happiness. The goals suggested included: developing emotional relationships, resizing your expectations, being productive doing activities that have meaning, eliminating negative feelings and problems, being good friends, not worrying, and being focused on the present. Though he knew the limits of the reliability of the instruments used to measure the outcomes of the intervention, at the end of these studies Fordyce suggested that the programmes aimed at the development of happiness: were possible and effective; could be intended for young people and adults; taught participants about the nature and factors of personal happiness; and favoured the development and the practical application of knowledge in this area.

MARTIN SELIGMAN: FROM POSITIVE PSYCHOLOGY TO POSITIVE PSYCHOTHERAPY. Before World War II, psychology had three missions: curing mental illness; making the lives of all people more rewarding; and enabling them to identify and develop talent. At the end of the 1990s, Seligman found that during the postwar period, psychology was mainly focused on the study and treatment of psychopathological states. In 1998, at the time of his appointment as president of the American Psychological Association, Seligman expressed the intention to guide research towards the factors that promote wellbeing and personal development and onto the psychological interventions aimed at improving the living conditions of the individual and the community. The first issue of *American Psychologist* in 2000 opens with an introduction by Seligman and Csikszentmihalyi on positive psychology. This publication shifted the focus of psychology from a sole emphasis on the "repair" aspects of the worst realities of life to the promotion of positive qualities. Although positive psychology had several illustrious predecessors and was not an original idea, until now it had not been possible to promote the formation of a large group of research and practitioners, such as to provide a solid empirical basis to theoretical elaborations. The successive contributions of research and reflection have led to a conceptual understanding of positive psychology as the scientific study of positive experiences, positive individual traits and the structures and social organizations that facilitate their development. The prospects of intervention already outlined in Fordyce's work has a more detailed exposition in "Positive psychology in clinical practice", where it is claimed that people want to be more satisfied, gratified and happy instead of being only less sad and worried. It also states that people aim to strengthen their own resources rather than focusing on solely correcting their weaknesses. On the basis of these guidelines, Seligman, Rashid and Parks treated depression by applying methods of intervention defined as "positive psychotherapy". These initiatives are aimed primarily at encouraging the development of positive emotions directly through the activation of personal psychological resources, and life enhancement, rather than addressing the mitigation of negative symptoms. The research, conducted in a variety of contexts, has demonstrated the efficacy of this approach: the development of internet exercises inspired by positive psychology has resulted in slightly depressed subjects, who had taken part in the trial, having a reduction of symptoms for at least six months. In addition, positive psychotherapy, balanced by a traditional approach attentive to psychopathological symptoms and conducted individually with depressed patients, proved equally effective. The authors do not exclude the possibility that this approach could be effective with other psychological disorders.

WELLBEING PSYCHOTHERAPY. The expectations that the authors mentioned above have expressed the usefulness of the positive approach with disorders other than depression are widespread and there is convincing confirmation in clinical trials conducted by Fava and his group. The wellbeing psychotherapy – as indicated by Fava's *Well-Being Therapy* – has been developed and applied during the last 90 years, initially with patients suffering from depression and, later, referring to other diagnoses, such as generalized anxiety disorder, panic and agoraphobia. For the setting and the development of this therapeutic strategy, aimed at facilitating the psychological wellbeing and quality of life, reference is made to the specific model of C. Ryff. This model conceptualizes psychological wellbeing in six dimensions: autonomy, self-acceptance, environmental control, personal growth, purpose in life and positive relationships. Using these techniques inspired by cognitive-behavioural psychotherapy – which among other things provides a template for self-observation, the systematic use of the diary, the performance of specific tasks, interaction between patient and therapist – has tended to improve the general level of psychological wellbeing, based upon Ryff's model.

The intervention is performed when the patient, after successfully completing the specific pharmacological or psychotherapeutic treatment still presented some form of residual discomfort, such as: irritability, anxiety, interpersonal problems and difficulty in experiencing pleasure. The acquisition of a higher state of wellbeing associated with a greater ability to face and overcome life's adversities, reduces vulnerability to possible future adversities and contributes markedly to prevent recurrence, as the path to lasting healing is not only about mitigating the negative, but also promoting the positive.

Among the latest developments in wellbeing psychotherapy, there is a growing emphasis on the possible future implementation of group interventions and the development of prevention programmes for children. Preliminary action research recently carried out with students in the first year of high school set out to promote positive emotions and psychological wellbeing through the use of concepts and techniques such as those set out above. The intervention, but not psychotherapy, aimed at adolescents of both sexes, has proved effective both in promoting psychological wellbeing and in alleviating psychological distress, especially anxiety and somatization.

CONCLUDING REMARKS. Fordyce and, initially, Seligman have turned their interventions to the use of the "non-clinical" population. In the case of positive psychotherapy, computer exercises were used based on intervention programmes offered via the internet. Later, Seligman and Fava were interested in clinical subjects who had mainly mood disorders, but also anxiety syndromes. The Fava group has, in recent times, trialled the promotion of psychological wellbeing with the use of school groups. The model being pursued by these authors presents common features and some differences: Fordyce proposes the achievement of a state of happiness, but it is not always clearly defined; Seligman sees wellbeing as an intrinsic human capacity for development and Fava enhances the proven model of Ryff's psychological wellbeing.

Patients with overt psychological disorders are treated in a personalized manner; this treatment is implemented within a specific therapeutic relationship. Fava and his team obtained the remission of symptoms by both pharmacological and psychological interventions, additionally implementing wellbeing psychotherapy in order to consolidate the achievements and prevent relapse and recurrence. On the other hand, Seligman believes that positive psychotherapy, not mentioning specific psychopathological symptoms, is required through direct action to stimulate positive emotions and existential involvement, as well as to discern meaning in life.

Thus, what has emerged is a consistent corpus of concepts and techniques for the promotion of psychological wellbeing in large "non-clinical" population groups, also demonstrating the use of the opportunities offered by the internet, which do not require a direct relationship between therapist and patient. In addition, these new procedures can both strengthen and make permanent the results obtained by conventional therapies, and integrate treatments traditionally oriented to treat symptomatic manifestations. *[Sirigatti, B. Giangrasso]*

REFERENCES. Duckworth A.L., Steen T.A., Seligman M.E.P., *Positive psychology in clinical practice*, in «Annual Review of Clinical Psychology», 2005, 1; Fava G.A., Ruini C., *Development and characteristics of a well-being enhancing psychotherapeutic strategy: Well-being therapy*, in «Journal of Behaviour Therapy and Experimental Psychiatry», 2003, 34; Fordyce M.W., *Development of a program to increase personal happiness*, in «Journal of Counselling Psychology », 1977, 24; Id., *Human happiness: The findings of psychological research*, 1974, in Id., *A program to increase happiness: Further studies*, in «Journal of Counselling Psychology», 1983, 30, 4; Seligman M.E.P, Csikszentmihalyi M., *Positive psychology: An introduction*, in «American Psychologist », 2000, 5; Seligman M.E.P., Rashid T., Parks A.C., *Positive psychotherapy*, in «American Psychologist», 2006, 61.

WILD PSYCHOANALYSIS

Expression introduced by Freud in 1910, the year of the foundation of the International Association of Psychoanalysis, that stigmatizes, in the treatment of a patient, "the recourse to psychoanalytic notions that are not based on a sufficient understanding of the theory and/or of the technique, that is not guided by 'tact' that helps the clinician to find the right words at the right time". This practice will cause harm to the patient as well as to psychoanalysis, constituting a form of "abuse". The term "wild" is applied by Freud to the analyst that does not have the proper training, as well as to an intervention that does not respect the patient as an individual and the process of treatment. In Freud's work, one can retrace the double preoccupation – deontological and political – that is the mark of a concept that marks the fortune and the limitations of a concept that is always at risk of transforming itself into an anathema. *[S. Nicasi]*

REFERENCES. Ferenczi S., *The elasticity of psycho-analytic technique*, in *Final contributions to the problems and methods of psycho-analysis*, 1928; Freud S. (1910), "Wild" psychoanalysis, in *The Standard Edition*, XI, 1953–1974; Napolitano F., *La filiazione e la trasmissione nella psicoanalisi*, 1999.

WILL

A regulatory function of voluntary conscious conduct directed to a purpose. Will is the synthesis between the emotional-affective, cognitive-rational and behavioural components of an individual. In this sense, it involves motivational elements, such as desires and emotions, cognitive elements, such as the representation and the strategic planning of goals, and behavioural-strategic elements, such as the selection and implementation of the most appropriate actions to achieve a goal. From a psychopathological perspective, the disorder of this regulatory function is immediately evident in addiction problems (where, for example, the conscious efforts to avoid taking a drug do not have any results), in obsessive-compulsive disorders (doubt, inner conflict, persistent and Ego-dystonic thoughts, rituals), in depressive disorders (aboulia or ipobulia, respectively lack or shortage of will, reduction of interest, concentration difficulties) and in loss of control over impulses (→ acting out). The concept of will is opposed to → spontaneity, understood as the free use of natural instances. → Common sense, but also some forms of psychotherapy, give this term a meaning analogous to health and freedom, whereas other approaches consider the acquiring of control of one's own → impulses as essential. In recent years, the most accredited position sees the achievement of psychological integration as based on a succession of will and spontaneity. In the light of the above considerations, the psychotherapeutic work addresses the issue of will in complex ways. The therapist considers whether patients are located at the level of perception and awareness of their own feelings or emotions, at a cognitive processing level or at the level of behavioural-strategic management of their feelings and emotions. *[R.]*

▷ In the psychodynamic field, will, in the terms conceived by Rank, is that instance which brings into play all activities and energies without repressing any of them. It essentially is the will to be born again, to self-generate, to create. It is a concept that seemed generic, elusive or, even, contradictory to most, and it has been criticized as "pre-psychoanalytic". As a consequence, it cannot be fruitfully approached without embracing multiple points of view. Rank, indeed, conceives will in relationship to constructs of → projection and creation, → birth trauma and → anguish, → separation and → sense of guilt. Since the "world is my projection" (that is how Rank retranslates A. Schopenhauer), one is born when becoming aware of this projection. Projection itself inhibits birth. The consequence is that the neurotic is a failed artist, to the extent to which one suffers because of an inhibited will. Analogously, Freud, in whose lexicon the term "will" is not considered, did not understand that the father is a symbol of the person's inhibited will and has interpreted it as resistance, which is, instead, the counter-will of the patient. Will substantiates itself in wanting birth and its trauma; that is to say: wanting separation and → individuation; putting up with anguish and guilt. That is what the myth of genesis and that of Prometheus would be about; an instance where, creating, it paradoxically produces guilt at the same time. That is what the → Oedipus complex is about, reconceived like a conflict of will: the child's will (of separation, self-generation) against the parents' counter-will. In this view, the hero doesn't aim at getting into their father's place, as Oedipus would like to, but it aspires to be a representative of the individual's creative will. Therapy, ultimately, consists in letting the creative will emerge in the patient. *[G. Antonelli]*

REFERENCES. Rank O., *Wahrheit und Wirklichkeit*, 1929; Id., *Die analytische Reaktion in ihren konstruktiven Elementen*, 1929.

WILL TO MEANING

One of the three pilars of → logotherapy and existential analysis according to V.E. Frankl, together with freedom of will and meaning of life. It represents the main motivational principle of the human person, which is mainly oriented to → self-transcendence: not striving for pleasure (Freud; → pleasure principle and reality principle) or power (Adler), but aiming at meaning. The will to meaning, rooted in the spiritual dimension of the human being, does not fit Maslow's hierarchy of needs because it is not a "need": it can be deeply frustrated even when every psycho-physical need is adequately satisfied (for instance in the phenomenon of "existential vacuum" and noogenic neurosis) and, on the other hand, expresses itself even when all the basic needs are systematically frustrated (for instance in concentration camps, where Frankl was imprisoned between 1942 until 1945). For this reason, it is an essential resource (→ resilience) in facing limits and extreme situations in life. Search for meaning is potentially inexhaustible and requires an unconditional object of intention (the so-called "ultimate meaning") that in the light of faith becomes the religious relationship to God. Experimental detection of the will to meaning has been operated through several psychometric tests, which measure existential gratification or frustration and goal orientation: PIL (Purpose in Life Questionnaire) by J.C. Crumbaugh and L.T. Maholick, SONG (Seeking of Noetic Goals Test) by Crumbaugh, Logotest by E. Lukas, Belfast Test by B. Giorgi, MIST (Meaning in Suffering Test) by P.L. Starck, and so on. *[D. Bruzzone]*

REFERENCES. Batthyany A., Guttmann D., *Empirical research on logotherapy and meaning-oriented psychotherapy*, 2005; Frankl V.E., *Man's search for meaning*, 1959; Id., *The will to meaning*, 1969.

WISH FULFILMENT

In Freudian psychoanalysis, the notion of "wish fulfilment" derives from the empirical datum of an infant's incapacity to provide for his/her own needs. In the absence of an adult to provide adequate care, there occurs a hallucinatory reinvestment of the mnestic traces of previous experiences of wish fulfilment. Therefore, wish fulfilment is primarily connected with a → drive and consists in the abatement of tension – potentially to a zero degree – also known as the principle of neuronic inertia or Nirvana principle; on the other hand, life pulsions determine only a relative abatement of the tension (principle of constance). The development of the Ego inhibits the intensity of the investment of the mnestic traces, thereby replacing a "hallucination" with a "representation" of the wish fulfilment under the guise of its desire. This developmental process involves the passage from a "perceptual identity" to a "thought identity" and leads to the acquisition of the "principle of Definitive Reality" (see also → pleasure principle and reality principle) *[F. Conrotto]*

REFERENCES. Breuer J., Freud S. (1893–1895), *Studies on hysteria*, in *The Standard Edition*, II, 1953–1974; Freud S. (1911), *Formulations on the two principles of mental functioning*, in The Standard Edition, XII, 1953–1974; Id. (1920), *Beyond the pleasure principle*, in *The Standard Edition*, XIV, 1953–1974.

WORST FANTASY TECHNIQUE

A technique used in brief strategic therapy, Nardone model, devised by G. Nardone at the end of the 1980s for the treatment of phobic disorders, panic attacks and obsessions. The patient is asked to isolate himself every day for half an hour and to try to imagine all the worst fantasies with regard to his fears, phobias or obsessions, forcing himself to try and provoke as much anxiety as possible in himself and to give vent to all the feelings that these fantasies evoke in him. This technique is based on paradoxical logic (→ logic of paradox): the more a person tries to voluntarily evoke anxiety in himself, which by its nature is spontaneous, the more this will be inhibited because of the → "be spontaneous" paradox. In this way, the person will experience for the first time an important → corrective emotional experience with regard to the management of his anxiety, discovering that he is able to quash it by trying to produce it. In the subsequent therapeutic sessions, the patient is instructed in using the same technique, this time, however, dividing the time spent conjuring up their worst fantasies through the course of the day (five minutes every three hours, five times a day), with the final aim of using this technique only when needed (five minutes every time it is needed), in other words, in situations where anxiety is experienced.

By learning how to use this technique, patients are able to discover how to manage their anxiety effectively and can, in this way, be guided in overcoming, in conjunction with the use of other techniques, the limits that their fear has introduced in their lives. *[R.Milanese]*

REFERENCES. Nardone G., *Brief strategic solution-oriented therapy of phobic and obsessive disorders*, 1996; Id., *La terapia degli attacchi di panico*, 2016; Nardone G., Watzlawick P., *The art of change*, 1993.

WRITTEN EMOTIONAL DISCLOSURE

A cognitive-behavioural psychotherapy method that requires the subject to produce a short, written description, in a limited period of time (typically 15 to 30 minutes), of a specific episode related to a very painful or traumatic personal experience. The report, varying in length from a half to two pages, asks for a description of one's own experience, without adding any other, previous or subsequent, elements. However, it is a requirement that the most painful emotions experienced are described, as well as more hidden thoughts, even those never shared with anyone. This mode of writing is considered "intensive"; shorter or longer descriptions, oral descriptions, or positive episodes do not fall within the definition of written emotional expression. *[L. Sibilia]*

REFERENCES. Lepore S.J., Smyth J.M. (eds.), *The writing cure: How expressive writing promotes health and emotional well-being*, 2002; Pennebaker J.W., *Expressive writing therapy*, in I. Marks (ed.), L. Sibilia, S. Borgo (eds.), *Common language for psychotherapy procedures*, 2010.

APPENDIX

Empirical research in psychotherapy

Gianluca Castelnuovo, Enrico Molinari, Giorgio Nardone, Alessandro Salvini

Introduction

Is there only one way to deal with psychological issues? A complex discipline such as psychotherapy can offer a number of different approaches to treatment and care, each characterized by a peculiar way of coping with patients' issues: past–present, individual–family, reflection–action, cause–goal are among the themes on which each psychology and psychotherapy school can assume points of view that can even be diametrically opposed. In the past half-century, research in psychotherapy has grown, with thousands of studies proving both the efficacy and efficiency of many psychotherapeutic treatments for a wide range of mental issues. Traditionally, clinicians believe that researchers, through the use of statistical analysis, have come to the same conclusions that had been reached years before only relying on clinical experience.

Today, research and clinical practice are in an ongoing dialogue; to bridge the gap between these two in psychotherapy, researchers have been focusing attention on the efficacy and efficiency of different treatments. In this investigation about mental health, two different approaches are the most common among researchers and practitioners.[1, 2] On one side, the development of empirically supported treatments (ESTs) based on randomized controlled trials[3, 4] (RCTs) in the evidence-based medicine (EBM) stream; on the other side, we underline the growth in the number of studies on the Common Factors Perspective, according to the confirmation of the so-called "Dodo Bird Verdict".[5, 6] The distinction between these two different approaches is mostly related to completely distinct epistemological and philosophical attitudes towards psychotherapy and research. These two different approaches are well described by Tracey[7] (2003):

> one view is that each model of therapy has distinctive effects on clients. This assumption of distinctiveness leads naturally to the inference that some models are more effective than others with particular client types. A competing and perhaps complementary view is that different theoretical approaches are comparably effective.
>
> (p. 401)

Modern research in psychotherapy can be traced back to the 1950s. In particular, in 1952, British psychologist Eysenck questioned the scientificity of psychotherapy, giving it no more efficacy than the absence of treatment: going to the therapist didn't work better than not going.[8] Psychotherapy was questioned throughout the following decade[9], until the publication of thousands of studies supporting the superiority of psychotherapy, compared to other treatments, related to some mental issues.[10,11] It even turned on its head the scenario described by Eysenck – from the Dodo Bird's pronouncement (contained in the novel *Alice in Wonderland*): "Everybody has won, and all must have prizes" –, namely, the efficacy of various techniques of psychotherapy appeared similar. A great merit in the field of research in psychotherapy should be given also to the Society of Psychotherapy Research that has promoted, since 1968, the creation of an international network of scholars on this topic (for further information please refer to www.psychotherapyresearch.org). Other international research networks later arise, like the brief psychotherapy ones that can be found at www.bsst.org and www.aabst.org

Empirically supported treatments: the evidence-based medicine movement in psychotherapy

The evidence-based medicine movement has determined profound changes, both at the research level and in clinical practice in health treatment. As Sanderson stated:

> the emergence of managed care and similar reimbursement systems that require greater accountability and the development of clinical practice guidelines have increased the importance of evidence-based clinical practice. As a result of these two trends, it appears as though the future of psychotherapy will require clinicians to deliver a psychological intervention that is supported by research.
>
> (p. 290)[12]

Some approaches in psychotherapy reacted defensively to this trend. For example, the psychoanalytic approach has traditionally been based on the assumption that theoretical principles can be developed only with single-case studies in uncontrolled clinical settings.[13] Existential and humanistic therapies perceive RCTs (randomized controlled trials that are the basis of EBM methods) as a dehumanizing procedure unable to capture the critical factors responsible for change, such as the therapist–client relationship.[14] Since the 1990s, the American Psychological Association (APA) has created a list of scientific (empirical) treatments tested for their efficacy:[12] these are empirically supported treatments, which are based on empirical studies. The birth of this new psychotherapy approach dates back to 1995, when the Task Force on Promotion and Dissemination of Psychological Procedures of Division 12 (Clinical Psychology) of the American Psychological Association (APA) identified "a number of psychological interventions as empirically validated treatments (EVTs), later called empirically supported treatments (ESTs).[14, 15]

The interest in promoting the importance of ESTs probably finds its origin in a broader movement, born in the United Kingdom, named evidence-based medicine (EBM).[16] In the 1995 report, the Task Force indicated the criteria to select an EST and reported a very preliminary list of 25 selected treatments that reached the amount of 71 in 1998[17, 18] and continued to increase in 2001.[15] A similar approach encountered much criticism, mostly because it doesn't seem comprehensive of the entire psychotherapies survey, representing only those that are best suited to certain research designs (we can speak of a distortion towards cognitive-behavioural therapies, more suitable for measurements and clinical trial protocols). Despite the APA's emphasis, these evidence-based psychotherapies are not widely used for those working in the field. Herbert noticed that "this effort has been met with criticism, however, both by practitioners, on one hand, and psychotherapy researchers on the other".[4] Moreover, a consensus regarding the criteria for determining what is empirically supported or not has not yet been reached.[19]

Many critical issues have been highlighted regarding the ESTs approach. A first general consideration allows it, first of all, to be noted that the development of evidence-based medicine has become a real "social phenomenon": "EBM has acquired a powerful role of making 'verdicts' about what is good treatment and what is not" (p. 278).[20] It is also important to consider that the standard EBM procedures are often not applicable in the field of psychotherapy, since they are based on observation and research, therefore never free from theories or values. However, the core assumption of EBM is scientific realism, "which postulates that there is an independently existing reality and that the truth about such reality is attainable through scientific investigation" (p. 279).[20] Some authors stated that, in the clinical field, can be found "a rejection of empirical epistemology in general and randomized clinical trials in particular, as legitimate methods for evaluating psychotherapies" (p. 413).[4] Therefore, can the status of the specific procedures for identifying ESTs be regarded as scientific? The ESTs approach is built on the medical model where the steps towards the improvement of the symptom are characterized by the diagnosis and the prescription of a treatment.[14] In this scenario, where the RCTs method is used to evaluate psychotherapy, hazardous, if not negative, effects can be obtained. A lucid description of these possible consequences is reported by Duncan:

> it meant that a study must include manualized therapies (to approximate drug protocols) and Diagnostic and Statistical Manual of Mental Disorders (4th Ed., DSM– IV; American Psychiatric Association, 1994) defined disorders to be eligible for an NIMH-sponsored research grant. The result: Funding for studies not related to specific disorders dropped nearly 200% from the late 1980s to 1990 [. . .]. In addition to these limiting effects, force fitting the RCT on psychotherapy research is empirical tyranny and bereft of scientific reasoning
>
> (p. 45)

The cognitive-behavioural model has benefited by imposing a certain supremacy in the ESTs lists.

Another negative effect, beside the omission of many non–cognitive-behavioural oriented treatments,[22] is the limitation of innovation in clinical practice and research in psychotherapy,[23] also emphasized by Jacobson: "moreover, randomized clinical trials can evaluate only currently existing treatments; they cannot develop new and better ones" (p. 1038).[24] In agreement with the current criteria, for a treatment to be "probably efficacious" it simply needs to show its superiority in comparison to the non-treatment condition (for example, a waiting-list condition). Many authors have criticized this approach;[25, 26] with the use of this dangerous criterion "virtually any intervention is superior to no-treatment, especially for mood and anxiety disorders" (p. 417),[4] thus even prayers and placebo could be included in the ESTs list.

There are other methodological issues in dispute. One is that a treatment can be considered effective only with the minimum standard of two supportive studies: "to make the EVT list, an approach needs only to prove its efficacy, or superiority over the placebo condition, in two studies" (p. 44),[21] "even if 50 other studies failed to find positive effects" (p. 418).[4] Thus, there is a bias against publication of null results.[27] Another issue is how to distinguish between seemingly similar treatments. Currently the border between different approaches, reported as ESTs, seems overly based on appearance (frequently it is only the name that is considered); a negative consequence of this might be that "a potentially infinite number of variations of established treatments may be added to the list" (p. 419).[4] For example, several studies have shown that the features that may distinguish eye movement desensitization and reprocessing (EMDR), included as EST, from imaginative exposure are negligible.[28] Moreover, the criteria currently in use do not include the possibility of a treatment to be removed from the list, even if alternative procedures have proven their superiority.[29]

Another important point to consider is the excessive focus on symptom reduction rather than on the patient's fulfilment-wellbeing and a perceived improvement in quality of life.[4, 30] In this regard, it should be emphasized that an improvement in psychotherapy can not only coincide with the symptom reduction or disappearance; the therapist works also on issues that don't correspond to psychopathology as inferred by the DSM-IV-TR (American Psychiatric Association, 2000). Not just relational, familiar, couple issues but existential, evolutionary issues as well, don't have a diagnostic label to be included in the official nosologic manuals, but they are also hardly considered and measured with traditional tools in the clinical trials research. Even personality disorders and comorbidities (co-occurring mental disorders) are little considered in a logic based on the symptoms typical of a clinical trial: the risk of this science is the loss of representativeness because, given the randomized procedures, patients tend to be so "pure" (with only one psychopathology from the DSM) that they may not be "real" anymore, namely, reliable samples.

To this end Lambert, one of the leading scholars on psychotherapy, suggested a "return to the origins" in the progress of research on psychotherapy[31] highlighting its past stages of development. Phase 0, clinical case studies: the first outcomes exploration methods in psychotherapy related to single-case studies. Although fascinating, from the clinical point of view, such cases could hardly be defined as rigorous from a scientific-methodological point of view. Phase 1, descriptive research: such studies, most popular between the 1940s and 1960s, consisted in measuring pre- and post-treatment outcomes of groups. It begins to spread the idea of the quantitative sample (it is important that the research has therefore a certain largeness), but still lack adequate control groups to compare results with experimental groups. Phase 2, naturalistic process research: that is, studies aimed at identifying the causal factors of psychotherapy (the "how and why it works"), rather than its efficacy (the "if it works" had already been partially demonstrated); a typical example of such process studies is the work of Carl Rogers and his students. Phase 3, randomized clinical trials: since the 1970s and with the development of evidence-based medicine (EBM) in the 1980s and 1990s, extensive research was conducted with clinical trials designed to confront different treatments (e.g. treatment A, previously validated, and treatment B, not yet "accepted" by the scientific and clinical community) or placebo and treatments. Despite the identified limitations, this kind of research led to definitively prove the absolute superiority of psychotherapy compared to placebo and the relative superiority (in certain circumstances) of the same compared to psychopharmacology.

In 2004[32] Lambert and Ogles argued that the efficacy of placebo allows an improvement of approximately 40% of patients, compared with 70% in the event of a psychotherapeutic treatment. Phase 4, clinical efficacy research: the need to improve treatment protocols in the context of different clinical settings (hospitals, services, clinics, etc.) has led to a broadening of the focus of research in psychotherapy from experimental efficacy to clinical efficacy. If efficacy respects the internal validity of an experimental design, it aims at external validity; thus in real clinical settings clients are often not pre-screened and have frequent comorbidities, and are usually "rejected" by strict clinical tests. Stage 5, patient-focused research: single-case studies return to be regarded through the use of research designs and sophisticated statistical methods, a bridge between clinical practice and research; studies such as these, as well as having real-time effects on the improvement of treatment outcomes, can even provide an estimation of the number of sessions required in order to achieve an improvement with regard to the health status of the patient: well-made research, therefore, does not necessarily need the use of a large number of subjects. From Lambert's analysis, it seems there is an actual "return to the origins" in psychotherapy research, given the flourishing of patient-focused subjects. In fact, to date, given the coexistence of different research paradigms, it is indispensable that each of them can be evolved and provide peculiar contributions. A well-made clinical trial can assure the empirical efficacy of a specific treatment but it is only with a process research (for example a single-case study) that it might be possible to reconstruct why and how that works.

Are randomized clinical trials the best approach in psychotherapy research?

About the use of RCTs, which are considered the best standard in psychotherapy research, clinical practitioners have advanced harsh critiques. An interesting description of the primary characteristics of this methodological procedure with relative critical areas has been carried out by Starcevic (see Table 1)[20].

Table 1 Features of RCTs and relative criticisms (modified by Starcevic, 2003[20])

Features of RCTs	*Critical areas of RCTs*
"Randomized controlled trials" (RCTs) are a methodological procedure that consists in the comparison of the group of patients in whom the usefulness of treatment is being examined (experimental group) with the group of patients who are receiving no active treatment (e.g. a ***placebo; control group***).	In the psychotherapy studies there is no counterpart to a placebo that is used in the pharmacotherapy studies. The non-specific (and presumably placebo-like) psychological treatments, administered to patients in control groups, are not "neutral" in the way that placebo is pharmacologically "neutral" because they produce psychological effects, regardless of whether these are clinically significant.
RCTs focus on ***strict diagnostic homogeneity*** of the groups of patients and place emphasis on diagnostic precision.	Psychiatric diagnosis is usually not the main factor that determines the use of psychotherapy and diagnostic precision is not emphasized in psychotherapy. As a result, psychotherapy patients are not as diagnostically homogeneous as patients in RCTs and often have additional disorders that would exclude them from RCTs.
Another key feature is represented by the ***randomization*** into experimental and control groups of patients.	Randomizing patients in the psychotherapy usefulness studies is troublesome because clinical practice is not randomized; also, randomization creates an artificial situation because it ignores the fact that psychotherapy patients actively choose their own treatment.
It is important to carry on double-blind–design research.	A double-blind design is impossible in psychotherapy research. Patients cannot be blind to what psychological treatment they are receiving because they actively participate in it; likewise, therapists cannot be blind, because they know what treatments they administer.
Another "gold standard" of the RCT procedure is the use of standardization of treatment procedures, so that all patients receive (or are presumed to receive) treatment in the same way.	Psychotherapy is extremely difficult to "standardize" so that its procedures and techniques are used in the same way by all the therapists, regardless of their training and personality. Every encounter between the patient and the therapist has some unique features, with the potential of producing "something" that cannot be predicted and entirely "standardized".

According to the critiques reported in Table 1, RCTs can be specified as a procedure to test any artificial treatment in an artificially controlled clinical setting with atypical patients[33]. Garfield[34] also pointed out that the use of the current ESTs approach may even be deleterious to the development of psychotherapy: ESTs underestimate many variables (e.g. the therapist's adherence to a certain model), are dependent on "manualized" therapies, do not represent therapeutic practice and can lead to the imposition of strict constraints on clinical manoeuvers through the clarification of specific treatments for specific diagnoses.[34, 35] Moreover, the efficacy proven in RCTs, does not correspond to efficacy in clinical settings; so the internal validity does not necessarily ensure the external validity.[21, 36] It can then be argued that RCTs are not the most appropriate methodological procedure for the empirical validation of psychotherapy in accordance with the practice in the real world.[37] Duncan[21] noted that

> unlike the RCT, in actual clinical practice manuals are not used, therapies are not ever purely practiced, clients are not randomly assigned to treatments and clients rarely, if ever, enter therapy for singular DSM-defined disorders or experience success solely as diagnostic symptom reduction.
>
> (p. 47)[2]

Last, but not least, is the problem related to RCTs regarding the possibility of generalizing the results obtained from clinical trials in which subjects (volunteers) are recruited through advertisements. "Investigators question whether these subjects are representative of the types of individuals who seek treatment in clinical practice" (p. 242).[38] The use of volunteers eager to participate in the research was analyzed and criticized in a study on the estimated usefulness of cognitive-behavioural treatments.[39] In the ESTs approach, studies on psychotherapy outcomes have used the double-blind randomized placebo control design in which, in order to exclude any possibility of falsification of results, not only patients, but also the "treatment administrators" should ignore the conditions in which patients are assigned to evaluate the effects of various therapeutic factors.[40] This methodological approach was originally developed in the medical field, from the 1930s, in the USA and in Great Britain,[41, 42] with the "purpose of maintaining constant all factors except the medication's active ingredient" (p. 973).[43] Only after it had been adopted in medicine did Rosenthal and Frank[44] suggest that the randomized double-blind placebo control group design could also be used in psychotherapy research. The consequence was that, for example, whether

> Cognitive-Behavioural Therapy (CBT) for depression was compared with an adequate placebo control group and found to produce superior outcomes, these results would support the contention that the purported active ingredients in CBT (e.g., altering the core schema and challenging irrational thoughts) were responsible for the benefits of the treatment.
>
> (p. 973)[43]

But in order to successfully apply this methodological design in psychotherapy, several conditions must be met, as evidenced Baskin (p. 974,[43]; see Table 2).

Table 2 Conditions to fruitfully apply the double-blind placebo control group design in psychotherapy research (p. 974, Baskin 2003 [43])

1) All factors other than those purporting to be the active ingredients of that treatment must be made equivalent (i.e. held constant). That is, the placebo control treatment must be structurally indistinguishable from the specific treatment (e.g. same number of sessions and same treatment modality).
2) The participants, study administrators and study examiners must all be blind to the treatment conditions.
3) Other psychological factors, such as participants' expectations, belief in treatment and the credibility of the treatment, need to be controlled (i.e. made comparable for the active and placebo treatments).

Unfortunately some problems reduce the positive impact of placebo control procedures in psychotherapy. First of all, psychotherapy studies cannot be blind to the same extent as placebo controlled medical studies (see, for example, pharmacological research).[43] The therapist, in fact, needs to know the nature of the treatment selected in order to follow and apply a clinical protocol.[37, 45] In addition, the placebo is often distinguishable from active treatment:

> If the study participants are informed that they will be randomly assigned to an active treatment or to a placebo treatment without active ingredients, the apparent differences between the groups would allow the participants to determine that they were assigned to the less desirable treatment. Therefore, the quality of the design is increased by informing the participants that both treatments are equally efficacious, thereby creating a deception
>
> (p. 974)[43]

But even using a deception, some differences between the placebo control and active treatment remain. For example, the treatment group protocol differs and thus the credibility of the active treatment and expectations of participants could be different, taking into account that a credible treatment protocol has a powerful beneficial effect.[41, 43, 45] Borkovec and Nau[46] found that the protocols for the control conditions were considered less credible than those for the different treatment conditions. Another key consideration is that a well-designed placebo control condition (according to the above criteria) is much more similar to an active treatment than to control conditions.

So, the placebo to be used in psychotherapy research has to become a real therapeutic treatment. In fact, in agreement with Baskin,[43] "when placebo controls are better designed, the present meta-analysis found that the benefits produced by such treatments were not substantially different from the active treatments to which they were compared" (p. 976). Another critical note, more connected to the waiting-list/no-treatment conditions, that is, when the patient waits for treatment, concerns more ethical issues. Wesley and Waring,[47] in a critical review of outcomes research in couples therapy, noted that "there is some evidence to indicate that future outcome research should avoid the use of 'waiting list control groups', since their use appears to be neither ethical nor humane" (p. 421). A harsh critique of the EST movement, which summarizes the main weaknesses exposed so far, has been expressed in a masterly article by Westen, Novotny and Thompson-Brenner (2004) in the leading journal "Psychological Bulletin"[48].

Has the evidence-based rationale really changed clinical practice?

Many authors have pointed out that the real impact of the lists of ESTs on clinical practice was not significant. For example, in the case of anxiety disorders, only a minority of the patients had received an EST despite the fact that a significant number of articles, reports and documents would support the efficiency of these treatments.[49, 50] It is also important to consider that, according to the RCT approach, EBM supporters consider efficacy studies as more appropriate in the clinical field, whereas psychotherapists evaluate efficacy studies as the most suitable, considering them to be a more adequate reflection of actual clinical practice.[20] With regard to the application of "manualized" or "free" protocols, treatment manuals are traditionally considered restrictive, not able to capture the different nuances of each patient and not useful in the most complex cases.[4] Moreover, the use of an EST approach tends to support cognitive-behavioural therapies (15 out of 16 treatments identified as efficacious in 1998 were behavioural or cognitive-behavioural) and to limit other models that are less amenable to a manual-based presentation.[35, 51] It is also important to consider that treatment manuals are not very flexible in comparison to the heterogeneity of each DSM-based category of disorders; indeed "there remains a wide degree of therapist and intertreatment variability within a given model of treatment, even when a manual is closely followed, and therapist effects are often quite large" (p. 151).[52] A possible conclusion of this review on the state of ESTs in psychotherapy could be a quotation from Lawson and Deegear: "Although there are political, societal and monetary enticements to accepting the current rendering of ESTs, sufficient evidence has cast doubt on the movement as it currently exists" (p. 276).[35]

The "common factors" perspective

Duncan[21] has recommended that, instead of assuming a medical model in psychopathology, "a call is made for a systematic application of the common factors based on a relation model of client competence" (p. 32).[21] The Dodo Bird Verdict (from *Alice in Wonderland* by Lewis Carrol: "Everybody has won, and all must have prizes") has become a fitting metaphor to represent the state of research in psychotherapy[5, 53] and "a symbol of a raging controversy regarding the privileging of specific approaches for specific disorders based on demonstrated efficacy in randomized clinical trials" (p. 33).[21] Weinberger[54] noticed that, after 1980, writings and significant proposals began to appear that connected to the "Common Factors"; [55–59] in 1992, Lambert, who for many years had written major reviews of psychotherapy research, identified four therapeutic factors as the key elements for achieving improvements in psychotherapy: *extratherapeutic factors, common ones, expectancy or placebo, techniques*[60]. A good summary of the main commonalities across therapeutic factors is reported in Tracey,[7] according to the original classification of Grencavage and Norcross[61] (see Table 3).

Duncan[21] and Miller *et al.* [57] extended the use of the term *common factors* from its traditional meaning of "non specific or relational factors" to include four specific factors: client (40%), relationship (30%), placebo (15%) and technique (15%); the percentages of influence indicated are reported in Assay and Lambert.[62] Although there is a general agreement about the above areas, "the specific factors within each of these categories vary considerably in nature and number with "little apparent agreement" (p. 373)[61] among researchers regarding what they are" (p. 402).[7] A possible critical point relative to this perspective is the belief about the limited influence of the techniques in the explanation of the improvement in psychotherapy: only 15% of all the common factors.[62] In fact, a specific technique may profoundly influence and characterize the role of the other three factors.

First of all, the possible and concrete action of the *client factors* is closely related to the particular type of epistemology (and the relative techniques) specific to each approach. Thus, to allow patients to contribute to the psychotherapic change,[21, 63, 64] the approach selected must give them the role of leading actors in the therapeutic process. This is possible only with a particular type of technique that influences the relationship and communication with patients, giving them the credit for any improvements. Not all approaches convey this idea to patients, especially if the underlying epistemology is more deterministic than constructivist. Thus, if the medical model characterizes the theoretical foundations of a particular approach, the patient is not the "heroic client"[21, 64] anymore, but only subjected to the action of external factors such as drugs or the ability-expertise of a famous psychotherapist or "guru".

At the same time, to allow the *relationship factors* to play a transformative role in psychotherapy, the therapist has to build a special relationship aimed at changing the dysfunctional situation of the client. The use of direct or indirect communication, a one-down or one-up position, open or closed questions, brief aphorisms or long reframings, suggestion or rationality in the prescription of homework, etc. could quickly accomplish that task. But in order to select the best type of communication and relationship, in accordance with both the specific patient and the different steps of psychotherapy, it is necessary to use peculiar techniques. In fact, only an advanced use of these techniques could allow

Table 3 Commonalities across therapeutic factors and five superordinate categories identified by Grencavage and Norcross [61] (1990) (as reported in Tracey 2003[7])

Superordinate category Commonality	*Superordinate category Commonality*
1. Client characteristics	1. Positive expectation/hope or faith
	2. Distressed or incongruent client
	3. Patient actively seeks help
2. Therapist qualities	4. General positive descriptors
	5. Cultivates hope/enhances expectancies
	6. Warmth/positive regard
	7. Empathic understanding
	8. Socially sanctioned healer
	9. Acceptance
3. Change processes	10. Opportunity for catharsis/ventilation
	11. Acquisition and practice of new behaviours
	12. Provision of rationale
	13. Foster insight/awareness
	14. Emotional and interpersonal learning
	15. Feedback/reality testing
	16. Suggestion
	17. Success and mastery experiences
	18. Persuasion
	19. Placebo effect
	20. Identification with the therapist
	21. Contingency management
	22. Tension reduction
	23. Therapist modelling
	24. Desensitization
	25. Education/information provision
4. Treatment structures	26. Use of techniques/rituals
	27. Focus on "inner world"/exploration of emotional issues
	28. Adherence to theory
	29. A healing setting
	30. There are participants/interaction
	31. Communication (verbal and nonverbal)
	32. Explanation of therapy and participants' roles
5. Relationship elements	33. Development of alliance/relationship (general)
	34. Engagement
	35. Transference

therapists to "tailor" the chosen approach to different patients' features and logics. "Some clients, for instance, will prefer a formal or professional manner to a casual or warmer one. Others might prefer more self-disclosure from their therapists, greater directiveness" (p. 39).[21]

Even for what concerns the *placebo, hopes and expectation factors*, Duncan[21] noted that the client's awareness of being treated is not the only element that could allow the placebo component to carry on a significant therapeutic improvement: to have a valid placebo effect"the assessment of the credibility of the therapy's rationale and related *techniques*"(p. 40)[21] is also necessary. Assay and Lambert[62] defined *model/technique factors* as beliefs and procedures unique to each specific treatment. Rosenzweig[65, 66] proposed that the critical point of techniques was the formal consistency with referential theory, whether the approach has to do with psychoanalysis or a religion. Another relevant point is that the main contribution of model/techniques to therapy is simply related to the enhancement of the other common factors[67]. In fact, theoretical-methodological issues referring to techniques and to the chosen model that heavily influence the realization of the effect of other common factors, are not the least relevant factors in the therapeutic process, but a fundamental constituent. Devoid of a functional technique, therefore, a therapist cannot easily build a relationship, a communication and a change-oriented strategy.

Before closing this section dedicated to the different common factors and the importance of *model/technique factors*, in particular, we would like to stress some reflections in order to avoid an excessive emphasis on technique and, therefore, the risk of falling into a possible new kind of reductionism: technique is important but it's not everything. During the training of a young therapist, learning a specific set of techniques and adherence to them is key; but, after many years of experience, the technique must be modified in accordance with the personal style of each therapist. Only through a personal evolution, can techniques be modified and/or improved to allow a more effective and efficient therapeutic process. Moreover, some steps in psychotherapy are more related to applications that are "tailored" on the basis of insight and perception (even with a percentage of "mystery" and unexplained and inexplicable issues) rather than the repetition of well-learned techniques.

Going back to methodological bias, the latter are not only present in EST studies, but also in research on common factors in psychotherapy. For example, the problem of control conditions is reported by Chambless[68] about Luborsky's studies. Chambless, in fact, underlining a significant number of problems found in Luborsky *et al.*'s meta-analysis[53] on the effects reported by some comparative studies on psychotherapy, noted that the "acceptance of the Dodo Bird verdict is dangerous. Despite my great respect for Lester Luborsky and his colleagues, I must disagree with their conclusion that there are no meaningful differences in outcomes of different approaches to psychotherapy".[68] The most important methodological criticisms about Luborsky's "Dodo Bird verdict" are well summarized by the same Chambless:[68]

> Luborsky et al.'s conclusion that there are no meaningful differences in the efficacy of various psychotherapies should be reconsidered for the following reasons: (a) errors in data analysis, (b) exclusion of research on many types of clients (e.g., children and adolescents), (c) faulty generalization to comparisons between therapies that have never been made, and (d) erroneous assumption that the average difference between all sorts of treatments for all sorts of problems can be assumed to represent the difference between any two types of treatment for a given problem. Concern for clients' welfare requires psychologists to be cautious to accept the Dodo Bird Verdict.[68]

Meta-analysis contributions in the "common factors" perspective

One of the main methodological resources used within the "common factors" perspective is the meta-analysis. For example, a recent large study designed to test the "Dodo Bird verdict" has once again confirmed that judgement.[21, 69] Wilson and Lipsey[70] in their synthesis of 319 meta-analyses of psychological, behavioural and educational treatment research, pointed out that "these results underscore the difficulty of detecting treatment outcomes, the importance of cautioning interpreting findings from a single study, and the importance of meta-analysis in summarizing results across studies" (p. 413). A good reflection on meta-analysis as a tool in psychotherapy can be found in Koch and Ziegler:[71]

> in these days, more than one clinical trial is mostly performed to evaluate a new treatment or therapeutic intervention. This necessitates a combined evaluation of their results. An integration of evidence from several trials it is also helpful to determine the actual knowledge.

These are the main goals of meta-analysis. Since the late 1980s, meta-analysis has been widely used in clinical research. At the beginning of a meta-analysis, it has to develop a protocol. Similar to the clinical trial protocol, inclusion and exclusion criteria for trials, the hypothesis and planned analysis have to be fixed. After a careful localization of the trials, a combined statistical analysis is performed. An investigation on heterogeneity (for example, the differences between results of the studies) is also essential. In recent years, the tool of meta-analysis has been criticized. These criticisms arise mainly from those poorly conducted meta-analyses that generated results without pre-specifying the hypotheses or that simply combined different studies. Well-planned meta-analyses, on the contrary, have an increasing influence in clinical research (Koch and Ziegler,[71] p. 109). The main positive features of the meta-analysis procedures are well summarized by Rosenthal:[72] "advantages of the meta-analytic procedures include seeing the 'landscape' of a research domain, keeping statistical significance in perspective, minimizing wasted data, becoming intimate with the data summarized, asking focused research questions, and finding moderator variables" (p. 59).

A more critical examination of this methodological tool considers that

> negative trials are often unreported, and hence can be missed by meta-analysts. And how much heterogeneity between trials is acceptable? A recent major criticism is that large randomized trials do not always agree with a prior meta-analysis. Neither individual trials nor meta-analyses, reporting as they do with population effects, tell how to treat the individual patient.
>
> (p. 123)[73]

O'Rourke[74] reported an interesting comment on the current difficulties in obtaining solid results based on meta-analysis, but emphasizing good expectations about its future applications in helping clinicians and policymakers to answer these questions. Although the conclusions of such meta-analyses have been promising, they often include studies with methodological shortcomings that might invalidate the obtained results: for example, the analysis of two major meta-analyses conducted on the study of the effects of psychotherapy with children and adolescents.[75] Furthermore, according to Shadish *et al.*,[76] "concern has arisen that meta-analyses overestimate the effects of psychological therapies and that these therapies may not work under clinically representative conditions" (p. 512).

Effective psychotherapies: better than placebo and superior to drug treatments

It has been previously pointed out that psychotherapy has largely demonstrated its utility through research carried out since the 1960s.[10, 11, 15, 18, 77, 78] In order to present the most effective psychotherapic interventions (see Table 4) we avoided the traditional diagnostic classifications because, although intended to be atheoretical, they are inevitably affected by the different underlying epistemologies. In this regard, as amply demonstrated, economic interests can influence and distort the outcome of scientific research[79–82] or the compilation of diagnostic manuals.[83] There is, in fact, today, a tendency to create psychodiagnostic manuals organized according to the underlying paradigm-approach (cognitive-behavioural, psychodynamic, systemic-relational, etc.) more than by psychopathologies and patient issues. For example, the DSM-IV-TR refers to the cognitive-behavioural tradition and is influenced by the medical-pharmacological approach. The use of PDM categories (*Psychodynamic Diagnostic Manual*, American Psychoanalytic Association, International Psychoanalytic Association, Division 39 (Psychoanalysis) American Psychological Association, American Academy of Psychoanalysis and Dynamic Psychiatry, National Membership Committee on Psychoanalysis in Clinical Social Work, 2006), instead, would mean to side with a psychodynamic approach. Therefore, the use of a single criterion, although founded, might be a questionable choice.

This need has also emerged in other areas, such as the evaluation of scientific production. In this field, the hegemony of the Impact Factor (IF) – an index of the scientific relevance of publications based on a circuit of international journals with specific criteria – might exclude from scientific validity a series of contributions, based on the fact that they are not included in those journals monitored by the IF circuit itself. Fields such as psychology and psychotherapy are not always suited to the diffusion of their knowledge through magazines. If Sigmund Freud, Carl Rogers or Milton Erickson had been evaluated based on the IF, they would not have reached a sufficient criterion of scientific validity. Fortunately, their books and manuals, despite not having an Impact Factor, had a strong impact on the scientific and clinical community. Milton Erickson, in particular, was able to be "heretical" (in the etymological sense of "someone who has the ability to choose"), innovating method in psychotherapy, thanks to the fact that he wasn't involved in the academic community of scientific excellence that could have restrained his creative and evolutionary spirit.

It is important to give space to authors and approaches that are spreading their knowledge without making use of the Impact Factor: science is disseminated along less official paths of diffusion and measures of knowledge. In clinicians' studies there are many texts and manuals of great authors rather than scientific articles with a high IF but a low clinical impact. Possible additional criteria, complementary to the Impact Factor, have been introduced in the evaluation of scientific production (for example the H index, which also evaluates texts and manuals, points of reference in psychotherapy), with the aim of creating a series of evaluation indices,[84,85] alternative circuits (articles, books, manuals, contributions, etc.) where authors have presented, distributed and cited thoughts and work in psychotherapy that have been valued. To avoid an epistemological monopoly, in which a classification is presented (with its epistemological background) that excludes others that are equally valid from an historical, theoretical, scientific and epistemological point of view, we have taken into account broad categories of psychopathology in which each, with its own model, may find itself. Pluralism has moved us in our work in the selection of both psychopathological categories and psychotherapeutic treatments of excellence. The following table shows the main psychotherapy or clinical psychology interventions that might have more effective results for each issue. References considered were, necessarily, many, in order to avoid being conditioned by a single source of information.

Regarding the superiority of psychotherapy over placebo, see the studies previously reported:[10, 11, 32] evidence of the superiority of psychotherapy over exclusively pharmacological intervention for many psychopathologies and organic disorders with psychological factors involved are more recent.[92–163] The EST approach in clinical psychology, referring to the previously discussed EBM model, is based on the integration between psychotherapy and pharmacotherapy; in some clinical trials of the previous generation, a combination of treatments was planned from the outset. For many psychopathological conditions or problems there are, however, clear indications for psychotherapy or pharmacological intervention as elective or preferential treatments; for example, in case of mood disorders and depression (other disorders could have been considered, such as anxiety disorders).[126, 127, and 164] The results of a recent meta-analysis of clinical trials on the use of antidepressants[165, 166] added more information to the debate, still alive in the scientific and clinical communities, on the best treatment for depression. The importance of recognizing plural factors (psychological variables, family and social environment, life styles, etc.) in the etiology and treatment of many disorders may be historically represented by one of the best-known Hippocratic principles – *similia similibus curantur*.

Table 4 Most effective psychotherapies or clinical psychology interventions for each problematic area

ABUSE AND ADDICTION

- Behaviour Therapy: brief educational interventions, including Motivational Interviewing (source APA, RF).
- Structural-Strategic Family Therapy (source PSY)
- Cognitive-Behavioural Therapy (source APA, RF)

EATING DISORDERS

- Family Therapy (source RF)
- Cognitive-Behavioural Therapy (source APA, RF, CE)
- Eclectic Therapy (source CE, RF and APA only for bulimia)
- Brief Strategic Therapy (source PSY, RF)

DEPRESSION

- Psychodinamic Therapy (with particular reference to the Interpersonal Psychotherapy) (source CE, RF, APA)
- Brief Strategic Therapy (source PSY, RF)
- Cognitive-Behavioural Therapy (source APA, RF, CE, PSY)
- Psychosocial Interventions (source PSY)

SEXUAL DYSFUNCTIONS (INDIVIDUAL AND COUPLE)

- Systemic Therapy (source PSY)
- Cognitive-Behavioural Therapy (source APA, RF)
- Brief Strategic Therapy (source PSY, RF)

PHOBIC and ANXIETY DISORDERS

- Cognitive Therapy (source APA) and Relaxation Training (source APA)
- Cognitive-Behavioural Therapy (source APA, RF)
- Behaviour Therapy (source APA)
- Brief Strategic Therapy (source PSY, RF)
- EMDR (source CE)
- Structured Psychodinamic Therapy (source RF)

OBSESSIVE-COMPULSIVE DISORDERS

- Cognitive-Behavioural Therapy (source CE, APA, RF)
- Behaviour Therapy (source APA)
- Brief Strategic Therapy (source PSY, RF)

PERSONALITY DISORDERS

- Psychodinamic Therapy (source RF)
- Dialectical Behaviour Therapy (source APA, RF)
- Systemic-Strategic therapy (source PSY)

PSYCHOSIS or PRESUMED PSYCHOSIS

- Family Therapy (source CE, APA, RF, PSY)
- Cognitive-Behavioural Therapy (source CE, APA, RF)
- Behaviour Therapy: Social Skills Training (source RF, APA); supported work placement (source APA); Psychoeducational Multifamily Groups (source PSY)

(continued)

Table 4 (continued)

DEVELOPMENTAL INTERVENTIONS

- Integration of different models (Behavioural, Analytical, Systemic-familiar model) (source RF)
- Brief Strategic Therapy (source PSY, RF)
- Cognitive-Behavioural Therapy (mild to moderate depression) (source CE)
- Psychodinamic Therapy (with particular reference to the Interpersonal Psychotherapy) (source CE)

MARITAL AND FAMILIAR INTERVENTIONS

- Strategic Family Therapy (source PSY)
- Brief Strategic Therapy (source PSY, RF)
- Functional Family Therapy (source PSY)
- Eclectic Therapy (source PSY)
- Systemic-Relational Paradigm (source PSY)
- Behavioural Couples Therapy (source PSY)
- Rational-Emotive Couples Therapy (source PSY)

REFERENCES

Clinical evidence from scientific medical literature from PubMed and Cochrane review (abbreviation CE)
Comprendre et traiter la souffrance psychique: Quel traitement pour quel trouble?, Mony Elkaïm, Seuil, Paris, 2007 (abbreviation RF)
Psicoterapie e prove di efficacia. Quale terapia per quale paziente, Anthony Roth, Peter Fonagy, Il Pensiero Scientifico, 1997 (original title: *What works for whom?: A critical review of psychotherapy research*, Guilford, New York (abbreviation RF)
The Society of Clinical Psychology (Division 12), American Psychological Association (abbreviation APA)
Psychotherapy manuals (see [86–90]) or other academic articles (see [91]) from psychological data base (EBSCO'S PBSC) non-overlapping medical data bases as PubMed or APA (abbreviation PSY)

These considerations, sometimes neglected by modern medicine, especially in the field of mental health, suggest that pathology should be considered as the product of several factors and the relative treatments should based on the same principle that "similar things are cured by similar things": if a problem is generated at a cultural, social, interpersonal, familiar level perhaps the best way to treat it is to provide care at the same level. There are, in fact, many different ways to treat a psychological or psychopathological issue; for example to work with individual patients, couples, and families, the social context, school. However, one of the main trends in official medicine is to provide an intervention limited to the individual and biological level (psychopharmacological). If a problem is generated at a biological, molecular, neurological level, as occurs in some forms of severe depression, an effective treatment should focus on that level; yet, if a person presents difficulties limited to particular and selected situations and contexts (such as at work but not in the family, or alone but not with other people), which would then be the most appropriate treatment? The bio-pharmacological approach can then be considered the best treatment with respect to the *similia similibus curantur* principle.[167, 168] It is also important to underline that bio-psychopharmacological reductionism might increase side effects:[169, 170, 171, 172] in a recent study on children and adolescents, the risk of attempted suicide was 1.52 times higher after an antidepressant therapy compared to a therapy without antidepressants.[173] The main concern with the use of psychotropic drugs in the mental health field is that the adolescent brain is still developing, so the effects of these drugs might have harmful long-term consequences, according to measures that have not yet been understood.[174]

Much criticism on the use and continued use of psychopharmacological treatments is expressed by psychiatrists.[175, 176] For instance, antidepressants are likely at times to create abnormal brain states that do not necessarily correspond to the cure:

> antidepressants are assumed to work on the specific neurobiology of depressive disorders according to a "disease-centered" model of drug action. However, little evidence supports this idea. An alternative, "drug-centered" model suggests that psychotropic drugs create abnormal states that may coincidentally relieve symptoms. Drug-induced effects of antidepressants vary widely according to their chemical class from sedation and cognitive impairment to mild stimulation and occasionally frank agitation. Results from clinical trials could be explained by drug-induced effects and placebo amplification. No evidence shows that antidepressants or any other drugs produce long-term elevation of mood or other effects that are particularly useful in treating depression
>
> (p. 961)[175]

The implication of these effects includes the possibility that much of the research on maintenance treatment is flawed. "If withdrawal induced adverse effects could be effectively managed, the success of drug discontinuation might be much greater than usually assumed and might outweight the disadvantages of continued treatment" (p. 517),[176] The use of drugs in the treatment of depression, desired and necessary, should be part of an integrated approach that does not neglect the aged but still functional Hippocratic principle. The international guidelines on the treatment of depression, published as reviews in the prestigious medical journal the "British Medical Journal",[177] argue that psychosocial treatments appear to be "first-line" interventions to deal with mild depression, while in moderate to severe depression psychological treatments such as cognitive-behavioural therapy or interpersonal therapy are chosen, together with psychopharmacological treatments. Significant experimental evidence indicates that psychotherapy integrated with antidepressants might be more effective than the sole psychopharmacological therapy in cases of mild, severe and chronic depression.

In 2004, the Cochrane Collaboration, responsible for the world's most authoritative reviews in the clinical field, stated that the differences between antidepressants and psychological treatments are minimal in terms of efficacy.[141] This "minimal difference in terms of efficacy" hides "a significant difference in terms of quality of life and therapeutic result". If clinical scales, on the level of depression perceived, show the same statistical result between psychotherapy and psychopharmacological intervention, there are other variables that, if taken into account, would shift significantly the advantage towards psychotherapy: lack of both short-term and long-term side effects (present in pharmacological treatment); activation of personal resources of the individual (who, instead, in the case of drugs use, relies passively on the "magic pill"); enhancement of the sense of personal self-esteem, as in "I have managed to get out of the situation" (while in psychopharmacology there is still a sense of dependence on the chemical factors); strengthening of an intimate sense of autonomy, as in "I can now go on with my own legs" (while in drug use there is a constant fear of relapse in case of treatment interruption).

With similar statistical effects, very different changes occur that are in favour of psychotherapy over psychopharmacological treatments, in an overall assessment of quality of life and self-esteem. These types of treatment could be seen as the cure for symptomatic aspects while a true change can only be achieved with psychotherapy. When dealing with drugs, the clinician has to ask the question: Does the "crutch" represented by chemicals represent a real therapeutic change in the long term? Is pharmacological symptom reduction a real sign of effective psychotherapic change? There is a substantial difference between alleviating a symptom with chemical inhibition, and working on the person to decrease psychological distress and lead the individual to transform their particular way of dealing with reality. In the first case (pharmacological) it is a simple symptomatic reduction: the distress, chemically inhibited but still unresolved, will tend to recur or will require a further increase in the pharmacological treatment; psychotherapy, instead, leads to a true change that the person is aware of and will tend to persist with over time. The purely psychological treatment, when effective, represents a real overcoming of the disorder, while the pharmacological treatment, even when capable of reducing the symptom, cannot be considered as effective.

There is also an economic aspect that should not be underestimated. Hansen, in 2005, used antidepressants together with neuroleptics as an example of non-superiority over psychotherapy in terms of both efficacy and costs[178] as previously demonstrated by the London Depression Intervention Trial,[179] where the pharmacological intervention resulted in being more expensive than the psychotherapeutic systemic approach. Similar examples might also be made for other psychopathologies such as anxiety disorders, which are among the most widespread psychiatric issues, affecting 400 million people. Relative to panic disorder, Isaac Marks' historical studies,[180–182] carried out in London and Toronto,[183] and a recent Cochrane review,[110] show that "first-line intervention" for this issue is psychotherapy compared to pharmacotherapy, especially with regard to long-term efficacy and absence of side effects.

In conclusion, it might be observed that among the methods considered most valid, cognitive-behavioural therapy is often cited. This frequent occurrence, due to historical and cultural reasons, should not be confused with an effective superiority over other approaches to personal care. This has been highlighted in some recent reviews[178, 184–186] that demonstrated the excellence of other psychotherapies, such as the interactional-strategic, systemic-relational and psychodynamic.[91, 179, 187–189] Psychodynamic therapy has also gained important recognition,[189–192] for instance, in the treatment of personality disorders[193]. As Assay and Lambert[62] stated, 50% of psychological and behavioural disorders can be resolved with a treatment limited to no more than ten sessions, thanks to the technical evolutions of psychotherapy; another 25% require a treatment that will last no more than 30 sessions while the remaining 25% of disorders require a prolonged period of time in therapy. This indicates the importance not only of the efficacy but also the efficiency of the treatment, with regard to psychotherapy outcomes. Treatment efficiency is a key factor in considering the costs to patients in both economic and existential terms. Recently, the psychotherapeutic community has increasingly agreed in differentiating two main approaches to the care of individuals, based on the problems they are facing: on one hand, there are treatments that deal with personal growth and developmental aspects of the individual, the so-called "long-term therapies"; on the other hand, there are treatments focused on the rapid extinction of issues, the so-called "short focal therapies". The apparent paradox is represented by the fact that we have a higher efficiency in working with diseases that show more limiting symptoms (such as panic, phobias or compulsions) compared to the treatment of disorders that are apparently less debilitating yet requiring longer time to be processed, such as the so-called "personality disorders". Therefore we should give equal dignity to various forms of psychotherapy, both short- and long-term; their application to specific and different forms of discomfort configures and legitimates their peculiar structure, process and duration.

Notes

1 Castelnuovo G., Faccio E., Molinari E., Nardone G., Salvini A., *A critical review of Empirically Supported Treatments (ests) and Common Factors perspective in Psychotherapy*, in «Brief Strategic and Systemic Therapy European Review», 208–224 (2004).

2 Castelnuovo G., Faccio E., Molinari E., Nardone G., Salvini A., *Evidence based approach in psychotherapy the limitations of current Empirically Supported Treatments paradigms and of similar theoretical approaches as regards establishing efficient and effective treatments in psychotherapy*, in «Brief Strategic and Systemic Therapy European Review», 229–248 (2005).

3 Morrison K.H., Bradley R., Westen D., *The external validity of controlled clinical trials of psychotherapy for depression and anxiety: A naturalistic study*, in «Psychology and Psychotherapy» 76, 109–132 (2003).
4 Herbert J.D., *The science and practice of empirically supported treatments*, in «Behavior Modification» 27, 412–430 (2003).
5 Luborsky L., Singer B., *Comparative studies of psychotherapies. Is it true that "Everywon has won and all must have prizes"?*, in «Archives of General Psychiatry» 32, 995–1008 (1975).
6 Luborsky L., *et al.*, *The Dodo bird verdict is alive and well – mostly*, in «Clinical Psychology: Science and Practice» 9, 1 (2004).
7 Tracey T.J.G., Lichtenberg J.W., Goodyear R.K., Claiborn C.D., Wampold B.E., *Concept mapping of therapeutic common factors*, in «Psychotherapy Research» 13, 401–413 (2003).
8 Eysenck H.J., *The effects of psychotherapy: An evaluation*, in «Journal of Consulting and Clinical Psychology», 319–324 (1952).
9 Frank J.D., *Critical evaluation of Strupp and Bergin: Common features account for effectiveness*, in «International Journal of Psychiatry» 7, 122–127 (1969).
10 Lambert M.J., Bergin A.E., *The effectiveness of psychotherapy*, in A.E. Bergin and S.L. Garfield (Eds.), *Handbook of psychotherapy and behaviour change (4th ed.)* 143–189 (1994).
11 Lambert M.J., *The status of empirically supported therapies: Comment on Westen and Morrison's (2001) multidimensional meta-analysis*, in « Journal of Consulting and Clinical Psychology» 69, 910–913 (2001).
12 Sanderson W.C., *Why empirically supported psychological treatments are important*, in «Behavior Modification» 27, 290–299 (2003).
13 Safran J.D., *When worlds collide: Psychoanalysis and the empirically supported treatment movement*, in «Psychoanalytic Dialogues», 11, 659–681 (2001).
14 Bohart A.C., O'Hara M., Leitner L.M., *Empirically violated treatment: Disenfranchisement of humanistic and other psychotherapies*, in «Psychotherapy Research», 141–157 (1998).
15 Chambless D.L., Ollendick T.H., *Empirically supported psychological interventions: Controversies and evidence*, in «Annual Review of Psychology» 52, 685–716 (2001).
16 Sackett D.L., *Evidence-based medicine*, in «Seminars in Perinatology» 21, 3–5 (1997).
17 Chambless D.L., *et al.*, *Update on empirically validated therapies: II*, in «The Clinical Psychologist» 51, 3–16 (1998).
18 Chambless D.L., Hollon S.D., *Defining empirically supported therapies*, in «Journal of Consulting and Clinical Psychology» 66, 7–18 (1998).
19 Beutler L.E., Clarkin J.F., Bongar B., *Guidelines for systematic treating of the depressed patient* (2000).
20 Starcevic V., *Psychotherapy in the era of evidence-based medicine*, in «Australian Psychiatry» 11, 278–281 (2003).
21 Duncan B.L., *The Legacy of Saul Rosenzweig: The Profundity of the Dodo Bird*, in «Journal of Psychotherapy Integration» 12, 32–57 (2002).
22 Brunswik E., *The conceptual framework of psychology* (1952).
23 Chwalisz K., *A Common Factors revolution: Let's not "cut off our discipline's nose to spite its face"*, in «Journal of Counseling Psychology» 48, 262–267 (2001).
24 Jacobson N.S., Christensen A., *Studying the effectiveness of psychotherapy: How well can clinical trials do the job?*, in «American Psychologist» 51, 1031–1039 (1996).
25 Herbert J.D., *Defining empirically supported treatments: Pitfalls and possible solutions*, in «The Behavior Therapist», 113–134 (2000).
26 Klein D.F., *Dodo deliberations*, in «Clinical Psychology: Science and Practice» 28–29 (2002).
27 Rosenthal R., *The "file drawer problem" and tolerance for null results*, in «Psychological Bullettin», 638–641 (1979).
28 Davidson P.R., Parker K.C.H., *Eye movement desensization and reprocessing (EMDR): A meta-analysis*, in «Journal of Consulting and Clinical Psychology», 305–316 (2001).
29 Dishion T.J., McCord J., Poulin F., *When interventions harm: Peer groups and problem behavior*, in «American Psychologist», 755–764 (1999).
30 Fensterheim H., Raw S.D., *Psychotherapy research is not psychotherapy practice*, in «Clinical Psychology: Science and Practice» 3, 168–171 (1996).
31 Lambert M.J., *Metodi ed obiettivi della ricerca in psicoterapia*, in G. Nicolò and S. Salvatore (Eds.), *La ricerca sui risultati e sui processi in psicoterapia*, 137–147 (2007).
32 Lambert M.J., Ogles B.M., *The efficacy and effectiveness of psychotherapy*, in M.J. Lambert (ed.), *Bergin and Garfield handbook of psychotherapy and behavior change (edition 5)*, 139–193 (2004).
33 Ablon J.S., Jones E.E., *Validity of controlled clinical trials of psychotherapy: Findings from the NIMH Treatment of Depression Collaborative Research Program*, in «American Journal of Psychiatry», 775–783 (2002).
34 Garfield S.L., *Some comments on empirically supported treatments*, in «Journal of Consulting and Clinical Psychology» 66, 121–125 (1998).

35 Deegear J., Lawson D.M., *The utility of empirically supported treatments*, in «Professional Psychology: Research and Practice» 54, 271–277 (2003).
36 Goldfried M., Wolfe B., *Toward a more clinically valid approach to therapy research*, in «American Psychologist» 66, 143–150 (1998).
37 Seligman M.E.P., *The effectiveness of psychotherapy: The Consumer Reports survey*, in «American Psychologist» 50, 965–974 (1995).
38 Rapaport M.H. *et al.*, *A comparison of descriptive variables for clinical patients and symptomatic volunteers with depressive disorders*, in «Journal of Clinical Psychopharmacology» 16, 242–246 (1996).
39 Stanley M.A., Novy D.M., *Cognitive-behavior therapy for generalized anxiety in late life: an evaluative overview*, in «Journal of Anxiety Disorders» 14, 191–207 (2000).
40 Goldfried M.R., Wolfe B.E., *Psychotherapy practice and research: Repairing a strained alliance*, in «American Psychologist» 51, 1007–1016 (1996).
41 Wampold B.E., *Contextualizing psychotherapy as a healing practice: Culture, history, and methods*, in «Applied and Preventive Psychology» 10, 69–86 (2001a).
42 Shapiro A.K. and Shapiro, E.S. *The powerful placebo: From ancient priest to modern medicine* (1997).
43 Baskin, T.W., Tierney S.C., Minami T., Wampold B.E., *Establishing specificity in psychotherapy: a meta-analysis of structural equivalence of placebo controls*, in «Journal of Consulting and Clinical Psychology» 71, 973–979 (2003).
44 Rosenthal D., Frank J.D., *Psychotherapy and the placebo effect*, in «Psychological Bulletin» 53, 294–302 (1956).
45 Wampold B.E., *The great psychotherapy debate: Model, methods, and findings* (2001).
46 Borkovec T.D., Nau S.D., *Credibility of analogue therapy rationales*, in «Journal of Behavior Therapy and Experimental Psychiatry» 3, 257–260 (1972).
47 Wesley S., Waring E.M., *A critical review of marital therapy outcome research*, in «Canadian Journal of Psychiatry» 41, 421–428 (1996).
48 Westen D., Novotny C., Thompson-Brenner H., *The empirical status of empirically supported therapies: Assumptions, methods, and findings*, in «Psychological Bulletin» 130, 631–663 (2004).
49 Goisman R.M. *et al.*, *Utilization of behavioural methods in a multicenter anxiety disorders study*, in «Journal of Clinical Psychiatry», 213–218 (1993).
50 Goisman R.M., Warshaw M.G., Keller M.B., *Psychosocial treatment prescriptions for generalized anxiety disorder, panic disorder, and social phobia, 1991–1996*, in «American Journal of Psychiatry», 1819–1821 (1999).
51 Beutler L.E., *Identifying empirically supported treatments: What if we didn't?*, in «Journal of Consulting and Clinical Psychology» 66, 113–120 (1998).
52 Malik M.L., Beutler L.E., Alimohamed S., Gallagher-Thompson D., Thompson L., *Are all cognitive therapies alike? A comparison of cognitive and noncognitive therapy process and implications for the application of empirically supported treatments*, in «Journal of Consulting and Clinical Psychology» 71, 150–158 (2003).
53 Luborsky L. *et al.*, *The Dodo bird verdict is alive and well-mostly*, in «Clinical Psychology: Science and Practice» 9, 2–12 (2002).
54 Weinberger J., *Common factors aren't so common: The common factors dilemma*, in «Clinical Psychology: Science and Practice» 2, 45–69 (1995).
55 Garfield S.L., *Some problems associated with "validated" forms of psychotherapy*, in «Clinical Psychology: Science and Practice» 3, 218–229 (1996).
56 Goldfried M.R., *Converging themes in psychotherapy* (1982).
57 Miller S.D., Duncan B.L., Hubble M.A., *Escape from Babel* (1997).
58 Patterson C.H., *Foundations for a systematic eclectic psychotherapy*, in «Psychotherapy» 26, 427–435 (1989).
59 Weinberger J., *Common factors in psychotherapy*, in G. Stricker and J. Gold (Eds.), *Comprehensive handbook of psychotherapy integration*, 43–56 (1993).
60 Lambert M.J., *Implications of outcome research for psychotherapy integration*, in C. Norcross and M.R. Goldfried (Eds.), *Handbook of psychotherapy integration*, 94–129 (1992).
61 Grencavage L., Norcross J., *Where are the commonalities among the therapeutic common factors?*, in «Professional Psychology: Research and Practice» 21, 372–378 (1990).
62 Assay T.P., Lambert M.J., *The empirical case for the common factors in therapy: Qualitative findings*, in M.A. Hubble, B.L. Duncan and S.D. Miller (Eds.), *The hearth and soule of change: What works in therapy*, 33–56 (1999).
63 Bohart A.C., Tallman K. *What clients do to make therapy work* (1999).
64 Duncan B.L., Miller S.D., *The heroic client* (2000).
65 Rosenzweig S., *Some implicit common factors in diverse methods of psychotherapy*, in «American Journal of Ortopsychiatry» 6, 412–415 (1936).

66 Rosenzweig S., *Areas of agreement in psychotherapy*, in «American Journal of Ortopsychiatry» 10, 703–704 (1940).
67 Hubble M.A., Duncan B.L., Miller S.D., *Directing attention to that works*, in M.A. Hubble, B.L. Duncan, S.D. Miller (Eds.), *The hearth and souls of change: What works in therapy* (1999).
68 Chambless D.L., *Beware the Dodo Bird: The Dangers of overgeneralization*, in «Clinical Psychology: Science and Practice» 9 (2002).
69 Wampold B.E., *Methodological problems in identifying efficacious psychotherapies*, in «Psychotherapy Research» 7, 21–44 (1997).
70 Wilson D.B., Lipsey M.W., *The role of method in treatment effectiveness research: evidence from meta-analysis*, in «Psychological Methods» 6, 413–429 (2001).
71 Koch A., Ziegler S. *Meta-analysis as a tool for evaluation of evidence* in «Med Klin (Munich)» 95, 109–116 (2000).
72 Rosenthal R., DiMatteo M.R., *Meta-analysis: recent developments in quantitative methods for literature reviews*, in «Annual Review of Psychology» 52, 59–82 (2001).
73 Lau J., Ioannidis J.P., Schmid C.H., *Summing up evidence: One answer is not always enough*, in «The Lancet» 351, 123–127 (1998).
74 O'Rourke K., Detsky A.S., *Meta-analysis in medical research: Strong encouragement for higher quality in individual research efforts*, in «Journal of Clinical Epidemiology» 42, 1021–1024 (1989).
75 Weiss B., Weisz J.R., *The impact of methodological factors on child psychotherapy outcome research: A meta-analysis for researchers*, in «Journal of Abnormal Child Psychology»18, 639–670 (1990).
76 Shadish W.R., Matt G.E., Navarro A.M., Phillips G., *The effects of psychological therapies under clinically representative conditions: a meta-analysis*, in « Psychological Bulletin» 126, 512–529 (2000).
77 Lambert M.J., *Early response in psychotherapy: Further evidence for the importance of common factors rather than "placebo effects"*, in «Journal of Clinical Psychology» 61, 855–869 (2005).
78 Chambless D.L. *et al.*, *An update on empirically validated therapies*, in «The Clinical Psychologist», 5–18 (1996).
79 Ioannidis J.P., *Why most published research findings are false*, in «PLoS Medicine» 2, e124 (2005).
80 Ioannidis J.P., *Why most discovered true associations are inflated*, in «Epidemiology» 19, 640–648 (2008).
81 Young N.S., Ioannidis J.P., Al-Ubaydli O., *Why current publication practices may distort science*, in «PLoS Med» 5, e201 (2008).
82 Perlis R.H. *et al.*, *Industry sponsorship and financial conflict of interest in the reporting of clinical trials in psychiatry*, in «American Journal of Psychiatry» 162, 1957–1960 (2005).
83 Cosgrove L., Krimsky S., Vijayaraghavan M., Schneider L., *Financial ties between DSM-IV panel members and the pharmaceutical industry*, in «Psychotherapy and Psychosomatics» 75, 154–160 (2006).
84 Castelnuovo G., *More on impact factors*, in «Epidemiology» 19, 762–763 (2008).
85 Castelnuovo G., *Ditching impact factors: Time for the single researcher impact factor*, in «British Medical Journal» 336, 789 (2008).
86 Elkaim M. (Ed.), *Comprendre et traiter la souffrance psychique: Quel traitement pour quel trouble?* (2007).
87 Nardone G., *Brief Strategic Solution-Oriented Therapy of phobic and obsessive disorders* (1996).
88 Nardone G. and Portelli C., *Knowing through changing: The evolution of Brief Strategic Therapy* (2005).
89 Nardone G. and Watzlawick P., *The art of change: Strategic therapy and hypnotherapy without trance* (1993).
90 Nardone G. and Watzlawick P., *Brief strategic therapy,* 2005.
91 Northey W.F. Jr., *Studying marriage and family therapists in the 21st century: Methodological and technological issues*, in «Journal of Marital and Family Therapy» 31, 99–105 (2005).
92 Abbass A.A., Hancock J.T., Henderson J., Kisely S., *Short-term psychodynamic psychotherapies for common mental disorders*, in «Cochrane Database of Systematic Reviews», CD004687 (2006).
93 Akechi T., Okuyama T., Onishi J., Morita T., Furukawa T.A., *Psychotherapy for depression among incurable cancer patients*, in «Cochrane Database of Systematic Reviews», CD005537 (2008).
94 Amato L. *et al.*, *Psychosocial and pharmacological treatments versus pharmacological treatments for opioid detoxification*, in «Cochrane Database of Systematic Reviews», CD005031 (2004).
95 Amato L. *et al.*, *Psychosocial combined with agonist maintenance treatments versus agonist maintenance treatments alone for treatment of opioid dependence*, in «Cochrane Database of Systematic Reviews», CD004147 (2004).
96 Anderson C.S., Hackett M.L., House A.O., *Interventions for preventing depression after stroke*, in «Cochrane Database of Systematic Reviews», CD003689 (2004).
97 Anie K.A., Green J., *Psychological therapies for sickle cell disease and pain*, in «Cochrane Database of Systematic Reviews», CD001916 (2000).
98 Anie K.A., Massaglia P., *Psychological therapies for thalassaemia*, in «Cochrane Database of Systematic Reviews», CD002890 (2001).

99 Bacaltchuk J., Hay P., Trefiglio R., *Antidepressants versus psychological treatments and their combination for bulimia nervosa*, in «Cochrane Database of Systematic Reviews», CD003385 (2001).

100 Barth J., Critchley J., Bengel J., *Psychosocial interventions for smoking cessation in patients with coronary heart disease*, in «Cochrane Database of Systematic Reviews», CD006886 (2008).

101 Bausewein C., Booth S., Gysels M., Higginson I., *Non-pharmacological interventions for breathlessness in advanced stages of malignant and non-malignant diseases*, in «Cochrane Database of Systematic Reviews», CD005623 (2008).

102 Bisson J., Andrew M., *Psychological treatment of post-traumatic stress disorder (PTSD)*, in «Cochrane Database of Systematic Reviews», CD003388 (2005).

103 Brazzelli M., Griffiths P., *Behavioural and cognitive interventions with or without other treatments for defaecation disorders in children*, in «Cochrane Database of Systematic Reviews», CD002240 (2001).

104 Brazzelli M., Griffiths P., *Behavioural and cognitive interventions with or without other treatments for the management of faecal incontinence in children*, in «Cochrane Database of Systematic Reviews», CD002240 (2006).

105 Buckley L.A., Pettit T., *Supportive therapy for schizophrenia*, in «Cochrane Database of Systematic Reviews», CD004716 (2007).

106 Cormac I., Jones C., Campbell C., *Cognitive behaviour therapy for schizophrenia*, in «Cochrane Database of Systematic Reviews», CD000524 (2002).

107 Dennis C.L., Creedy D., *Psychosocial and psychological interventions for preventing postpartum depression*, in «Cochrane Database of Systematic Reviews», CD001134 (2004).

108 Eccleston C., Yorke L., Morley S., Williams A.C., Mastroyannopoulou K., *Psychological therapies for the management of chronic and recurrent pain in children and adolescents*, in «Cochrane Database of Systematic Reviews», CD003968 (2003).

109 Edwards A.G., Hailey S., Maxwell M., *Psychological interventions for women with metastatic breast cancer*, in «Cochrane Database of Systematic Reviews», CD004253 (2004).

110 Furukawa T.A., Watanabe N., Churchill R., *Combined psychotherapy plus antidepressants for panic disorder with or without agoraphobia*, in «Cochrane Database of Systematic Reviews», CD004364 (2007).

111 Glazener C.M., Evans J.H., *Simple behavioural and physical interventions for nocturnal enuresis in children*, in «Cochrane Database of Systematic Reviews», CD003637 (2004).

112 Glazener C.M., Evans J.H., Peto R.E., *Complex behavioural and educational interventions for nocturnal enuresis in children*, in «Cochrane Database of Systematic Reviews», CD004668 (2004).

113 Gold C., Heldal T.O., Dahle T., Wigram T., *Music therapy for schizophrenia or schizophrenia-like illnesses*, in «Cochrane Database of Systematic Reviews», CD004025 (2005).

114 Grimshaw G.M., Stanton A., *Tobacco cessation interventions for young people*, in «Cochrane Database of Systematic Reviews», CD003289 (2006).

115 Guzman J. *et al.*, *Multidisciplinary bio-psycho-social rehabilitation for chronic low back pain*, in «Cochrane Database of Systematic Reviews», CD000963 (2002).

116 Guzman J. *et al.*, *WITHDRAWN: Multidisciplinary bio-psycho-social rehabilitation for chronic low-back pain*, in «Cochrane Database of Systematic Reviews», CD000963 (2006).

117 Hackett M.L., Anderson C.S., House A., Halteh C., *Interventions for preventing depression after stroke*, in «Cochrane Database of Systematic Reviews», CD003689 (2008).

118 Hawton K. *et al.*, *Psychosocial versus pharmacological treatments for deliberate self harm*, in «Cochrane Database of Systematic Reviews», CD001764 (2000).

119 Hay P., Bacaltchuk J., Claudino A., Ben-Tovim D., Yong P.Y., *Individual psychotherapy in the outpatient treatment of adults with anorexia nervosa*, in «Cochrane Database of Systematic Reviews», CD003909 (2003).

120 Hay P.J., Bacaltchuk J., *Psychotherapy for bulimia nervosa and binging*, in «Cochrane Database of Systematic Reviews», CD000562 (2000).

121 Hay P.J., Bacaltchuk J., *Psychotherapy for bulimia nervosa and binging*, in «Cochrane Database of Systematic Reviews», CD000562 (2003).

122 Hay P.J., Bacaltchuk J., Stefano S., *Psychotherapy for bulimia nervosa and binging*, in «Cochrane Database of Systematic Reviews», CD000562 (2004).

123 Huertas-Ceballos A., Logan S., Bennett C., Macarthur C., *Psychosocial interventions for recurrent abdominal pain (RAP) and irritable bowel syndrome (IBS) in childhood*, in «Cochrane Database of Systematic Reviews», CD003014 (2008).

124 Huibers, M.J., Beurskens, A.J., Bleijenberg, G., van Schayck, C.P. The effectiveness of psychosocial interventions delivered by general practitioners, in «Cochrane Database of Systematic Reviews», CD003494 (2003).

125 Huibers M.J., Beurskens A.J., Bleijenberg G., van Schayck C.P., *Psychosocial interventions by general practitioners*, in «Cochrane Database of Systematic Reviews», CD003494 (2007).

126 Hunot V., Churchill R., Silva de Lima M., Teixeira V., *Psychological therapies for generalised anxiety disorder*, in «Cochrane Database of Systematic Reviews», CD001848 (2007).
127 James A., Soler A., Weatherall R., *Cognitive behavioural therapy for anxiety disorders in children and adolescents*, in «Cochrane Database of Systematic Reviews», CD004690 (2005).
128 Jones C., Cormac I., Mota J., Campbell C., *Cognitive behaviour therapy for schizophrenia*, in «Cochrane Database of Systematic Reviews», CD000524 (2000).
129 Jones C., Cormac I., Silveira da Mota Neto J.I., Campbell C., *Cognitive behaviour therapy for schizophrenia*, in «Cochrane Database of Systematic Reviews», CD000524 (2004).
130 Joy C.B., Adams C.E., Rice K., *Crisis intervention for people with severe mental illnesses*, in «Cochrane Database of Systematic Reviews», CD001087 (2000).
131 Kisely S., Campbell L.A., Skerritt P., *Psychological interventions for symptomatic management of non-specific chest pain in patients with normal coronary anatomy*, in «Cochrane Database of Systematic Reviews», CD004101 (2005).
132 Koger S.M., Brotons M., *Music therapy for dementia symptoms*, in «Cochrane Database of Systematic Reviews», CD001121 (2000).
133 Lancaster T., Stead L.F., *Individual behavioural counselling for smoking cessation*, in «Cochrane Database of Systematic Reviews», CD001292 (2000).
134 Lancaster T., Stead L.F., *Individual behavioural counselling for smoking cessation*, in «Cochrane Database of Systematic Reviews», CD001292 (2002).
135 Lip G.Y., Lane D.A., Millane T.A., Tayebjee M.H., *Psychological interventions for depression in adolescent and adult congenital heart disease*, in «Cochrane Database of Systematic Reviews», CD004394 (2003).
136 Macdonald G.M., Higgins J.P., Ramchandani P., *Cognitive-behavioural interventions for children who have been sexually abused*, in «Cochrane Database of Systematic Reviews», CD001930 (2006).
137 Macdonald G.M., Turner W., *Treatment foster care for improving outcomes in children and young people*, in «Cochrane Database of Systematic Reviews», CD005649 (2008).
138 Martinez Devesa P., Waddell A., Perera R., Theodoulou M., *Cognitive behavioural therapy for tinnitus*, in «Cochrane Database of Systematic Reviews», CD005233 (2007).
139 Melnik T., Soares B.G., Nasselo A.G., *Psychosocial interventions for erectile dysfunction*, in «Cochrane Database of Systematic Reviews», CD004825 (2007).
140 Moher M., Hey K., Lancaster T., *Workplace interventions for smoking cessation*, in «Cochrane Database of Systematic Reviews», CD003440 (2003).
141 Moncrieff J., Wessely S., Hardy R., *Active placebos versus antidepressants for depression*, in «Cochrane Database of Systematic Reviews», CD003012 (2004).
142 Montgomery P., *Media-based behavioural treatments for behavioural disorders in children*, in «Cochrane Database of Systematic Reviews», CD002206 (2001).
143 Montgomery P., Dennis J., *Cognitive behavioural interventions for sleep problems in adults aged 60+*, in «Cochrane Database of Systematic Reviews», CD003161 (2002).
144 O'Kearney R.T., Anstey K.J., von Sanden C., *Behavioural and cognitive behavioural therapy for obsessive compulsive disorder in children and adolescents*, in «Cochrane Database of Systematic Reviews», CD004856 (2006).
145 Panton J., Barley E.A., *Family therapy for asthma in children*, in «Cochrane Database of Systematic Reviews», CD000089 (2000).
146 Proctor M.L., Murphy P.A., Pattison H.M., Suckling J., Farquhar C.M., *Behavioural interventions for primary and secondary dysmenorrhoea*, in «Cochrane Database of Systematic Reviews», CD002248 (2007).
147 Roe B., Williams K., Palmer M., *Bladder training for urinary incontinence in adults*, in «Cochrane Database of Systematic Reviews», CD001308 (2000).
148 Smith C.A., Collins C.T., Cyna A.M., Crowther C.A., *Complementary and alternative therapies for pain management in labour*, in «Cochrane Database of Systematic Reviews», CD003521 (2003).
149 Sola I., Thompson E., Subirana M., Lopez C., Pascual A., *Non-invasive interventions for improving well-being and quality of life in patients with lung cancer*, in «Cochrane Database of Systematic Reviews», CD004282 (2004).
150 Soo C., Tate R., *Psychological treatment for anxiety in people with traumatic brain injury*, in «Cochrane Database of Systematic Reviews», CD005239 (2007).
151 Soo S. *et al.*, *Psychological interventions for non-ulcer dyspepsia*, in «Cochrane Database of Systematic Reviews», CD002301 (2001).
152 Soo S. *et al.*, *Psychological interventions for non-ulcer dyspepsia*, in «Cochrane Database of Systematic Reviews», CD002301 (2004).
153 Stead L.F., Lancaster T., *Group behaviour therapy programmes for smoking cessation*, in «Cochrane Database of Systematic Reviews», CD001007 (2000).

154 Stead L.F., Lancaster T., *Group behaviour therapy programmes for smoking cessation*, in «Cochrane Database of Systematic Reviews», CD001007 (2002).
155 Stead L.F., Lancaster T., *Group behaviour therapy programmes for smoking cessation*, in «Cochrane Database of Systematic Reviews», CD001007 (2005).
156 Terplan M., Lui S., *Psychosocial interventions for pregnant women in outpatient illicit drug treatment programs compared to other interventions*, in «Cochrane Database of Systematic Reviews», CD006037 (2007).
157 Thomas P.W., Thomas S., Hillier C., Galvin K., Baker R., *Psychological interventions for multiple sclerosis*, in «Cochrane Database of Systematic Reviews», CD004431 (2006).
158 Turner W., Macdonald G.M., Dennis J.A., *Cognitive-behavioural training interventions for assisting foster carers in the management of difficult behaviour*, in «Cochrane Database of Systematic Reviews», CD003760 (2005).
159 Uman L.S., Chambers C.T., McGrath P.J., Kisely S., *Psychological interventions for needle-related procedural pain and distress in children and adolescents*, in «Cochrane Database of Systematic Reviews», CD005179 (2006).
160 van der Meer R.M., Wagena E.J., Ostelo R.W., Jacobs J.E., van Schayck C.P., *Smoking cessation for chronic obstructive pulmonary disease*, in «Cochrane Database of Systematic Reviews», CD002999 (2003).
161 van Tulder M.W.*, et al.*, *Behavioural treatment for chronic low back pain*, in «Cochrane Database of Systematic Reviews», CD002014 (2000).
162 Woolfenden S.R., Williams K., Peat J., *Family and parenting interventions in children and adolescents with conduct disorder and delinquency aged 10–17*, in «Cochrane Database of Systematic Reviews», CD003015 (2001).
163 Yorke J., Shuldham C., *Family therapy for chronic asthma in children*, in «Cochrane Database of Systematic Reviews», CD000089 (2005).
164 Manzoni G.M., Pagnini F., Castelnuovo G., Molinari E., *Relaxation training for anxiety: A ten-years systematic review with meta-analysis*, in «BMC Psychiatry» 8, 41 (2008).
165 Kirsch I. *et al.*, *Initial severity and antidepressant benefits: A meta-analysis of data submitted to the Food and Drug Administration*, in «PLoS Medicine» 5, e45 (2008).
166 Mayor S., *Study shows difference between antidepressants and placebo is only significant in severe depression*, in «in «British Medical Journal»», 7642 (2008).
167 Ahn A.C., Tewari M., Poon C.S., Phillips R.S., *The limits of reductionism in medicine: Could systems biology offer an alternative?*, in «PLoS Medicine» 3, e208 (2006).
168 Longino C.F., Jr. *The limits of scientific medicine:Paradigm strain and social policy*, in «Journal of Health and Social Policy» 9, 101–116 (1998).
169 Hammad T.A., Laughren T.P., Racoosin J.A., *Suicide rates in short-term randomized controlled trials of newer antidepressants*, in «Journal of Clinical Psychopharmacology» 26, 203–207 (2006).
170 Hammad T.A., Laughren T.P., Racoosin J.A., *Suicidality in pediatric patients treated with antidepressant drugs*, in «Archives of General Psychiatry» 63, 332–339 (2006).
171 Mosholder A.D., Gelperin, K., Hammad T.A., Phelan K., Johann-Liang R., *Hallucinations and other psychotic symptoms associated with the use of attention-deficit/hyperactivity disorder drugs in children*, in «Pediatrics» 123, 611–616 (2009).
172 Stein R.E. *et al.*, *Attention-deficit/hyperactivity disorder: How much responsibility are pediatricians taking?*, in «Pediatrics» 123, 248–255 (2009).
173 Olfson M., Marcus S.C., Shaffer D., *Antidepressant drug therapy and suicide in severely depressed children and adults: A case-control study*, in «Archives of General Psychiatry» 63, 865–872 (2006).
174 Friedman R.A., *The changing face of teenage drug abuse: the trend toward prescription drugs*, in «New England Journal of Medicine» 354, 1448–1450 (2006).
175 Moncrieff J., Cohen D., *Do antidepressants cure or create abnormal brain states?*, in «PLoS Medicine» 3, e240 (2006).
176 Moncrieff J., *Why is it so difficult to stop psychiatric drug treatment? It may be nothing to do with the original problem*, in «Medical Hypotheses» 67, 517–523 (2006).
177 Timonen M., Liukkonen T., *Management of depression in adults*, in «British Medical Journal» 336, 435–439 (2008).
178 Hansen B., *The Dodo Manifesto*, in «Australian and New Zealand Journal of Family Therapy» 26, 210–218 (2005).
179 Jones E., Asen E., *Systemic Couple Therapy and Depression* (2000).
180 Marks I., O'Sullivan G., *Drugs and psychological treatments for agoraphobia/panic and obsessive-compulsive disorders: A review*, in «British Journal of Psychiatry» 153, 650–658 (1988).
181 Marks I.M. *et al.*, *Drug treatment of panic disorder. Further comment*, in «British Journal of Psychiatry» 162, 795–796 (1993).

182 Marks I.M. *et al.*, *The "efficacy" of alprazolam in panic disorder and agoraphobia: A critique of recent reports*, in «Archives of General Psychiatry» 46, 668–672 (1989).
183 Marks I.M. *et al.*, *Alprazolam and exposure alone and combined in panic disorder with agoraphobia: A controlled study in London and Toronto*, in «British Journal of Psychiatry» 162, 776–787 (1993).
184 Parker G., Roy K., Eyers K., *Cognitive behavior therapy for depression? Choose horses for courses*, in «American Journal of Psychiatry» 160, 825–834 (2003).
185 Shear M.K., Pilkonis P.A., Cloitre M., Leon A.C., *Cognitive behavioral treatment compared with nonprescriptive treatment of panic disorder*, in «Archives of General Psychiatry» 51, 395–401 (1994).
186 McIntosh V.V. *et al.*, *Three psychotherapies for anorexia nervosa: A randomized, controlled trial*, in «American Journal of Psychiatry» 162, 741–747 (2005).
187 Wallis A., Rhodes P., Kohn M., Madden S., *Five-years of family-based treatment for anorexia nervosa: The Maudsley Model at the Children's Hospital at Westmead*, in «International Journal of Adolescent Medicine and Health» 19, 277–283 (2007).
188 Bergh C. *et al.*, *How effective is family therapy for the treatment of anorexia nervosa?*, in «European Eating Disorders Review» 14, 371–373 (2006).
189 Leichsenring F., Rabung S., *Effectiveness of long-term psychodynamic psychotherapy: A meta-analysis*, in «Journal of the Americal Medical Association» 300, 1551–1565 (2008).
190 Leichsenring F., Leibing E., *Psychodynamic psychotherapy: A systematic review of techniques, indications and empirical evidence*, in «Psychology and Psychotherapy» 80, 217–228 (2007).
191 Leichsenring F., *Are psychodynamic and psychoanalytic therapies effective?: A review of empirical data*, in «International Journal of Psychoanalysis» 86, 841–868 (2005).
192 Leichsenring F., Rabung S., Leibing E., *The efficacy of short-term psychodynamic psychotherapy in specific psychiatric disorders: A meta-analysis*, in «Archives of General Psychiatry» 61, 1208–1216 (2004).
193 Verheul R., Herbrink M., *The efficacy of various modalities of psychotherapy for personality disorders: A systematic review of the evidence and clinical recommendations*, in «International Review of Psychiatry», 25–38 (2007).

For Product Safety Concerns and Information please contact our EU
representative GPSR@taylorandfrancis.com
Taylor & Francis Verlag GmbH, Kaufingerstraße 24, 80331 München, Germany

www.ingramcontent.com/pod-product-compliance
Ingram Content Group UK Ltd.
Pitfield, Milton Keynes, MK11 3LW, UK
UKHW050055200926
475702UK00019B/2855
* 9 7 8 0 3 6 7 1 1 0 9 3 2 *